Clinical Handbook of Psychotropic Drugs

Adil Virani, BSc (Pharm), PharmD, FCSHP[A] (Principal Editor)
Kalyna Z. Bezchlibnyk-Butler, BScPhm, FCSHP (Co-Editor)
J. Joel Jeffries, MB, FRCPC[B] (Co-Editor)

Chapter Editors:
Leslie Phillips BSc (Pharm), PharmD[C] and Carla Dillon BSc (Pharm), Pharm D[C] (Antipsychotics)
Adil Virani, BSc (Pharm), PharmD, FCSHP[A] (Mood Stabilizers, Psychostimulants)
Sylvia Zerjav, BSc (Pharm), PharmD, BCPP[D] (Antidepressants)

The Editors wish to acknowledge contributions from the following chapter co-editors:

Andrius Baskys, MD, PhD[E] (Drugs for Treatment of Dementia)
Robert Dickey, MD, FRCPC[B] (Sex-Drive Depressants)
Jane Dumontet BSc (Pharm), PharmD (Mood Stabilizers)[A]
Gary Hasey, MD, FRCPC, MSc[F] (Repetitive Transcranial Magnetic Stimulation)
Barry A. Martin, MD, FRCPC[B] (Electroconvulsive Therapy)
Roger S. McIntyre, MD, FRCPC[G] (Mood Stabilizers)
Myroslava Romach, MSc, MD, FRCPC[H] (Drugs of Abuse, Treatment of Substance Use Disorders)
Edward M. Sellers, MD, PhD, FRCPC, FACP[H] (Drugs of Abuse, Treatment of Substance Use Disorders)
Margaret Weiss, MD, PhD[I] (Psychostimulants)

[A] Fraser Health Authority and University of British Columbia, Vancouver, BC, Canada
[B] Centre for Addiction and Mental Health and Department of Psychiatry, University of Toronto, Toronto, ON, Canada
[C] School of Pharmacy, Health Sciences Centre, Memorial University, St. John's, NL, Canada
[D] Provincial Health Services Authority, and University of British Columbia, Vancouver, BC, Canada
[E] Department of Psychiatry and Human Behavior, University of California, Irvine, CA, USA
[F] St. Joseph's Healthcare Hamilton, and Department of Psychiatry and Neurosciences, McMaster University, Hamilton, ON, Canada
[G] Toronto Western Hospital, University Health Network, and Department of Psychiatry, University of Toronto, Toronto, ON, Canada
[H] Kendle Early Stage, Toronto, ON, Canada
[I] Provincial ADHD Program, Children's and Women's Health Centre, Vancouver, BC, Canada

HOGREFE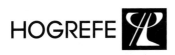

Library of Congress Cataloging-in-Publication Data

is available via the Library of Congress Marc Database under the
LC Control Number 2009922908

Canadian Cataloging-in-Publication Data

Main entry under title:

Clinical handbook of psychotropic drugs
18th rev. ed.
Includes bibliographical references and index

ISBN 978-0-88937-369-3

1. Psychotropic drugs – Handbooks, manuals, etc.
I. Bezchlibnyk-Butler, Kalyna Z., 1947–.
II. Jeffries, J. Joel, 1939–.
III. Virani, Adil, 1969–.
RM315.C55   2009   615'.788   C93-094102-0

18th completely revised edition

ISBN 978-0-88937-369-3
Hogrefe & Huber Publishers

INTRODUCTION

The *Clinical Handbook of Psychotropic Drugs* is intended to be a user-friendly and practical resource guide for using psychotropic drugs in any setting. Its content is derived from various forms of published literature (including randomized controlled trials, scientific data such as pharmacokinetic trials, cohort trials, case series, and case reports) as well as from leading clinical experts. We endeavor to continually update this handbook as the psychiatric literature evolves so we can continue to provide evidence-based clinically relevant information that is easily accessed and utilized to aid with patient care decisions. New sections, periodically added, reflect changes in therapy and in current practice.

As in previous editions, charts and tables of comparisons are employed whenever possible to enable the reader to have quick access to information.

Both American and Canadian trade names are used throughout the text. Though plasma levels are given in SI units, conversion rates to Imperial U.S. units are available in the text.

Given that changes may occur in a medication's indications, and differences are seen among countries, specific "indications" listed in this text as "approved" should be viewed in conjunction with product monographs approved in your jurisdiction of interest.

Dose comparisons and plasma levels are based on scientific data. However, it is important to note that some patients will respond to doses outside the reported ranges. Age, sex, and the medical condition of the patient must always be taken into consideration when prescribing any psychotropic agent.

Patient Information Sheets have been included for most drug categories, to facilitate education/counselling of patients receiving these medications.

I would like to sincerely thank Kalyna for her leadership and continued efforts in meticulously keeping this handbook current and relevant to readers' needs. I would also like to thank Joel, the chapter editors, and the chapter co-editors (whose names are listed on the previous page) for their extremely useful contributions to this edition of the handbook. Lastly, I would like to thank my wife Ashifa for her continued support and my children Sophia and Keyan for the lessons they teach me.

Over the years, many readers have asked many interesting questions and provided useful comments and suggestions regarding the content and format of the handbook. I feel this input is essential to keeping this handbook current, accurate, and relevant. Please feel free to e-mail me at the address below with your comments and questions for the editors and authors.

Dr. Adil S. Virani
E-mail: avirani@interchange.ubc.ca

Information on how to obtain future editions of this handbook is given at the end.

TABLE OF CONTENTS

ANTIDEPRESSANTS

Classification

- Antidepressants can be classified as follows:

Chemical Class	Agent	Page
Cyclic Antidepressants[A]		
Selective Serotonin Reuptake Inhibitors (SSRI)	Example: Citalopram, fluoxetine, paroxetine	See p. 3
Norepinephrine Dopamine Reuptake Inhibitor (NDRI)	Bupropion	See p. 16
Selective Serotonin-Norepinephrine Reuptake Inhibitor (SNRI)	Example: Venlafaxine	See p. 21
Serotonin-2 Antagonists/Serotonin Reuptake Inhibitors (SARI)	Example: Trazodone	See p. 27
Noradrenergic/Specific Serotonergic Agent (NaSSA)	Mirtazapine	See p. 33
Non-Selective Cyclic Agents (Mixed Reuptake Inhibitor/Receptor Blockers)	Example: Desipramine, amitriptyline	See p. 37
Monoamine Oxidase Inhibitors		
Reversible MAO-A Inhibitor (RIMA)	Moclobemide	See p. 46
Irreversible MAO-A-B Inhibitors (MAOIs)	Example: Phenelzine	See p. 50
Monoamine Oxidase B Inhibitor	Selegiline	See p. 56

[A] Cyclic antidepressants are currently classified on the basis of their specificity on the reuptake of brain neurotransmitters. This specificity confers a pharmacologic profile on the drugs that determines their spectrum of activity and adverse effects (see table p. 59).

General Comments

- **Antidepressants can cause restlessness or psychomotor agitation before improving core symptoms of depression. This agitation may be associated with hostility or suicidal thoughts and behavior. Risk for suicide should be closely monitored during the first weeks of antidepressant therapy**
- Though there are some randomized double-blind, controlled trials to the contrary, on average, all antidepressants are equally efficacious at reducing symptoms of depression. Overall effects of antidepressants appear to be overstated when the effects of publication bias are considered. After considering the latter, the overall effect size of treatment is reported as being a modest 0.31[16]
- Different classes of antidepressants can be combined for additive efficacy in refractory cases, but caution must be exercised – see Interactions
- Prophylaxis of depression is most effective if the therapeutic dose is maintained; continued therapy with all classes of antidepressants shown to significantly reduce risk of relapse
- Tolerance (tachyphylaxis or "poop-out" syndrome) has been reported in 10–20% of patients on various antidepressants, despite compliance with therapy. Possible explanations include adaptations in the CNS, increase in disease severity or pathogenesis, loss of placebo effect, accumulation of a detrimental metabolite, unrecognized rapid-cycling or prophylactic inefficacy. [Check compliance with therapy; dosage adjustment may help; switching to an alternate antidepressant (p. 66) or augmentation strategies (p. 68) have also been tried]
- Certain non-selective cyclic and MAOI antidepressants are toxic in overdose; limited quantities should be prescribed to patients with suicidal propensities

Therapeutic Effects

- Elevation of mood, improved appetite and sleep patterns, increased physical activity, improved clarity of thinking, better memory; decreased feelings of guilt, worthlessness, helplessness, inadequacy, decrease in delusional preoccupation and ambivalence

Selective Serotonin Reuptake Inhibitors (SSRI)

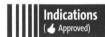 **Product Availability**

Chemical Class	Generic Name	Trade Name[A]	Dosage Forms and Strengths
Phthalane derivative	Citalopram	Celexa	Tablets: 10 mg, 20 mg, 40 mg Oral solution[B]: 10 mg/5 ml
	Escitalopram	Lexapro[B], Cipralex[C]	Tablets: 5 mg[B], 10 mg, 20 mg Oral solution: 5 mg/5 ml
Bicyclic	Fluoxetine	Prozac, Sarafem[B]	Capsules: 10 mg, 20 mg, 40 mg Enteric-coated tablets: 90 mg Delayed-release pellets 90 mg[B] Oral solution: 20 mg/5 ml
Monocyclic	Fluvoxamine[D]	Luvox	Tablets: 25 mg[B], 50 mg, 100 mg
Phenylpiperidine	Paroxetine hydrochloride	Paxil	Tablets: 10 mg, 20 mg, 30 mg, 40 mg[B] Oral suspension[B]: 10 mg/5 ml
		Paxil CR	Controlled-release tablets: 12.5 mg, 25 mg, 37.5 mg[B]
	Paroxetine mesylate[B]	Paxeva	Tablets[B]: 10 mg, 20 mg, 30 mg, 40 mg
Tetrahydronaphthylmethylamine	Sertraline	Zoloft	Capsules/Tablets: 25 mg, 50 mg, 100 mg Oral solution: 20 mg/ml[B]

[A] Generic preparations may be available, [B] Not marketed in Canada, [C] Not marketed in USA, [D] Not approved for depression in USA

Indications
(Approved)

- Major depressive disorder (MDD)
- Prophylaxis of recurrent MDD
- Treatment of secondary depression in other mental illnesses, e.g., schizophrenia, dementia
- Depressed phase of bipolar disorder (see Precautions)
- Bulimia nervosa (approved for fluoxetine and sertraline)
- Obsessive-compulsive disorder (OCD) (approved for fluvoxamine, fluoxetine, paroxetine and sertraline)
- Panic disorder with or without agoraphobia (paroxetine, sertraline, fluoxetine)
- Social anxiety disorder (paroxetine, sertraline)
- Posttraumatic stress disorder (paroxetine, sertraline – USA)
- Premenstrual dysphoric disorder (fluoxetine, paroxetine, sertraline – USA)
- Generalized anxiety disorder (paroxetine, escitalopram); response reported with sertraline
- Bipolar depression and maintenance treatment of bipolar disorder (olanzapine/fluoxetine combination – Symbyax – USA)
- Dysthymia
- Atypical depression
- MDD in patients with comorbid medical disorder (i.e., poststroke depression and crying, myocardial infarction) or Alzheimer's disease
- Double-blind studies suggest efficacy of fluvoxamine and citalopram in binge-eating disorder
- Self-injurious behavior, aggression, impulsive behavior and behavior disturbances of dementia and borderline personality disorder
- May aid in smoking cessation, and withdrawal from drugs, including alcohol – variable response reported
- Benefit reported in chronic fatigue syndrome, body dysmorphic disorder

Selective Serotonin Reuptake Inhibitors (SSRI) (cont.)

- Open trial suggests sertraline may prevent recurrence of postpartum depression after childbirth in women with a prior history
- Preliminary data suggest efficacy in pervasive developmental disorder (autism) and elective mutism
- Pain management (e.g., diabetic neuropathy, arthritis), phantom limb pain (fluoxetine, sertraline), Raynaud's phenomenon (fluoxetine), fibrositis, and fibromyalgia (fluoxetine) – data conflicting as to efficacy
- Trichotillomania
- May reduce episodes of cataplexy
- Premature ejaculation
- Data contradictory as to efficacy in the treatment of functional enuresis – case reports of bedwetting in children treated with SSRIs
- Open label and double-blind studies have found a variable response to SSRIs in the treatment of hot flashes in women in menopause. About 30% of women showed a 30% reduction in hot flashes, one third had less than 30% reduction and 37% showed an increase in hot flashes. A larger percentage of women with a history of breast cancer appear to have greater reductions in hot flashes.
- Overview of studies and clinical experience is contradictory in terms of efficacy of SSRIs in the treatment of paraphilias and paraphilia-related disorders. Use of these agents in high-risk patients should be approached with caution

General Comments

- Suggested that premenopausal women may respond better to SSRIs (compared to tricyclics)
- SSRIs have been associated with increased suicidal ideation, hostility, and psychomotor agitation in clinical trials involving children, adolescents, and young adults (up to 24 years old). Monitor all patients for worsening of depression and suicidal thinking
- In a STAR*D trial, approximately 30% of patients with a history of chronic depression reached remission after 10 weeks of therapy on citalopram (average dose = 42 mg) and 50% had a response[15]

Pharmacology

- Exact mechanism of antidepressant action unknown; SSRIs, through inhibition of serotonin uptake, increase concentrations of serotonin in the synapse, which causes downregulation of post-synaptic receptors (e.g., $5-HT_2$); other neurotransmitter systems may also be influenced

Dosing

- See p. 65
- SSRIs have flat dose-response curves, i.e., most patients respond to the initial (low) dose. Do not increase the dose till steady state is reached (4 weeks for fluoxetine and 1–2 weeks for other drugs)
- Dosage should be decreased (by 50%) in patients with hepatic impairment as plasma levels can increase up to 3-fold
- In kidney impairment sertraline levels may increase 1.5-fold; use 50% of the standard dose of paroxetine if creatinine clearance is 10–50 ml/min, and 25% of the standard dose if creatinine clearance is < 10ml/min
- Higher doses are usually required in the treatment of OCD; treatment should be continued for at least 10 weeks
- Lower starting dose may be required in panic disorder due to patient sensitivity to stimulating effects
- Dosing interval of every 2 to 7 days has been used with fluoxetine in prophylaxis of depression; once weekly dosing used in the maintenance treatment of panic disorder
- Intermittent dosing (during luteal phase of menstrual cycle) found effective for the treatment of premenstrual dysphoric disorder

Pharmacokinetics

- Rapidly absorbed; undergo little first-pass effect
- Highly bound to plasma protein; all SSRIs (least – escitalopram and fluvoxamine) will displace other drugs from protein binding and elevate their plasma level (see Interactions, p. 10)
- Metabolized primarily by the liver; all SSRIs affect cytochrome P-450 metabolizing enzyme (least – citalopram and escitalopram) and will affect the metabolism of other drugs metabolized by this system (see Interactions, p. 10). Fluoxetine and paroxetine have been shown to decrease their own metabolism over time
- Peak plasma level of sertraline is 30% higher when drug taken with food, as first-pass metabolism is reduced
- Fluoxetine as well as its active metabolite, norfluoxetine, have the longest half-lives (up to 70 h and 330 h, respectively); this has implications for reaching steady-state drug levels as well as for drug withdrawal

- Controlled-release paroxetine is enteric-coated and formulated for controlled dissolution; it appears to be better tolerated than the regular release preparations in regards to GI effects, especially at start of therapy
- Once weekly dose of enteric-coated fluoxetine 90 mg results in mean steady state plasma concentration of fluoxetine and norfluoxetine, achieved with a daily dose of 10–20 mg; peak to trough differences vary (rates of nausea appear to be similar with immediate-release and controlled-release preparations)
- Clearance of all SSRIs reduced in patients with liver cirrhosis
- Clearance of sertraline and paroxetine greatly reduced in renal disease; caution with escitalopram if CrCl < 20 ml/min

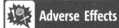
Onset & Duration of Action

- SSRIs are long-acting drugs and can be given in a single daily dose, usually in the morning; fluvoxamine may cause sedation and can be prescribed at night
- Therapeutic effect seen after 7–28 days; most patients with depression respond to the initial (low) dose; increasing the dose too rapidly due to absence of therapeutic effect or adverse effects can ultimately result in an overshoot of the therapeutic range
- Tolerance to effects seen in some patients after months of treatment ("poop-out syndrome" or tachyphylaxis) (see p. 2)

Adverse Effects

- The pharmacological and side effect profile of SSRIs is dependent on their in vivo affinity for and activity on neurotransmitters/receptors (see Table p. 59)
- See accompanying chart (p. 62) for incidence of adverse effects at therapeutic doses
- Incidence may be greater in early days of treatment; patients adapt to many side effects over time
- Rule out withdrawal symptoms of previous antidepressant – can be misattributed to side effects of current drug

CNS Effects

- A result of antagonism at histamine H_1-receptors and α_1-adrenoreceptors
- Headache common, worsening of migraines [Management: analgesics prn]
- Seizures reported, primarily in patients with underlying seizure disorder (risk 0.04–0.3%)
- Both activation and sedation can occur early in treatment
- Activation, excitement, impulse dyscontrol, anxiety, agitation, and restlessness; more frequent at higher doses [may respond to lorazepam]; psychosis or panic reactions may occur; isolated reports of antidepressants causing motor activation, aggression, depersonalization, **suicidal urges**, and potential to harm others. CAUTION in children and adolescents (see p. 8)
- Insomnia: decreased REM sleep, prolonged sleep onset latency, reduced sleep efficacy, and increased awakenings with all SSRIs; increased dreaming, nightmares, sexual dreams and obsessions reported with fluoxetine [may respond to clonazepam or cyproheptadine 2–4 mg]; case reports of somnambulism with paroxetine
- Drowsiness – more common with fluvoxamine; prescribe bulk of dose at bedtime; sedation with fluoxetine may be related to high concentration of metabolite norfluoxetine
- Precipitation of hypomania or mania (up to 30% of patients with a history of bipolar disorders – less frequent if patient receiving mood stabilizers); increased risk in patients with comorbid substance abuse
- Lethargy, apathy or amotivational syndrome (asthenia) reported – may be dose-related [prescribe bulk of dose at bedtime; bromocriptine 2.5–20 mg/day (rarely up to 60 mg/day), amantadine (100–200 mg/day), bupropion, buspirone, olanzapine (2.5–10 mg/day), modafinil (100–400 mg/day), or psychostimulant (e.g., methylphenidate 5–20 mg bid) may be helpful]
- Case reports of cognitive impairment, decreased attention and short-term memory [early data suggest donepezil 2.5–10 mg/day may be of benefit]
- Case reports of visual hallucinations with fluoxetine, fluvoxamine, paroxetine, and sertraline
- Fine tremor [may respond to dose reduction or to propranolol]
- Akathisia [may respond to dose reduction, to propranolol or to a benzodiazepine]
- Dystonia, dyskinesia, parkinsonism or tics; more likely in older patients
- Tinnitus
- Myoclonus (e.g., periodic leg movements during sleep) [may respond to lamotrigine, gabapentin or bromocriptine]; may increase spasticity; recurrence of restless legs syndrome
- Dysphasia, stuttering
- May induce or worsen extrapyramidal effects when given with antipsychotics (see Interactions p. 10)

Selective Serotonin Reuptake Inhibitors (SSRI) (cont.)

- Increased extrapyramidal symptoms reported in patients with Parkinson's disease
- Impaired balance reported, especially in the elderly
- Case reports of tardive dyskinesia following chronic fluoxetine, sertraline and paroxetine use; more likely in older patients
- Nocturnal bruxism reported – may result in morning headache or may lead to damage to teeth or bridgework [may respond to buspirone up to 50 mg/day]
- Paresthesias; may be caused by pyridoxine deficiency [Management: pyridoxine 50–150 mg/day]; "electric-shock" sensations
- Joint pain
- Cerebrovascular disease and case reports of stroke (high doses of high-affinity SSRIs can increase risk of bleeding or vasospasm due to antiplatelet effect or serotenergic overstimulation)

Anticholinergic Effects

- Sweating most likely with paroxetine (also a result of NE-reuptake inhibition) [Management: daily showering, talcum powder; in severe cases: Drysol solution, terazosin: 1–10 mg daily, oxybutynin up to 5 mg bid, clonidine 0.1 mg bid, guanfacine 2 mg hs, benztropine 0.5 mg hs; drug may need to be changed]
- Case reports of urinary retention, urgency, incontinence or cystitis
- Case report of acute angle-closure with paroxetine in patient with narrow angle glaucoma

Cardiovascular Effects

- Suggested by some to have a protective effect on cardiovascular function related to reduced platelet aggregation
- Rare reports of tachycardia, palpitations, hypertension, and atrial fibrillation
- Bradycardia occurs more frequently
- Dizziness
- May cause coronary vasoconstriction; caution in patients with angina/ischemic heart disease
- Slowing of sinus node reported with fluoxetine; caution in sinus node disease and in patients with serious left ventricular impairment; case reports of QT prolongation with fluoxetine (two mechanisms proposed: Direct blockade of the hERG potassium ion channels and disruption of hERG protein expression on the cell membrane)[17]
- Increased LDL cholesterol levels reported with paroxetine and sertraline

Endocrine & Metabolic Effects

- Can induce SIADH (syndrome of inappropriate secretion of antidiuretic hormone) with hyponatremia; can result in nausea, fatigue, headache, cognitive impairment, and seizures; risk increases with age (up to 32% incidence), female sex, low body weight, smoking and concomitant diuretic use
- Elevated prolactin – risk increased in females (up to 22% reported in women on fluoxetine); cases of galactorrhea reported; breast enlargement; case of gynecomastia in a male on paroxetine – not related to dose
- Up to 30% decrease in fasting blood glucose has been reported
- Weight gain reported: up to 18% of individuals gain more than 7% of body weight with chronic use – reported more frequently in females (more common with paroxetine); [bupropion, topiramate (100–250 mg/day)]

GI Effects

- A result of inhibition of 5-HT reuptake (activation of 5-HT$_3$ receptors)
- Nausea; vomiting – generally decreases over time due to gradual desensitization of 5-HT3 receptors [may respond to taking drug with meals or switching to the delayed/controlled-release preparation; cyproheptadine 2 mg or lactobacillus acidophilus (e.g., yogurt)]
- Diarrhea, bloating – usually transient and dose-related; may be more frequent with fluoxetine 90 mg given weekly
- Anorexia and weight loss frequently reported during early treatment – more pronounced in overweight patients and those with carbohydrate cravings
- 2–4 times higher risk of upper GI bleeding, with SSRIs, especially if combined with NSAIDs (risk increased 12-fold) or ASA
- Case reports of stomatitis with fluoxetine; glossodynia (burning mouth syndrome) reported during treatment with fluoxetine, sertraline

Urogenital and Sexual Effects

- A result of increased serotonergic transmission by way of the 5-HT$_2$ receptor which results in reduced dopaminergic transmission, acetylcholine (ACh) blockade, and reduced nitric oxide levels – appears to be dose-related; risk increased with age and concomitant drug use

- Decreased libido, impotence, ejaculatory disturbances occur relatively frequently [Management: sildenafil (25–100 mg prn), amantadine (100–400 mg prn), bethanechol (10 mg tid or 10–50 mg prn), cyproheptadine (4–16 mg prn – sedation and/or loss of antidepressant response reported occasionally), neostigmine (7.5–15 mg prn), yohimbine (5.4–16.2 mg prn or 5.4 mg tid – may cause anxiety/agitation), buspirone (15–60 mg od or prn), bupropion (75–300 mg/day – results contradictory), granisetron (1–2 mg prn), loratidine (2.5–15 mg/day), or "drug holidays" (i.e., skip dose for 24 h prior to sexual activity; not effective with fluoxetine]
- Genital anesthesia (fluoxetine, sertraline) [Management: ginkgo biloba 240–900 mg]
- Anorgasmia or delayed orgasm [Management: amantadine (100–400 mg prn); cyproheptadine (4–16 mg prn – sedation and/or loss of antidepressant response reported occasionally), buspirone (15–60 mg od or prn), bupropion (75–300 mg od – results contradictory); mirtazapine (15–45 mg od), yohimbine (5.4–10.8 mg od or prn – may cause anxiety/agitation); methylphenidate (5–40 mg od), dextroamphetamine (5–40 mg od), ginseng, ginkgo biloba (180–900 mg), granisetron (1–2 mg prn – results contradictory); sildenafil (25–150 mg prn), loratidine (2.5–15 mg/day)]
- Spontaneous orgasm with yawning
- Cases of priapism in both males and females reported with citalopram, fluoxetine and sertraline

Allergic Reactions	

- Rare
- Rash (up to 1% incidence), urticaria, psoriasis, pruritus, edema, photoallergy/photosensitivity (cross-sensitivity between SSRIs has been suggested); rare cases of Stevens-Johnson syndrome
- Serum sickness, toxic epidermal necrolysis (fluvoxamine)
- Increased hepatic enzyme levels, bilirubinemia, jaundice, hepatitis
- Rare blood dyscrasias including neutropenia and aplastic anemia
- Bleeding disorders including petechiae, purpura (1% risk with fluoxetine); thrombocytopenia with fluoxetine; bruising, nosebleeds and bleeding after surgery reported with all SSRI drugs; increased bleeding attributed to inhibition of serotonin-uptake by platelets; risk increased in older individuals, those with a history of GI bleed or in combination with drugs such as NSAIDs or ASA (see Interactions p 10–15) [suggested that ascorbic acid 500 mg may ameliorate bleeding]

Other Adverse Effects	

- Case reports of alopecia
- Rhinitis common
- Case reports of exacerbation of Raynaud's syndrome
- Several cases of decreased thyroid indices reported with sertraline
- Nocturia (in up to 16% of patients)
- Osteoporosis: Rate of bone loss 1.6-fold higher in SSRI users; increased risk of fractures in women and older adults [screen women > age 65 routinely for osteoporosis][13]

D/C Discontinuation Syndrome	

- Abrupt discontinuation of high doses may cause a syndrome consisting of *somatic symptoms*: dizziness (exacerbated by movement), lethargy, nausea, vomiting, diarrhea, headache, fever, sweating, chills, malaise, incoordination, insomnia, vivid dreams; *neurological symptoms*: myalgia, paresthesias, dyskinesias, "electric-shock-like" sensations, visual discoordination; *psychological symptoms*: anxiety, agitation, crying, irritability, confusion, slowed thinking, disorientation; rarely aggression, impulsivity, hypomania, and depersonalization; cases of mania reported following antidepressant taper, despite adequate concomitant mood-stabilizing treatment
- Most likely to occur within 1–7 days after drug stopped or dose drastically reduced, and typically disappears within 3 weeks
- Incidence (of 2–78%) is related to half-life of antidepressant – reported most frequently with paroxetine, least with fluoxetine; attributed to rapid decrease in 5-HT availability
- ☞ THEREFORE THESE MEDICATIONS SHOULD BE WITHDRAWN GRADUALLY AFTER PROLONGED USE. Taper antidepressant no more rapidly than by 25% per week (or nearest dose possible) and monitor for recurrence of depressive symptoms

Management	

- Re-institute drug and taper more slowly
- Report that ginger can mitigate nausea and disequilibrium effects; substitution with one dose of fluoxetine (10–20 mg) also recommended to help in the withdrawal process

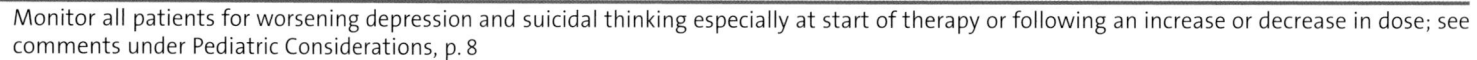

Selective Serotonin Reuptake Inhibitors (SSRI) (cont.)

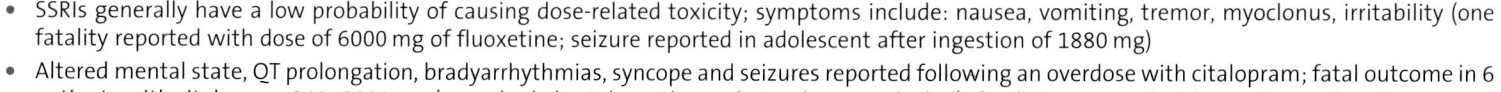 **Precautions**	• Monitor all patients for worsening depression and suicidal thinking especially at start of therapy or following an increase or decrease in dose; see comments under Pediatric Considerations, p. 8
	• May impair the mental and physical ability to perform hazardous tasks (e.g., driving a car or operating machinery)
	• May induce manic reactions in up to 20% of patients with bipolar disorders (BD) – reported more frequently with fluoxetine; because of risk of increased cycling, BD is a relative contraindication unless a mood stabilizer is added
	☞ **Use of SSRIs** with other serotonergic agents may result in a hypermetabolic **serotonin syndrome – usually occurs within 24 hours of medication initiation, overdose or change in dose. Symptoms include: nausea, diarrhea, chills, sweating, dizziness, elevated temperature, elevated blood pressure, palpitations, increased muscle tone with twitching, tremor, myoclonic jerks, hyperreflexia, unsteady gait, restlessness, agitation, excitation, disorientation, confusion and delirium; may progress to rhabdomyolysis, coma and death (see Interactions) [Treatment: stop medication and administer supportive care, cyproheptadine 4–16 mg may reduce duration of symptoms]**
	• Fluoxetine, paroxetine and sertraline will displace drugs from protein binding and elevate their plasma levels
	• Fluoxetine, fluvoxamine, and paroxetine affect cytochrome P-450 and will inhibit the metabolism (and elevate the levels) of drugs metabolized by this system; sertraline will inhibit metabolism in higher doses (over 100 mg/day) (see Interactions, pp. 10–15)
	• Combination of SSRIs with other cyclic antidepressants can lead to increased plasma level of other antidepressant. Combination therapy has been used in the treatment of resistant patients. Caution when switching from fluoxetine to another antidepressant (see Interactions). Caution when switching from one SSRI to another
	• Lower doses should be used in patients with renal or hepatic disease

Toxicity	• SSRIs generally have a low probability of causing dose-related toxicity; symptoms include: nausea, vomiting, tremor, myoclonus, irritability (one fatality reported with dose of 6000 mg of fluoxetine; seizure reported in adolescent after ingestion of 1880 mg)
	• Altered mental state, QT prolongation, bradyarrhythmias, syncope and seizures reported following an overdose with citalopram; fatal outcome in 6 patients with citalopram 840–3920 mg (some had also taken other sedative drugs or alcohol); fatalities reported with overdoses of citalopram and moclobemide
	• Case of serotonin syndrome reported after overdose of 8 g of sertraline
Management	• Treatment: symptomatic and supportive

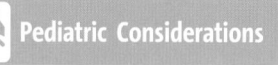 **Pediatric Considerations**	• For detailed information on the use of SSRIs in this population, please see the *Clinical Handbook of Psychotropic Drugs for Children and Adolescents* (2007)
	• Fluoxetine approved for use in children and adolescents with depression (age 8–17) or OCD (age 7–17) (USA)
	• Fluvoxamine, and sertraline approved for the treatment of OCD (in children and adolescents > 7 years and > 6 years of age, respectively) (USA)
	• Efficacy for major depressive disorder (MDD) in children and adolescents NOT demonstrated in controlled trials with sertraline, paroxetine, and citalopram; no data with fluvoxamine and escitalopram
	• CAUTION: Episodes of self-harm and potential suicidal behavior reported to be 1.5–3.2 times higher in patients under age 18 who were taking paroxetine, than those receiving placebo; may also apply to other SSRIs (fluoxetine appears to be safer)
	• SSRIs have been used in the treatment of depression, dysthymia, social phobia, anxiety, panic disorder, bulimia, OCD, autism, selective mutism, Gilles de la Tourette syndrome, and attention deficit hyperactivity disorder (ADHD); preliminary data suggest efficacy in some children with pervasive developmental disorders (autism) and elective mutism
	• Children are more prone to behavioral adverse effects including: agitation, restlessness (32–46%), activation, hypomania (up to 13%), insomnia (up to 21%), irritability and social disinhibition (up to 25%)

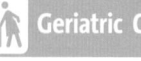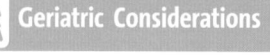 **Geriatric Considerations**	• SSRIs generally have a low risk of CNS, anticholinergic, and cardiovascular effects
	• Initiate dose lower and increase more slowly; higher doses of fluoxetine have been associated with delirium
	• Elderly patients may take longer to respond and may need trials of at least 12 weeks before treatment response noted; data contradictory as to efficiency in older patients

- Half-life of paroxetine increased by 170% and mean plasma level increased 4-fold in the elderly; clearance of sertraline decreased; citalopram plasma level and $T_{1/2}$ increased, C_{max} AUC and $T_{1/2}$ of escitalopram increased by 35%, 50%, and 50%, respectively
- Monitor for drug-drug interactions
- Improvement in cognitive functioning in elderly depressed patients has been noted
- Impaired balance and falls reported; tend to occur early in treatment and are more likely with higher doses
- Both weight gain and weight loss reported; monitor for excessive weight loss in debilitated patients
- Neurological side effects more likely
- Monitor serum electrolytes (sodium and urea nitrogen levels); hyponatremia reported with all SSRIs (e.g., in 12% of elderly on paroxetine) usually within 2 weeks of drug initiation; can present with confusion, somnolence, fatigue, delirium, hallucinations, urinary incontinence, hypotension and vomiting

Use in Pregnancy

- Increased risk of heart defects (1.5–2%) with paroxetine taken in early pregnancy, as compared to the general population (1%) – Category D drug
- AVOID; fetal echocardiography should be considered for women exposed to paroxetine in early pregnancy (Level B evidence).[1] Other SSRIs have not been demonstrated to have teratogenic effects in humans; possible increased risk of miscarriage (Category C drugs); with escitalopram, teratogenic effects have been reported in animal studies
- If possible, avoid during first trimester; when stopping the SSRI, taper the dose gradually to minimize adverse fetal outcome; with fluoxetine be aware of long half-life of metabolite, norfluoxetine
- Reports of an increase in premature births and poor neonatal adaptation when drug taken in the third trimester
- Neonates exposed to SSRIs (especially paroxetine) in the third trimester (after 20th week) have developed complications upon delivery including: jitteriness, restlessness, irritability, tremors, feeding difficulties, changes in muscle tone, respiratory distress, persistent pulmonary hypertension (6-fold risk), temperature instability, seizures (with fluoxetine is related to blood level of fluoxetine and norfluoxetine)
- Higher plasma levels of paroxetine reported in infants whose mothers also received clonazepam

Breast Milk

- Fluoxetine and citalopram appear in breast milk in therapeutic levels; caution: infant can receive up to 17% of maternal dose of fluoxetine and up to 9% of dose of citalopram
- Paroxetine and fluvoxamine are present in very low concentrations in plasma of breast-fed infants; sertraline detected in breast milk especially if mother on dose of 100 mg or higher
- The American Academy of Pediatrics considers SSRIs as "drugs whose effect on nursing infants is unknown but may be of concern."

Nursing Implications

- Psychotherapy and education are also important in the treatment of depression
- Monitor therapy by watching for adverse effects, mood and activity level changes including worsening of suicidal thoughts especially at start of therapy or following an increase or decrease in dose
- Be aware that the medication reduces the degree of depression and may increase psychomotor activity; this may create concern about suicidal behavior
- Watch for increased bruising, nosebleeds, or evidence of GI bleed, especially in patients also taking ASA or NSAIDs, steroids or anticoagulants
- Excessive ingestion of caffeinated foods, drugs, or beverages may increase anxiety and agitation and confuse the diagnosis
- Fluvoxamine tablets should be swallowed whole, with water, without chewing
- Sertraline should be given with food (increases peak plasma level); food reduces incidence of nausea with all SSRIs
- Ingestion of grapefruit juice while taking fluvoxamine and sertraline may increase the plasma level of these drugs
- SSRIs should not be stopped suddenly due to risk of precipitating withdrawal reactions

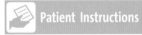
Patient Instructions

- For detailed patient instructions on SSRI antidepressants, see the Patient Information Sheet on p. 317

Selective Serotonin Reuptake Inhibitors (SSRI) (cont.)

➡️⬅️ Drug Interactions

- Clinically significant interactions are listed below

Class of Drug	Example	Interaction Effects
Analgesic	Acetylsalicylic acid (see NSAID, p. 14)	Increased risk of upper GI bleed with combined use
Anorexiant	Phentermine	Case reports of mania and psychosis in combination
Antiarrhythmic	Propafenone, flecainide, mexiletine	Increased plasma level of antiarrhythmic with fluoxetine and paroxetine due to inhibited metabolism via CYP2D6
	Quinidine, lidocaine	Increased plasma level of antiarrhythmic possible with fluoxetine, fluvoxamine, sertraline, and paroxetine due to inhibited metabolism via CYP3A4
Antibiotic	Clarithromycin	Case of delirium with fluoxetine; case of serotonin syndrome with citalopram
	Erythromycin	Increased plasma level of citalopram due to inhibited metabolism via CYP3A4 is possible but not confirmed; case of serotonin syndrome with sertraline in a 12-year-old
	Linezolid	Monitor for increased serotonergic effects due to linezolid's weak MAO inhibition
Anticoagulant	Warfarin	Increased risk of bleeding; increased prothrombin ratio or INR response due to decreased platelet aggregation secondary to depletion of serotonin
		Loss of anticoagulant control with fluoxetine – data contradictory 65% increase in plasma level of warfarin with fluvoxamine due to accumulation of R-warfarin through inhibited metabolism (via CYP1A2 and 3A4) and decreased clearance of S-isomer (via CYP2C9)
Anticonvulsant	Barbiturates	Barbiturate metabolism inhibited by fluoxetine; reduced plasma level of SSRIs due to enzyme induction
	Carbamazepine, phenytoin, phenobarbital	Decreased plasma level of SSRIs; half-life of paroxetine decreased by 28% Increased plasma level of carbamazepine or phenytoin due to inhibition of metabolism with fluoxetine and fluvoxamine; elevated phenytoin level with sertraline and paroxetine Increased nausea with fluvoxamine and carbamazepine
	Valproate, valproic acid, divalproex	Increased plasma level of valproate (up to 50%) with fluoxetine Valproate may increase plasma level of fluoxetine
	Topiramate	Two case reports of angle-closure glaucoma in females on combination
Antidepressant Cyclic (non-selective)	Amitriptyline, desipramine, imipramine	Elevated plasma level of cyclic antidepressant with fluoxetine, fluvoxamine and paroxetine due to release from protein binding and inhibition of oxidative metabolism; can occur with higher doses of sertraline Increased desipramine level (by 50%) with citalopram and escitalopram
	Clomipramine	Additive antidepressant effect in treatment-resistant patients Increased serotonergic effects
Irreversible MAOI	Phenelzine, tranylcypromine	Hypermetabolic syndrome ("serotonin syndrome" – see p. 8) and death reported with combined use. Suggest waiting 5 weeks when switching from fluoxetine to MAOI and vice versa. Increased plasma level of tranylcypromine (by 15%) reported with paroxetine

Class of Drug	Example	Interaction Effects
RIMA	Moclobemide	Combined therapy may have additive antidepressant effect in treatment-resistant patients; use caution and monitor for serotonergic effects; case reports of serotonin syndrome especially with citalopram and escitalopram
NDRI	Bupropion	Additive antidepressant effect in refractory patients. Bupropion may reverse SSRI-induced sexual dysfunction. Case of hypersexual behavior in combination with fluoxetine Reports of unsteadiness and ataxia in elderly subjects in combination with paroxetine Cases of anxiety, panic, delirium, tremor, myoclonus and seizure reported with fluoxetine due to inhibited metabolism of bupropion and/or fluoxetine (via CYP3A4 and 2D6), competition for protein binding, and additive pharmacological effects
NaSSA	Mirtazapine	Combination reported to alleviate insomnia and augment antidepressant response May mitigate SSRI-induced sexual dysfunction and "poop-out" syndrome through 5-HT$_3$ blockade Increased serotonergic effects possible Increased sedation and weight gain reported with combination Increased mirtazapine level (up to 4-fold) reported in combination with fluvoxamine due to inhibited metabolism
SARI	Trazodone, nefazodone	Additive antidepressant effect Elevated plasma level of SARI; increased serotonergic effects Increased level of MCPP metabolite of trazodone and nefazodone, with paroxetine (via inhibition of CYP2D6) resulting in increased anxiogenic potential Nefazodone may reverse SSRI-induced sexual dysfunction and enhance REM sleep
SNRI	Venlafaxine	Reports that combination with SSRIs that inhibit CYP2D6 (e.g., paroxetine, fluoxetine) can result in increased levels of venlafaxine, with possible increase in blood pressure, anticholinergic effects, and serotonergic effects
Antiemetic (5-HT$_3$ antagonists)	Dolasetron, granisetron, ondansetron Alosetron	Reports of serotonin syndrome with paroxetine and sertraline DO NOT USE with fluvoxamine as plasma level of alosetron increased 6-fold and half-life life increased 3-fold due to inhibited metabolism via CYP3A4
Antifungal	Ketoconazole, fluconazole	Decreased C_{max} of ketoconazole by 21% with citalopram 2 cases of life-threatening serotonin syndrome reported with citalopram[10]
Antihistamine	Diphenhydramine	Increased plasma levels of fluoxetine and paroxetine possible, due to inhibited metabolism via CYP2D6 Additive CNS effects
Antiparkinsonian	Benztropine Procyclidine	Increased plasma level of benztropine with paroxetine Increased plasma level of procyclidine with paroxetine (by 40%)

Selective Serotonin Reuptake Inhibitors (SSRI) (cont.)

Class of Drug	Example	Interaction Effects
Antipsychotic	General	May worsen extrapyramidal effects and akathisia, especially if antidepressant added early in the course of anti-psychotic therapy May be useful for negative symptoms of schizophrenia Additive effect in treatment of OCD
	Risperidone, ziprasidone, olanzapine	Case reports of dose-related mania when risperidone or ziprasidone added to SSRI Increased AUC by 119% and decreased clearance (by 50%) of olanzapine with fluvoxamine; 2.8-fold increase in risperidone level with fluoxetine as well as with paroxetine Increased risk of weight gain with chronic use of olanzapine + fluoxetine
	Chlorpromazine, fluphenazine, haloperidol, perphenazine	Increased serum level of antipsychotic (up to 100% increase in haloperidol level with fluvoxamine or fluoxetine and 4-fold increase with sertraline) (up to 21-fold increase in peak plasma level of perphenazine with paroxetine)
	Pimozide	40% increase in pimozide AUC and C_{max} with sertraline; AUC and C_{max} increased with paroxetine by 151% and 62%, respectively; pimozide level also increased when combined with citalopram, escitalopram or fluvoxamine, increasing risk of QT_c prolongation – DO NOT COMBINE
	Thioridazine	3-fold increase in thioridazine levels with fluvoxamine DO NOT COMBINE fluvoxamine, fluoxetine or paroxetine with thioridazine, due to risk of cardiac conduction disturbances
	Clozapine	Fluvoxamine increases steady-state plasma clozapine levels 5–10 fold, decreases the norclozapine/clozapine ratio, and inhibits its metabolism (via multiple CYP isoenzymes); this results in a reduction of metabolic side effects (attributed to norclozapine) and a need to use a lower dose of clozapine to achieve therapeutic effects 76% increase in clozapine level with fluoxetine, and 40–45% increase with paroxetine and sertraline; potentially significant increase reported with citalopram
Anxiolytic Benzodiazepine	Alprazolam, diazepam, bromazepam	Increased plasma level of alprazolam (by 100%), bromazepam, triazolam, midazolam and diazepam with fluvoxamine and fluoxetine, due to inhibited metabolism; small (13%) decrease in clearance of diazepam reported with sertraline Increased sedation, psychomotor and memory impairment
Buspirone		May potentiate anti-obsessional effects Anxiolytic effects of buspirone may be antagonized Increased plasma level of buspirone (3-fold) with fluvoxamine May mitigate SSRI-induced sexual dysfunction Case report of possible serotonin syndrome with fluoxetine
β-Blocker	Propranolol, metoprolol	Decreased heart rate and syncope (additive effect) reported Increased side effects, lethargy, and bradycardia with fluoxetine, fluvoxamine, and paroxetine due to decreased metabolism of the β-blocker via CYP2D6 (five-fold increase in propranolol level reported with fluvoxamine) Increased metoprolol level with citalopram (by 100%) and with escitalopram (by 50%)
	Pindolol	Increased concentration of serotonin at post-synaptic sites; faster onset of therapeutic response Increased half-life of pindolol (by 28%) with fluoxetine; increased plasma level with paroxetine due to inhibited metabolism via CYP2D6
Caffeine		Increased caffeine levels with fluvoxamine due to inhibited metabolism via CYP1A2; half-life increased from 5 to 31 h Increased jitteriness and insomnia
Ca-channel blocker	Nifedipine, verapamil, nicardapine	Increased side effects (headache, flushing, edema) due to inhibited clearance of Ca-channel blocker with fluoxetine, fluvoxamine, sertraline, and paroxetine via CYP3A4
	Diltiazem	Bradycardia in combination with fluvoxamine

Class of Drug	Example	Interaction Effects
CNS depressant	Alcohol, antihistamines	Potentiation of CNS effects; low risk Rate of fluvoxamine absorption increased by ethanol
	Chloral hydrate	Increased sedation and side effects with fluoxetine due to inhibited metabolism of chloral hydrate
Corticosteroid		Increased risk of GI bleed
Cyclobenzaprine		Increased side effects of cyclobenzaprine with fluoxetine, due to inhibited metabolism; observe for QT prolongation
Cyproheptadine		Report of reversal of antidepressant and antibulimic effects of fluoxetine and paroxetine
Digoxin		Decreased level (area under curve) of digoxin by 18% reported with paroxetine
Ergot alkaloid	Dihydroergotamine	Increased serotonergic effects with intravenous use – **AVOID**. Oral, rectal and subcutaneous routes can be used, with monitoring
	Ergotamine	Elevated ergotamine levels possible due to inhibited metabolism, via CYP3A4, with fluoxetine and fluvoxamine
Ginkgo biloba		Possible increased risk of petechiae and bleeding due to combined anti-hemostatic effects
Grapefruit juice		Decreased metabolism of fluvoxamine and sertraline resulting in increased plasma levels
H$_2$ antagonist	Cimetidine	Inhibited metabolism and increased plasma level of sertraline (by 25%), paroxetine (by 50%), citalopram and escitalopram
	Tizanidine	Increased AUC of tizanidine (14- to 103-fold), increased Cmax (5- to 32-fold), and half-life (3-fold) with fluvoxamine due to inhibition of metabolism via CYP1A2
Hallucinogen	LSD	Recurrence or worsening of flashbacks reported with fluoxetine, sertraline, paroxetine Grand mal seizure
Hormone	Oral contraceptive	Increased activity of combined oral contraceptive possible with fluoxetine and fluvoxamine due to inhibited metabolism
Immunosuppressant	Cyclosporin	Decreased clearance of cyclosporin with sertraline due to competition for metabolism via CYP3A4
Insulin		Increased insulin sensitivity reported
Lithium		Increased serotonergic effects Changes in lithium level and clearance reported Caution with fluoxetine and fluvoxamine; neurotoxicity and seizures reported Increased tremor and nausea reported with sertraline and paroxetine Additive antidepressant effect in treatment-resistant patients
L-Tryptophan		May result in central and peripheral toxicity, hypermetabolic syndrome ("serotonin syndrome" – see p. 8)
MAO-B inhibitor	Selegiline (L-deprenyl)	Case reports of serotonin syndrome, hypertension, and mania when combined with fluoxetine
Melatonin		Increased levels of melatonin with fluvoxamine due to inhibited metabolism via CYP1A2 or 2C9; endogenous melatonin secretion increased
Metoclopramide		Report of increased extrapyramidal and serotonergic effects with sertraline

Selective Serotonin Reuptake Inhibitors (SSRI) (cont.)

Class of Drug	Example	Interaction Effects
Narcotic	Codeine, oxycodone, hydrocodone	Decreased analgesic effect with fluoxetine and paroxetine due to inhibited metabolism to active moiety – morphine, oxymorphone and hydromorphone, respectively (interaction may be beneficial in the treatment of dependence by decreasing morphine and analog formation and opiate reinforcing properties)
	Pentazocine, tramadol	Report of excitatory toxicity (serotonergic) with fluoxetine and pentazocine; and with paroxetine, sertraline and tramadol
	Dextromethorphan	Visual hallucinations reported with fluoxetine
	Methadone	Elevated plasma level of methadone by 10–100% reported with fluvoxamine
	Morphine, fentanyl	Enhanced analgesia
NSAID		Increased risk of upper GI bleed with combined use (risk increased 12-fold) CAUTION
Proguanil		Increased plasma level of proguanil with fluvoxamine due to inhibited metabolism via CYP2C19
Protease inhibitor	Ritonavir	Increased plasma level of sertraline due to competition for metabolism; moderate increase in level of fluoxetine and paroxetine. Serotonin syndrome reported in combination with high dose of fluoxetine Cardiac and neurological side effects reported with fluoxetine, due to elevated ritonavir level (19% increase AUC)
	Fosamprenavir/ritonavir	Decreased plasma level of paroxetine
Proton pump inhibitor	Omeprazole	Increased plasma level of citalopram due to inhibited metabolism via CYP2C19
Sibutramine		Reports of serotonin syndrome (see p. 8) Case report of hypomania with citalopram
Sildenafil		Possible enhanced hypotension due to inhibited metabolism of sildenafil via CYP3A4 with fluoxetine and fluvoxamine
Smoking – cigarettes		Increased metabolism of fluvoxamine by 25% via CYP1A2
Statin	Lovastatin	Increased plasma level of statin with fluoxetine, fluvoxamine, sertraline, and paroxetine due to inhibited metabolism via CYP3A4
St. John's Wort		May augment serotonergic effects – several reports of serotonin syndrome (see p. 8)
Stimulant	Amphetamine, methylphenidate	Potentiated effect in depression, dysthymia, and OCD, in patients with comorbid ADHD; may improve response in treatment-refractory paraphilias and paraphilia-related disorders Plasma level of antidepressant may be increased
Sulfonylurea antidiabetic agent	Glyburide, tolbutamide	Increased hypoglycemia reported in diabetics Increased plasma level of tolbutamide due to reduced clearance (up to 16%) with sertraline
Tacrine		Increased plasma level of tacrine with fluvoxamine; peak plasma level increased 5-fold and clearance decreased by 88% due to inhibited metabolism via CYP1A2
Tamoxifen		Inhibitors of CYP2D6 (paroxetine, fluoxetine) appear to reduce the conversion of tamoxifen to its active metabolite (endoxifen) and may decrease the therapeutic efficacy of this drug
Theophylline		Increased plasma level of theophylline with fluvoxamine due to decreased metabolism via CYP1A2
Thyroid drug	Triiodothyronine (T_3-liothyronine)	Antidepressant effect potentiated Elevated serum thyrotropin (and reduced free thyroxine concentration) reported with sertraline
Tolterodine		Decreased oral clearance of tolterodine by up to 93% with fluoxetine

Class of Drug	Example	Interaction Effects
Triptan	Sumatriptan, rizatriptan, zolmitriptan, eletriptan, almotriptan, naratriptan, frovatriptan	Increased risk of serotonin syndrome (see p. 8) Exacerbation of migraine headache reported with combination
Zolpidem		Case reports of hallucinations and delirium when combined with sertraline, fluoxetine and paroxetine Chronic (5-night) administration of sertraline resulted in faster onset of action and increase in peak plasma concentration of zolpidem

Norepinephrine Dopamine Reuptake Inhibitor (NDRI)

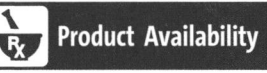 **Product Availability**

Chemical Class	Generic Name	Trade Name(A)	Dosage Forms and Strengths
Monocyclic agent (aminoketone)	Bupropion (amfebutamone)	Wellbutrin Wellbutrin-SR, Zyban(D) Wellbutrin XL	Tablets: 75 mg(B), 100 mg Sustained-release tablets: 100 mg, 150 mg, 200 mg(B) Extended-release tablets: 150 mg, 300 mg

(A) Generic preparations may be available, (B) Not marketed in Canada, (D) Marketed as aid in smoking cessation (as 150 mg)

Indications
(👍 Approved)

- 👍 Major depressive disorder (MDD)
- 👍 Prophylaxis of recurrent MDD
- 👍 Depressed phase of bipolar disorder
- 👍 Aid in smoking cessation (Zyban)[6]
- May play a role in treating addictive disorders (e.g., cocaine)
- Efficacy reported in seasonal affective disorder, dysthymia and chronic fatigue syndrome; case reports of efficacy in social phobia
- Controlled studies suggest benefit in ADHD in adults and children; primarily in individuals with simple ADHD, or with comorbid depression, cigarette smoking or active substance use disorder
- Mitigates sexual dysfunction (reduced sexual desire, anorgasmia, erectile problems) induced by SSRIs and SNRI (sustained-release preparations may be less effective than regular-release products)
- Randomized control studies suggest benefit in neuropathic pain
- Case report of benefit in trichotillomania

General Comments

- May have a lower switch rate (to hypomania or mania) than other antidepressants
- May enhance energy and motivation early in treatment due to effects on norepinephrine and dopamine; reported to improve neurocognitive function in patients with depression[7]
- SR preparation appears to be better tolerated and is associated with a decreased risk of seizures and lower risk of sexual dysfunction
- Monitor patients for worsening of depression and suicidal thinking
- Superior to placebo for smoking cessation at 3 months and 12 months. May be superior to nicotine replacement therapy.[8] >30 RCTs for bupropion (n > 7000). Abstinence rates at 12 months: BUP 19% (vs. 9% on placebo).[6,12]
- Bupropion does not potentiate the sedative effects of alcohol
- Rarely impairs sexual functioning or behavior; some improvement noted
- There is no evidence of increased abuse potential

Pharmacology

- Inhibits the re-uptake of primarily norepinephrine (and dopamine to a lesser extent) into presynaptic neurons
- Antidepressant activity is not well understood. It may be mediated primarily through noradrenergic and/or dopaminergic pathways

Dosing

- See p. 64
- Regular bupropion and SR preparation should be prescribed in divided doses, with a maximum of 150 mg per dose; XL preparation formulated for once daily dosing
- In adults with ADHD: begin at 150 mg/day and titrate dose gradually to a maximum of 450 mg/day in divided doses; up to 4 weeks may be required for maximum drug effect
- In renal impairment reduce dosing frequency and monitor for adverse effects

- In mild to moderate hepatic impairment begin at 100 mg/day and monitor for adverse effects; use with caution in severe hepatic impairment; dose should not exceed 150 mg q 2 days

 Pharmacokinetics

- Rapid absorption with peak concentration occurring within 3 h (mean = 1.5 h); peak plasma concentration of sustained-release preparation is 50–85% of the immediate-release tablets after single dosing, and 25% after chronic dosing
- Highly bound to plasma protein (80–85%)
- Metabolized predominantly by the liver primarily via CYP2B6 and to a lesser extent by other isoenzymes – 6 metabolites; 3 are active
- Bupropion and hydroxybupropion inhibit CYP2D6 isoenzyme
- Elimination half-life: 11–14 h; with chronic dosing: 21 h (mean); increased half-life of bupropion and its metabolites and decreased clearance reported in the elderly
- Weak inducer of its own metabolism, as well as that of other drugs
- Use cautiously in patients with hepatic impairment – reduce dose or frequency of administration

 Onset & Duration of Action

- Therapeutic effect seen after 7–28 days

Adverse Effects

- See chart on p. 62 for incidence of adverse effects

CNS Effects

- A result of antagonism at histamine H_1-receptors and α_1-adrenoreceptors
- Insomnia; vivid dreams and nightmares reported; decreased REM latency and increased REM sleep
- Agitation, anxiety, irritability, dysphoria, aggression, hostility, depersonalization, coupled with urges of self-harm or harm to others
- Precipitation of hypomania or mania felt to be less likely than with other cyclic antidepressants; increased risk in bipolar patients with comorbid substance abuse
- Can exacerbate psychotic symptoms
- Very high doses can result in CNS toxicity including delirium, confusion, impaired concentration, hallucinations, delusions, EPS and seizures
- Reported to exacerbate symptoms of obsessive compulsive disorder
- Short-term memory loss reported
- Seizures can occur after abrupt dose increases, or use of daily doses above 450 mg; use divided doses (maximum single dose no greater than 150 mg) – anorexic and bulimic patients may be at higher risk. Risk of seizures at doses of 100–300 mg = 0.1%; at 300–450 mg = 0.4%; above 450 mg risk increases 10-fold; risk with SR preparation = 0.15% (doses up to 300 mg)
- Disturbance in gait, fine tremor, myoclonus
- Headache, arthralgia (4%), neuralgias (5%), myalgia [Management: analgesics prn]
- Tinnitus reported
- Reversible dyskinesia reported; may aggravate neuroleptic-induced tardive dyskinesia

Anticholinergic Effects

- Occur rarely
- Dry mouth
- Sweating (also due to NE-reuptake inhibition)

Cardiovascular Effects

- Modest sustained increases in blood pressure reported in adults and children (more likely in patients with pre-existing hypertension) – caution in patients with ischemic heart disease
- Orthostatic hypotension, dizziness occurs occasionally, especially when bupropion added to SSRI – caution in the elderly
- Palpitations
- Case of transient ischemic attacks reported
- Rare cases of myocarditis, myocardial infarction, and cardiac death

Norepinephrine Dopamine Reuptake Inhibitor (NDRI) (cont.)

Endocrine & Metabolic Effects	• Menstrual irregularities reported (up to 9% risk) • Cases of hypoglycemia reported
Other Adverse Effects	• Urticarial or pruritic rashes have been reported; rare cases of erythema multiforme and Stevens-Johnson syndrome • Reports of serum sickness • Clitoral priapism reported • Urinary frequency • Anorexia • Rarely febrile neutropenia • Alopecia • Case report of rhabdomyolysis in a patient with hepatic dysfunction • Anaphylactoid reactions with pruritus, urticaria, angioedema, and dyspnea (up to 0.3%) • Case reports of liver failure • Delayed hypersensitivity reactions with arthralgia, myalgia, fever and rash

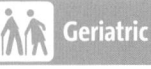 **Discontinuation Syndrome**

• Case of mania reported 2 weeks after abrupt discontinuation of bupropion 300 mg/day taken for 5 weeks to aid in smoking cessation

 Precautions

• Monitor all patients for worsening depression and suicidal thoughts, especially at the start of therapy and following an increase or decrease in dose
• May lower the seizure threshold; therefore administer cautiously to patients with a history of convulsive disorders, organic brain disease and when combining with other drugs that may lower the seizure threshold; contraindicated in patients with a current seizure disorder. To minimize seizures with regular-release bupropion, do not exceed a dose increase of 100 mg in a 3-day period. No single dose should exceed 150 mg for the immediate-release or the sustained-release preparation
• Contraindicated in patients with history of anorexia, bulimia, undergoing alcohol or benzodiazepine withdrawal, or with other conditions predisposing to seizures
• Use with caution (i.e., use lower dose and monitor regularly) in patients with hepatic impairment
• Zyban, marketed for smoking cessation, contains bupropion – DO NOT COMBINE with Wellbutrin

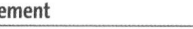 **Toxicity**

• Reports of QTc interval prolongation following overdose[17]
• Rare reports of death following massive overdose, preceded by uncontrolled seizures, bradycardia, cardiac failure and cardiac arrest

Management

• Induce vomiting
• Activated charcoal given every 6–12 h
• Supportive treatment
• Monitor ECG and EEG

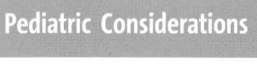 **Pediatric Considerations**

• Exacerbation of tics reported in ADHD and Tourette's syndrome
• Dosage in children: initiate at 1 mg/kg/day, in divided doses, and increase gradually to maximum of 6 mg/kg/day (divided doses)
• Rash reported in up to 17% of youths

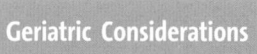 **Geriatric Considerations**

• The elderly are at risk for accumulation of bupropion and its metabolites due to decreased clearance
• Orthostatic hypotension or dizziness reported; may predispose to falls
• Prior to prescribing bupropion, screen for factors that may predispose an elderly patient to seizures

Use in Pregnancy

- No harm to fetus reported in animal studies; no teratogenic effects reported in humans following use of bupropion in the first trimester[2]

Breast Milk

- Bupropion and metabolites are secreted in breast milk; infant can receive up to 2.7% of maternal dose
- Case report of possible infant seizure

Nursing Implications

- Risk of seizures increases if any single dose exceeds 150 mg (immediate-release or sustained-release), or if total daily dose exceeds 300 mg; doses above 150 mg daily should be given in divided doses, preferably 8 h or more apart
- Crushing or chewing the sustained-release preparation destroys the slow-release activity of the product; cutting or splitting the SR preparation in half will increase the rate of drug release in the first 15 minutes. If the tablet is split, the unused half should be discarded unless used within 24 h
- Bupropion degrades rapidly on exposure to moisture, therefore tablets should not be stored in an area of high humidity
- Monitor therapy by watching for adverse effects, mood and activity level changes including worsening depression and suicidal thoughts, especially at the start of therapy or following an increase or decrease in dose
- If the patient has difficulty sleeping, ensure that the last dose of bupropion is no later than 1500 h
- Ensure the patient is not currently being treated for smoking cessation with Zyban (also contains bupropion)

Patient Instructions

- For detailed patient instructions on bupropion, see the Patient Information Sheet on p. 319

Drug Interactions

- Clinically significant interactions are listed below

Class of Drug	Example	Interaction Effects
Amantadine		Increased side effects, including excitement, restlessness and tremor due to increased dopamine availability Case reports of neurotoxicity in elderly patients; delirium
Antiarrhythmic (Type 1c)	Propafenone, flecainide	Increased plasma level of antiarrhythmic due to inhibited metabolism via CYP2D6
Antibiotic – Quinolone	Ciprofloxacin Linezolid	Seizure threshold may be reduced Due to weak MAOI activity, monitor for increased serotonergic effects
Anticholinergic	Antiparkinsonian agents, antihistamines, etc. Orphenadrine	Increased anticholinergic effect Altered levels of either drug due to competition for metabolism via CYP2B6
Anticonvulsant	Carbamazepine, phenytoin, phenobarbital Valproate	Decreased plasma level of bupropion and increased level of its metabolite hydroxybupropion due to increased metabolism by the anticonvulsant Increased level of hydroxybupropion due to inhibited metabolism; level of bupropion not affected
Antidepressant Cyclic (non-selective) Irreversible MAOI SSRI SNRI	Imipramine, desipramine, nortriptyline Phenelzine Fluoxetine Venlafaxine	Elevated imipramine level (by 57%) and nortriptyline level (by 200%) with combination; desipramine peak plasma level and half-life increased up to 5-fold due to decreased metabolism (via CYP2D6) Seizure threshold may be reduced Additive antidepressant effect in treatment-refractory patients DO NOT COMBINE – dopamine metabolism inhibited Case of delirium, anxiety, panic and myoclonus with fluoxetine due to inhibited metabolism of bupropion and/or fluoxetine (via CYP3A2 and 2D6), competition for protein binding and additive pharmacological effects Additive antidepressant effect in treatment-refractory patients; bupropion may mitigate SSRI-induced sexual dysfunction 3-fold increase in venlafaxine level due to inhibited metabolism via CYP2D6, and reduction of level of OD-metabolite Potentiation of noradrenergic effects

Norepinephrine Dopamine Reuptake Inhibitor (NDRI) (cont.)

Class of Drug	Example	Interaction Effects
Antimalarial	Mefloquine, chloroquine	Seizure threshold may be reduced
Antipsychotic	Thioridazine	Increased plasma level of thioridazine due to decreased metabolism via CYP2D6; increased risk of thioridazine-related ventricular arrhythmias and sudden death. DO NOT COMBINE. Washout of 14 days recommended between drugs
	Chlorpromazine	Seizure threshold may be reduced
β-Blocker	Metoprolol	Increased plasma level of b-blocker possible due to inhibited metabolism via CYP2D6
Corticosteroid (systemic)		Seizure threshold may be reduced
Ginkgo biloba		Seizure threshold may be reduced
Hormone	Estrogen/Progesterone	Decreased metabolism (hydroxylation) of bupropion via CYP2B6
L-Dopa		Increased side effects, including excitement, restlessness, nausea, vomiting and tremor due to increased dopamine availability; case reports of neurotoxicity
Lithium		Additive antidepressant effect
Nicotine transdermal		Combination reported to promote higher rates of smoking cessation than either drug alone Increased risk of hypertension with combination
Nitrogen mustard analog	Cyclophosphamide, ifosfamide	Altered levels of either drug due to competition for metabolism via CYP2B6
Protease inhibitor	Ritonavir, nelfinavir, efavirenz	Increased plasma level of bupropion due to decreased metabolism via CYP2B6; risk of seizure
Stimulant	Methylphenidate, dextroamphetamine	Additive effect in ADHD
Sympathomimetic	Pseudoephedrine	Report of manic-like reaction with pseudoephedrine Seizure threshold may be reduced
Theophylline		Seizure threshold may be reduced
Tramadol		Seizure threshold may be reduced
Zolpidem		Case reports of visual hallucinations with combination

Selective Serotonin Norepinephrine Reuptake Inhibitor (SNRI)

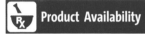 **Product Availability**

Chemical Class	Generic Name	Trade Name[A]	Dosage Forms and Strengths
Bicyclic agent (phenethylamine)	Venlafaxine	Effexor Effexor XR	Tablets: 25 mg[B], 37.5 mg, 50 mg[B], 75 mg, 100 mg[B] Sustained-release tablets: 37.5 mg, 75 mg, 150 mg
	Duloxetine	Cymbalta	Delayed-release capsules: 20 mg[B], 30 mg, 60 mg
	Desvenlafaxine[B]	Pristiq	Extended-release tablets: 50 mg, 100 mg

[A] Generic preparations may be available, [B] Not marketed in Canada

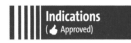 **Indications**
(Approved)

- Major depressive disorder (MDD)
- Generalized anxiety disorder (GAD)
- Social anxiety disorder (venlafaxine)
- Pain due to diabetic peripheral neuropathy (duloxetine); efficacy reported with venlafaxine
- Depressed phase of bipolar disorder
- Preliminary data suggest efficacy of venlafaxine in treatment-resistant depression, dysthymia, postpartum depression and melancholic depression
- Double-blind studies and open trials report efficacy of venlafaxine in OCD, in the higher dose range; efficacy reported with duloxetine
- Preliminary studies suggest efficacy of venlafaxine in panic disorder, premenstrual dysphoric disorder, borderline personality disorder, and in children and adults with ADHD
- Treatment of fibromyalgia (randomized studies in patients with or without MDD); more effective in females
- Preliminary studies suggest efficacy of duloxetine in premenstrual dysphoric disorder and generalized anxiety disorder.
- Anecdotal reports of efficacy of venlafaxine in alleviating sexual dysfunction induced by SSRIs
- Double-blind and open-label studies have shown that venlafaxine and duloxetine reduce hot flashes in menopausal women.
- Management of chronic pain syndromes
- Migraine and tension headaches
- Stress urinary incontinence (duloxetine)
- Open-label study suggests benefit of venlafaxine in pervasive developmental disorders (autism)

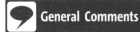 **General Comments**

- Dosing is similar for MDD and GAD; some patients with GAD, however, may require a slower titration
- Suggested that postmenopausal females show better response to venlafaxine than to SSRIs
- May have a faster onset of action, may increase energy; meta-analysis and clinical trials suggests that SNRIs have higher remission rates when compared to some other classes of antidepressants (i.e., most SSRIs)
- Venlafaxine XR preparation may be better tolerated, especially at start of therapy
- Duloxetine should not be given to individuals with chronic hepatic disease or excessive alcohol consumption
- Desvenlafaxine is the major active metabolite of venlafaxine, therefore does not undergo metabolism via CYP2D6
- Venlafaxine has been associated with increased suicidal ideation, hostility, and psychomotor agitation in clinical trials involving children and adolescents. Monitor all patients for worsening depression and suicidal thinking

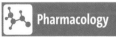 **Pharmacology**

- Potent uptake inhibitors of serotonin and norepinephrine; venlafaxine affects NE at doses above 150 mg, while duloxetine has equal affinity to both NE and serotonin; inhibition of dopamine reuptake occurs at high doses

Selective Serotonin Norepinephrine Reuptake Inhibitor (SNRI) (cont.)

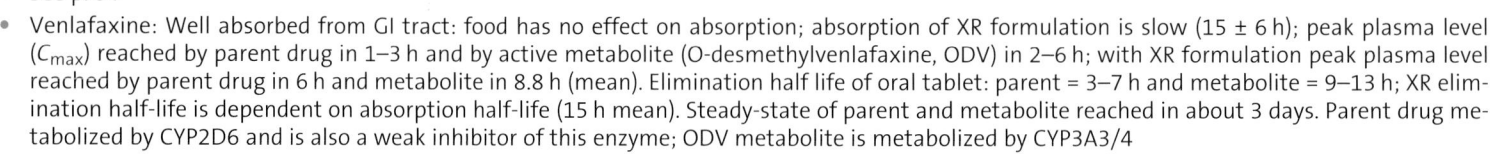 **Dosing**	<ul><li>See p. 64</li><li>Venlafaxine: Initiate drug at 37.5–75 mg (once daily for XR preparation and twice daily for regular preparation), and increase after 1 week in increments no greater than 75 mg q 4 days, up to 225 mg/day (in divided doses); severely depressed patients may require up to 375 mg/day (in divided doses). Decrease dose by 50% in hepatic disease and by 25–50% in renal disease</li><li>Duloxetine: Initiate drug at 30 mg daily and increase to 60 mg bid. Studies have initiated doses at 60 mg daily but a higher incidence of nausea may occur. AVOID in severe renal insufficiency as AUC increased 100% and metabolites increase up to 9-fold; in hepatic disorders AUC increased 5-fold and half-life increased 3-fold</li><li>Desvenlafaxine: Initiate drug at 50 mg once daily – usual maintenance dose; dose may be increased to 100 mg/day if needed. In patients with renal insufficiency (CrCl 30–50 ml/min), use maximum of 50 mg/day; if < 30 ml/min, use 50 mg every other day)</li><li>Have a linear dose-response relationship</li></ul>
Pharmacokinetics	<ul><li>See p. 64</li><li>Venlafaxine: Well absorbed from GI tract: food has no effect on absorption; absorption of XR formulation is slow (15 ± 6 h); peak plasma level (C_{max}) reached by parent drug in 1–3 h and by active metabolite (O-desmethylvenlafaxine, ODV) in 2–6 h; with XR formulation peak plasma level reached by parent drug in 6 h and metabolite in 8.8 h (mean). Elimination half life of oral tablet: parent = 3–7 h and metabolite = 9–13 h; XR elimination half-life is dependent on absorption half-life (15 h mean). Steady-state of parent and metabolite reached in about 3 days. Parent drug metabolized by CYP2D6 and is also a weak inhibitor of this enzyme; ODV metabolite is metabolized by CYP3A3/4</li><li>Duloxetine: Can be given with or without meals, although food delays T_{max} by 6–10 h. There is a 3 h delay in absorption and a 30% increase in clearance with an evening dose as compared to a morning dose. Bioavailability is reduced by about 30% in smokers. Duloxetine is metabolized by CYP1A2 and 2D6 and is an inhibitor of CYP2D6; elimination $T_{1/2}$ increased to 47.8 h (mean) in patients with liver impairment</li><li>Desvenlafaxine: Well absorbed from GI tract; food has no effect on absorption; peak plasma concentration reached in about 7.5 h and mean half-life is about 11 h. Metabolized primarily in the liver by UGT conjugation and to a lesser extent by CYP3A4</li></ul>
Onset & Duration of Action	<ul><li>Therapeutic effect seen after 7–28 days</li></ul>
Adverse Effects	<ul><li>Generally dose-related; see chart p. 62 for incidence of adverse effects</li></ul>
CNS Effects	<ul><li>Both sedation and insomnia reported; prolonged sleep onset latency, disruption of sleep cycle, decreased REM sleep, increased awakenings, reduced sleep efficiency, vivid nightmares</li><li>Headache common</li><li>Nervousness, agitation, hostility, suicidal urges</li><li>Asthenia, fatigue, difficulty concentrating, decreased memory – more likely on higher doses of venlafaxine</li><li>Risk of hypomania/mania estimated to be 0.5% with venlafaxine (no data on duloxetine); caution in bipolar patients with comorbid substance abuse</li><li>10–30% of patients on venlafaxine who improve initially can have breakthrough depression after several months ("poop-out syndrome") – an increase in dosage or augmentation therapy may be of benefit</li><li>Seizures reported rarely (0.3%) with venlafaxine</li><li>Mydriasis; caution in patients with narrow angle glaucoma</li><li>Case reports of restless legs syndrome and myoclonus with venlafaxine</li></ul>
Anticholinergic Effects	<ul><li>May be mediated through NE-reuptake inhibition</li><li>Dry mouth common</li><li>Sweating (in > 10%)</li></ul>

- Urinary retention; cases of urinary frequency and incontinence in females on venlafaxine
- Constipation
- Mydriasis; cases of elevated ocular pressure in patients with narrow angle glaucoma

Cardiovascular Effects

- Venlafaxine: modest, sustained increase in blood pressure can occur, usually within two months of dose stabilization; seen in over 3% of individuals on less than 100 mg/day of venlafaxine and up to 13% of individuals on doses above 300 mg/day of immediate-release drug, and 3–4% with sustained-release product.[3] Sustained increases in blood pressure and heart rate also noted with desvenlafaxine. Caution in patients with history of hypertension or ischemic heart disease [recommended that patients have BP monitored for 2 months at each dose level]. Duloxetine has small changes in blood pressure but these are not considered to be clinically significant with doses up to 120 mg daily.
- Tachycardia; increase by 4 beats/min – more likely in the elderly
- Dizziness common, hypotension occasionally reported
- Duloxetine has no effect on QTc interval

Endocrine & Metabolic Effects

- No weight gain reported

GI Effects

- Nausea occurs frequently at start of therapy and tends to decrease after 1–2 weeks; less frequent with XR formulation of venlafaxine
- Case report of glossodynia (burning mouth syndrome) in a female on venlafaxine

Urogenital and Sexual Effects

- Sexual side effects reported include: decreased libido, delayed orgasm/ejaculation, anorgasmia, no ejaculation, and erectile dysfunction (see SSRIs p. 6 for suggested treatments)
- Risk increased with increasing age, use of higher doses, and concomitant medication
- Priapism reported[11]

Other Adverse Effects

- Duloxetine has been associated with a risk of severe hepatic injury. Cases of hepatitis accompanied by abdominal pain, hepatomegaly, and serum transaminase concentrations more than 20 times the upper limit of normal, with or without jaundice, have been reported during postmarketing surveillance. Elevation in serum transaminase concentrations has in some cases required the discontinuation of duloxetine. Laboratory findings suggestive of severe hepatic injury with evidence of cholestasis were reported in 3 patients who received duloxetine in clinical studies
- Cases of elevated hepatic enzyme levels, hepatitis, bilirubinemia, and jaundice with venlafaxine
- Epistaxis
- Mean increase in serum cholesterol of 3 mg/dL with venlafaxine; elevations in fasting serum total cholesterol, LDL and triglycerides reported with desvenlafaxine [monitor serum lipids during treatment]
- Case report of breast engorgement and pain with venlafaxine
- Case reports of SIADH with hyponatremia with venlafaxine
- Case of Stevens-Johnson syndrome with venlafaxine

D/C Discontinuation Syndrome

- Discontinuation syndrome can occur within 8–16 h of abrupt discontinuation, even after several weeks' therapy, and can last for 8 days
- Symptoms include: asthenia, dizziness, headache, insomnia, tinnitus, nausea, nervousness, confusion, agitation, irritability, nightmares, auditory hallucinations, "electric-shock" sensations, chills, cramps, and diarrhea
- Cases of inter-dose withdrawal reported with regular-release tablet; withdrawal reactions also reported with XR product
- Case of mania reported following venlafaxine taper, despite adequate concomitant mood stabilizing treatment
- ☞ **THEREFORE THIS MEDICATION SHOULD BE WITHDRAWN GRADUALLY AFTER PROLONGED USE**

Management

- Suggested to taper slowly over a two-week period (some suggest over 6 weeks)
- Substituting one dose of fluoxetine (10 or 20 mg) near the end of the taper may help in the withdrawal process; ondansetron 8–12 mg/day over 10 days suggested to be helpful during the taper

⚠ Precautions

- Monitor all patients for worsening depression and suicidal thoughts, especially at start of therapy and following an increase or decrease in dose
- AVOID duloxetine in patients with severe renal insufficiency (CrCl < 30 ml/min)

Selective Serotonin Norepinephrine Reuptake Inhibitor (SNRI) (cont.)

- AVOID duloxetine in patients with underlying liver disease; DO NOT USE in patients with substantial alcohol use, chronic liver disease or hepatic insufficiency
- Do not use in patients with uncontrolled hypertension, as SNRIs can cause modest, sustained increases in blood pressure [blood pressure monitoring recommended for all patients]
- May induce manic reaction in patients with BD and rarely in unipolar depression
- Case report of serotonin-syndrome induced by monotherapy with venlafaxine

Toxicity

- Symptoms of toxicity include vomiting, excess adrenergic stimulation, mydriasis, tachycardia, hypotension, arrhythmias, increase in QTc interval, bowel dysmobility, decreased level of consciousness, seizures – increased risk of fatal outcomes following overdose[4]
- Delayed onset of rhabdomyolysis or serotonin-syndrome possible

Pediatric Considerations

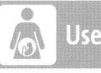

- For detailed information on the use of SNRIs in this population, please see the *Clinical Handbook of Psychotropic Drugs for Children and Adolescents* (2007)
- CAUTION: No approved indications in children and adolescents; recommend against using venlafaxine in pediatric patients due to lack of efficacy and concerns about increased hostility and suicide ideation (rate 2% vs placebo 1%)
- May cause behavior activation and aggravate symptoms of hyperactivity; monitor all patients for worsening depression and suicidal thinking

Geriatric Considerations

- Dosage adjustments in healthy elderly patients are not usually required; 14% increase in metabolite level and 24% increase in half-life reported with venlafaxine
- Can increase heart rate in frail elderly, related to its noradrenergic activity; increased cardiovascular and cerebrovascular adverse effects reported
- Clearance of desvenlafaxine decreased in the elderly

Use in Pregnancy

- Category C drugs – animal studies show a decrease in offspring weight, as well as stillbirths with high doses
- No teratogenic effects reported in humans with venlafaxine, to date; may be a trend toward higher rates of spontaneous abortion; no data on duloxetine
- Neonates exposed to venlafaxine and desvenlafaxine in third trimester have developed complications upon delivery including respiratory distress, temperature instability, feeding difficulties, agitation, irritability, changes in muscle tone, seizures

Breast Milk

- The total dose of venlafaxine and its ODV metabolite ingested by a breast-fed infant can be as high as 9.2% of the maternal dose

Nursing Implications

- A gradual titration of dosage at start of therapy will minimize nausea
- Psychotherapy and education are also important in the treatment of depression
- Monitor therapy by watching for adverse effects as well as mood and activity level changes including worsening of suicidal thoughts especially at start of therapy or following an increase or decrease in dose; keep physician informed
- Be aware that the medication may increase psychomotor activity; this may create concern about suicidal behavior
- Excessive ingestion of caffeinated foods, drugs, or beverages may increase anxiety and agitation and confuse the diagnosis
- Instruct patient not to chew or crush the sustained-release Effexor XR tablet, the extended-release desvenlafaxine tablet or the delayed-release duloxetine capsules, but swallow them whole
- If a dose is missed, do not attempt to make it up; continue with regular daily schedule (divided doses)
- SNRIs should not be stopped suddenly due to risk of precipitating a withdrawal reaction

Patient Instructions

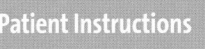

- For detailed patient instructions on venlafaxine, see the Patient Information Sheet on p. 321

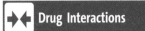

Drug Interactions

- Clinically significant interactions are listed below

Class of Drug	Example	Interaction Effects
Analgesic	Acetylsalicylic acid (see NSAID)	Increased risk of upper GI bleeding with combined use
Antiarrhythmic (type 1c)	Propafenone, flecainide	Increased plasma level of venlafaxine and duloxetine due to inhibited metabolism via CYP2D6
	Quinidine	Increased plasma level of duloxetine due to inhibited metabolism
Antibiotic	Ciprofloxacin, enoxacin	Increased plasma level of duloxetine due to inhibition of metabolism via CYP1A2
	Linezolid	Due to its weak MAOI activity, monitor for increased serotonergic and noradrenergic effects
Anticholinergic	Antiparkinsonian agents, antipsychotics, etc.	Increased anticholinergic effects
Anticoagulant	Warfarin, acenocoumarol	Case reports of significant decreases in international normalized ratio (INR) with duloxetine
		Increased risk of bleeding
Antidepressant NDRI	Bupropion	3-fold increase in venlafaxine plasma level due to inhibited metabolism via CYP2D6 and reduction in level of ODV metabolite Potentiation of noradrenergic effects Bupropion may mitigate SNRI-induced sexual side effects
SSRI	Paroxetine, fluoxetine	Reports that combination with SSRIs that inhibit CYP2D6 can result in increased levels of venlafaxine and duloxetine, with possible increases in blood pressure, anticholinergic effects and serotonergic effects
	Fluvoxamine	5-fold increase in AUC and 2.5-fold increase in half-life of duloxetine due to inhibited metabolism via CYP1A2
Irreversible MAOI	Phenelzine	**AVOID**; possible hypertensive crisis and serotonergic reaction
RIMA	Moclobemide	Enhanced effects of norepinephrine and serotonin; caution – no data on safety with combined use
SARI	Trazodone	Case report of serotonin syndrome with venlafaxine
Tricyclic	Imipramine	C_{max} and AUC of imipramine increased by 40% with venlafaxine
	Desipramine	Desipramine (metabolite) clearance reduced by 20% with venlafaxine; desipramine level increased 3-fold with duloxetine Increased levels of cyclic antidepressants metabolized by CYP2D6 possible with duloxetine
	Trimipramine	Case report of seizure in combination with venlafaxine – postulated to be a result of inhibited metabolism via CYP2D6
NaSSA	Mirtazapine	Case report of serotonin syndrome with venlafaxine
Antipsychotic	General	Increased levels of antipsychotics metabolized by CYP2D6 possible with duloxetine
	Haloperidol	Increased peak plasma level and AUC of haloperidol with venlafaxine; no change in half-life
	Thioridazine	Increased plasma level of venlafaxine and decreased concentration of ODV metabolite Possible increased plasma level of thioridazine and arrhythmias – AVOID with duloxetine
	Risperidone	Increased AUC of risperidone by 32% and decreased renal clearance by 20% with venlafaxine
β-Blocker	Propranolol	Increased plasma level of venlafaxine due to competition for metabolism via CYP2D6
H₂ antagonist	Cimetidine	Increased plasma level of venlafaxine due to decreased clearance by 43%; peak concentration increased by 60% Increased plasma level of duloxetine due to inhibited metabolism
Lithium		Case report of serotonin syndrome with venlafaxine (see p. 8)
MAO-B inhibitor	Selegiline (L-deprenyl)	Case reports of serotonergic reaction with venlafaxine
Metoclopramide		Case report of extrapyramidal and serotonergic effects with venlafaxine

Selective Serotonin Norepinephrine Reuptake Inhibitor (SNRI) (cont.)

Class of Drug	Example	Interaction Effects
NSAID		Increased risk of upper GI bleed with combined use. CAUTION
Protease inhibitor	Ritonavir Indinavir	Moderate decrease in clearance of venlafaxine with ritonavir Both increases (by 13%) and decreases (by 60%) in total concentration (AUC) of indinavir reported with venlafaxine
Stimulant	Dextroamphetamine Methylphenidate	Case report of serotonin syndrome with venlafaxine Potentiated effect in the treatment of depression and ADHD
Tolterodine		C_{max} and half-life of tolterodine increased; no effect on active metabolites
Zolpidem		Case report of delirium and hallucinations with venlafaxine

Serotonin-2 Antagonists/Reuptake Inhibitors (SARI)

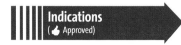 Product Availability

Chemical Class	Generic Name	Trade Name[A]	Dosage Forms and Strengths
Phenylpiperidine	Nefazodone[B]	(generic)	50 mg, 100 mg, 150 mg, 200 mg, 250mg
Triazolopyridine	Trazodone	Desyrel Desyrel Dividose	Tablets: 50 mg, 100 mg, 150 mg, 300 mg Tablets: 150 mg, 300 mg

[A] Generic preparations may be available, [B] Nefazodone withdrawn in Canada November 2003

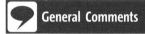

Indications
(👍 Approved)

- 👍 Major depressive disorder (MDD)
- 👍 Prophylaxis of recurrent MDD
- 👍 Depressed phase of bipolar disorder (see Precautions)
- Treatment of secondary depression in other mental illnesses, e.g., schizophrenia, dementia
- Chronic depression (nefazodone)
- Agoraphobia associated with panic disorder
- Efficacy in dysthymia reported
- Bulimia nervosa
- Benefit reported in social phobia (nefazodone)
- Open trials suggest efficacy of nefazodone in posttraumatic stress disorder, including alleviation of sleep problems
- Insomnia
- Premenstrual syndrome (nefazodone)
- Preliminary data suggest benefit in generalized anxiety disorder (nefazodone)
- Erectile impotence (trazodone), anorgasmia (nefazodone)
- Trazodone reported to decrease disturbed behavior in patients with dementia and improve delirium (case reports); open trials suggest efficacy in treatment of aggression in children
- Preliminary data suggest nefazodone decreases nonparaphilic compulsive sexual behavior
- Open trials suggest nefazodone improves fatigue, sleep disturbances and mood in patients with chronic fatigue syndrome
- Open trials report benefit of nefazodone in alleviating chronic (daily) headaches; anecdotal reports suggest benefit for neuropathic pain
- Efficacy in reducing symptoms of pathological gambling reported in open trial with trazodone

General Comments

- Nefazodone withdrawn in Canada due to risk of hepatotoxicity
- Trazodone increases slow-wave (stage 3–4) sleep
- Monitor all patients for worsening depression and/or suicidal thoughts

Pharmacology

- Exact mechanism of action unknown; equilibrate the effects of biogenic amines through various mechanisms; cause downregulation of β-adrenergic receptors
- Nefazodone blocks 5-HT$_{2A}$ receptors, antagonizes 5-HT$_{2C}$ receptors, inhibits reuptake of 5-HT (at higher doses) and serves as an adrenergic antagonist

Dosing

- See p. 64 See p. 64

Serotonin-2 Antagonists/Reuptake Inhibitors (SARI) (cont.)

- Initiate drug at a low dose and increase dose every 3 to 5 days to a maximum tolerated dose based on side effects; there is a wide variation in dosage requirements; prophylaxis is most effective if therapeutic dose is maintained
- Trazodone doses of 25–100 mg hs used in chronic sleep disorders
- Trazodone should be taken on an empty stomach as food delays absorption and decreases drug effect
- Regular ingestion of grapefruit juice while on nefazodone may affect the antidepressant plasma level (see Interactions below)
- Once stabilized, the patient can be placed on a once-daily dose of nefazodone

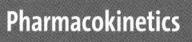 **Pharmacokinetics**

- See. p. 64
- Completely absorbed from the gastrointestinal tract; food significantly delays and decreases peak plasma effect of trazodone
- Large percentage metabolized by first-pass effect
- Highly bound to plasma protein
- Metabolized primarily by the liver; half-life of nefazodone is dose-dependent varying from 2 h at 100 mg/day to 4–5 h at 600 mg/day; half-life and AUC of nefazodone and hydroxy metabolite doubled in patients with severe liver impairment
- Trazodone metabolized by CYP3A4 to active metabolite m-chlorophenylpiperazine (MCPP); elimination half-life 4–9 h in adults and 11.6 h (mean) in the elderly; steady state reached in about 3 days
- Nefazodone is a potent inhibitor of CYP3A4 and may decrease the metabolism of drugs metabolized by this isoenzyme (see Interactions pp. 31–32)

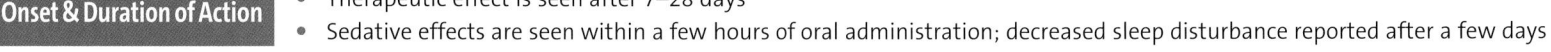 **Onset & Duration of Action**

- Therapeutic effect is seen after 7–28 days
- Sedative effects are seen within a few hours of oral administration; decreased sleep disturbance reported after a few days

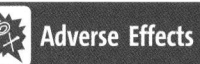 **Adverse Effects**

- The pharmacological and side effect profile of SARI antidepressants is dependent on their affinity for and activity on neurotransmitters/receptors (see table p. 59)
- See chart p. 62 for incidence of adverse effects at therapeutic doses; incidence of adverse effects may be greater in early days of treatment; patients adapt to many side effects over time

CNS Effects

- A result of antagonism at histamine H_1-receptors and α_1-adrenoreceptors
- Occur frequently
- Drowsiness (most common adverse effect; reported in 20–50%) [Management: prescribe bulk of dose at bedtime]
- Weakness, lethargy, fatigue
- Conversely, excitement, agitation and restlessness have occurred
- Confusion, disturbed concentration, disorientation
- Nefazodone increases REM sleep and sleep quality
- Improved psychomotor and complex memory performance reported with nefazodone after single doses; dose-related impairment noted after repeated doses
- Precipitation of hypomania or mania, increased risk in bipolar patients with comorbid substance abuse
- Psychosis, panic reactions, anxiety, or euphoria may occur
- Fine tremor
- Akathisia (rare – check serum iron for deficiency)
- Seizures can occur rarely following abrupt drug increase or after drug withdrawal; risk increases with high plasma levels
- Tinnitus
- Paresthesias reported with nefazodone (approximate risk 4%)
- Myoclonus; includes muscle jerks of lower extremities, jaw, and arms, and nocturnal myoclonus – may be severe in up to 9% of patients [If severe, clonazepam, valproate or carbamazepine may be of benefit]

- Dysphasia, stuttering
- Disturbance in gait, parkinsonism, dystonia
- Headache; worsening of migraine reported with trazodone and nefazodone

Anticholinergic Effects	

- A result of antagonism at muscarinic receptors (ACh)
- Occur occasionally; more frequently in elderly patients on nefazodone
- Include dry eyes, blurred vision, constipation, dry mouth [see Cyclic Antidepressants p. 39 for treatment suggestions]

Cardiovascular Effects	

- A result of antagonism at α_1-adrenoreceptors, muscarinic, 5-HT$_2$, and H$_1$-receptors, and inhibition of sodium fast channels
- More common in elderly
- Risk increases with high plasma levels
- Bradycardia seen with nefazodone
- Dizziness (10–30%) orthostatic hypotension and syncope [Management: sodium chloride tablets, caffeine, fludrocortisone (0.1–0.5 mg), midodrine (2.5–10 mg tid), use of support stockings]
- Trazodone can exacerbate ischemic attacks; arrhythmias reported (with doses > 200 mg/day) including torsades de pointes
- Cases of prolonged conduction time with trazodone and nefazodone (by inhibiting hERG potassium ion channels)[17]; contraindicated in heart block or post-myocardial infarction

Endocrine & Metabolic Effects	

- Decreases in blood sugar levels reported (nefazodone)
- Can induce syndrome of SIADH with hyponatremia; risk increased with age
- Weight gain reported with trazodone; rare with nefazodone

GI Effects	

- A result of inhibition of 5-HT uptake and ACh antagonism
- Peculiar taste, "black tongue," glossitis
- Reports of upper GI bleeding

Urogenital and Sexual Effects	

- A result of altered dopamine (D$_2$) activity, 5-HT$_2$ blockade, inhibition of 5-HT reuptake, α_1-blockade, and ACh blockade
- Occur rarely
- Testicular swelling, painful ejaculation, retrograde ejaculation, increased libido; spontaneous orgasm with yawning (trazodone)
- Priapism with trazodone and nefazodone due to prominent α_1-blockade in the absence of anticholinergic activity

Allergic Reactions	

- Rare
- Rash, urticaria, pruritus, edema, blood dyscrasias

Other Adverse Effects	

- Jaundice, hepatitis, hepatic necrosis and hepatic failure reported with therapeutic doses of nefazodone (laboratory evidence includes: increased levels of ALT, AST, GGT, bilirubin and increased prothrombin time) – Cases of liver failure and death reported. Recommend baseline and periodic liver function tests with nefazodone. Monitor for signs of hepatotoxicity.
- Cases of palinopsia with both trazodone and nefazodone and scotoma with nefazodone – may be dose related
- Rare reports of alopecia with nefazodone.
- Case reports of burning sensations, in various parts of the body, with nefazodone.

D/C Discontinuation Syndrome	

- Reported incidence 20–80% – likely due to serotonergic and adrenergic rebound
- Abrupt withdrawal from high doses may occasionally cause a "flu-like" syndrome consisting of fever, fatigue, sweating, coryza, malaise, myalgia, headache; anxiety, insomnia, nightmares, panic; as well as dizziness, nausea, vomiting, akathisia, dyskinesia, and priapism
- Most likely to occur 24–48 h after withdrawal, or after a large dosage decrease
- Rebound depression can occur (even in individuals not previously depressed – such as patients with obsessive-compulsive disorders)
- Paradoxical mood changes reported on abrupt withdrawal, including hypomania or mania
- ☞ **THEREFORE THESE MEDICATIONS SHOULD BE WITHDRAWN GRADUALLY AFTER PROLONGED USE**

Serotonin-2 Antagonists/Reuptake Inhibitors (SARI) (cont.)

Management	• Reinstitute the drug at a lower dose and taper gradually over several days

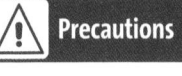

Precautions

- Trazodone is a substrate of CYP3A4 and its metabolism can be inhibited by CYP3A4 inhibitors; nefazodone is a potent inhibitor of CYP3A4 (see Interactions pp. 31–32)
- Use caution in combination with drugs that prolong the QT interval
- Use nefazodone cautiously in patients in whom excess anticholinergic activity could be harmful (e.g., prostatic hypertrophy, urinary retention, narrow-angle glaucoma)
- Use nefazodone with caution in patients with respiratory difficulties, since antidepressants with anticholinergic properties can dry up bronchial secretions and make breathing more difficult
- May lower the seizure threshold; therefore, administer cautiously to patients with a history of convulsive disorders, organic brain disease, or a predisposition to convulsions (e.g., alcohol withdrawal)
- May impair the mental and physical ability to perform hazardous tasks (e.g., driving a car or operating machinery); will potentiate the effects of alcohol
- May induce manic reactions in patients with bipolar disorder and rarely in unipolar depression; because of risk of increased cycling, bipolar disorder is a relative contraindication
- Use caution in prescribing nefazodone for patients with a history of alcoholism or liver disorder. Monitor liver function tests at baseline and periodically during treatment, and at first symptom or clinical sign of liver dysfunction
- Combination with SSRIs can lead to increased plasma level of trazodone. Combination therapy has been used in the treatment of resistant patients; use caution and monitor for serotonin syndrome
- Use caution when switching from trazodone to fluoxetine and vice versa (see Interactions pp. 31–32, and Switching Antidepressants p. 66)

Toxicity

- Acute poisoning results in drowsiness, ataxia, nausea, vomiting; deep coma as well as arrhythmias (including torsade de pointes) and AV block reported; no seizures reported

Pediatric Considerations

- For detailed information on the use of trazodone in this population, please see the *Clinical Handbook of Psychotropic Drugs for Children and Adolescents* (2007)
- Trazodone used in acute and chronic treatment of insomnia and night terrors, and in major depressive disorder and behavior disturbances in children (agitation, aggression)
- Start drug at a low dose (10–25 mg) and increase gradually by 10–25 mg every 4–5 days

Geriatric Considerations

- Initiate dose lower and slower than in younger patients; elderly patients may take longer to respond and may require trials of up to 12 weeks before response is noted
- AUC increased in elderly; highest in elderly females
- Monitor for excessive CNS and anticholinergic effects
- Caution when combining with other drugs with CNS and anticholinergic properties; additive effects can result in confusion, disorientation, and delirium; elderly are sensitive to anticholinergic effects
- Caution regarding cardiovascular side effects: orthostatic hypotension (can lead to falls). Can potentiate effects of antihypertensive drugs
- Cognitive impairment can occur

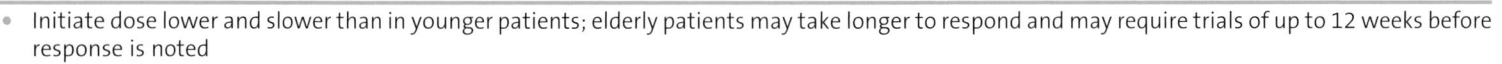

Use in Pregnancy

- Trazodone in high doses was found to be teratogenic and toxic to the fetus in some animal species; trazodone and nefazodone found not to increase rates of malformations in humans above the baseline of 1–3%
- If possible, avoid during first trimester

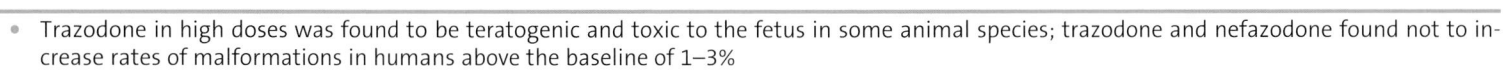

Breast Milk	• SARI antidepressants are secreted into breast milk
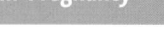	• The American Academy of Pediatrics classifies SARI antidepressants as drugs "whose effects on nursing infants are unknown but may be of concern."

Nursing Implications

- Psychotherapy and education are also important in the treatment of depression
- Monitor therapy by watching for adverse side effects, mood and activity level changes including worsening of suicidal thoughts; keep physician informed
- Be aware that the medication reduces the degree of depression and may increase psychomotor activity; this may create concern about suicidal behavior
- Expect a lag time of 7–28 days before antidepressant effects will be noticed
- Reassure patient that drowsiness and dizziness usually subside after first few weeks; if dizzy, patient should get up from lying or sitting position slowly, and dangle legs over edge of bed before getting up
- Instruct patient to avoid ingestion of grapefruit juice, as the blood level of trazodone and nefazodone may increase
- Excessive use of caffeinated foods, drugs, or beverages may increase anxiety and agitation and confuse the diagnosis
- These drugs should not be stopped suddenly due to risk of precipitating withdrawal reactions
- Because these drugs can cause drowsiness, caution patient that activities requiring mental alertness should not be performed until response to the drug has been determined
- With nefazodone monitor for signs of hepatatoxicity, including nausea, vomiting, fatigue, pruritus, jaundice, dark urine

 Patient Instructions

- For detailed patient instructions on SARI, see the Patient Information Sheet on p. 323
- Avoid ingestion of grapefruit juice while taking nefazodone, as the blood level of the antidepressant may increase

▶◀ Drug Interactions

- Clinically significant interactions are listed below

Class of Drug	Example	Interaction Effects
Alcohol		Short-term or acute use reduces first-pass metabolism of antidepressant and increases its plasma level; chronic use induces metabolizing enzymes and decreases its plasma level
Antibiotic	Linezolid	Monitor for increased serotonergic effects due to weak MAOI activity of linezolid
Anticholinergic	Antiparkinsonian agents, antihistamines	Increased anticholinergic effect; may increase risk of hyperthermia, confusion, urinary retention, etc.
Anticonvulsant	Carbamazepine, phenytoin	Increased plasma level of carbamazepine or phenytoin due to inhibition of metabolism with trazodone Increased plasma level of carbamazepine with nefazodone due to inhibited metabolism via CYP3A4
	Carbamazepine, barbiturates, phenytoin	Decreased plasma level of trazodone and its MCPP metabolite (by 76% and 60%, respectively with carbamazepine) and of nefazodone, due to enzyme induction via CYP3A4
Anticoagulant	Warfarin	Case reports of decreased prothrombin time and INR with trazodone
Antidepressant Irreversible MAOI	Phenelzine, tranylcypromine	Low doses of trazodone (25–50 mg) used to treat antidepressant-induced insomnia Combined therapy with MAOI has additive antidepressant effects; monitor for serotonergic effects
RIMA	Moclobemide	Additive antidepressant effect in treatment-resistant patients; monitor for serotonergic effects
NDRI	Bupropion	Additive antidepressant effect in treatment-resistant patients
SSRI	Fluoxetine, fluvoxamine, paroxetine, sertraline	Elevated SSRI plasma level (due to release from protein binding and inhibition of oxidative metabolism); monitor plasma level and for signs of toxicity Nefazodone metabolite (mCPP) level increased 4-fold with fluoxetine; case report of serotonin syndrome with combination Additive antidepressant effect in treatment-resistant patients Nefazodone may reverse SSRI-induced sexual dysfunction and may enhance sleep
Antifungal	Ketoconazole	Increased plasma level of trazodone due to inhibited metabolism via CYP3A4

Serotonin-2 Antagonists/Reuptake Inhibitors (SARI) (cont.)

Class of Drug	Example	Interaction Effects
Antihypertensive	Bethanidine, debrisoquin, methyldopa, guanethidine, reserpine Clonidine Acetazolamide, thiazide diuretics	Decreased antihypertensive effect due to inhibition of α-adrenergic receptors Additive hypotension and sedation Hypotension augmented
Antipsychotic	Chlorpromazine, haloperidol, perphenazine, clozapine	Increased plasma level of either agent Potentiation of hypotension
Ca-channel blocker	Amlodipine	Elevated amlodipine level due to inhibited metabolism by nefazodone, via CYP3A4
CNS depressant	Hypnotics, antihistamines, benzodia-zepines, alcohol	Increased sedation, CNS depression
Cholestyramine		Decreased absorption of antidepressant, if given together
Digoxin		Increased digoxin plasma level, with possible toxicity
Ginkgo biloba		Case report of coma with trazodone (postulated to be due to excess stimulation of GABA receptors)
Grapefruit juice		Decreased metabolism of trazodone and nefazodone via CYP3A4
Lithium		Additive antidepressant effect
L-Trypophan		Additive antidepressant effect; monitor for serotonergic effects
MAO-B inhibitor	Selegiline (L-deprenyl)	Reports of serotonergic reactions
Protease inhibitor	Ritonavir, indinavir	Increased plasma levels of trazodone and nefazodone due to decreased metabolism (with ritonavir, trazodone clearance decreased 52%)
Sildenafil		Possible enhanced hypotension due to inhibited metabolism of sildenafil by nefazodone via CYP3A4
Statins	Simvastatin, pravastatin, atorvastatin	Inhibited metabolism of statins by nefazodone (via CYP3A4); increased plasma level and adverse effects – myositis and rhabdomyolysis reported
St. John's Wort		May augment serotonergic effects – case reports of serotonergic reactions
Sulfonylurea	Tolbutamide	Increased hypoglycemia
Thyroid drug	Triiodothyronine (T_3-liothyronine), L-thyroxine (T_4)	Additive antidepressant effect in treatment-resistant patients

Noradrenergic/Specific Serotonergic Antidepressants (NaSSA)

Product Availability

Chemical Class	Generic Name	Trade Name[A]	Dosage Forms and Strengths
Tetracyclic agent	Mirtazapine	Remeron Remeron SolTab[B], Remeron RD[C]	Tablets: 7.5 mg[B], 15 mg[B], 30 mg, 45 mg[B] Oral disintegrating tablets: 15 mg, 30 mg, 45 mg

[A] Generic preparation may be available, [B] Not marketed in Canada, [C] Not marketed in USA

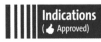

Indications
(Approved)

- Major depressive disorder (MDD) (with or without comorbid anxiety)
- Mirtazapine may mitigate SSRI-induced sexual dysfunction and "poop-out" syndrome (see p. 2)
- Preliminary reports of efficacy in panic disorder, generalized anxiety disorder, OCD, PTSD, dysthymia and premenstrual dysphoric disorder
- Open-label study suggests improvement in symptoms of aggression, self-injury, irritability, hyperactivity, anxiety, depression and insomnia in pervasive developmental disorders (autism)
- Mirtazapine may benefit negative symptoms of schizophrenia and psychotic depression
- Double-blind study showed improvement in akathisia with addition of low-dose (15 mg) mirtazapine
- Early data suggests benefit in treating chronic pain (e.g., tension, headache)
- Has been found helpful in alcohol withdrawal; may help maintain abstinence

General Comments

- Reduces sleep latency and prolongs sleep duration due to H_1 and $5-HT_{2A+C}$ blockade – may be helpful in treating depression with prominent insomnia or agitation
- Has mild anxiolytic effects at lower doses
- Suggested that mirtazapine may have a faster onset of antidepressant action than some other classes of antidepressants (e.g., most SSRIs) – may be secondary to early restoration of sleep and decrease of anxiety
- Monitor all patients for worsening depression and suicidal thinking

Pharmacology

- Selective antagonist at α_2-adrenergic auto- and heteroreceptors which are involved in regulation of neuronal release of norepinephrine and serotonin (increases noradrenergic and serotonergic transmission via blockade of α-adrenoreceptors; increases the release of norepinephrine and serotonin, and blocks $5-HT_{2A+C}$ and $5-HT_3$ receptors)

Dosing

- See p. 64
- Initiate at 15–30 mg daily for 4 days; increase to 30 mg and maintain for at least 10 days; if ineffective, can increase to 60 mg daily

Pharmacokinetics

- Bioavailability is approximately 50% due to gut wall and hepatic first-pass metabolism; food slightly decreases absorption rate
- Remeron SolTabs dissolve on the tongue within 30 seconds; can be swallowed with or without water, chewed, or allowed to dissolve
- Peak plasma level achieved in 2 h
- Protein binding of 85%
- Females and the elderly show higher plasma concentrations than males and young adults
- Extensively metabolized via CYP1A2, 2D6 and 3A4; desmethyl metabolite has some clinical activity
- Half-life 20–40 h – half-life significantly longer in females than in males
- Hepatic clearance decreased by 40% in patients with cirrhosis
- Clearance reduced by 30–50% in patients with renal impairment

Noradrenergic/Specific Serotonergic Antidepressants (NaSSA) (cont).

 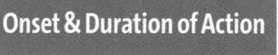 **Onset & Duration of Action**

- Therapeutic effects seen after 7–28 days

Adverse Effects

- See p. 62

CNS Effects

- Fatigue, sedation in over 30% of patients; less sedation at doses above 15 mg due to increased effect on α_2-receptors and increased release of NE
- Shown to impair driving performance and decreased psychomotor functioning during the acute treatment phase
- Insomnia, agitation, hostility, depersonalization, restlessness, and nervousness reported occasionally coupled with urges of selfharm or harm to others
- Increases slow-wave sleep and decreases stage 1 sleep. Reported to shorten sleep onset latency, improve sleep efficiency and increase total sleep time; vivid dreams reported; case reports of REM sleep behavior disorder with hallucinations and confusion
- Case report of panic attack during dose escalation
- Rarely delirium, hallucinations, psychosis
- Seizures (very rare – 0.04%)

Anticholinergic Effects

- Dry mouth frequent; constipation [for treatment suggestions see Non-Selective Cyclic Antidepressants, p. 39)]
- Increased sweating, blurred vision and urinary retention reported rarely

Cardiovascular Effects

- Hypotension, hypertension, vertigo, tachycardia, and palpitations reported rarely
- Edema 1–2%
- No significant ECG changes reported

Endocrine & Metabolic Effects

- Carbohydrate craving, increased appetite and leptin concentrations, and weight gain (of over 4 kg) reported in >16% of patients (due to potent antihistaminic properties); occur primarily in the first 4 weeks of treatment and may be dose-related – may be of benefit in depressed patients with marked anorexia

GI Effects

- Rare reports of bitter taste, dyspepsia, nausea, vomiting and diarrhea
- Decreased appetite and weight loss occasionally reported

Other Adverse Effects

- Sexual dysfunction occurs occasionally; risk increased with age, use of higher doses, and concomitant medication
- Case reports of erotic dream-related ejaculation in elderly patients
- Rare reports of tremor, hot flashes
- Transient elevation of ALT reported in about 2% of patients; cases of hepatitis
- Febrile neutropenia (1.5% risk) and agranulocytosis (0.1%) reported; monitor WBC if patient develops signs of infection [some recommend doing baseline and annual CBC]
- Increases in plasma cholesterol, to over 20% above the upper limit of normal, seen in 15% of patients; increases in nonfasting triglyceride levels (7%)
- Cases of joint pain or worsening of arthritis reported
- Myalgia and flu-like symptoms in 2–5% of patients
- Case of palinopsia reported
- Cases of pancreatitis and of gall-bladder disorder
- Cases of rhabdomyolysis reported with mirtazapine used alone, in combination with risperidone, and in overdose

D/C Discontinuation Syndrome	• Case report of dizziness, nausea, anxiety, insomnia, and paresthesia following abrupt withdrawal • Case report of hypomania and of panic attack ☞ **THEREFORE THESE MEDICATIONS SHOULD BE WITHDRAWN GRADUALLY AFTER PROLONGED USE**
Management	• Reinstitute drug at a lower dose and taper gradually over several days
⚠ Precautions	• Monitor all patients for worsening depression and suicidal thoughts especially at start of therapy or following an increase or decrease in dose; see Pediatric Considerations (p. 35) • Caution in patients with compromised liver function or renal impairment • Monitor WBC if patient develops signs of infection; a low WBC requires discontinuation of therapy • May induce manic reactions in patients with BD and rarely in unipolar depression
☠ Toxicity	• Low liability for toxicity in overdose if taken alone; no changes in vital signs, with dose of 900 mg, reported • No fatalities when drug used alone
Pediatric Considerations	• For detailed information on the use of mirtazapine in this population, please see the *Clinical Handbook of Psychotropic Drugs for Children and Adolescents* (2007) • CAUTION: Episodes of self-harm and potential suicidal behaviors have been reported with certain serotonergic antidepressants in patients under age 18
Geriatric Considerations	• Clearance reduced in elderly males by up to 40%, and in elderly females by up to 10% • Dosing: start at 7.5 mg hs and increase to 15 mg after 1–2 weeks, depending on response and side effects; monitor for sedation, hypotension and anticholinergic effects
Use in Pregnancy	• Early data suggests no teratogenic effects in humans • Higher rate of spontaneous abortions and preterm births reported[5]
Breast Milk	• Mirtazapine and its metabolite are secreted into breast milk in low concentrations[9]
Nursing Implications	• Psychotherapy and education are also important in the treatment of depression • Monitor therapy by watching for adverse effects, mood and activity level changes including worsening of suicidal thoughts • Signs and symptoms of infections (e.g., sore throat, fever, mouth sores, elevated temperature) should be reported to the physician as soon as possible • Because mirtazapine can cause drowsiness, caution patient not to perform activities requiring mental alertness, until response to this drug has been determined • Mirtazapine should not be stopped suddenly due to risk of precipitating a withdrawal reaction
Patient Instructions	• For detailed patient instructions on mirtazapine, see Patient Information Sheet on p. 325

Noradrenergic/Specific Serotonergic Antidepressants (NaSSA) (cont).

►◄ Drug Interactions	• Clinically significant interactions are listed below	

Class of Drug	Example	Interaction Effects
Anticonvulsant	Carbamazepine	Decreased plasma level of mirtazapine by 60% due to induction of metabolism via CYP3A4
Antidepressant Irreversible MAOI	Phenelzine, tranylcypromine	Possible serotonergic reaction; DO NOT COMBINE
SSRI	Fluoxetine, sertraline	Combination reported to alleviate insomnia and augment antidepressant response; may have activating effects May mitigate SSRI-induced sexual dysfunction and "poop-out" syndrome
	Fluvoxamine	Increased serotonergic effects possible Increased sedation and weight gain reported with combination
SNRI	Venlafaxine	Increased plasma level of mirtazapine (3- to 4-fold) due to inhibited metabolism Case report of serotonin syndrome (see p. 8)
Antiemetics (5-HT$_3$ antagonists)	Dolasetron, granisetron, ondansetron	Case reports of serotonin syndrome
CNS depressant	Alcohol, benzodiazepines	Impaired cognition and motor performance
Narcotic	Tramadol	Case of lethargy, hypotension and hypoxia in elderly patient
Stimulant	Phentermine, dextroamphetamine, methylphenidate	May increase agitation and risk of mania, especially in patients with bipolar disorder

Non-Selective Cyclic Antidepressants

Product Availability

Chemical Class	Generic Name	Trade Name[A]	Dosage Forms and Strengths
Tricyclic antidepressant (TCA)	Amitriptyline	Elavil, Endep[B]	Tablets: 10 mg, 25 mg, 50 mg, 75 mg, 100 mg[B], 150 mg[B] Oral suspension[C]: 10 mg/5 ml
	Clomipramine[E]	Anafranil	Tablets[C]: 10 mg, 25 mg, 50 mg Capsules[B]: 25 mg, 50 mg, 75 mg
	Desipramine	Norpramin	Tablets: 10 mg, 25 mg, 50 mg, 75 mg, 100 mg, 150 mg[B]
	Doxepin	Sinequan, Adapin[B]	Capsules: 10 mg, 25 mg, 50 mg, 75 mg, 100 mg, 150 mg Oral solution[B]: 10 mg/ml
	Imipramine HCl	Tofranil	Tablets: 10 mg, 25 mg, 50 mg, 75 mg[C]
	Imipramine pamoate	Tofranil PM[B]	Capsules[B]: 75 mg, 100 mg, 125 mg, 150 mg
	Nortriptyline	Aventyl[C], Pamelor[B]	Capsules: 10 mg, 25 mg, 50 mg[B], 75 mg[B] Syrup[B]: 10 mg/5 ml
	Protriptyline[B]	Vivactil	Tablets: 5 mg, 10 mg
	Trimipramine	Surmontil	Tablets[C]: 12.5 mg, 25 mg, 50 mg, 100 mg Capsules: 25 mg[B], 50 mg[B], 75 mg[C], 100mg[B]
Dibenzoxazepine	Amoxapine[B]	Asendin	Tablets: 25 mg, 50 mg, 100 mg, 150 mg
Tetracyclic	Maprotiline	Ludiomil	Tablets: 10 mg[C], 25 mg, 50 mg, 75 mg

[A] Generic preparations may be available, [B] Not marketed in Canada, [C] Not marketed in USA, [D] Includes NE-reuptake inhibitors, mixed NE/5-HT reuptake inhibitors, serotonin reuptake inhibitors, [E] Not approved for depression in USA

Indications (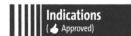 Approved)

- Major depressive disorder (MDD)
- Prophylaxis of recurrent MDD
- Treatment of secondary depression in other mental illnesses, e.g., schizophrenia, dementia
- Depressed phase of bipolar disorder (see Precautions, p. 41)
- Obsessive-compulsive disorder (clomipramine)
- Treatment of enuresis (imipramine)
- Depression and/or anxiety associated with alcoholism or organic disease (doxepin – USA)
- Psychoneuroses with MDD (doxepin – USA)
- Panic disorder prophylaxis (imipramine, desipramine)
- Agoraphobia associated with panic disorder
- Efficacy in dysthymia reported (imipramine, desipramine)
- Bulimia
- Post-stroke depression (nortriptyline)
- Efficacy against intrusive symptoms of posttraumatic stress disorder reported
- Generalized anxiety disorder (imipramine)
- Attention deficit hyperactivity disorder not responsive to other agents
- Premenstrual dysphoric disorder (clomipramine, nortriptyline)

Non-Selective Cyclic Antidepressants (cont.)

- Cataplexy (protriptyline)
- Insomnia (doxepin)
- Premature ejaculation (clomipramine)
- Sialorrhea induced by clozapine (amitriptyline)
- Anti-ulcer effect (doxepin)
- Pain management, including migraine headache, diabetic neuropathy, postherpetic neuralgia, chronic oral-facial pain, and adjuvant analgesic; may help with sleep problems associated with fibromyalgia and other pain syndromes (especially amitriptyline)
- Antipsychotic effect reported with low dose amoxapine
- Smoking cessation (nortriptyline), alone or in combination with nicotine patch. Nortriptyline appears to be as effective as bupropion for smoking cessation and has been recommended as second line therapy for treating smoking dependence (25–75 mg/day)[6]

General Comments

- Suggested that men respond better to tricyclics (and less well to SSRIs) than premenopausal women; postmenopausal women respond well
- Studies suggest improved outcomes in panic disorder with combination of imipramine and psychotherapy
- Presence of hallucinations or delusions are negative predictors of response to TCAs

Pharmacology

- Exact mechanism of action unknown; equilibrate the effects of biogenic amines through various mechanisms (such as reuptake blockade); cause downregulation of β-adrenergic receptors
- The action in the treatment of enuresis may involve inhibition of urination due to the anticholinergic effect and CNS stimulation, resulting in easier arousal by the stimulus of a full bladder
- Tricyclics may exert analgesic effects through blockade of sodium channels

Dosing

- Initiate drug at a low dose and increase dose every 3 to 5 days to a maximum tolerated dose based on side effects – TCAs demonstrate a dose-response relationship
- There is a wide variation in dosage requirements (partially dependent on plasma levels) (see p. 64)
- Once steady-state is reached, give drug as a single bedtime dose; use divided doses if patient develops nightmares
- Prophylaxis is most effective if therapeutic dose is maintained
- Usual route of administration is oral – IM injection has no advantage except with patients unwilling or unable to receive drug orally

Pharmacokinetics

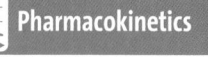

- Completely absorbed from the gastrointestinal tract
- Large percentage metabolized by first-pass effect
- Peak plasma levels occur more rapidly with tertiary tricyclics, like amitriptyline (1–3 h) than with secondary tricyclics like desipramine and nortriptyline (4–8 h)
- Highly lipophilic; concentrated primarily in myocardial and cerebral tissue
- Highly bound to plasma protein
- Metabolized primarily by the liver
- Most tricyclics have linear pharmacokinetics, i.e., a change in dose leads to a proportional change in plasma concentration
- Elimination half-life: see p. 64; steady state reached in about 5 days
- Pharmacokinetics may vary between males and females; data suggest that plasma levels of tricyclic antidepressants may dip in female patients prior to menstruation

Onset & Duration of Action

- Tricyclics and related drugs are long-acting; they may be given in a single daily dose, usually at bedtime (except protriptyline, which is usually given in the morning)
- Therapeutic effect is seen after 7–28 days
- Sedative effects are seen within a few hours of oral administration, with lessened sleep disturbance after a few days
- Occasionally patients may lose response to antidepressant after several months ("poop-out syndrome") [Check compliance with therapy; optimize dose (plasma level may be useful); may need to change drug]

Adverse Effects

- The pharmacological and side effect profile of cyclic antidepressants is dependent on their affinity for and activity on neurotransmitters/receptors (see table p. 59)
- See chart p. 61 for incidence of adverse effects at therapeutic doses of specific agents; incidence of adverse effects may be greater in early days of treatment; patients adapt to many side effects over time

CNS Effects

- A result of antagonism at histamine H_1-receptors and α_1-adrenoreceptors
- Occur frequently
- Drowsiness (most common adverse effect) [Management: prescribe bulk of dose at bedtime]
- Weakness, lethargy, fatigue
- Conversely, excitement, agitation, restlessness, and insomnia have occurred
- Secondary amines reduce sleep efficiency and increase wake time after sleep onset; tertiary amines improve sleep continuity; decrease REM sleep (except for trimipramine); vivid dreaming or nightmares can occur, especially if all the medication is given at bedtime
- Confusion, disturbed concentration, disorientation
- Precipitation of hypomania or mania (in patients with a history of BD – less frequent in patients receiving mood stabilizers), episode acceleration (in up to 67% of patients), psychosis, panic reactions, anxiety, or euphoria may occur
- Fine tremor
- Akathisia (rare – check serum iron for deficiency); can occur following abrupt drug withdrawal; reported with amoxapine, imipramine and desipramine
- Tardive dyskinesia (reported primarily with amoxapine, but also seen on rare occasions with other antidepressants)
- Seizures (more common in children with autism and patients with eating disorder) can occur following abrupt drug increase or after drug withdrawal; risk increases with high plasma levels
- Tinnitus – more likely with serotonergic agents
- Paresthesias reported with tricyclics (approximate risk 4%)
- Myoclonus – more likely with serotonergic agents; includes muscle jerks of lower extremities, jaw, and arms, and nocturnal myoclonus – may be severe in up to 9% of patients [If severe, clonazepam, valproate or carbamazepine may be of benefit]
- Dysphasia, stuttering
- Disturbance in gait, parkinsonism, dystonia

Anticholinergic Effects

- A result of antagonism at muscarinic receptors (ACh)
- Occur frequently, especially in elderly patients
- Dry mucous membranes; may predispose patient to monilial infections [Management: sugar-free gum and candy, oral lubricants (e.g., MoiStir, Ora-Care D), pilocarpine tablets (10–15 mg/day) or mouthwash (4 drops 4% solution to 12 drops water swished in mouth and spat out), bethanechol]
- Blurred vision [Management: pilocarpine 0.5% eye drops]
- Dry eyes; may be of particular difficulty in the elderly or those wearing contact lenses [Management: artificial tears, but employ caution with patients wearing contact lenses; these patients should have their dry eyes managed with their usual wetting solutions or comfort drops]
- Constipation (frequent in children on therapy for enuresis) [Management: increase bulk and fluid intake, fecal softener, bulk laxative]
- Urinary retention, delayed micturition [Management: bethanechol 10–30 mg tid]
- Excessive sweating [Management: daily showering, talcum powder; in severe cases: Drysol solution, terazosin 1–10 mg daily, oxybutynin up to 5 mg bid, clonidine 0.1 mg bid; drug may need to be changed]

Non-Selective Cyclic Antidepressants (cont.)

- Confusion, disorientation, delirium, delusions, hallucinations (more common in the elderly, especially with higher doses)
- Dental caries due to decreased salivation, changes in buffer capacity of saliva, and bacterial environment [Management: maintain oral hygiene]

Cardiovascular Effects

- A result of antagonism at α_1-adrenoreceptors, muscarinic, 5-HT$_2$, and H$_1$-receptors and inhibition of sodium fast channels
- More common in elderly
- Risk increases with high plasma levels
- Tachycardia; may be more pronounced in younger patients
- Orthostatic hypotension [Management: sodium chloride tablets, caffeine, fludrocortisone (0.1–0.5 mg/day), midodrine (2.5–10 mg tid), use of support stockings]
- Prolonged conduction time by delaying the inward sodium current into cardiomyocytes, thereby slowing cardiac depolarization and lengthening the QTc interval[17]; contraindicated in heart block or post-myocardial infarction
- Arrhythmias, syncope, thrombosis, thrombophlebitis, stroke, and congestive heart failure have been reported on occasion
- May cause hypertension in patients with bulimia

Endocrine & Metabolic Effects

- Both increases and decreases in blood sugar levels reported
- Carbohydrate craving reported in up to 87% of patients on maintenance therapy – may result in weight gain
- Menstrual irregularities, amenorrhea and galactorrhea (amoxapine)
- Can induce syndrome of SIADH with hyponatremia; risk increased with age
- Weight gain (up to 30% patients with chronic use; average gain of up to 7 kg – weight gain is linear over time and is often accompanied by a craving for sweets) [Management: nutritional counseling, exercise, dose reduction, changing antidepressant]

GI Effects

- A result of inhibition of 5-HT uptake and ACh antagonism
- Anorexia, nausea, vomiting, diarrhea
- Constipation (see anticholinergic effects)
- Peculiar taste, "black tongue," glossitis

Urogenital and Sexual Effects

- A result of altered dopamine activity, 5-HT$_2$ blockade, inhibition of 5-HT reuptake, α_1-blockade, and ACh blockade
- Decreased libido, impotence [Management: amantadine (100–400 mg prn), bethanechol (10 mg tid or 10–25 mg prn), neostigmine (7.5–15 mg prn), cyproheptadine (4–16 mg prn), yohimbine (5.4–16.2 mg prn]
- Testicular swelling, painful ejaculation, retrograde ejaculation, increased libido, and priapism; spontaneous orgasm with yawning (clomipramine)
- Breast engorgement and breast tissue enlargement in males and females
- Anorgasmia [Management: amantadine (100–400 mg prn), cyproheptadine (4–16 mg prn), yohimbine (5.4–10.8 mg od or prn), ginseng, ginkgo biloba (180–900 mg)]

Allergic Reactions

- Rare
- Jaundice, hepatitis, rash, urticaria, pruritus, edema, blood dyscrasias
- Photosensitivity, skin pigmentation (imipramine, desipramine)
- Case reports of thrombocytopenia

Other Adverse Effects

- Rare reports of alopecia with tricyclics

D/C Discontinuation Syndrome

- Reported incidence: 20–100% most frequently with clomipramine; likely due to cholinergic and adrenergic rebound
- Abrupt withdrawal from high doses may cause a "flu-like" syndrome consisting of fever, fatigue, sweating, coryza, malaise, myalgia, headache; anxiety, agitation, hypomania or mania, insomnia, vivid dreams, as well as dizziness, nausea, vomiting; akathisia and dyskinesia also reported

- Most likely to occur 24–48 h after withdrawal, or after a large dosage decrease
- Rebound depression can occur (even in individuals not previously depressed – such as patients with obsessional disorders)
- Paradoxical mood changes reported on abrupt withdrawal, including hypomania or mania
- ☞ **THESE MEDICATIONS SHOULD THEREFORE BE WITHDRAWN GRADUALLY AFTER PROLONGED USE**

Management	

- Reinstitute drug (at slightly lower dose) and gradually taper dose over several days (e.g., by 25 mg every 3–5 days)
- Alternatively, can treat specific symptoms:
  - Cholinergic rebound (e.g., nausea, vomiting, sweating) – ginger, benztropine 0.5–4 mg prn, atropine 1–4 mg tid to qid
  - Anxiety, agitation, insomnia – benzodiazepine (e.g., lorazepam 0.5–2 mg prn)
  - Dizziness – meclizine 12.5–25 mg q6h prn, dimenhydrinate 25–50 mg q6h prn
  - Neurological symptoms: akathisia – propranolol 10–20 mg tid–qid; dyskinesia – clonazepam 0.5–2 mg prn; dystonia – benztropine 0.5–4 mg prn

 Precautions

- Use cautiously in patients in whom excess anticholinergic activity could be harmful (e.g., prostatic hypertrophy, urinary retention, narrow-angle glaucoma)
- Use with caution in patients with respiratory difficulties, since antidepressants with anticholinergic properties can dry up bronchial secretions and make breathing more difficult
- May lower the seizure threshold; therefore, administer cautiously to patients with a history of convulsive disorders, organic brain disease, or a predisposition to convulsions (e.g., alcohol withdrawal)
- May impair the mental and physical ability to perform hazardous tasks (e.g., driving a car or operating machinery); will potentiate the effects of alcohol
- May induce manic reactions in up to 50% of patients with bipolar disorder; because of risk of increased cycling, bipolar disorder is a relative contra-indication
- Combination of cyclic antidepressants with SSRIs can lead to increased plasma level of the cyclic antidepressant. Combination therapy has been used in the treatment of resistant patients; use of serotonergic cyclic antidepressants with SSRIs can cause a serotonin syndrome (see p. 8)
- Use caution when switching from a cyclic antidepressant to fluoxetine and vice versa (see Interactions, pp. 43–45 and Switching Antidepressants, p. 66)
- Concurrent ingestion of a cyclic antidepressant with high fiber foods or laxatives (e.g., bran, psyllium) can decrease absorption of the antidepressant

 Toxicity

- The therapeutic margin is low (lethal dose is about 3 times the maximum therapeutic dose); prescribe limited quantities
- Symptoms of toxicity are extensions of the common adverse effects: anticholinergic, CNS stimulation followed by CNS depression, myoclonus, hallucinations, respiratory depression and seizures
- Cardiac irregularities occur and are most hazardous; duration of QRS complex on the electrocardiogram (ECG) reflects the severity of the overdose; if it equals or exceeds 0.12 s, it should be considered a danger sign (normal range 0.08–0.11 s)

Management	

- Activated charcoal (1–2 g/kg initially followed by 2 or 3 more doses several hours apart) decreases tricyclic antidepressant absorption and lowers its blood level
- Cathartics (sorbitol or magnesium citrate) will aid in drug evacuation. Give together with charcoal. Monitor bowel sounds to avoid impaction
- DO NOT GIVE IPECAC due to possibility of rapid neurological deterioration and high incidence of seizures
- Supportive treatment, with patient closely monitored in hospital
- Physostigmine salicylate injection (Antilirium) 1 mg im counteracts both central and peripheral anticholinergic effects; use only in patients with coma or those with arrhythmias or convulsions resistant to standard treatment, since associated risks often outweigh the benefits
- Diazepam IV is the drug of choice for convulsions
- Forced diuresis and dialysis are of little benefit

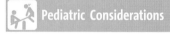 **Pediatric Considerations**

- For detailed information on the use of non-selective cyclic antidepressants in this population, please see the *Clinical Handbook of Psychotropic Drugs for Children and Adolescents* (2007)

Non-Selective Cyclic Antidepressants (cont.)

- Antidepressants are used in enuresis, insomnia and parasomnias, attention deficit hyperactivity disorder (ADHD), major depressive disorder, obsessional disorder, panic disorder, school phobia, separation anxiety disorder, bulimia, and Tourette's syndrome (clomipramine); value of tricyclics in treating depression in children is questioned
- Start drug at a low dose (10–25 mg) and increase gradually by 10–25 mg every 4–5 days to a maximum dose of 3–5 mg/kg (tricyclics)
- Prior to treatment, a baseline ECG is sometimes recommended. When an effective daily dose is reached, a steady state serum level and ECG should be done. Do a follow-up ECG at any dose change and a plasma level every few months
- The U.S. FDA defines the following ECG and examination values as unsafe in children treated with tricyclics: (a) PR interval > 200 ms, (b) QRS interval > 30% above a baseline (or > 120 ms), (c) BP > 140 mmHg systolic or 90 mmHg diastolic, (d) Heart rate > 130 beats/min at rest
- Sudden death (rarely) reported with desipramine, even with therapeutic plasma levels; plasma levels may be higher by 42% in children than adults, at the same dose

 Geriatric Considerations

- Initiate dose lower and slower than in younger patients; elderly patients may take longer to respond and may require trials of up to 12 weeks before response is noted
- Monitor for excessive CNS and anticholinergic effects; use an antidepressant least likely to cause these effects (e.g., nortriptyline, desipramine)
- Caution when combining with other drugs with CNS and anticholinergic properties; additive effects can result in confusion, disorientation, and delirium; elderly are sensitive to anticholinergic effects
- Caution regarding cardiovascular side effects: orthostatic hypotension (can lead to falls), tachycardia, and conduction slowing
- Cognitive impairment can occur, including decreased word-recall and facial recognition

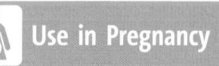 **Use in Pregnancy**

- Cyclic antidepressants have not been demonstrated to have teratogenic effects
- If possible, avoid during first trimester
- Dosage required to achieve therapeutic plasma level may increase during the third trimester of pregnancy
- Urinary retention in neonate has been associated with antidepressant use in third trimester

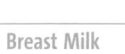 Breast Milk

- Cyclic antidepressants are secreted into breast milk and it is estimated that the baby will receive up to 4% of the mother's dose; half-life of antidepressant increased in neonate 3–4-fold
- Doxepin metabolite concentration reported to reach similar plasma level in infant as in mother; case report of respiratory depression
- The American Academy of Pediatrics classifies antidepressants as drugs "whose effects on nursing infants are unknown but may be of concern"

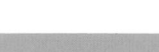 **Nursing Implications**

- Psychotherapy and education are also important in the treatment of MDD
- Monitor therapy by watching for adverse side effects, mood and activity level changes; keep physician informed
- Be aware that the medication reduces the degree of depression and may increase psychomotor activity; this may create concern about suicidal behavior
- Expect a lag time of 7–28 days before antidepressant effects will be noticed
- Check for constipation; increase fluids and increase bulk in diet to lessen constipation; instruct the patient to avoid ingesting high fiber foods or laxatives (e.g., bran) concurrently with medication, as this may reduce the antidepressant level
- Check for urinary retention; if required the physician may order bethanechol orally or by sc injection
- Reassure patient that drowsiness and dizziness usually subside after first few weeks; if dizzy, patient should get up from lying or sitting position slowly, and dangle legs over edge of bed before getting up
- Because these drugs can cause sedation, caution patient not to perform activities requiring alertness until response to the drug has been determined
- Excessive use of caffeinated foods, drugs, or beverages may increase anxiety and agitation and confuse the diagnosis
- Expect a dry mouth; suggest frequent mouth rinsing with water, and sour or sugarless hard candy or gum
- Artificial tears may be useful for patients who complain of dry eyes (or wetting solutions for those wearing contact lenses)
- Caution patient not to stop the drug suddenly due to risk of precipitating a withdrawal reaction

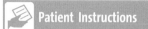
Patient Instructions

- For detailed patient instructions on cyclic antidepressants, see the Patient Information Sheet on p. 326

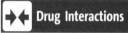
Drug Interactions

- Clinically significant interactions are listed below

Class of Drug	Example	Interaction Effects
ACE inhibitor	Enalapril	Increased plasma level of clomipramine due to decreased metabolism
Alcohol		Short-term or acute use reduces first-pass metabolism of antidepressant and increases its plasma level; chronic use induces metabolizing enzymes and decreases its plasma level Increased sedation, CNS depression
Anesthetic	Enflurane	Report of seizures with amitriptyline
Antiarrhythmic	Quinidine, procainamide Propafenone, quinidine	Prolonged cardiac conduction Increased plasma level of desipramine (by 500%) and imipramine (by 30%)
Antibiotic	Linezolid	Monitor for increased serotonergic and noradrenergic effects due to linezolid's weak MAO inhibition
Anticholinergic	Antiparkinsonian agents, antihist-amines, antipsychotics	Increased anticholinergic effect; may increase risk of hyperthermia, confusion, urinary retention, etc.
Anticoagulant	Warfarin	Increased prothrombin time with tricyclics
Anticonvulsant	Carbamazepine, barbiturates, phenytoin Valproate, divalproex, valproic acid Phenobarbital	Decreased plasma level of tricyclics due to enzyme induction Increased plasma level of tricyclic antidepressant Increased plasma level of phenobarbital with clomipramine
Antidepressant Irreversible MAOI RIMA NDRI SSRI	Phenelzine, tranylcypromine, isocarboxazid Moclobemide Bupropion Fluoxetine, fluvoxamine, paroxetine, sertraline (less likely with citalopram or escitalopram)	If used together, do not add cyclic antidepressants to MAOI: start cyclic antidepressant first or simultaneously with MAOI; for patients already on MAOI, discontinue MAOI 10–14 days before starting combination therapy Combined cyclic and MAOI therapy has additive antidepressant effects in treatment-resistant patients Additive antidepressant effect in treatment-resistant patients Additive antidepressant effect in treatment-resistant patients Elevated imipramine level (by 57%), desipramine level (by 82%), and nortriptyline level (by 200%) with combination Elevated tricyclic plasma level (due to release from protein binding and inhibition of oxidative metabolism); monitor plasma level and for signs of toxicity Additive antidepressant effect in treatment-resistant patients
Antifungal	Ketoconazole, fluconazole Terbinafine	Increased plasma level of antidepressant due to inhibited metabolism (89% with amitriptyline; 70% with nortriptyline); 20% increase with imipramine and no increase with desipramine Prolonged increase in plasma level of amitriptyline and its metabolite nortriptyline, due to inhibited metabolism via CYP2D6
Antihistamine	Diphenhydramine	Increased plasma level of antidepressants metabolized via CYP2D6 is possible (e.g., amitriptyline, desipramine, clomipramine, imipramine) due to inhibited metabolism Additive CNS effects
Antihypertensive	Bethanidine, clonidine, debrisoquin, methyldopa, guanethidine, reserpine Acetazolamide, thiazide diuretics Labetalol	Decreased antihypertensive effect due to inhibition of α-adrenergic receptors Hypotension augmented Increased plasma level of imipramine (by 54%) and desipramine

Non-Selective Cyclic Antidepressants (cont.)

Class of Drug	Example	Interaction Effects
Antipsychotic	Chlorpromazine, haloperidol, perphenazine	Increased plasma level of either agent
	Clozapine	Possible serotonin syndrome reported in a patient taking clomipramine following the withdrawal of clozapine
Ca-channel blocker	Nifedipine	May antagonize the efficacy of antidepressant drugs
	Diltiazem, verapamil	Increased imipramine plasma level by 30% and 15%, respectively; increased level of trimipramine
Cannabis/marihuana		Case reports of tachycardia, lightheadedness, confusion, mood lability and delirium with nortriptyline and desipramine; may evoke cardiac complications in youth
CNS depressant	Hypnotics, antihistamines, alcohol, benzodiazepines	Increased sedation, CNS depression
Cholestyramine		Decreased absorption of antidepressant, if given together
Evening primrose oil		May lower the seizure threshold
Grapefruit juice		Decreased conversion of clomipramine to metabolite due to inhibition of CYP3A4
H₂ antagonist	Cimetidine	Increased plasma level of antidepressant; for desipramine, inhibition of hydroxylation occurs only in rapid metabolizers
Hormone	Estrogen/progesterone oral contraceptive	Increased plasma level of antidepressant due to decreased metabolism Reduced clearance of combined oral contraceptive possible with amitriptyline due to inhibited metabolism
Insulin		Decreased insulin sensitivity reported with amitriptyline
Lithium		Additive antidepressant effect
L-Tryptophan		Additive antidepressant effect
MAO-B inhibitor	Selegiline (L-deprenyl)	Reports of serotonergic reactions
Narcotic	Methadone	Increased plasma level of desipramine (by about 108%)
	Morphine	Enhanced analgesic effect
	Codeine	Marked inhibition of conversion of codeine to morphine (active moiety) with amitriptyline, clomipramine, desipramine, imipramine and nortriptyline
Oxybutynin		Increased metabolism of clomipramine (may be due to induction of CYP3A4)
Phenylbutazone		Decreased gastric emptying with desipramine leading to impaired absorption of phenylbutazone
Propoxyphene		Increased plasma level of doxepin due to decreased metabolism
Protease inhibitor	Ritonavir	Increased plasma levels of tricyclic antidepressant due to decreased metabolism (AUC of desipramine increased by 145%; peak plasma level increased 22%)
Proton pump inhibitor	Omeprazole	Increased plasma level of antidepressant due to inhibited metabolism
Rifampin		Decreased plasma level of antidepressant due to increased metabolism
Smoking – cigarettes		Increased clearance of antidepressant due to induction of CYP1A2

Class of Drug	Example	Interaction Effects
Stimulant	Methylphenidate	Plasma level of antidepressant may be increased Used together to augment antidepressant effect and response to symptoms of ADHD Cardiovascular effects increased with combination, in children – monitor Case reports of neurotoxic effects with imipramine, but considered rare – monitor
Sulfonylurea	Tolbutamide	Increased hypoglycemia
Sympathomimetic	Epinephrine, norepinephrine (levarterenol), phenylephrine Isoproterenol	Enhanced pressor response from 2- to 8-fold; benefit may outweigh risks in anaphylaxis May increase likelihood of arrhythmias
Tamoxifen		Decreased plasma level of doxepin by 25% due to induced metabolism via CYP3A4
Thyroid drug	Triiodothyronine (T_3-liothyronine), L-thyroxine (T_4)	Additive antidepressant effect in treatment-resistant patients
Triptan	Sumatriptan, zolmitriptan	Possible serotonergic reaction when combined with antidepressants with serotonergic activity (e.g., clomipramine)
Zolpidem		Case report of visual hallucinations in combination with desipramine

Monoamine Oxidase Inhibitors

● General Comments	• Monoamine oxidase inhibitors can be classified as follows:	

Chemical Class	Agent	Page
Reversible Inhibitor of MAO-A (RIMA)	Moclobemide	See p. 46
Irreversible MAOIs	Isocarboxazid[B] Phenelzine Tranylcypromine	See p. 50 See p. 50 See p. 50
MAO-B inhibitor	Selegiline (L-deprenyl)[B]	See p. 56

[B] Not marketed in Canada

Reversible Inhibitor of MAO-A (RIMA)

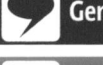 **Product Availability**

Chemical Class	Generic Name	Trade Name[A]	Dosage Forms and Strengths
Reversible Inhibitor of MAO-A (RIMA)	Moclobemide[C]	Manerix	Tablets: 100 mg, 150 mg, 300 mg

[A] Generic preparations may be available, [B] Not marketed in Canada, [C] Not marketed in USA

Indications
(👍 Approved)

- 👍 Major depressive disorder
- 👍 Chronic dysthymia
- Weak evidence suggests efficacy in seasonal affective disorder, chronic fatigue syndrome and obsessive compulsive disorder
- Suggested to modulate impulsivity/aggression and affective instability in borderline personality disorder
- Social anxiety disorder

General Comments

- Increases REM sleep

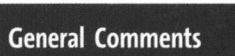 **Pharmacology**

- Benzamide derivative chemically distinct from irreversible MAOIs
- Inhibits the action of MAO-A enzyme that metabolizes the neurotransmitters serotonin, norepinephrine, and dopamine; in chronic doses over 400 mg daily, will produce 20–30% inhibition of MAO-B in platelets
- Inhibition is reversible (within 24 h)
- Combined therapy with cyclic antidepressants or lithium may increase antidepressant effect

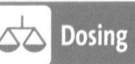 **Dosing**

- Starting dose, 300–450 mg daily given in divided dose; usual dose range, 300–600 mg daily; some patients respond to 150 mg daily, but most require doses above 450 mg/day
- Dosing is not affected by age or renal function; should be decreased in patients with liver disorder

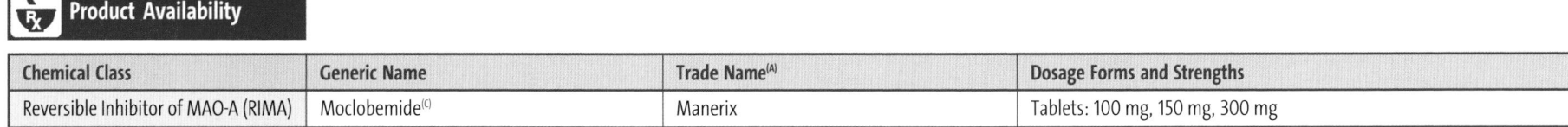
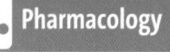
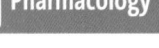

- Should be taken after meals to minimize tyramine-related responses (e.g., headache)
- Preliminary data suggest once daily dosing as effective as divided dosing

Pharmacokinetics

- See p. 64
- Relatively lipophilic, but at low pH is highly water-soluble
- Rapidly absorbed from gut, high first-pass effect; peak effect seen between 0.7 and 3 h
- Has low plasma-protein binding (50% – albumin)
- Plasma level increases in proportion to dose; blockade of MAO-A correlates with plasma concentration
- Metabolized by oxidation primarily via CYP2C19; elimination half-life 1–3 h; clearance decreased as dosage increased because of auto-inhibition or metabolite-induced inhibition
- Age has no effect on pharmacokinetics

Onset & Duration of Action

- Therapeutic effects seen after 7–28 days

Adverse Effects

- See table p. 63

CNS Effects

- Most common: insomnia, headache and sedation
- Increased stimulation (restlessness, anxiety, agitation, and aggressivity) can occur – dose related
- Hypomania reported especially in patients with bipolar disorder

Anticholinergic Effects

- Dry mouth
- Blurred vision

Cardiovascular Effects

- Hypotension
- Tachycardia

Endocrine & Metabolic Effects

- Reports of galactorrhea in females
- Both weight loss and weight gain

GI Effects

- Nausea, abdominal pain
- Constipation

D/C Discontinuation Syndrome

- None known

Precautions

- Hypertensive patients should avoid ingesting large quantities of tyramine-rich foods
- Hypertensive reactions may occur in patients with thyrotoxicosis or pheochromocytoma
- Patients prescribed doses above 600 mg/day should minimize the use of tyramine-rich foods
- Use caution when combining with serotonergic drugs as "serotonin syndrome" has been reported (see p. 7) with CNS irritability, increased muscle tone, myoclonus, diaphoresis, and elevated temperature (see Interactions, pp. 48–49)
- Reduce dose by 1/2 to 2/3 in patients with severe liver impairment

Toxicity

- Symptoms same as side effects, but intensified: drowsiness, disorientation, stupor, hypotension, tachycardia, hyperreflexia, grimacing, sweating, agitation and hallucinations; serotonin syndrome reported
- Fatalities have occurred when combined with citalopram or clomipramine in overdose

Management

- Gastric lavage, emesis, activated charcoal may be of benefit
- Monitor vital functions, supportive treatment

Reversible Inhibitor of MAO-A (RIMA) (cont.)

Pediatric Considerations	• For detailed information on the use of moclobemide in this population, please see the *Clinical Handbook of Psychotropic Drugs for Children and Adolescents* (2007)
Geriatric Considerations	• Dosing not affected by age or renal function • Improvement in cognitive functioning in elderly depressed patients has been noted
Use in Pregnancy	• Data on safety in pregnancy is lacking • Animal studies have not shown any particular adverse effects on reproduction
Breast Milk	• Moclobemide is secreted into breast milk at about 1% of maternal dose
Nursing Implications	• If patient has difficulty sleeping, ensure last dose of moclobemide is no later than 1700 h • It is not necessary to maintain a special diet when on moclobemide; however, excessive amounts of foods with high tyramine content can lead to headache • Administer moclobemide after food to minimize side effects; a big meal should not be consumed after taking moclobemide • Warn patient not to self-medicate with over-the-counter drugs or herbal preparations, but to consult physician or pharmacist to prevent drug-drug interactions
Patient Instructions	• For detailed patient instructions on moclobemide, see the Patient Information Sheet on p. 328
Food Interactions	• No particular precautions are required; however, excessive consumption of tyramine-containing food should be avoided to minimize hypertension risk
Drug Interactions	• Clinically significant interactions are listed below

Class of Drug	Example	Interaction Effects
Anticholinergic	Antiparkinsonian drugs	Increased atropine-like effects
Antidepressant Cyclic (non-selective)	Desipramine, nortriptyline	Additive antidepressant effect in treatment-resistant patients Potentiation of weight gain, hypotension, and anticholinergic effects
	Clomipramine	Enhanced serotonergic effects – **AVOID**
NDRI	Bupropion	Enhanced neurotoxic (central adrenergic) effect
SNRI, SARI	Venlafaxine, nefazodone	Enhanced effects of serotonin and/or norepinephrine; no data on safety with combination
SSRI	Fluoxetine, citalopram	Use cautiously and monitor for serotonergic adverse effects, especially with citalopram and escitalopram Higher incidence of insomnia may occur; increased headache reported with fluvoxamine Fluoxetine and fluvoxamine can inhibit the metabolism of moclobemide
Anxiolytic	Buspirone	Serotonergic reaction possible
Atomoxetine		Enhanced neurotoxic (central adrenergic) effect
H₂ antagonist	Cimetidine	Decreased metabolism of moclobemide; plasma level can double
Lithium		Additive antidepressant effect in treatment-resistant patients
L-Tryptophan		"Serotonin syndrome" possible (see p. 8)

Class of Drug	Example	Interaction Effects
MAO-B inhibitor	Selegiline (L-deprenyl)	Caution – dietary restrictions recommended as both A + B MAO enzymes inhibited with combination
Narcotic	Meperidine, pentazocine, dextropropoxyphene, dextromethorphan	Serotonergic reaction, increased restlessness, potentiation of analgesic effect – **AVOID**
NSAID	Ibuprofen	Enhanced effect of ibuprofen
Stimulant	Amphetamine, methylphenidate	See indirect-acting sympathomimetic amines
Sympathomimetic amine Indirect-acting	Ephedrine, amphetamine, methylphenidate, L-dopa, etc.	Increased blood pressure and enhanced effects if used over prolonged periods or at high doses
Direct-acting	Salbutamol, epinephrine, etc.	As above
Triptan	Sumatriptan, zolmitriptan Rizatriptan	Possibly increased serotonergic effects Decreased metabolism of rizatriptan; AUC and peak plasma level increased by 119% and 41%, respectively, and AUC of metabolite increased by 400%

Irreversible Monoamine Oxidase Inhibitors

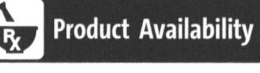 **Product Availability**

Chemical Class	Generic Name	Trade Name[A]	Dosage Forms and Strengths
Hydrazine derivative	Isocarboxazid[B] Phenelzine	Marplan Nardil	Tablets: 10 mg Tablets: 15 mg
Non-hydrazine derivative	Tranylcypromine	Parnate	Tablets: 10 mg

[A] Generic preparations may be available, [B] Not marketed in Canada

Indications
(Approved)

- 👍 "Atypical" depression
- 👍 Major depressive disorder (MDD) unresponsive to other antidepressants
- 👍 Phobic anxiety states or social phobia
- • Atypical (anergic) bipolar depression
- • Panic disorder prophylaxis
- • Obsessive-compulsive disorder
- • MDD in patients with borderline personality disorder
- • Chronic dysthymia
- • Efficacy in posttraumatic stress disorder reported
- • May improve negative symptoms in chronic schizophrenia
- • Possible antiherpetic effect

General Comments
- • Premenopausal women may respond better to MAOIs than to tricyclics
- • Ability of patient to adhere to dietary and drug restrictions should be assessed before prescribing

Pharmacology
- • Inhibit the action of MAO-A and B enzymes that metabolize the neurotransmitters responsible for stimulating physical and mental activity (serotonin, norepinephrine, dopamine); cause down-regulation of β-adrenoceptors
- • Inhibition is irreversible and lasts about 10 days
- • Combined therapy with cyclic antidepressants or lithium may increase antidepressant effect
- • Best response to MAOIs occurs at dosages that reduce MAO enzyme activity by at least 80%; may require up to 2 weeks to reach maximum MAO inhibition

Dosing
- • See p. 64
- • Due to short half-life, bid dosing required; give doses in the morning and mid-day to avoid overstimulation and insomnia (occasionally cause sedation)
- • Percentage of MAO enzyme inhibited is related to dose

Pharmacokinetics
- • See p. 64
- • Rapidly absorbed from the GI tract, metabolized by the liver and excreted almost entirely in the urine
- • Peak plasma level of tranylcypromine occurs within 1–2 h and correlates with elevations in supine blood pressure, orthostatic drop of systolic blood pressure, and rise in pulse rate. Blood pressure elevation correlates with dose
- • With long-term use, irreversible MAOIs can impair own metabolism resulting in nonlinear pharmacokinetics and potential for drug accumulation

| **Onset & Duration of Action** | • May require up to 2 weeks to reach maximum MAO inhibition
• Energizing effect often seen within a few days
• Tolerance to antipanic effects reported |

| **Adverse Effects** | • See p. 63 |

| **CNS Effects** | • Drowsiness
• Stimulant effect (insomnia, restlessness, anxiety) can occur [trazodone 50 mg beneficial as a hypnotic]
• Increased sleep onset latency and reduced sleep efficiency; REM sleep decreased and may be eliminated at start of therapy-rebound REM of up to 250% above baseline reported on drug withdrawal
• Headache
• Hypomania and mania: in patients with bipolar disorder, risk up to 35%; lower risk with concomitant use of a mood stabilizer; in unipolar disorder, risk about 4%; episode acceleration in up to 67% of patients
• Paresthesias or "electric shock-like" sensations; carpal tunnel syndrome (numbness) reported; may be due to vitamin B6 deficiency [Management: pyridoxine 50–150 mg/day]
• Myoclonic jerks, especially during sleep (10–15%), tremor, muscle tension, cramps, akathisia (dose-related) [cyproheptadine may be helpful for cramps or jerks; clonazepam or valproate are useful for nocturnal myoclonus] |

| **Anticholinergic Effects** | • Constipation common [Management: increase bulk and fluid intake, fecal softener, bulk laxative]
• Dry mouth
• Urinary retention |

| **Cardiovascular Effects** | • Dizziness, weakness, orthostatic hypotension [Management: fludrocortisone 0.1–0.5 mg/day]
• Occasionally, hypertensive patients may experience a rise in blood pressure
• Edema in lower extremities restrict sodium; support hose; amiloride 5–10 mg bid, hydrochlorothiazide up to 50 mg/day] |

| **Endocrine & Metabolic Effects** | • Hyponatremia and SIADH reported
• Increased appetite and weight gain |

| **GI Effects** | • The most common are anorexia, nausea and vomiting |

| **Urogenital and Sexual Effects** | • Impotence, anorgasmia, decreased libido, ejaculation difficulties [Management: see SSRIs, p. 6]
• May diminish sperm count
• Rarely priapism |

| **Other Adverse Effects** | • Rare reports of liver toxicity
• Rare reports of hair loss with tranylcypromine
• Case reports of thrombocytopenia |

| **Hypertensive Crisis** | • Can occur with irreversible MAOIs due to ingestion of incompatible foods (containing substantial levels of tyramine) or drugs (see lists pp. 53–54)
• Not related to dose of drug |

| **Signs and Symptoms** | • Occipital headache, neck stiffness or soreness, nausea, vomiting, sweating (sometimes with fever and sometimes with cold, clammy skin), dilated pupils and photophobia, sudden nose bleed, tachycardia, bradycardia, and constricting chest pain |

| **Management** | • Withhold medication and notify physician immediately
• Monitor vital signs, ECG
• Sublingual captopril 25 mg, or nifedipine 10 mg bitten and swallowed, may decrease blood pressure (occasionally drastically – monitor) |

Irreversible Monoamine Oxidase Inhibitors (cont.)

- Phentolamine is an alternative parenteral treatment
- Patient should stand and walk, rather than lie down, during a hypertensive reaction; BP will drop somewhat

D/C Discontinuation Syndrome	• Occur occasionally 1–4 days after abrupt withdrawal • Reports of muscle weakness, agitation, vivid nightmares, headache, palpitations, nausea, sweating, irritability, and myoclonic jerking; acute organic psychosis with hallucinations reported • REM rebound occurs (up to 250% above baseline) • Maintain dietary and drug restrictions for at least 10 days after stopping MAOI
⚠ Precautions	• Should not be administered to patients with cerebrovascular disease, cardiovascular disease, or a history of hypertension • Should not be used alone in patients with marked psychomotor agitation • When changing from one MAOI to another, or to a tricyclic antidepressant, allow a minimum of 10 medication-free days • Need 10–14 days before an incompatible drug or food is given, or before surgery or ECT • Hypertensive crisis can occur if given concurrently with certain drugs or foods (see lists below) • Use caution when combining with serotonergic drugs as "serotonin syndrome" has been reported (see p. 8)
☠ Toxicity	• Symptoms same as side effects but intensified • Severe cases progress to extreme dizziness and shock • Overdose, whether accidental or intentional, can be fatal: patient may be symptom-free up to 6 h, then progress to restlessness-coma-death – therefore, close medical supervision is indicated for 48 h following an overdose
Pediatric Considerations	• For detailed information on the use of MAOIs in this population, please see the *Clinical Handbook of Psychotropic Drugs for Children and Adolescents* (2007) • MAOIs are prescribed in panic disorder/agoraphobia, separation anxiety, major depressive disorder, selective mutism, and attention-deficit hyperactivity disorder • Dose should be carefully titrated and maintained between 0.3 and 1 mg/kg • Ability to comply with restrictions as to diet and drugs should be assessed before prescribing
Geriatric Considerations	• Suggested that MAOIs may have particular efficacy in the elderly, as monoamine oxidase activity in the brain increases with age • Orthostatic hypotension may be problematic, use divided doses [Management: support stockings, sodium chloride tablets, fludrocortisone]
Use in Pregnancy	• Avoid; increased incidence of malformations demonstrated with use in first trimester
Breast Milk	• The American Academy of Pediatrics considers tranylcypromine compatible with breast feeding • No data on phenelzine or isocarboxazid
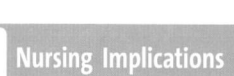 **Nursing Implications**	• The incidence of orthostatic hypotension is high, especially in the elderly and at the start of treatment: tell patient to get out of bed slowly • Educate patient regarding foods and drugs to avoid; a diet sheet should be provided for each patient • Warn patient not to self-medicate with over-the-counter drugs or herbal preparations, but to consult physician or pharmacist to prevent drug-drug interactions • Educate patient to report headache; measure pulse and blood pressure, and report increases to physician immediately • If patient has difficulty sleeping, ensure last dose of MAOI is no later than 1500 h

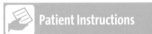

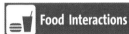 **Patient Instructions**

- For detailed patient instructions on MAOIs, see the Patient Information Sheet on p. 330

Food Interactions

There are many serious food and drug interactions that may precipitate a hypertensive crisis; maintain dietary and drug restrictions for at least 10 days after stopping MAOI

Foods to avoid as they are high in tyramine content:

- All matured or aged cheeses (e.g., cheddar, brie, blue, stilton, Roquefort, camembert)
- Broad bean pods (e.g., Fava) – contain dopamine
- Concentrated yeast extracts (e.g., Marmite)
- Dried salted fish, pickled herring
- Packet soup (especially miso)
- Sauerkraut
- Aged/smoked meats – sausage (especially salami, mortadella, pastrami, summer sausage), other unrefrigerated fermented meats, game meat that has been hung, liver
- Soy sauce or soybean condiments, tofu
- Tap (draft) beer, alcohol-free beer
- Improperly stored or spoiled meats, poultry or fish

It is SAFE to use in moderate amounts (only if fresh):

- Cottage cheese, cream cheese, farmer's cheese, processed cheese, Cheez Whiz, ricotta, Havarti, Boursin, brie without rind, gorgonzola
- Liver (as long as it is fresh), fresh or processed meats, poultry or fish (e.g., hot dogs, bologna)
- Spirits (in moderation)
- Sour cream
- Soy milk
- Salad dressings
- Worcestershire sauce
- Yeast-leavened bread

Reactions have also been reported with the following as they contain moderate amounts of tyramine – use moderately with caution:

- Smoked fish, caviar, snails, tinned fish, shrimp paste
- Yogurt
- Meat tenderizers
- Homemade red wine, Chianti, canned/bottled beer, sherry, champagne
- Cheeses (e.g., Parmesan, muenster, Swiss, gruyere, mozzarella, feta)
- Pepperoni
- Overripe fruit: bananas, avocados, raspberries, plums, tomatoes, canned figs or raisins, orange pulp
- Meat extract (e.g., Bovril, Oxo)
- Asian foods
- Spinach, eggplant
- ☞ **MAKE SURE ALL FOOD IS FRESH, STORED PROPERLY, AND EATEN SOON AFTER BEING PURCHASED** – products stored even under refrigeration will show an increase in tyramine content after several days
- Never touch food that is fermented or possibly "off"
- Avoid restaurant sauces, gravy, and soup

Over-the-counter drugs: DO NOT USE without prior consultation with doctor or pharmacist:

- Cold remedies, decongestants (including nasal sprays and drops), some antihistamines and cough medicines

Irreversible Monoamine Oxidase Inhibitors (cont.)

- Narcotic painkillers (e.g., products containing codeine)
- All stimulants including pep-pills (Wake-ups, Nodoz)
- All appetite suppressants
- Anti-asthma drugs (Primatine P)
- Sleep aids and sedatives (Sominex, Nytol)
- Yeast, dietary supplements (e.g., Ultrafast, Optifast)

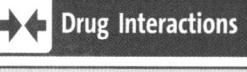 **Drug Interactions**

- Clinically significant interactions are listed below

Class of Drug	Example	Interaction Effects
Anesthetic, general		May enhance CNS depression
Anorexiant	Fenfluramine, dexfenfluramine	"Serotonin syndrome" (see p. 8); AVOID
Anticholinergic	Antiparkinsonian agents, antihistamines	Increased atropine-like effects
Anticonvulsant	Carbamazepine	Possible decrease in metabolism and increased plasma level of carbamazepine with phenelzine
Antidepressant Cyclic (non-selective)	Amitriptyline, desipramine	If used together, do not add cyclic antidepressants to MAOI. Start cyclic antidepressant first or simultaneously with MAOI. For patients already on MAOI, discontinue the MAOI for 10–14 days before starting combination therapy Combined cyclic and MAOI therapy has increased antidepressant effects and will potentiate weight gain, hypotension and anticholinergic effects
	Clomipramine	"Serotonin syndrome" reported; AVOID (see p. 8)
SARI	Trazodone	Low doses of trazodone (25–50 mg) used to treat antidepressant-induced insomnia Combined therapy has additive antidepressant effects; monitor for serotonergic effects
SNRI	Venlafaxine	Metabolism of serotonin and norepinephrine inhibited; AVOID
SSRI	Fluoxetine, paroxetine, sertraline	"Serotonin syndrome" and death reported with serotonergic antidepressants; AVOID
NDRI	Bupropion	Metabolism of dopamine inhibited; AVOID
NaSSA	Mirtazapine	Possible serotonergic reaction; AVOID
Antihypertensive	ACE-inhibitors, α-blockers, β-blockers Guanethidine	Enhanced hypotension Antihypertensive effects of guanethidine decreased
Antipsychotic	Phenothiazines, clozapine	Additive hypotension and anticholinergic effects
Atropine		Prolonged action of atropine
Anxiolytic	Buspirone	Several cases of increased blood pressure reported
Bromocriptine		Increased serotonergic effects
CNS depressant	Barbiturates, sedatives, alcohol	May enhance CNS depression
Ginseng		May cause headache, tremulousness or hypomania; case report of irritability and visual hallucinations with combination
Insulin		Enhanced hypoglycemic response through stimulation of insulin secretion and inhibition of gluconeogenesis

Class of Drug	Example	Interaction Effects
L-Dopa		Increase in storage and release of dopamine and/or norepinephrine Increased blood pressure
L-Tryptophan		Reports of "serotonin syndrome," with hyperreflexia, tremor, myoclonic jerks, and ocular oscillations (see p. 8); **AVOID**
Lithium		Increased serotonergic effects Additive antidepressant effect in treatment-resistant patients
MAO-B inhibitor	Selegiline (L-deprenyl)	Increased serotonergic effects
Muscle relaxant	Succinylcholine	Phenelzine may prolong muscle relaxation by inhibiting metabolism
Narcotics and related drugs	Meperidine, dextromethorphan, diphenoxylate, tramadol	Excitation, sweating, and hypotension reported; may lead to development of encephalopathy, convulsions, coma, respiratory depression, and "serotonin syndrome." If a narcotic is required, meperidine should not be used; other narcotics should be instituted cautiously
	Propoxyphene	Potentiation of catecholamine-release reported, resulting in anxiety, confusion, ataxia, hypotension
Nicotine		Low doses of tranylcypromine reported to inhibit nicotine metabolism by competitive inhibition via CYP2A6
Reserpine		Central excitatory syndrome and hypertension reported due to central and peripheral release of catecholamines
Sibutramine		Increased noradrenergic and serotonergic effects possible. DO NOT COMBINE
Stimulants	MDMA ("Ecstasy"), MDA	Case reports of "serotonin syndrome" (see p. 8) and hypertensive crisis
Sulfonylureas		Enhanced hypoglycemic response
Sympathomimetic amine	*Indirect acting:* amphetamine, methylphenidate, ephedrine, pseudoephedrine, phenylpropanolamine, dopamine, tyramine	Release of large amounts of norepinephrine with hypertensive reaction; **AVOID**
	Direct acting: epinephrine, isoproterenol, norepinephrine (levarterenol), methoxamine, salbutamol	No interaction
	Phenylephrine	Increased pressor response
Tetrabenazine		Central excitatory syndrome and hypertension reported due to central and peripheral release of catecholamines
Triptan	Sumatriptan, zolmitriptan, rizatriptan	"Serotonin syndrome" (see p. 8); **AVOID**; recommend that 2 weeks elapse after discontinuing an irreversible MAOI before using sumatriptan

Monoamine Oxidase B Inhibitor

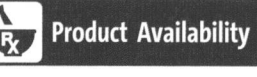 **Product Availability**

Chemical Class	Generic Name	Trade Name	Dosage Forms and Strengths
Levo-acetylenic derivative of phenethylamine	Selegiline (deprenyl) transdermal[B]	EMSAM	Transdermal patch: 20 mg/20 cm^2, 30 mg/30 cm^2, 40 mg/40 cm^2

[B] Not available in Canada

Indications (✋ Approved)

- ✋ Treatment of MDD in adults
- Selegiline may reduce physiological and subjective effects of cocaine

General Comments

- Approved in low doses of oral formulation (in Canada and USA) for the treatment of Parkinson's disease; higher doses required for treatment of MDD
- Transdermal patches contain 1 mg of selegiline per cm^2 and deliver approximately 0.3 mg of selegiline per cm^2 over 24 hours. EMSAM systems are available in three sizes: 20 mg/20 cm^2, 30 mg/30 cm^2, and 40 mg/40 cm^2

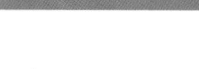 **Pharmacology**

- Transdermal selegiline leads to sustained plasma concentrations of the parent compound, increasing the amount of drug delivered to the brain and decreasing metabolite production. At low doses, selegiline irreversibly inhibits MAO-B, which is involved in oxidative deamination of dopamine in the brain and also inhibits the uptake of dopamine. At higher doses, it inhibits both MAO-A and B. The transdermal format allows for targeted inhibition of central nervous system monoamine A (MAO-A) and monoamine B isoenzymes with minimal effects on MAO-A in the gastrointestinal (gut wall) and hepatic systems (avoids first-pass effect), thereby reducing the risk of interactions with tyramine-rich foods
- Induces antioxidant enzymes and decreases the formation of oxygen radicals; it interferes with early apoptotic signaling events induced by various kinds of insults in cell cultures, thus protecting cells from apoptotic death

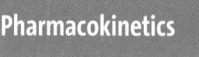 **Dosing**

- EMSAM should be applied to dry, intact skin on the upper torso (below the neck and above the waist), upper thigh or the outer surface of the upper arm once every 24 hours
- 20 mg/20 cm^2 delivers 6 mg/24 h – found effective in MDD without the need for dietary restrictions; if dose increases are indicated for individual patients, they should occur in dose increments of 3 mg/24 h (up to a maximum dose of 12 mg/24 h) at intervals of no less than two weeks
- The recommended dose for elderly patients is 6 mg/24 h
- No adjustment in dosage necessary in moderate hepatic or renal insufficiency

Pharmacokinetics

- Following dermal application of EMSAM to humans, 25–30% of the selegiline content, on average, is delivered systemically over 24 h (range ~10–40%). Transdermal dosing results in substantially higher exposure to selegiline and lower exposure to metabolites compared to oral dosing, where extensive first-pass metabolism occurs. Absorption of selegiline is similar when EMSAM is applied to the upper torso or upper thigh; it is not metabolized in human skin
- Selegiline is approximately 90% bound to plasma protein
- Steady-state selegiline plasma concentrations achieved within five days of daily dosing
- Extensively metabolized by several CYP450 enzymes including: CYP2B6, CYP2C9, and CYP3A4/5 and CYP2A6
- Selegiline and N-desmethylselegiline cause a concentration dependent inhibition of CYP2D6 at 10–250 µM and CYP3A4/5 at 25–250 µM and have a minor effect on CYP2C19 and CYP2B6
- The mean half-lives of selegiline and its three metabolites, R(–)-N-desmethylselegiline, R(–)-amphetamine, and R(–)-methamphetamine range from 18–25 h
- No pharmacokinetic information is available on selegiline or its metabolites in patients with renal or hepatic impairment

Adverse Effects	• Insomnia common [can be lessened by taking the patch off before bedtime]
	• Dermatological reactions common at site of application of patch (24%) [rotate sites of application]
	• Diarrhea, pharyngitis, dizziness, lightheadedness, headache (18%); hypotension (10%); dry mouth
	• Increased blood pressure at doses above 6 mg/24 h possible
	• Increased anxiety, agitation, irritability, increase in suicidal thoughts; activation of mania/hypomania (0.4%)
	• Weight loss > 5% body weight (5%)
Contraindications	• Simultaneous administration of drugs with serotonergic properties (see interactions)
	• Combination with sympathomimetic amines, including amphetamines as well as cold products and weight-reducing preparations that contain vasoconstrictors
Precautions	• Though dietary restrictions are not required for the 6 mg/24 h dose, use of higher doses can negate drug selectivity and pressor response can occur to tyramine-rich foods – patients should observe dietary and drug restrictions (as per irreversible MAO inhibitors pp. 53–54)
	• A 14-day washout is required between termination of selegiline and starting an antidepressant with serotonergic activity, to prevent serotonin syndrome (see Interaction p. 58 and Switching Antidepressants pp. 66–67)
	• Both adults and children may experience worsening of their MDD, unusual changes in their behavior, and/or the emergence of suicidal ideation and behavior
	• Patients should be evaluated carefully for a history of drug abuse, and such patients should be observed closely for signs of EMSAM misuse or abuse (e.g., development of tolerance, increases in dose, or drug-seeking behavior)
Toxicity	• CNS and cardiovascular toxicity likely
	• Delays of up to 12 h between ingestion of drug and the appearance of signs may occur, and peak effects may not be observed for 24–48 h. Since death has been reported following overdosage with MAOI agents, hospitalization with close monitoring during this period is essential
Management	• Symptomatic and supportive
Pediatric Considerations	• Not recommended
	• **Antidepressants shown to increase the risk of suicidal thinking and behavior (suicidality) in short-term studies in children and adolescents with major depressive disorder and other psychiatric disorders (4% risk vs. placebo risk of 2%).**
Geriatric Considerations	• The recommended dose for elderly patients is 6 mg/24 h
	• Patients age 50 and older appeared to be at higher risk for rash (4.4% versus 0% placebo) than younger patients
Use in Pregnancy	• Pregnancy Category C drug
Breast Milk	• It is not known whether selegiline hydrochloride is excreted in human milk
Nursing Implications	• Dietary restrictions are not necessary at a dose of 6 mg/24 h; however, patients should be informed about the signs and symptoms associated with MAOI induced hypertensive crisis and urged to seek immediate medical attention if these symptoms occur
	• Patients should be advised to report immediately, any severe headache, neck stiffness, palpitations or other atypical or unusual symptoms not previously experienced
	• Advise patient to avoid exposing the application site of patches to external sources of direct heat, such as heating pads or electric blankets, heat lamps, saunas, hot tubs, heated water beds, and prolonged direct sunlight as this may result in an increase in the amount of selegiline absorbed from the patch and produce elevated serum levels of selegiline.
	• **All patients being treated with antidepressants should be observed closely for clinical worsening, suicidality, and unusual changes in behavior, especially during the initial few months of therapy, or following an increase or decrease in dose**

Monoamine Oxidase B Inhibitor (cont.)

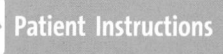 **Patient Instructions**

- For detailed patient instruction on transdermal selegiline, see the Patient Information Sheet on p. 332

 Drug Interactions

Class of Drug	Example	Interaction Effects
Anticonvulsants	Carbamazepine, oxcarbazepine	Increased level of selegiline and its metabolite (2-fold)
Antidepressants SSRI, SNRI, SARI, NaSSA, RIMA, MAOI, tricyclics		Increased serotonergic effects with possibility of serotonin syndrome
Anxiolytic	Buspirone	Several cases of elevated blood pressure have been reported
Narcotics	Meperidine	Stupor, muscular rigidity, severe agitation, and elevated temperature has been reported in some patients receiving the combination of selegiline and meperidine
St. John's Wort		Increased serotonergic effects with possibility of serotonin syndrome
Sympathomimetics	Amphetamines, pseudoephedrine, phenylephrine, phenylpropanolamine, and ephedrine	Risk of hypertensive crisis

Effects of Antidepressants on Neurotransmitters/Receptors*

	Amitriptyline	Clomipramine	Desipramine	Doxepin	Imipramine	Nortriptyline	Protriptyline	Trimipramine	Amoxapine	Maprotiline	Bupropion
NE reuptake block	+++	+++	+++++	+++	+++	++++	+++++	++	++++	++++	+
5-HT reuptake block	+++	++++	++	++	+++	++	++	+	++	+	+−
DA reuptake block	+	+	+	+	+	+	+	+	+	+	++
5-HT$_1$ blockade	++	+	+	++	+	++	+	+	++	+−	+−
5-HT$_2$ blockade	+++	+++	++	+++	+++	+++	+++	+++	+++++	++	+
M$_1$(ACh) blockade	+++	+++	++	+++	+++	++	+++	+++	++	++	+−
H$_1$ blockade	++++	+++	+++++	+++	+++	+++	+++	+++++	+++	++++	+
α_1 blockade	+++	+++	++	+++	+++	+++	++	+++	+++	+++	+
α_2 blockade	++	+	+	+	+	+	+	+	+	+	+−
D$_2$ blockade	+	++	+	+	+	+	+	++	++	++	−
Selectivity	NE > 5-HT	NE < 5-HT	NE > 5-HT	NE > 5-HT	NE > 5-HT	NE > 5-HT	NE > 5-HT	NE > 5-HT	NE > 5-HT	NE > 5-HT	NE > 5-HT

	Trazodone	Nefazodone	Venlafaxine$^{(A)}$	Duloxetine	Citalopram	Escitalopram	Fluoxetine	Fluvoxamine	Paroxetine	Sertraline	Mirtazapine
NE reuptake block	+	++	++	+++++	+	+	++	++	+++	++	++
5-HT reuptake block	++	++	++++	+++++++	++++	++++	++++	++++	+++++	++++	+
DA reuptake block	+−	+		+++	−	−	+	+−	+	+	−
5-HT$_1$ blockade	+++	+++	+−	−	+−	+−	+−	+−	+−	+−	−
5-HT$_2$ blockade	++++	+++	+−	−	+	+	++	+	+−	+	++++
M$_1$(ACh) blockade	−	+−	−	+	+	+	++	+−	++	++	++
H$_1$ blockade	++	+−	−	+	++	+	+	−	+	+−	+++++
α_1 blockade	+++	+++	−	+	+	+	+	+	+	++	++
α_2 blockade	++	++	+−	−	+−	?	+−	+	+	+	+++++
D$_2$ blockade	+	++	−	−	+−	+	+	+	++	+−	+−
Selectivity	NE < 5-HT	NE < 5-HT	NE < 5-HT	NE < 5-HT	NE < 5-HT	NE < 5-HT	NE < 5-HT	NE < 5-HT	NE < 5-HT	NE < 5-HT	NE = 5-HT

* The ratio of K_i values (intrinsic dissociation constant) between various neurotransmitters/receptors determines the pharmacological profile for any one drug

$^{(A)}$ Desvenlafaxine has similar effects on neurotransmitters as venlafaxine

Key: K_i (nM) > 100,000 = −; 10,000–100,000 = ++−; 1000–10,000 = ++; 100–1000 = +++; 10–100 = ++++; 1–10 = +++++; 0.1–1 = +++++++
$1/K_i$ (M) < 0.001 = −; 0.001–0.01 = ++−; 0.01–0.1 = ++; 0.1–1 = +++; 1–10 = ++++; 10–100 = +++++; 100–1000 = +++++++

Adapted from Seeman P. Receptor Tables Vol. 2: Drug Dissociation Constants for Neuroreceptors and Transporters. Toronto: SZ Research, 1993; Richelson E. Synaptic effects of antidepressants. J Clin Psychopharmacol. 1996; 16 (3 Suppl. 2): 1–9.

Pharmacological Effects of Antidepressants on Neurotransmitters/Receptors

NE Reuptake Blockade

- Antidepressant effect
- Side effects: tremors, tachycardia, hypertension, sweating, insomnia, erectile and ejaculation problems
- Potentiation of pressor effects of NE (e.g., sympathomimetic amines)
- Interaction with guanethidine (blockade of antihypertensive effect)

5-HT Reuptake Blockade

- Antidepressant, anti-anxiety, anti-panic, anti-obsessional effect
- Can increase or decrease anxiety, depending on dose
- Side effects: dyspepsia, nausea, headache, nervousness, akathisia, extrapyramidal effects, anorexia, sexual side effects
- Potentiation of drugs with serotonergic properties (e.g., L-tryptophan); caution regarding "serotonin syndrome"

DA Reuptake Blockade

- Antidepressant, antiparkinsonian effect; may enhance motivation, cognition and mitigate against prolactin elevation
- Side effects: psychomotor activation, aggravation of psychosis

$5\text{-}HT_1$ Blockade

- Antidepressant, anxiolytic and antiaggressive action

$5\text{-}HT_2$ Blockade

- Anxiolytic ($5\text{-}HT_{2C}$), antidepressant ($5\text{-}HT_{2A}$), antipsychotic, antimigraine effect, improved sleep
- Side effects: hypotension, ejaculatory problems, sedation, weight gain ($5\text{-}HT_{2C}$)

M_1(ACh) Blockade

- Second most potent action of cyclic antidepressants
- Side effects: dry mouth, blurred vision, constipation, urinary retention, sinus tachycardia, QRS changes, memory disturbances, sedation, exacerbation/attack of narrow angle glaucoma
- Potentiation of effects of drugs with anticholinergic properties

H_1 Blockade

- Most potent action of cyclic antidepressants
- Side effects: sedation, postural hypotension, weight gain
- Potentiation of effects of other CNS drugs

α_1 Blockade

- Side effects: postural hypotension, dizziness, reflex tachycardia, sedation
- Potentiation of antihypertensives acting via α_1 blockade (e.g., prazosin, doxazosin, labetalol)

α_2 Blockade

- CNS arousal; possible decrease in depressive symptoms
- Side effect: sexual dysfunction, priapism
- Antagonism of antihypertensives acting as α_2 stimulants (e.g., clonidine)

D_2 Blockade

- Antipsychotic effect
- Side effects: extrapyramidal (e.g., tremor, rigidity), endocrine changes, sexual dysfunction (males)

Frequency of Adverse Reactions to Cyclic Antidepressants at Therapeutic Doses

Reaction	Amitriptyline	Clomipramine	Desipramine	Doxepin	Imipramine	Nortriptyline	Protriptyline	Trimipramine	Amoxapine	Maprotiline
CNS Effects										
Drowsiness, sedation	> 30%	> 2%	> 2%	> 30%	> 10%	> 2%	< 2%	> 30%	> 10%	> 10%
Insomnia	> 2%	> 10%	> 2%	> 2%	> 10%	< 2%	> 10%	> 2%[b]	> 10%	< 2%
Excitement, hypomania*	< 2%	< 2%	> 2%	< 2%	> 10%	> 2%	> 10%	< 2%	> 2%	> 2%
Disorientation/confusion	> 10%	> 2%	–	< 2%	> 2%	> 10%	–	> 10%	> 2%	> 2%
Headache	> 2%	> 2%	< 2%	< 2%	> 10%	< 2%	–	> 2%	> 2%	< 2%
Asthenia, fatigue	> 10%	> 2%	> 2%	> 2%	> 10%	> 10%	> 10%	> 2%	> 2%	> 2%
Anticholinergic Effects										
Dry mouth	> 30%	> 30%	> 10%	> 30%	> 30%	> 10%	> 10%	> 10%	> 30%	> 30%
Blurred vision	> 10%	> 10%	> 2%	> 10%	> 10%	> 2%	> 10%	> 2%	> 2%	> 10%
Constipation	> 10%	> 10%	> 2%	> 10%	> 10%	> 10%	> 10%	> 10%	> 30%	> 10%
Sweating	> 10%	> 10%	> 2%	> 2%	> 10%	< 2%	> 10%	> 2%	> 2%	> 2%
Delayed micturition**	> 2%	> 2%	–	< 2%	> 10%	< 2%	< 2%	< 2%	> 10%	> 2%
Extrapyramidal Effects										
Unspecified	> 2%[a]	< 2%[a]	< 2%	> 2%[a]	< 2%	–	–	< 2%	> 2%[a]	> 2%
Tremor	> 10%	> 10%	> 2%	> 2%	> 10%	> 10%	> 2%	> 10%	> 2%	> 10%
Cardiovascular Effects										
Orthostatic hypotension/dizziness	> 10%	> 10%	> 2%	> 10%	> 30%	> 2%	> 10%	> 10%	> 10%	> 2%
Tachycardia, palpitations	> 10%	> 10%	> 10%	> 2%	> 10%	> 2%	> 2%	> 2%	> 10%	> 2%
ECG changes***	> 10%[e]	> 10%[e]	> 2%[e]	> 2%[e]	> 10%[e]	> 2%[e]	> 10%[e]	> 10%[e]	< 2%[e]	< 2%[e]
Cardiac arrhythmia	> 2%	> 2%	> 2%	> 2%	> 2%	> 2%	> 2%	> 2%	< 2%	< 2%
GI distress	> 2%	> 10%	> 2%	< 2%	> 10%	< 2%	–	< 2%	> 2%	> 2%
Dermatitis, rash	> 2%	> 2%	> 2%	< 2%	> 2%	< 2%	< 2%	< 2%	> 10%	> 10%
Weight gain (over 6 kg)	> 30%	> 10%	> 2%	> 10%	> 10%	> 2%	< 2%	> 10%	< 2%	> 10%
Sexual disturbances	> 2%	> 30%	> 2%	> 2%	> 30%	< 2%	< 2%	< 2%	> 2%	< 2%
Seizures[c]	< 2%	< 2%[d]	< 2%	< 2%	< 2%	< 2%	< 2%	< 2%	< 2%[d]	< 2%[d]

– None reported in literature perused, * More likely in bipolar patients, ** Primarily in the elderly, *** ECG abnormalities usually without cardiac injury

[a] Tardive dyskinesia reported (rarely), [b] No effect on REM sleep, [c] In non-epileptic patients, [d] Higher incidence if dose above 250 mg daily clomipramine, 225 mg daily maprotiline, or 300 mg daily amoxapine, [e] Conduction delays: increased PR, QRS, or QTc interval

Frequency of Adverse Reactions to Cyclic Antidepressants at Therapeutic Doses (cont.)

	SARI		NDRI	SNRI			SSRI						NaSSA
Reaction	Trazo-done	Nefazo-done	Bupro-pion	Venlafax-ine	Desvenla-faxine	Duloxe-tine	Citalopram	Escitalo-pram	Fluoxetine	Fluvoxa-mine	Paroxetine	Sertraline	Mirtazapine
CNS Effects													
Drowsiness, sedation	>30%	>30%	>2%	>10%	>10%	>10%	>10%	>2%	>10%	>10%	>10%	>10%	>30%[t]
Insomnia	>2%	>2%	>10%	>10%[o]	>10%	>10%	>10%	>10%	>10%[o]	>10%	>10%	>10%	>2%
Excitement, hypomania*	–[k]	>2%	>10%[k]	>10%[k]	>3%	<2%	>2%	<2%	>2%	>10%	>2%	>10%	>2%
Disorientation/confusion	<2%	>10%	>2%	>2%	?	–	<2%	<2%	>10%	>2%	<2%	<2%	>2%
Headache	>2%	>30%	>10%	>10%	>3%	>10%	>10%	>10%	>10%	>10%	>10%	>10%	>10%
Asthenia, fatigue	>10%	>10%	>2%	>10%	>10%	>10%	>10%	>2%	>10%	>10%	>10%	>2%	>10%
Anticholinergic Effects													
Dry mouth	>10%	>10%	>10%	>10%	>10%	>10%	>10%	>10%	>10%	>10%	>10%	>10%	>30%
Blurred vision	>2%[i]	>10%	>10%	>2%	>3%	>2%	>2%	<2%	>2%	>2%	>2%	>2%	>10%
Constipation	>2%	>10%	>10%	>10%	>10%	>10%	>2%	>2%	>2%	>10%	>10%	>2%	>10%
Sweating	–	>2%	>10%	>10%	>10%	>10%	>10%	>2%	>2%	>10%	>10%	>2%	>2%
Delayed micturition**	<2%	<2%	>2%	<2%	?	<2%	>2%	–	>2%	>2%	>2%	<2%	>2%
Extrapyramidal Effects													
Unspecified	>2%[g]	<2%	<2%	>2%	?	<2%	>2%	<2%	<2%	>2%[g]	>2%	>2%	>2%
Tremor	>2%	<2%	>10%	>2%	?	>2%	>2%	<2%	>10%	>10%	>10%	>10%	>2%
Cardiovascular Effects													
Orthostatic hypotension/dizziness	>10%[l]	>10%	>2%[s]	>10%[s]	>10%[s]	>10%[s]	>2%	>2%	>10%	>2%	>10%	>10%	>2%
Tachycardia, palpitations	>2%	<2%[p]	>2%	>2%[x]	>3%	>2%	>2%[p]	>2%[p]	<2%[p]	<2%[p]	>2%[p]	>2%[p]	>2%
ECG changes***	>2%	<2%	<2%	<2%[x]	<2%	–	<2%	<2%	<2%	<2%	<2%	<2%	<2%
Cardiac arrhythmia	>2%[m]	<2%	<2%	<2%	<2%	–	<2%	<2%	<2%[u]	<2%	<2%	<2%	<2%
GI distress	>10%	>10%	>10%	>30%	>30%	>10%	>10%	>10%	>10%	>30%	>10%	>30%	>2%
Dermatitis, rash	<2%	<2%	>2%	>2%	?	>2%	<2%	>2%	>2%	>2%	<2%	>2%	<2%
Weight gain (over 6 kg)[p]	>2%	>2%	>2%[r]	>2%[r]	?	>2%	>2%	>2%	>2%[r]	>2%[r]	>10%[r]	>2%[r]	>30%
Sexual disturbances	<2%[n]	>2%	>2%[n][v]	>30%[n]	>3%	>30%	>30%	>10%	>30%[n]	>30%	>30%[n]	>30%[n]	>2%
Seizures[a]	<2%	<2%	<2%[h]	<2%	?	<2%	<2%	<2%	<2%	<2%	<2%	<2%	<2%

– None reported in literature perused, * More likely in bipolar patients, ** Primarily in the elderly, *** ECG abnormalities usually without cardiac injury.

[f] In non-epileptic patients; risk increased with elevated plasma levels, [g] Tardive dyskinesia reported (rarely), [h] Higher incidence if doses used above 450 mg/day of bupropion or in patients with bulimia, [i] Found to lower intraocular pressure, [k] Less likely to precipitate mania, [l] Less frequent if drugs given after meals, [m] Patients with pre-existing cardiac disease have a 10% incidence of premature ventricular contractions, [n] Priapism reported, [o] Especially if given in the evening, [p] Decreased heart rate reported, [r] Weight loss reported initially, [s] Hypertension reported; may be more common in patients with pre-existing hypertension, [t] Sedation decreased at higher doses (above 15 mg), [u] Slowing of sinus node and atrial dysrhythmia, [v] Improved sexual functioning, [w] With chronic treatment, [x] Increased risk with higher doses

Frequency (%) of Adverse Reactions to MAOI Antidepressants at Therapeutic Doses

Reaction	Isocarboxazid	Phenelzine	Tranylcypromine	Moclobemide	Selegiline Transdermal
CNS Effects					
Drowsiness, sedation	> 2%	> 10%	> 10%	> 2%	< 2%
Insomnia	> 2%[a]	> 10%[a]	> 10%[a]	> 10%[a]	> 10%
Excitement, hypomania**	> 2%	> 10%	> 10%	> 10%	> 2%
Disorientation/confusion	> 2%	> 2%	> 2%	> 2%	< 2%
Headache	> 10%	> 2%	> 10%	> 10%	> 10%
Asthenia	> 2%	< 2%	< 2%	< 2%	< 2%
Anticholinergic Effects					
Dry mouth	> 10%	> 30%	> 10%	> 10%	> 2%
Blurred vision	> 2%	> 10%	> 2%	> 10%	< 2%
Constipation	> 2%	> 10%	> 2%	> 2%	> 2%
Sweating	< 2%	–	> 2%	> 2%	> 2%
Delayed micturition*	> 2%	> 2%	> 2%	< 2%	< 2%
Extrapyramidal Effects					
Unspecified	> 2%	> 10%	< 2%	< 2%	< 2%
Tremor	> 10%	> 10%	> 2%	> 2%	< 2%
Cardiovascular Effects					
Orthostatic hypotension/dizziness	> 10%	> 10%	> 10%	> 10%	> 2%[i]
Tachycardia	–	> 10%[d]	> 10%[d]	> 2%	< 2%
ECG changes***	> 2%	< 2%[e]	< 2%[e]	> 2%	< 2%
Cardiac arrhythmia	> 2%	< 2%	< 2%	> 2%	< 2%
GI distress (nausea)	> 10%	> 10%	> 2%	> 10%	> 2%
Dermatitis, rash	> 2%	< 2%	> 2%	> 2%	> 10%[g]
Weight gain (over 6 kg)	> 2%	> 10%	> 2%	< 2%	> 2%[h]
Sexual disturbances	> 2%	> 30%[f]	> 2%[f]	> 2%	< 2%
Seizures[c]	–	< 2%	–[b]	< 2%	–

* Primarily in the elderly, ** More likely in bipolar patients, *** ECG abnormalities usually without cardiac injury

[a] Especially if given in the evening, [b] May have anticonvulsant activity, [c] In non-epileptic patients, [d] Decreased heart rate reported, [e] Shortened QTc interval, [f] Priapism reported, [g] At site of patch application, [h] Weight loss reported, [i] Hypertension reported

Antidepressant Doses and Pharmacokinetics

Drug	Therapeutic Dose Range (mg)	Comparable Dose (mg)	Suggested Plasma Level (nmol/L**)	Bioavail-ability (%)	Protein Binding (%)	Peak Plasma Level (h) (T_{max})	Elimination Half-life (h) ($T_{1/2}$)	Metabolizing Enzymes[g] (CYP-450; other)	Enzyme Inhibition[h] (CYP-450; other)
SSRIs									
Citalopram (Celexa)	10–60	10		80	80	4	23–45**(L)**	2D6[i,m], 2C19[m], 3A4[m]	2D6[w], 2C9[w], 2C19[w]
Escitalopram (Lexapro)[b]	10–20	2.5		80	56	4–5 (metabolite = 14)	27–32**(L)(R)**	2D6[m], 3A4[m], 2C19[m]	2D6[w], 2C9[w], 2C19[w]
Fluoxetine (Prozac)	10–80[c]	10		72–85	94	6–8 (immediate release)	24–144 (parent)**(L)** 200–330 (metabolite)	1A2[w], 2B6[w], **2D6**[i,p], 3A4[w], **2C9**[p], **2C19**[p], 2E1	1A2[m], 2B6[w], **2D6**[p], 3A4[i,w], 2C9[w], 2C19[m]; P-gp
Fluvoxamine (Luvox)	50–300[c]	50		60	77–80	1.5–8	9–28**(L)**	1A2[w], 2D6	**1A2**[p], 2B6[w], 2D6[m], 3A4[w], 2C9[m], **2C19**[p]; P-gp
Paroxetine (Paxil) Paroxetine CR (Paxil CR)	10–60[c] 12.5–75	10 12.5		> 90	95	5.2 (immediate release)	3–65**(L)(R)**	**2D6**[p]; P-gp	1A2[w], **2B6**, **2D6**[p], 3A4[w], 2C9[w], 2C19[m]; P-gp
Sertraline (Zoloft)	50–200[c]	25		70	98	6	22–36 (parent) **(L)(R)** 62–104 (metabolite)	2B6, 2D6, **3A4**[p],2C9, 2C19[m]; UGT2B7	1A2[w], 2B6[m], 2D6[w], 3A4[w], 2C9(w), **2C19**[p]; P-gp
NDRI									
Bupropion (Wellbutrin)[b]	225–450[d]	200[d]	75–350*	> 90	80–85	1.6 (immediate release)	10–14 (parent)**(L)**	1A2[w], **2B6**[p], 2D6[i], 3A4[w], 2C9[w], 2E1[m]	2D6[w]
Bupropion SR (Wellbutrin SR, Zyban)	150–300 mg[d]	150[d]					20–27 (metabo-lites)		
SNRI									
Venlafaxine (Effexor)	75–375	50		13	27	2 (immediate release) XR = 5.5	3–7 (parent)**(L)(R)** 9–13 (metabolite) 9–12 (absorption half-life)	**2D6**[p], 3A4[i,w], 2C9, 2C19	2D6[w], 3A4[w]
Venlafaxine XR (Effexor XR)									
Desvenlafaxine	50–100	50	–	80	30	7.5	11**(R)**	**UGT**[p], 3A4	2D6
Duloxetine (Cymbalta)[a]	60–120	?		70	> 95	6	8–19**(L)(R)**	1A2, 2D6	2D6[m]
SARI									
Nefazodone	100–600	100		99	15–23	2	2–5[e] (parent) 3–18 (metabolites)	2D6[i], **3A4**[p]	1A2[w], 2D6[w], 3A4[p]; P-gp (acute dos-ing); inducer of P-gp
Trazodone (Desyrel)	150–600	100		70–90	93	2	4–9	2D6[i], **3A4**[p]	2D6[w]; inducer of P-gp
NaSSA									
Mirtazapine (Remeron)	15–60	15		50	85	2	20–40**(L)(R)**	**1A2**[p], **2D6**[i,p], **3A4**[p], 2C9	–

Drug	Therapeutic Dose Range (mg)	Comparable Dose (mg)	Suggested Plasma Level (nmol/L**)	Bioavail-ability (%)	Protein Binding (%)	Peak Plasma Level (h) (T_{max})	Elimination Half-life (h) ($T_{1/2}$)	Metabolizing Enzymes[g] (CYP-450; other)	Enzyme Inhibition[h] (CYP-450; other)
NON-SELECTIVE CYCLIC AGENTS–Tricyclic									
Amitriptyline (Elavil)	75–300	50	250–825*[f]	43–48	92–96	2–8	10–46**(L)**	1A2[w], 2B6[w], 2D6[m], **3A4**[p], 2C9[p], 2C19[p] 1A2[w], 2D6, 3A4[w], 2C9[w], 2C19[w]; P-gp	1A2, 2D6[m], 3A4, 2C9[w], 2C19[m], 2E1; P-gp; UGT
Clomipramine (Anafranil)	75–300	50	300–1000	98	98	2–6	17–37**(L)**	1A2, **2D6**[p]	2D6[m]; UGT
Desipramine (Norpramin)	75–300	50	400–1000[f]	73–92	73–92	2–6	12–76**(L)**	1A2, **2D6**[p], 3A4, 2C9[w], **2C19**[p]	2D6[m], 2C19[w], 2E1; P-gp
Doxepin (Sinequan, Triadapin)	75–300	50	500–950*	89	89	2–6	8–36**(L)**	1A2[w], 2B6[w], **2D6**[p], 3A4[m], 2C9[w], 2C19[w]; UGT1A3; UGT1A4	–
Imipramine (Tofranil)	75–300	50	500–800*[f]	89	89	2–6	4–34**(L)**	**2D6**[p], 3A4[m], 2C9[w], 2C19[m]; UGT1A4	1A2, 2D6[m], 2C19[m], 2E1; P-gp; UGT1A3
Nortriptyline (Aventyl, Pamelor)	40–200	25	150–500[f]	89–92	89–92	2–6	13–88**(L)**	1A2, 2D6[m], 3A4[m], 2C19; P-gp	2D6, 2C19[w], 2E1
Protriptyline (Vivactil)[b]	20–60	15	350–700	90–96	90–96	12	54–124**(L)**	?	?
Trimipramine (Surmontil)	75–300	50	500–800	95	95	2–6	7–30**(L)**	2D6, 2C9, 2C19	2D6; P-gp
Dibenzoxazepine									
Amoxapine (Asendin)[b]	100–600	100		46–82	?	1–2	8–14**(L)**	–	2D6
Tetracyclic									
Maprotiline (Ludiomil)	100–225	50	200–950*	66–100	88	9–16	27–58**(L)**	1A2, **2D6**[p]	2D6; P-gp
RIMA									
Moclobemide (Manerix)[a]	300–600	150	–	50–80	50	?	1–3**(L)**	**2C19**[p]	1A2[m], 2D6[m], 2C9, 2C19[m]
MAOI (irreversible)									
Isocarboxazid (Marplan)[b]	30–50	10	–	?	?	?	2.5	–	–
Phenelzine (Nardil)	45–90	15	–	?	?	?	1.5–4	2E1	–
Tranylcypromine (Parnate)	20–60	10	–	?	?	?	2.4**(L)**	–	1A2[w], **2A6**[p], 2D6[w], 2C9[w], 2C19[w], 3A4[w], 2E1[m]
MAO-B Inhibitor									
Selegiline Transdermal[b]	6 mg/24 h to 12 mg/24 h	?	–	10–40	90	4	18–25	2A6, 2B6, 2C9, 3A4/5	2B6, 2D6, 3A4/5

Monograph doses are just a guideline, and each patient's medication must be individualized. CYP activity data from www.gentest.com/human_p450_database/srchh450.asp (Dec. 03) and Oesterheld JR, Osser DN. P450 Drug Interactions: http://www.mhc.com/Cytochromes/

* Includes sum of drug and its metabolites. ** Approximate conversion: nmol/L = 3.5 × ng/ml.

(L) Increased in liver disorders – consider dose adjustment, **(R)** Increased in moderate to severe renal impairment – consider dose adjustment

[a] Not marketed in USA, [b] Not marketed in Canada, [c] SSRIs have a flat dose response curve. For depression most patients respond to the initial (low) dose. Higher doses are used in the treatment of OCD, [d] Give in divided doses (maximum of 150 mg per dose), [e] Dose-dependent, [f] Established ranges for efficacy in major depressive disorder, [g] Cytochrome P450 isoenzymes involved in drug metabolism, [h] CYP-450 isoenzymes inhibited by the drug; magnitude may be influenced by drug dose and plasma concentration, and by genotype and basal metabolic capacity of each patient, [i] Specific to metabolite, [p] Potent activity, [m] Moderate activity, [w] Weak activity

P-gp = p-glycoprotein – a transporter of hydrophobic substances in or out of specific body organs (e.g., block absorption in the gut); UGT = uridine diphosphate glucuronosyl transferase – involved in Phase 2 reactions (conjugation)

Switching Antidepressants

Antidepressant Non-Response	• Ascertain diagnosis is correct; ascertain patient is compliant with therapy • Ensure dosage prescribed is therapeutic; measure plasma level; ensure there has been an adequate trial period, i.e., up to 6 weeks at a reasonable dose

Factors Complicating Response	• Concurrent medical or psychiatric illness, e.g., hypothyroidism, obsessive compulsive disorder • Concurrent prescription drugs may interfere with efficacy, e.g., calcium channel blockers • Metabolic enhancers (e.g., carbamazepine) or inhibitors (e.g., erythromycin) will affect plasma level of antidepressant • Drug abuse may make management difficult, e.g., cocaine • Psychosocial factors may affect response • Personality disorders lead to poor outcome; however, depression may evoke personality problems which may disappear when the depression is alleviated

Switching Antidepressants	• Switching from one SSRI to another can offer enhanced response in previously non-responsive patients • 20–25% remission rate when switching from SSRI to another class of antidepressant or a different SSRI after failure of first SSRI (STAR*D studies) • Use caution when switching to or from irreversible MAOIs (see Switching Antidepressants pp. 66–67) • Switching between tricyclic agents is of questionable benefit

Advantages of Switching	• Minimizes polypharmacy • Second agent may be better tolerated • Less costly

Disadvantages of Switching	• Time required to taper first agent or need for a washout (risk of relapse) • Lose partial efficacy of first agent • Delayed onset of action

Switching from		Switching to	Washout Period[a]
Non-selective cyclic	→	Non-selective Cyclic	No washout – use dose equivalents for switching (pp. 64–65)
	→	SSRI	5 half-lives of cyclic antidepressant (caution: see Interactions, p. 10)[b]
	→	NDRI	5 half-lives of cyclic antidepressant
	→	SNRI or SARI, NaSSA	No washout – taper[b]
	→	Irrev. MAOI, MAO-B	5 half-lives of cyclic antidepressant
	→	RIMA	5 half-lives of cyclic antidepressant
SSRI or SARI	→	Non-selective Cyclic	5 half-lives of SSRI or SARI (caution: with fluoxetine due to long half-life of active metabolite)[b]
	→	NDRI	No washout – taper (caution: with fluoxetine)[b]
	→	SNRI	No washout – taper (caution: with fluoxetine)[b], monitor for serotonergic effects
	→	Irrev. MAOI, MAO-B	5 half-lives of SSRI or SARI (caution: with fluoxetine) – DO NOT COMBINE
	→	RIMA	5 half-lives of SSRI or SARI (caution: with fluoxetine)
	→	SSRI or SARI, NaSSA	No washout – taper first drug over 2–5 days then start second drug (use lower doses of second drug if switching from fluoxetine; longer taper may be necessary if higher doses of fluoxetine used); monitor for serotonergic effects

Switching from		Switching to	Washout Period[a]
NDRI	→	Non-selective Cyclic	2 days
	→	SSRI or SARI	No washout – taper (caution with fluoxetine)[b]
	→	SNRI , NaSSA	No washout – taper[b]; monitor for noradrenergic effects
	→	RIMA	5 half-lives of NDRI (3–5 days) – DO NOT COMBINE
	→	Irrev. MAOI, MAO-B	5 half-lives of NDRI (3–5 days) – DO NOT COMBINE
SNRI or NaSSA	→	Non-selective Cyclic	No washout – taper[b]
	→	SSRI or SARI	No washout – taper[b]; monitor for serotonergic effects
	→	NDRI	No washout – taper[b]; monitor for noradrenergic effects
	→	NaSSA, SNRI	No washout – taper[b]; monitor for serotonergic and noradrenergic effects
	→	Irrev. MAOI, MAO-B	5 half-lives of SNRI (3 days) or NaSSA (5–7 days) – DO NOT COMBINE
	→	RIMA	5 half-lives of SNRI (3 days) or NaSSA (5–7 days) – CAUTION
Irrev. MAOI	→	Non-selective Cyclic	10 days – CAUTION
	→	SSRI or SARI	10 days – DO NOT COMBINE
	→	NDRI	10 days – DO NOT COMBINE
	→	SNRI	Minimum of 14 days – DO NOT COMBINE. Caution: case reports of serotonin syndrome after 14 days washout
	→	NaSSA	10 days – DO NOT COMBINE
	→	RIMA	Start the next day if changing from low to moderate dose; taper from a high dose. Maintain dietary restrictions for 10 days
	→	Irrev. MAOI, MAO-B	10 days – DO NOT COMBINE
RIMA	→	Non-selective Cyclic	2 days – CAUTION
	→	SSRI, SARI or NaSSA	2 days – CAUTION
	→	NDRI	2 days – CAUTION
	→	SNRI	2 days – CAUTION
	→	Irrev. MAOI	Can start the following day at a low dose
	→	MAO-B	2 days – CAUTION
MAO-B	→	Non-selective Cyclic	5 days – CAUTION
	→	SSRI or SARI	5 days – CAUTION
	→	NDRI	5 days – CAUTION
	→	NaSSA, SNRI	5 days – CAUTION
	→	Irrev. MAOI	5 days – CAUTION
	→	RIMA	5 days – CAUTION

[a] Recommendations pertain to outpatients. More rapid switching may be used in inpatients (except from an irreversible MAOI or RIMA) with proper monitoring of plasma levels and synergistic effects; [b] Taper first drug over 3 to 7 days prior to initiating second antidepressant; consider starting second drug at a reduced dose.

Antidepressant Augmentation Strategies

Augmentation Strategies

Advantages of Augmentation	• May have rapid onset of response • Response > 50% with most combinations[15] • No need to taper first agent or have a washout
Disadvantages of Augmentation	• Increased potential for side effects • Increased risk for drug interactions • Increased cost • Decreased compliance possible due to need to take an increased number of tablets/capsules
Antidepressant Combinations	• Combining antidepressants which affect different neurotransmitter systems may produce a better antidepressant response than either drug alone; consider potential drug-drug interactions (pharmacokinetic and pharmacodynamic)
MAOI + Cyclic	• Six open series cases report response rates of 54–100% • Combination therapy should be started together, or MAOI can be added to the cyclic drug. Use caution with serotonergic agents (see Drug Interactions p. 54) • Require 6 weeks at adequate doses ☞ **DO NOT COMBINE AN IRREVERSIBLE MAOI WITH (1) SSRI, (2) SNRI, (3) NDRI, (4) SARI, (5) RIMA, or (6) NaSSA**
SSRI + Cyclic	• Up to 50% of patients may respond to combination of SSRI and noradrenergic TCA (e.g., desipramine, nortriptyline) • Use lower doses of TCA and monitor TCA levels to prevent toxicity (see Interactions, p. 10) • Combination of an SSRI and a noradrenergic cyclic drug (e.g., desipramine) reported to cause greater downregulation of β-adrenergic receptors, a more rapid response, and higher remission rates
RIMA + Cyclic	• Up to 57% response rate in open trials • Monitor for serotonergic adverse effects
RIMA + SSRI	• Up to 67% of refractory patients may respond to combination • Monitor for serotonergic adverse effects
NDRI + SSRI NDRI + SNRI	• STAR*D studies: 30% remission rate when bupropion was added to citalopram after failure of SSRI[15] • Up to 85% of partial responders reported to have clinically significant benefit from the combination in open trials and case series; adverse effects (e.g., tremor, panic attacks, increased seizure risk) may limit dosage (see Interactions p. 19) • Bupropion may improve sleep efficacy, energy, fatigue, and executive functions, and mitigate SNRI- or SSRI-induced sexual dysfunction
NaSSA + SSRI	• Response reported in 64% of refractory patients after mirtazapine 15–30 mg was added to SSRI treatment in an open trial • Reported to alleviate insomnia; may have an activating effect; weight gain and sedation also reported
SARI + SSRI	• Nefazodone (100–200 mg bid) used to augment antidepressant response and alleviate SSRI-induced sexual dysfunction • Up to 55% response reported when nefazodone (100 –200 mg bid) used to augment SSRIs in patients with treatment-refractory depression • Low dose trazodone (25–50 mg) used to alleviate insomnia • Monitor for serotonergic effects; combination may increase anxiety and irritability
SNRI + Cyclic	• 64% of patients achieved full clinical remission

Thyroid Hormone (T_3)(T_4)	• Dosage: 25–50 mg/day of liothyronine or 0.15–0.5 mg/day levothyroxine – if ineffective, discontinue after 3 weeks; T3 considered to be more effective than T_4 (T_3 augmentation may be more effective in women than in men) (see p. 297)
	• Mixed results reported – may be more effective in combination with TCAs than with SSRIs
Lithium	• Meta-analysis of controlled studies suggests that lithium augmentation of conventional antidepressants is effective in treatment-resistant depression; up to 60% of patients may respond to combined treatment (lower response rates reported with SSRIs); response may occur within 48 h, but usually within 3 weeks. May be less effective in the elderly
	• Unclear if there is a correlation between lithium level and clinical improvement when used as augmentation therapy; however, plasma level above 0.4 mmol/l is suggested for efficacy; usual dose: 600–900 mg/day
	• Response more likely in probable bipolar patients (with a first-degree relative with bipolar disorder or with a history of hypomania)
Anticonvulsants, e.g., Carbamazepine	• Combination reported to benefit patients with refractory depression or OCD (case reports)
	• Monitor TCA levels due to increased metabolism with carbamazepine; with SSRI, monitor carbamazepine level (see Interactions p. 10)
	• There is no significant correlation between anticonvulsant plasma level and clinical improvement
Buspirone	• Effect observed within 2–4 weeks
	• Remission rate = 30% when added to citalopram in people who failed SSRI in STAR*D trial
	• 43–100% of depressed patients reported to respond to combination with antidepressant in open-label trials – data contradictory with double-blind studies
	• May treat persistent anxiety and help alleviate SSRI-induced sexual dysfunction
	• Monitor for adverse effects due to serotonergic excess
	• Usual dose: 15–60 mg/day
Psychostimulants	• Methylphenidate (10–40 mg) or *d*-amphetamine (5–30 mg) used as augmentation therapy with cyclic agents, SSRIs, SNRI or irreversible MAOIs
	• Rapid symptom resolution reported in up to 78% of patients in open trials; response was sustained (no tolerance observed)
	• Improve residual symptoms of sleepiness, fatigue, and executive dysfunction in MDD
	• Caution: observe for activation and blood pressure changes
	• Irritability, anxiety and paranoia reported – use caution in patients who are anxious or agitated
Electroconvulsive Treatment	• See p. 72
	• May be used with antidepressant for acute treatment; maintenance therapy with antidepressant or with lithium may be required
Tryptophan	• See p. 179
	• Usual dose: 1.5–12 g/day
	• Data suggests efficacy when combined with cyclics, SSRIs or MAOIs; monitor for increased serotonergic effects
Pindolol	• Blocks β-adrenoreceptors and serotonin (5-HT$_{1A}$ and 5-HT$_{1B/1D}$) autoreceptors and increases serotonin concentration at postsynaptic sites (see p. 296)
	• Data contradictory, most recent data does not support using pindolol as an adjunctive agent. Some controlled studies show mixed results with regard to a more rapid antidepressant response when pindolol used in combination with antidepressants
	• Usual dose: 2.5 mg tid
	• Monitor blood pressure and heart rate; caution in patients with asthma or cardiac conduction problems
Second-Generation Antipsychotics	• 5-HT$_{2c}$ blockade suggested to increase NE and dopamine and acetylcholine levels in the prefrontal cortex; blockade of 5-HT$_{2A}$ and 5-HT$_{2C}$ receptors may improve the efficacy and side effect profile of SSRIs and enhance sleep; reported to improve cognition in MDD

Antidepressant Augmentation Strategies (cont.)

- Low doses of risperidone (0.5–2 mg/day), olanzapine (2.5–10 mg/day), quetiapine, ziprasidone, or aripiprazole can augment SSRIs in patients with MDD or OCD; reported to decrease anxiety, irritability and insomnia, improve cognition, and remission rates
- Fluoxetine/olanzapine combination (Symbyax) approved in USA for treatment of bipolar depression

| **Repetitive Transcranial Magnetic Stimulation** | - See p. 79
- Double-blind study reports that combined treatment using low-frequency rTMS for 10 sessions, with an antidepressant, was superior to an antidepressant alone in patients with partially responsive depression |

| **Modafinil** | - See p. 299
- Placebo-controlled and open label studies suggest modafinil can decrease daytime sleepiness and fatigue in patients with MDD and improve response and quality of life in patients treated with SSRI antidepressants
- Modafinil induces CYP3A4 and may decrease the plasma level of drugs metabolized by this isoenzyme (e.g., citalopram). *In vitro* studies suggest it also inhibits CYP2C19 and 2C9, and can increase the plasma level of drugs metabolized by this isoenzyme (e.g. fluoxetine, moclobemide) |

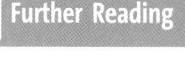 **Further Reading**

References

1. ACOG Committee on Practice Bulletins – Obstetrics. ACOG Practice Bulletin: Clinical management guidelines for obstetrician-gynecologists number 92, April 2008 (replaces practice bulletin number 87, November 2007). Use of psychiatric medications during pregnancy and lactation. *Obstet Gynecol* 2008;111(4):1001–1020.
2. Cole JA, Modell JG, Haight BR, et al. Bupropion in pregnancy and the prevalence of congenital malformations. Pharmacoepidemiol Drug Saf. 2007;16(5):474–484.
3. Deneys ML, Ahearn EP. Exacerbation of PTSD symptoms with use of duloxetine. J Clin Psychiatry. 2006;67(3):496–497.
4. Deshauer D. Venlafaxine (Effexor): Concerns about increased risk of fatal outcomes in overdose. CMAJ. 2007;176(1):39–40.
5. Djulus J, Koren G, Einarson TR, et al. Exposure to mirtazapine during pregnancy: a prospective, comparative study of birth outcomes. J Clin Psychiatry. 2006;67(8):1280–1284.
6. Fiore MC, Jaén CR, Baker TB, et al. Treating tobacco use and dependence: 2008 update. US Department of Health and Human Services, 2008. Available from http://www.ncbi.nlm.nih.gov/books/bv.fcgi?rid=hstat2.chapter.28163 (Accessed March 16, 2009).
7. Gualtieri CT, Johnson LG. Bupropion normalizes cognitive performance in patients with depression. Med Gen Med. 2007;9(1):22.
8. Jorenby DE, Leischow SJ, Nides MA, et al. A controlled trial of sustained-release bupropion, a nicotine patch, or both for smoking cessation. N Engl J Med. 1999;340:685–691.
9. Kristensen JH, Ilett KF, Rampono J, et al. Transfer of the antidepressant mirtazapine into breast milk. Br J Clin Pharmacol. 2007;63(3):322–327.
10. Levin TT, Cortes-Ladino A, Weiss M, et al. Life-threatening serotonin toxicity due to a citalopram-fluconazole drug interaction: Case reports and discussion. Gen Hosp Psychiatry. 2008;30(4):372–377.
11. Mago R, Anolik R, Johnson RA. Recurrent priapism associated with use of aripiprazole. J Clin Psychiatry. 2006;67(9):1471–1472.
12. National Institute for Health and Clinical Excellence (NICE). Smoking cessation – bupropion and nicotine replacement therapy: The clinical effectiveness and cost effectiveness of bupropion (Zyban) and nicotine replacement therapy for smoking cessation. Technology Appraisal Guidance No. 39 (March 2002). London: National Institute for Health and Clinical Excellence. Available from www.nice.org.uk/Guidance/TA39 (Accessed February 5, 2009).
13. SSRIs and osteoporosis. Med Lett Drugs Ther. 2007;49(1274):95–96
14. Talwar A, Jain M, Vijayan VK. Pharmacotherapy of tobacco dependence. Med Clin North Am. 2004;88(6):1517–1534.
15. Trivedi MH, Rush AJ, Wisniewski SR, et al. Evaluation of outcomes with citalopram for depression using measurement-based care in STAR*D: Implications for clinical practice. Am J Psychiatry 2006;163(1):28–40.
16. Turner EH, Matthews AM, Linardatos E, et al. Selective publication of antidepressant effectiveness and its influence on apparent efficacy. N Engl J Med. 2008;358(3):252–260.
17. Zemrak WR, Kenna GA. Association of antipsychotic and antidepressant drugs with Q-T interval prolongation. Am J Health Syst Pharm. 2008;65(11):1029–1038.

Additional Suggested Reading

- Alvarez Jr W, Pickworth KK. Safety of antidepressant drugs in the patient with cardiac disease: A review of the literature. Pharmacotherapy. 2003;23(6):754–771.
- American Hospital Formulary Service. AHFS Drug Information: Duloxetine. Bethesda, MD: American Society of Health-System Pharmacists; 2006.
- American Psychiatric Association. Practice guideline for the treatment of patients with obsessive-compulsive disorder. Arlington, VA: American Psychiatric Association, 2007. Available from http://www.psychiatryonline.com/pracGuide/loadGuidelinePdf.aspx?file=OCDPracticeGuidelineFinal05-04-07 (Accessed March 16, 2009).
- American Psychiatric Association. Practice guideline for the treatment of patients with panic disorder (2nd ed). Arlington, VA: American Psychiatric Association, 2008. Available from http://www.psychiatryonline.com/pracGuide/loadGuidelinePdf.aspx?file=PanicDisorder_2e_PracticeGuideline (Accessed March 16, 2009).
- Baldwin DS, Anderson IM, Nutt DJ, et al. Evidence-based guidelines for the pharmacological treatment of anxiety disorders: Recommendations from the British Association for Psychopharmacology. J Psychopharmacol. 2005;19(6):567–596. Available from http://www.bap.org.uk/consensus/Anxiety_Disorder_Guidelines.pdf (Accessed March 16, 2009).
- Bonnot O, Warot D, Cohen D. Priapism associated with sertraline. J Am Acad Child Adolesc Psychiatr. 2007;46(7):790–791.
- Burry L, Kennie N. Withdrawal reactions. Pharmacy Practice. 2000;16(4):46–54.
- Caccia S. Metabolism of the newer antidepressants; an overview of the pharmacological and pharmacokinetic implications. Clin Pharmacokinet. 1998;34(4):281–302.

- Carbone JR. The neuroleptic malignant and serotonin syndromes. Emerg Med Clin North Am. 2000;18(2):317–325.
- Carpenter JS, Storniolo AM, Johns S, et al. Randomized, double-blind, placebo-controlled crossover trials of venlafaxine for hot flashes after breast cancer. Oncologist. 2007;12(1):124–35.
- Endicott J, Russell JM, Raskin J, et al. Duloxetine treatment for role functioning improvement in generalized anxiety disorder: three independent studies. J Clin Psychiatr. 2007;68(4):518–524.
- Gerber PE, Lynd LD. Selective serotonin-reuptake inhibitor-induced movement disorders. Ann Pharmacother. 1998;32(6):692–698.
- Glueck CJ, Khalil Q, Winiarska M, et al. Interaction of duloxetine and warfarin causing severe elevation of international normalized ratio. JAMA. 2006;295(13):1517–1518.
- Greenblatt DJ, von Moltke LL, Harmatz JS, et al. Drug interactions with newer antidepressants: Role of human cytochromes P450. J Clin Psychiatry. 1998;58 Suppl 15:S19–S27.
- Haberfellner EM. Priapism with sertraline-risperidone combination. Pharmacopsychiatry. 2007;40(1):44–45.
- Hanje AJ, Pell LJ, Votolato NA, et al. Case report: Fulminant hepatic failure involving duloxetine hydrochloride. Clin Gastroenterol Hepatol. 2006;4(7):912–917.
- Hartford J, Kornstein S, Liebowitz M, et al. Duloxetine as an SNRI treatment for generalized anxiety disorder: Results from a placebo and active-controlled trial. Int Clin Psychopharmacol. 2007;22(3):167–174.
- Hirschfeld RMA, Montgomery S, Aguglia E, et al. Partial response or nonresponse to antidepressant therapy: Current approaches and treatment options. J Clin Psychiatry. 2002;63(9):826–837.
- Hughes JR, Stead LF, Lancaster T. Antidepressants for smoking cessation. Cochrane Database Syst. Rev. 2003:CD000031.
- Institute for Clinical Systems Improvement. Health care guideline: Major depression in adults in primary care (11th ed.). Bloomington, MN: ICSI; May 2008. Available from http://www.icsi.org/depression_5/depression__major__in_adults_in_primary_care_3.html (Accessed March 16, 2009). Summary available from http://www.guideline.gov/summary/pdf.aspx?doc_id=12617&stat=1&string= (Accessed March 16, 2009).
- Joffe H, Soares CN, Petrillo LF, et al. Treatment of depression and menopause-related symptoms with the serotonin-norepinephrine reuptake inhibitor duloxetine. J Clin Psychiatr. 2007;68(6):943–950.
- Kapczinski F, Lima MS, Souza JS, et al. Antidepressants for generalized anxiety disorder. Cochrane Database Syst. Rev. 2003;2:CD003592.
- Kerwin JP, Gordon PR, Senf JH. The variable response of women with menopausal hot flashes when treated with sertraline. Menopause. 2007;14:841–845.
- Klinkman MS. The role of algorithms in the detection and treatment of depression in primary care. J Clin Psychiatry. 2003;64 Suppl 2:S19–S23.
- Kornstein SG, McEnany G. Enhancing pharmacologic effects in the treatment of depression in women. J Clin Psychiatry. 2000;61 Suppl 11:S18–S27.
- Labbale LA, Croft HA, Oleshansky MA. Antidepressant-related erectile dysfunction: Management via avoidance, switching antidepressants, antidotes, and adaptation. J Clin Psychiatry. 2003;64 Suppl 10:S11–S19.
- Loibl S, Schwedler K, von Minckwitz G, et al. Venlafaxine is superior to clonidine as treatment of hot flashes in breast cancer patients: A double-blind, randomized study. Ann Oncol. 2008;18(4):689–693.
- Loprinzi CL, Levitt R, Barton D, et al. Phase III comparison of depomedroxyprogesterone acetate to venlafaxine for managing hot flashes: North Central Cancer Treatment Group Trial N99C7. J Clin Oncol. 2006;24(9):1409–1414.
- Machado M, Iskedjian M, Ruiz I, et al. Remission dropouts and adverse drug reaction rates in major depressive disorder: A meta-analysis of head-to-head trials. Curr Med Res Opin. 2006;22(9):1825–1837.
- Mazza M, Harnic D, Catalano V, et al. Duloxetine for premenstrual dysphoric disorder: A pilot study. Expet Opin Pharmacother. 2008;9(4):517–521.
- Monastero R, Camarda R, Camarda C. Potential drug-drug interaction between duloxetine and acenocoumarol in a patient with Alzheimer's disease. Clin Ther. 2007;29(12):2706–2709.
- National Institute for Health and Clinical Excellence. Depression: Management of depression in primary and secondary care (amended) [Clinical Guideline 23]. London: NICE; 2007. Available from http://www.nice.org.uk/nicemedia/pdf/CG23NICEguidelineamended.pdf (Accessed March 16, 2009).
- National Institute for Health and Clinical Excellence. Post-traumatic stress disorder (PTSD): The management of PTSD in adults and children in primary and secondary care [Clinical Guideline 26]. London: NICE; 2005. Available from http://www.nice.org.uk/nicemedia/pdf/CG026NICEguideline.pdf (Accessed March 16, 2009).
- Qaseem A, Snow V, Denberg TD, et al. Using second generation antidepressants to treat depressive disorders: A clinical practice guideline from the American College of Physicians. Ann Intern Med. 2008;149(10):725–733.
- Ramasubbu R. Cerebrovascular effects of selective serotonin reuptake inhibitors: A systematic review. J Clin Psychiatry. 2004;65(12):1642–1653.
- Thase ME, Tran PV, Wiltse C, et al. Cardiovascular profile of duloxetine, a dual reuptake inhibitor of serotonin and norepinephrine. J Clin Psychopharmacol. 2005;25(2):132–140.
- Tong IL. Treatment of menopausal hot flashes. Med Health. 2008;91(3):73–76.
- Westanmo AD, Gayken J, Haight R. Duloxetine: A balanced and selective norepinephreine and serotonine-reuptake inhibitor. Am J Health Syst Pharm. 2005;62(23):2481–2490.
- Wu P, Wilson K, Dimoulas P, et al. Effectiveness of smoking cessation therapies: A systematic review and meta-analysis. BMC Public Health. 2006;6:300.

ELECTROCONVULSIVE THERAPY (ECT)

Definition	• The induction of seizures, by means of an externally applied electric stimulus, for the treatment of certain mental disorders • **Not** to be confused with the administration of subconvulsive electric stimuli, referred to as cranial electrostimulation or electrosleep therapy; nor the administration of aversive electric stimuli as a behavior modification protocol; and not repetitive transcranial magnetic stimulation (rTMS; preliminary comparison of rTMS with ECT indicates that rTMS may be effective for major depression, but not with psychotic symptoms) • Sometimes called electro-shock therapy and, in the animal research literature, referred to as electroconvulsive shock (ECS)
Indications (Approved)	• Major depressive disorder; especially when associated with high suicide risk, inanition/dehydration, severe agitation, depressive stupor, catatonia, delusions, non-response to one or more adequate trials of antidepressants or intolerance of therapeutic dosages • Prophylaxis or attenuation of recurrent major depression; i.e., "maintenance" ECT after response to an acute/index course of ECT, if previous antidepressants have not prevented recurrence • Prevention of relapse of major depression, i.e., "continuation" ECT for up to 6 months after response to an acute/index course of ECT, if previous antidepressants have not prevented rapid relapse; may provide better outcome than antidepressants alone following an acute/index course; one small randomized trial found that treating patients with psychotic depression for 2 years with ECT plus nortriptyline was more effective than nortriptyline alone. • Depressed phase of bipolar disorder • Atypical depression; a randomized trial found that patients with atypical depression were 2.6 times more likely to have remission with ECT treatment than those with other types of depression. • Agitated depression • Manic phase of bipolar disorder; adjunct to mood stabilizers and antipsychotics for severe mania (manic "delirium") and rapidcycling illness • Dysphoric mania ("mixed bipolar") • Prophylaxis of depressed and manic phases of bipolar disorder if mood stabilizers have been ineffective • Post-partum psychoses; secondary line of treatment after non-response to antidepressants and/or antipsychotics • Schizophrenia; especially with concurrent catatonic and/or affective symptoms; adjunct to adequate dosage of antipsychotics for non-responsive "positive" symptoms; after failed clozapine trial • Schizoaffective disorder, first-episode psychosis; after non-response to one or more adequate drug trials • Reports of effectiveness for Parkinson's disease ("on-off" phenomenon), neuroleptic malignant syndrome, status epilepticus, tardive dyskinesia and affective/psychotic disorders associated with mental retardation • Efficacy in refractory obsessive compulsive disorder reported (probably indicated only when concurrent depression warrants ECT)
General Comments	• Consider ECT early in the treatment algorithm, in the presence of very severe illness (do not regard as treatment of last resort); may be first-line treatment for very severe depression or mania, however very chronic episodes may reduce effectiveness
Therapeutic Effects	• Vegetative symptoms of depression, such as insomnia and fatigue, and catatonic symptoms may respond initially; later improvement of affective symptoms, such as depressed mood and anhedonia; followed by improvement of cognitive symptoms, such as impaired self-esteem, helplessness, hopelessness, suicidal and delusional ideation • Manic symptoms which respond include agitation, euphoria, motor overactivity, and thought disorder • Some "positive" symptoms of schizophrenia and other psychoses may respond • Most effective treatment for severe depression in that a substantial proportion of non-responders to antidepressants do recover with ECT; "melancholic" and "psychotic" presentations respond best
Mechanism of Action	• Exact mechanism unknown • Affects almost all neurotransmitters implicated in the pathogenesis of the mental disorders (norepinephrine, serotonin, acetylcholine, dopamine, GABA)

- Neurophysiological effects include increased permeability of the blood-brain barrier, suppression of regional cerebral blood flow and neurometabolic activity; "anticonvulsant" effects may be related to outcome (inhibitory neurotransmitters are increased by ECT)
- Affects neuroendocrine substances (CRF, ACTH, TRH, prolactin, vasopressin, metenkephalins, β-endorphins)

 Dosage

- "Dosage" may be some combination of the electrical energy/charge of the stimulus, electrode placement, seizure duration and the total number of convulsions induced; the precise duration of seizure required is unknown (perhaps must be at least 15 s) because there is no clear correlation between seizure duration and outcome; augmenting agents (e.g., caffeine) are rarely necessary
- Minimum stimulus energy/charge necessary to induce a convulsion is the "threshold stimulus"; a multiple of this "threshold" stimulus is recommended for effective treatment (most accurate estimate of "threshold" is by "titration" technique)
- Bilateral stimulus electrode placement (1.5 times "threshold" stimulus energy/charge) has been found more effective than unilateral placement; "high-energy" bilateral (2.5 times threshold stimulus) may be effective for non-response to 1.5 times "threshold" bilateral treatment
- Unilateral electrode placement is effective for many patients but, when used, the stimulus energy/charge should be substantially greater than the "threshold" stimulus; if no response after 4 to 6 treatments, recommend switch to bilateral (preliminary evidence suggests that unilateral treatment with a multiple of 5 to 6 times the "threshold" stimulus may be as effective as bilateral and cause fewer cognitive side effects)
- Ultrabrief stimulus pulse width may be effective with reduced cognitive side effects
- Gender, age and electrode placement affect seizure threshold: males have higher thresholds than females, thresholds increase with age and are greater with bilateral than unilateral ECT
- Total number of treatments required for a full therapeutic effect may range from approximately 6 to 20; if there is absolutely no therapeutic effect after 12 to 15 treatments, it is unlikely that further treatments will be effective

Onset & Duration of Action

- Therapeutic effect may be evident within three treatments but onset may require as many as 12 treatments in some cases
- Relapse rate following discontinuation is high (30–70%) within 1 year, partly dependent on degree of medication resistance pre-ECT; prophylactic antidepressants should be administered in almost all cases; "continuation" ECT for up to 6 months if antidepressant prophylaxis of rapid relapse ineffective; lithium plus antidepressant may be the most effective medications to decrease relapse of major depression following ECT

Procedure

- Administer three times per week on alternate days; decrease frequency to twice weekly, if possible, to reduce cognitive side effects
- ECT must always be administered under general anesthesia with partial neuromuscular blockade
- Induce light "sleep" anesthesia with sodium thiopental; little clinical advantage seen with newer agents such as propofol (more expensive and almost always results in much briefer convulsions; may also raise the seizure threshold; reserve for patients with post-treatment delirium or severe nausea unresponsive to antinauseants)
- Induce neuromuscular blockade with succinylcholine or a short-acting non-depolarizing agent. Post-ECT myalgia may be due to insufficient relaxation or fasciculations (attenuate the latter if necessary with adjunctive non-depolarizing muscle relaxant (e.g., rocuronium) which necessitates a higher dosage of succinylcholine)
- Pretreat with atropine or glycopyrrolate if excess oral secretions and/or significant bradycardia anticipated (i.e., during "threshold" titration, patient on a β-blocker); post-treat with atropine if bradycardia develops
- Pretreat any concurrent physical illness which may complicate anesthesia (i.e., antihypertensives, gastric acid/motility suppressants, hypoglycemics); special circumstances require anesthesia and/or internal medicine consultation
- If possible, discontinue all psychotropics with anticonvulsant properties (i.e., benzodiazepines, carbamazepine, valproate) during the course of treatment
- Continue all other psychotropics, except MAOIs (see Contraindications), when clinically necessary
- Outpatient treatment can be administered if warranted by the clinical circumstances if there is no medical/anesthesia contraindication and if the patient can comply with the pre- and post-treatment procedural requirements

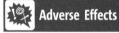 **Adverse Effects**

- Memory loss occurs to some degree during all courses of ECT
  - Significant, patchy amnesia for the period during which ECT is administered; may persist indefinitely
  - Retrograde amnesia for some events up to a number of months pre-ECT; may be permanent; uncommonly, longer periods of retrograde amnesia
  - Patchy anterograde amnesia for 3–6 months post-ECT; no evidence of permanent anterograde amnesia
  - Patients may rarely complain of permanent anterograde memory impairment; unknown if this is a residual effect of the ECT or an effect of residual symptoms of the illness for which ECT was prescribed [liothyronine may protect against memory impairment]

Electroconvulsive Therapy (ECT) (cont.)

- Mortality rate; between two and four deaths per 100,000 treatments; higher risk in those with concurrent cardiovascular disease
- Post-treatment delirium uncommon; usually of short duration
  - Reported in elderly patients; when more than one electric stimulus is used to induce a convulsion; after prolonged seizures
  - Due to concurrent drug toxicity (e.g., lithium carbonate; clozapine – see Drug Interactions p. 76)
  - May occur with too rapid pre-ECT discontinuation of some antidepressants
  - If occurs consider propofol anesthesia for subsequent treatments
- Tachycardia and hypertension may be pronounced; duration several minutes post-treatment
- Bradycardia (to the point of asystole) and hypotension may be pronounced if stimulus is subconvulsive
  - Increased risk if patient on a β-blocker
  - Attenuated by the subsequent convulsion, atropine and medication with anticholinergic effect
- Prolonged seizures and status epilepticus rare; monitor treatment with EEG until convulsion ends; seizures should be terminated after 3 min duration (with anesthetic dosage of the induction agent, repeated if necessary, or with a benzodiazepine – IV diazepam more rapidly effective than lorazepam)
- Spontaneous seizures
  - Incidence of post-ECT epilepsy is approximately that found in the general population
- Headache and muscle pain common but not usually severe
  - Pretreat with rocuronium bromide (approximately 3 mg) for severe muscle pain
- Temporo-mandibular joint pain; may be reduced with bifrontal electrode placement (compared to standard bitemporal placement); hold jaw closed (teeth firmly against bite block) during electric stimulus

⚠ Precautions

- Obtain pretreatment anesthesia and/or internal medicine consultation for all patients with significant pre-existing cardiovascular disease, potential gastro-esophageal reflux, compromised airway, and other circumstances which may complicate the procedure (i.e., personal or family history of significant adverse effects, or delay in recovery from general anesthesia); treat as indicated
- Monitor by ECG, pulse oximetry and blood pressure, before and after ECT; EEG during treatment
- Patients with insulin-dependent diabetes mellitus may have a reduced need for insulin after ECT, as ECT reduces blood glucose levels for several hours (may be related to pretreatment fasting)
- 10–30% of bipolar depressed patients can switch to hypomania or mania following ECT

🛑 Contraindications

Note: all contraindications should be regarded in the context of, and relative to, the risks of withholding ECT
- Rheumatoid arthritis complicated by erosion of the odontoid process
- Recent myocardial infarction
- Increased intracranial pressure
- Recent intracerebral hemorrhage/unstable aneurysm
- Extremely loose teeth which may be aspirated if dislodged
- Threatened retinal detachment
- Other disorders associated with increased anesthetic risk (American Society of Anesthesiologists level 3 or 4)
- Concurrent administration of an irreversible MAOI, which may interact with anesthetic agents (although most reports have implicated meperidine as the interacting drug). Severe impairment in cardiac output and hypotension during ECT may require resuscitation with a pressor agent; the choice may be limited in the presence of an irreversible MAOI. The literature therefore recommends that MAOIs be discontinued 14 days prior to elective anesthesia; if there are compelling reasons to continue the MAOI, or start ECT prior to this waiting period, obtain anesthesia consultation. The potential for a hypertensive response is much less in the presence of a selective, reversible MAOI (RIMA) such that their concurrent administration is acceptable
- Concurrent drug toxicity
- Clozapine (see Drug Interactions p. 76)

Lab Tests/Monitoring	• Assess and document patient's capacity to consent to treatment; answer patient's questions about ECT; obtain signed and witnessed consent form (valid consent requires full disclosure to the patient of the nature of the procedure, all material risks and expected benefit of ECT and those of alternative available treatments, and the prognosis if no treatment is given); if patient incapable, get written consent from eligible substitute
	• Assess memory pre-treatment if there is evidence of significant cognitive impairment; reassess if treatment-emergent loss is unduly severe
	• Physical examination
	• Hb, WBC and differential for all patients over age 60 and when clinically indicated
	• Electrolytes and creatinine for all patients on any diuretic, on lithium, or with insulin-dependent diabetes, and as clinically indicated, including patients with a history of water intoxication
	• ECG for all patients over age 45, those being treated for hypertension, or with a history of cardiac disease and as clinically indicated
	• Chest x-rays for patients with myasthenia gravis and spinal x-rays for those patients with a history of compression fracture or other injury, significant back pain, and as clinically indicated; cervical spine x-rays for all patients with rheumatoid arthritis
	• Sickle cell screening of all patients of African descent; infectious hepatitis screening as clinically indicated
	• Blood glucose on day of each treatment for patients with diabetes mellitus or taking antidiabetic medication
	• Prothrombin time and partial thromboplastin time for all patients on anticoagulants
Pediatric Considerations	• For detailed information on the use of ECT in this population, please see the *Clinical Handbook of Psychotropic Drugs for Children and Adolescents* (2007)
	• May be necessary for childhood or early adolescent onset of severe affective disorder with suicide risk, if antidepressants are ineffective
	• Should never be prescribed without consultation by a specialist in child and adolescent psychiatry
Geriatric Considerations	• No specific risks, benefits, or contraindications attributable to age
	• Concurrent early dementia is not a contraindication; ECT may be administered for any concurrent diagnostic indication
	• Suggestions that response to ECT is more favorable than in younger patients. Evidence on use of ECT in elderly suggests it is safe and effective at reducing symptoms of depression
Use in Pregnancy	• Safe in all trimesters; obtain obstetrical consultation
	• Fetal monitoring recommended
	• Precaution: increased risk of gastro-esophageal reflux
Nursing Implications	• Patients must be kept NPO (especially for solid food) for approximately 8 h before treatment; continuous observation may be required
	• Dentures must be removed before treatment
	• Observe and monitor vital signs until patient is recovered, oriented and alert before discharge from recovery room; patient should be advised not to operate a motor vehicle or potentially dangerous equipment/machinery/tools, until the day after each treatment. Outpatients should be escorted home after treatment
	• When possible avoid prn benzodiazepines the night prior to and the morning of treatment
	• Limit the use of prn sedatives and hypnotics the night before and the morning of treatment
Patient Instructions	• For detailed patient instructions on ECT, see the Patient Information Sheet on p. 334

Electroconvulsive Therapy (ECT) (cont.)

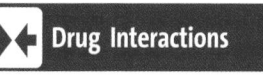 **Drug Interactions**

- Clinically significant interactions are listed below

Class of Drug	Example	Interaction Effects
Anesthetic	Propofol	Decreased seizure duration (may be very substantial); may increase seizure threshold
Anticonvulsant	Carbamazepine, valproate	Increased seizure threshold with potential adverse effects of subconvulsive stimuli; it is possible to over-ride the anticonvulsant effect with a modest increase in energy/charge of electric stimulus
Antidepressant Irreversible MAOI SARI, NDRI, SSRI	Phenelzine Trazodone, bupropion, fluoxetine Trazodone	Possible need for a pressor agent for resuscitation requires that this combination be avoided Prolonged seizures reported; clinical significance unknown. Concurrent administration not contraindicated Rare case reports of cardiovascular complications in patients with and without cardiac disease – more likely to occur at high dosages (i.e., > 300 mg/day)
Antihypertensive	β-blockers, e.g., propranolol	May potentiate bradycardia and hypotension with subconvulsive stimuli Confusion reported with combined use
Antipsychotic	Clozapine	Increased seizure duration reported in 16.6% of patients; spontaneous (tardive) seizures reported following ECT Delirium reported with concurrent, or shortly following clozapine treatment; however, there are many case reports of uncomplicated concurrent use
Benzodiazepine	Lorazepam, diazepam	Increased seizure threshold with potential adverse effects of subconvulsive stimuli or abbreviated seizure
Caffeine		Increased seizure duration Reports of hypertension, tachycardia, and cardiac dysrhythmia
Lithium		Lithium toxicity may occur, perhaps due to an increased permeability of the blood-brain barrier; decrease or discontinue lithium and monitor patient. Concurrent administration not contraindicated if lithium level within the therapeutic range
L-Tryptophan		Increased seizure duration
Theophylline		Increased seizure duration, status epilepticus. Concurrent administration not contraindicated if serum level within the therapeutic range

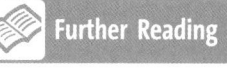 **Further Reading**

- American Psychiatric Association. The practice of electroconvulsive therapy: Recommendations for treatment, training, and privileging. 2nd ed. Washington, DC: APA;2001.
- Dombrovski AY, Mulsant BH. The evidence for electroconvulsive therapy (ECT) in the treatment of severe late-life depression. ECT: The preferred treatment for severe depression in late life. Int Psychogeriatr. 2007;19(1):10–14, 24–35.
- Husain MM, McClintock SM, Rush AJ, et al. The efficacy of acute electroconvulsive therapy in atypical depression. J Clin Psychiatry. 2008;69(3):406–411.
- Kellner CH, Knapp RG, Petrides G, et al. Continuation electroconvulsive therapy vs pharmacotherapy for relapse prevention in major depression: A multisite study from the Consortium for Research in Electroconvulsive Therapy (CORE). Arch Gen Psychiatry. 2006 Dec;63(12):1337–1344.
- Navarro V, Gasto C, Torres X, et al. Continuation/Maintenance treatment with nortriptyline vs. combined nortriptyline and ECT in late-life psychotic depression: A two year randomized study. Am J Geriatr Psychiatry. 2008;16(6):498–505.
- Petrides G, Fink M, Husain MM, et al. ECT remission rates in psychotic versus nonpsychotic depressed patients: A report from CORE. J ECT 2001;17:244–253.
- Sackeim HA, Prudic J, Devanand DP, et al. A prospective randomized, double-blind comparison of bilateral and right unilateral electroconvulsive therapy at different stimulus intensities. Arch Gen Psychiatry. 2000;57:425–434.
- Sackeim HA, Prudic J, Devanand DP, et al. Effect of stimulus intensity and electrode placement on the efficacy and cognitive effects of electroconvulsive therapy. N Engl J Med. 1993;328:839–846.
- Sackeim HA, Prudic J, Nobles MS, et al. Effects of pulse width and electrode placement on the efficacy and cognitive effects of electroconvulsive therapy. Brain Stimulat. 2008;1:78–83.
- Taylor S. Electroconvulsive therapy: A review of history, patient selection, technique, and medication management. South Med J. 2007;100(5):494–498.
- Wilkins KM, Ostroff R, Tampi RR. Efficacy of electroconvulsive therapy in the treatment of nondepressed psychiatric illness in elderly patients: A review of the literature. J Geriatr Psychiatry Neurol. 2008;21(1):3–11.

BRIGHT-LIGHT THERAPY (BLT)

 Definition
- Regular daily exposure to ultraviolet-filtered visible light. For standard light boxes, this involves at least 5000 lux-hours (units of illumination per unit time) per day of exposure

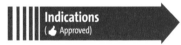 **Indications** (Approved)
- Seasonal affective disorder (SAD)
- Adjunctive therapy for some patients with bulimia nervosa
- Early data suggests possible efficacy in the treatment of premenstrual dysphoric disorder, postpartum depression and some sleep disorders
- Promising for nonseasonal depression, especially if administered in the morning during the first week of treatment, or as an adjunctive treatment
- Shown to be effective alone, or in combination with antidepressant for bipolar depression and chronic depression
- Open trial of BLT in combination with sleep deprivation, added to existing antidepressant and lithium, found useful in treatment-refractory patients
- Open label study concluded that two evenings of bright light exposure (2500-lux white light) induced a phase delay in circadian rhythms of insomniacs with early-morning awakenings
- Open trial suggests BLT during fall/winter may be a beneficial adjunct in adults with ADHD; improvement seen in core pathology, mood symptoms, and circadian shift

General Comments
- Acceptable light boxes must filter out potentially harmful ultraviolet rays
- The wavelength of visible light used is not of great importance
- Because they are used closer to the eyes, light visors produce much lower levels of light than do standard light boxes (which produce 2500–10,000 lux). Brightness appears to be less important for visors than for light boxes
- "Atypical" depressive symptoms such as hypersomnia and craving for carbohydrates are the best predictors of response to BLT
- Symptoms that respond least include: melancholy, psychomotor retardation, suicidality, depersonalization, typical diurnal variation, anxiety, insomnia, loss of appetite and guilt
- Patients with chronic depression and a seasonal worsening respond much less well to light than do patients with a history of full natural remission in the spring/summer months
- Standard antidepressants may enhance the effects of bright-light therapy

Therapeutic Effects
- The therapeutic effect of light is mediated by the eyes and retinas, not the skin. Notwithstanding, patients do not need to glance directly at the light source to experience a therapeutic effect
- The specific mechanism of BLT remains unknown. While light is a potent suppressor of melatonin, this is not the primary mechanism of action in most patients
- The ability of light to phase-advance circadian rhythms may be important in some patients, but does not account for the overall effectiveness of light in SAD
- BLT usually works within several days

 Dosage
- The standard "dose" of light is 5000 lux-hours per day. The most popular method to achieve this is exposure for 30 minutes per day using a 10,000-lux light unit. Morning exposure, shortly after awakening, appears to offer the maximum benefit. Estimating each patient's circadian rhythm phase can optimize timing

 Adverse Effects
- Cumulative exposure to light therapy over 6 years has shown no ocular damage. Notwithstanding, overuse of light may be problematic
- Nausea, headache and nervousness can occur
- Eye irritation (itching, stinging) – gradually disappears with time (may need to sit further from the light source, or initiate exposure gradually)
- Skin irritation – rare
- Hypomania can occur, particularly if light is overused or in patients with bipolar disorder
- Paranoid delusions reported in patients with Alzheimer's disease; case report of induced psychotic episode in 38-year-old female

Bright-Light Therapy (BLT) (cont.)

- Rarely, menstrual disturbances

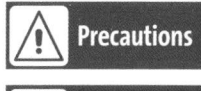 **Precautions**	• Patients with unidentified retinal conditions may be at risk • The effect of bright light on cataracts is unclear. Consult an ophthalmologist if needed for such cases
STOP Contraindications	• Patients with glaucoma, cataracts, retinal detachment or retinopathy • Light therapy is contraindicated in patients taking photosensitizing medications
Use in Pregnancy	• Only one small study of light therapy in pregnancy has been done; while no adverse effects on the pregnancy were found, some caution is required until more data are available
Patient Instructions	• For detailed patient instructions on Bright Light Therapy, see the Patient Information Sheet on p. 335 • Prior to initiating bright-light therapy, verify with your physician and/or pharmacist whether other drugs which you are taking (including over-the-counter and herbal preparations) may interact with the therapy • It is not necessary to glance directly at the light source
Drug Interactions	• Clinically significant interactions are listed below

Class of Drug	Example	Interaction Effects
Acne preparations	Benzoyl peroxide, retinoids (e.g., isotretinoin)	May cause photosensitivity reaction
Antibiotic	Tetracycline, doxycycline	May cause photosensitivity reaction
Antidepressant SSRI/SNRI MAOIs	Fluoxetine, citalopram, paroxetine, sertraline, venlafaxine Tranylcypromine	May augment the effects of bright-light therapy Rarely used in SAD. May augment the effect of bright-light therapy. Standard MAOI precautions needed
Antipsychotic	Chlorpromazine	May cause photosensitivity reaction
Diuretic	Hydrochlorothiazide	May cause photosensitivity reaction
Hypoglycemic	Chlorpropamide	May cause photosensitivity reaction
L-Tryptophan		May augment the effects of bright-light therapy
St. John's Wort		May cause photosensitivity reaction

Further Reading

- Singer EA. Seasonal affective disorder: Autumn onset, winter gloom. Clinician Reviews. 2001;11(11):49–54.
- Tuunainen A, Kripke DF, Ento T. Light therapy for non-seasonal depression. Cochrane Database Syst. Rev. 2004;2:CD004050.

Definition

- rTMS (repetitive transcranial magnetic stimulation) is a procedure which employs magnetic energy to alter cortical neuronal activity. TMS has been approved for the treatment of depression in several countries, including the United States, Canada, Mexico, and Israel; however, because of uncertainties related to the treatment parameters including treatment site, pulse frequency, number of treatments, etc., this technology should still be regarded as experimental

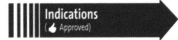

Indications
(♠ Approved)

- ♠ Medication-resistant major depressive disorder (MDD) (reported response rates vary from 18% to 50%; remission rates are much lower at about 10–15% in the RCTs). Left high-frequency or right low-frequency or bilateral (left high- plus right low-frequency) rTMS used
- Several double-blind placebo-controlled studies show benefit of rTMS in refractory major depression
- Small double-blind study suggests rTMS can hasten the response to antidepressants (amitriptyline) in patients with severe MDD
- Small double-blind studies suggest that left low frequency temporoparietal rTMS may reduce auditory hallucinations in schizophrenia; effects on other positive symptoms not established
- Open-label study suggests that maintenance rTMS to the left prefrontal cortex may be a safe and effective treatment for some patients with unipolar depression
- Open trials suggest that some patients with treatment-resistant OCD showed improvement after low frequency rTMS delivered to the supplementary motor cortex
- Double-blind study suggests positive response to high-frequency rTMS in patients with PTSD
- Open trial reports antimanic effects following high-frequency rTMS of the right prefrontal cortex (finding not supported in controlled trial)
- Case reports describe use of very high-frequency rTMS to induce seizures in patients with depression as an alternative to ECT; 5 out of 8 studies reported equivalence between rTMS and ECT, and relapse rates did not differ at 6 months
- Preliminary findings suggest rTMS may be effective and safe treatment alternative for patients with refractory depression and stroke

General Comments

- Response to rTMS varies depending on individual patient pathophysiology, on stimulus frequency and intensity, coil orientation, and brain region treated
- Non-invasive outpatient treatment that does not require anesthesia or sedation
- Labour-intensive procedure as treatment is administered 5 days/week and a course has 10–30 sessions
- The neuronal depolarization and other changes in brain activity can be detected by positron emission tomography (PET) imaging
- Most metaanalyses of rTMS in mood disorders report modest, statistically significant antidepressant effects after 2 weeks of daily treatment of high frequency repetitive left dorsolateral prefrontal cortex stimulation; randomized controlled studies suggest that longer courses of higher-intensity threshold, and greater number of pulses/day may be more effective than 2 weeks of daily rTMS
- Depressive symptoms may continue to decrease following cessation of a course of rTMS treatment
- In 301 medication-refractory MDD patients randomized to receive real or pretend TMS 5 times/week for 4–6 weeks, a response (50% decrease in MADRS scores) occurred after 6 weeks in 24% of patients with real TMS and 12% with pretend treatment ($P < 0.05$). Remission occurred in 14% with real TMS and 6% with sham stimulation. Both results were statistically significant.

Therapeutic Effect

- The therapeutic effect of rTMS remains unknown, however, there is some evidence suggesting rTMS may improve depression by restoring left-to-right balance of cerebral activity
- Some open-label randomized trials found no significant differences between rTMS and ECT in nonpsychotic patients with MDD. In other trials, ECT has been shown to be superior in both psychotic and nonpsychotic patients
- Clinical gains reported to last at least as long as those obtained following ECT
- Robust antidepressant effects reported with combined ECT and rTMS with fewer cognitive adverse effects than ECT alone
- Comparative study of rTMS and fluoxetine 20 mg/day showed similar response in depression in patients with Parkinson's disease, with additional improvement in motor function and cognition with rTMS. Early data suggest that rTMS may slow the development of Parkinson's disease

rTMS (cont.)

Mechanism of Action	• Studies suggest that rTMS may downregulate α-adrenergic receptors, increase dopamine and serotonin levels in the striatum, frontal cortex, and hippocampus, or alter the levels of brain proteins such as brain-derived neurotrophic factor, which can influence neuronal growth; increased pre-frontal cortex metabolism and blood flow has been noted in patients responding to high-frequency rTMS. • Low- and high-frequency rTMS may exert opposite neurophysiological effects. High-frequency pulses (> 1 pulse/s) may increase cortical excitability while low-frequency pulses (< 1 pulse/s) may reduce cortical excitability. These effects have been likened to the processes of "kindling" and "quenching" described in animals • The effects of rTMS appear to depend on the side of the brain treated, e.g., depression may respond to either high-frequency rTMS to the left dorso-lateral prefrontal cortex (DLPFC) or to low-frequency rTMS to the right DLPFC; high-frequency rTMS to the right DLPFC may lessen mania while the same frequency to the left DLPFC may make it worse; low frequency rTMS may increase cortical inhibition
Dosing	• Dose is determined by the stimulus intensity setting (typically 90–120% of the intensity required to elicit a muscle twitch by activating the motor cortex), and total number of stimuli administered (120–1800 pulses) over a single treatment session. When used to treat depression, rTMS is usually administered daily (time period for single treatment is dependent on frequency of pulses [1–20 Hz]) for at least 10 days; some studies recommend up to 30 days of treatment for some patients with depression
Procedure	• A wire coil (encased in insulated plastic) is held over the skull and an electrical current is pulsed through the coil to generate a transient magnetic field of up to 2 Tesla in intensity. Through the principle of Faraday induction a secondary electrical current is generated in cortical neurons lying beneath the coil. Neurons at this site and other sites in the brain may become more or less excitable depending upon whether the magnetic pulses are delivered at high or low frequency. The procedure is usually painless and no anesthetic is required. The patient is awake and alert throughout and there is no post-procedure recovery required • The psychological effects, including those upon mood, depend on the pulse frequency and the region of the brain treated. Mood seems to be most influenced when rTMS is administered over the DLPFC. Pilot studies suggest that the antidepressant effect is greater with more lateral coil placement over the DLPFC • Higher stimulus intensity, and longer courses of rTMS, may lead to greater improvement
Adverse Effects	• Usually very well tolerated; a minority of patients feel pain at the site of stimulation • Over 50% of patients experience muscle tension headache which can continue beyond treatment [analgesics are of benefit] • Some cases of nausea and tremor after rTMS have been reported • Transient increase in auditory thresholds [foam ear plugs during treatment minimize or eliminate this problem] • No deterioration in memory or cognitive performance reported • Case reports of seizures with use of high-frequency rTMS • Case reports of switches to mania in patients with Bipolar I and Bipolar II disorders, when treated with high-frequency rTMS of the left DLPFC; one case report with high frequency treatment of the right DLPFC • Case of psychotic symptoms in patient after 3 sessions • Very rarely transient dysphasia may occur during stimulation (depends on coil placement) • Minimal deficits in short-term memory reported following treatment; some studies report enhanced cognitive functioning
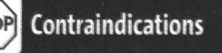 **Contraindications**	• Metallic implants in the head, cardiac pacemaker, personal history of seizures, or history of seizures in first degree relative
Pediatric Considerations	• rTMS has been used in children and adolescents for various diagnoses including ADHD, with and without Tourette's, and depression • One study reports response in 5 of 7 youth with depression treated with rTMS to the left DLPFC • No significant adverse effects or seizures reported

Geriatric Considerations	• rTMS applied to the right DLPFC has been shown to improve motor performance in patients with Parkinson's Disease • Early data suggests response in late-onset vascular depression
Use in Pregnancy	• Case report of successful treatment of female with depression in second trimester
Patient Instructions	• For detailed patient instructions on rTMS, see the Patient Information Sheet on p. 336
Drug Interactions	• Clinically significant interactions are listed below

Class of Drug	Example	Interaction Effects
Anticonvulsant	Valproate, clonazepam Gabapentin	May theoretically reduce the efficacy of high-frequency rTMS; however, this has not been well studied One report suggests that gabapentin may prolong duration of the antidepressant effect of rTMS
Antidepressants	Bupropion	Drugs that lower the seizure threshold may increase the risk of seizure during high-frequency rTMS rTMS has been used successfully combined with various antidepressants including SSRIs, MAOIs and amitriptyline
Antipsychotics	Haloperidol, clozapine	Drugs that lower the seizure threshold may increase the risk of seizure during high-frequency rTMS In one reported case a person seized during high-frequency rTMS after taking amitriptyline in combination with haloperidol; other studies have combined low frequency rTMS with various antipsychotics without adverse effects

 Further Reading

- Bretlau LG, Lunde M, Lindberg L, et al. Repetitive transcranial magnetic stimulation (rTMS) in combination with escitalopram in patients with treatment-resistant major depression: A double-blind, randomised, sham-controlled trial. Pharmacopsychiatry. 2008;41(2):41–47.
- CME Institute of Physicians Postgraduate Press, Inc. Transcranial magnetic stimulation: Potential new treatment for resistant depression. J Clin Psychiatry. 2007;68(2):315–330.
- Dowd SM, Janicak PG. Transcranial magnetic stimulation for major depression Part 1 and 2. Int Drug Ther Newsl. 2006;41(11):83–88, and 2007;42(1):1–8.
- Eranti S, Mogg A, Pluck G, et al. A randomized, controlled trial with 6-month follow-up of repetitive transcranial magnetic stimulation and electroconvulsive therapy for severe depression. Am J Psychiatry. 2007;164(1):73–81.
- Fitzgerald P, Brown TL, Marston NA, et al. Transcranial magnetic stimulation in the treatment of depression: A doubleblind, placebo-controlled trial. Arch Gen Psychiatry. 2003;60(10):1002–1008.
- Garcia-Toro M, Salva J, Daumal J, et al. High (20-Hz) and low (1-Hz) frequency transcranial magnetic stimulation as adjuvant treatment in medication-resistant depression. Psychiatry Res. 2006;146(1):53–57.
- Hasey G. Transcranial magnetic stimulation in the treatment of mood disorders: A review and comparison with electroconvulsive therapy. Can J Psychiatry. 2003;46:720–727.
- Hausmann A, Pascual-Leone A, Kemmler G, et al. No deterioration of cognitive performance in an aggressive unilateral and bilateral antidepressant rTMS add-on trial. J Clin Psychiatry. 2004;65(6):772–782.
- Janicak PG, O'Reardon JP, Sampson SM, et al. Transcranial magnetic stimulation in the treatment of major depressive disorder: A comprehensive summary of safety experience from acute exposure, extended exposure, and during reintroduction treatment. J Clin Psychiatry 2008; 69(2):222–232.
- Kaptsan A, Yaroslavsky Y, Applebaum J, et al. Right prefrontal TMS versus sham treatment of mania: A controlled study. Bipolar Disord. 2003;5(1):36–39.
- Mantovani A, Lisanby SH, Pieraccini F, et al. Repetitive transcranial magnetic stimulation (rTMS) in the treatment of obsessive-compulsive disorder (OCD) and Tourette's syndrome (TS). Int J Neuropsychopharmacol. 2006;9(1):95–100.
- O'Reardon JP, Solvason H, Janicak PG, et al. Efficacy and safety of transcranial magnetic stimulation in the acute treatment of major depression: A multisite randomized controlled trial. Biol Psychiatry. 2007;62(11):1208–1216.
- Paus T, Barrett J. Transcranial magnetic stimulation (TMS) of the human frontal cortex: Implications for repetitive TMS treatment of depression. J Psychiatry Neurosci. 2004;29(4):268–279.
- Quintana H. Transcranial magnetic stimulation in persons younger than the age of 18. J ECT. 2005;21(2):88–95.
- Simons W, Dierick M. Transcranial magnetic stimulation as a therapeutic tool in psychiatry. World J Biol Psychiatry. 2005;6(1):6–25.

ANTIPSYCHOTICS

Classification*

• Antipsychotics can be classified as follows:

Chemical Class	Agent	Page
"Second-Generation" Antipsychotics (SGAs)[A]		See p. 88
Benzisoxazole	Risperidone, paliperidone	
Dibenzodiazepine	Clozapine	
Dibenzothiazepine	Quetiapine	
Thienobenzodiazepine	Olanzapine	
Benzothiazolylpiperazine	Ziprasidone	
"Third-Generation" Antipsychotic (TGA)		
Dihydrocarbostyril	Aripiprazole[C]	See p. 107
"First-Generation" Antipsychotics (FGAs)[B]		See p. 112
Butyrophenone	Haloperidol	
Dibenzoxazepine	Loxapine	
Dihydroindolone	Molindone[C]	
Diphenylbutylpiperidine	Pimozide	
Phenothiazines – aliphatic – piperazine – piperidine	Example: chlorpromazine Example: trifluoperazine Example: pericyazine[D]	
Thioxanthenes	Example: thiothixene	

* This classification system is under review.

[A] Formerly called "atypical," which describes antipsychotics that have a decreased incidence of EPS at therapeutic doses; the boundaries, however, between "typical" and "atypical" antipsychotics are not definitive. "Atypical" antipsychotics (1) may have low affinity for D_2 receptors and are readily displaced by endogenous dopamine in striatum (e.g., clozapine, quetiapine); (2) may have high D_2 blockade and high muscarinic blockade-anticholinergic activity; (3) may block both D_2 and $5\text{-}HT_2$ receptors (e.g., risperidone, clozapine, olanzapine, quetiapine); (4) may have high D_4 blockade (e.g., clozapine, olanzapine, loxapine); (5) may lack a sustained increased prolactin response (e.g., clozapine, quetiapine, olanzapine); (6) show mesolimbic selectivity (e.g., olanzapine, clozapine, quetiapine).

[B] Formerly called "typical". [C] Not marketed in Canada; available through Special Access Program. [D] Not available in USA.

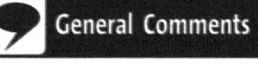

General Comments

• Significant pharmacological characteristics of antipsychotics:
  – Antipsychotic activity
  – Absence of physical or psychic dependence
• All classes have demonstrated efficacy in the treatment of positive symptoms of psychosis including hallucinations and delusions in addition to hostility and aggression
• No antipsychotics have proven (in a clinically significant manner) efficacy to decrease primary negative symptoms of psychosis (i.e., affective flattening, alogia, amotivation, social withdrawal)

- Results of studies comparing the beneficial effects of FGAs vs SGAs on cognitive function have yielded inconsistent results[11]
- Therapy needs to be individually optimized as different antipsychotics are associated with different efficacy and adverse effect profiles
- Accumulating evidence from studies suggests a correlation between early treatment of psychotic disorders with better prognosis. Second and third generation antipsychotics shown (in-vitro studies) to provide neuroprotection in the CNS
- Nonadherence (including partial adherence) to antipsychotic medication is a frequently occurring problem that has been associated with increased rates of relapse, hospitalization, and suicide in individuals with schizophrenia. Adherence is influenced by multiple factors (insight, adverse effects, cost, stigma, homelessness). Nonadherences are difficult to estimate as definitions vary. Some studies[4] have estimated nonadherence to antipsychotics to be 15–35% in inpatients and up to 80% in outpatients with oral medication after 18 months of therapy; with long-acting (depot) agents 10–15% nonadherance within 2 years and 40% within 7 years
- Droperidol is available only as an injectable and is marketed as an adjunct to anesthesia; it is used for sedation/behavior control of acutely psychotic patients; use with caution due to reports of QT prolongation, serious arrhythmias (torsade de pointes) and sudden death. Avoid in individuals at risk for QT prolongation, the elderly and in combination with drugs known to prolong cardiac conduction
- Long-acting (depot) formulations have been proven to improve concordance with medications and reduce consequences of missed doses; depending on the reasons for nonadherence, long-acting antipsychotic formulations may be a viable strategy to reduce relapse rates and progression of illness[6]

 Pharmacology

- See pp. 90, 107, and 114 for specific pharmacological statements
- Exact mechanism of action unknown – primary action has been attributed to D_2 blockade, although "second- and third-generation" compounds have suggested a role for antagonism of a combination of dopamine receptors (e.g., D_3, D_4) and other neurotransmitters (e.g., serotonin, glutamate)
- In contrast to FGAs, SGAs and TGA are reported to facilitate (through various mechanisms) dopamine transmission in the prefrontal cortex and striatum. This may explain the lower incidence of EPS and the potentially beneficial improvement on negative symptoms.
- Receptor specificity varies with different antipsychotics: e.g., clozapine, olanzapine, quetiapine, risperidone and ziprasidone have greater 5-HT_2 blockade than D_2 blockade (see p. 129). The relative lower affinity for the D_2 receptor by these agents appears to be determined by their faster rate of dissociation (i.e., unbinding) from the D_2 receptor (speed is determined by the fat solubility of the antipsychotic). Fast dissociation from the D_2 receptor, allowing it to periodically accommodate endogenous dopamine, has also been postulated as an explanation for how novel agents may be more effective for negative symptoms and less likely to cause EPS
- Recent PET data on long-acting risperidone showed considerable variability of D_2 receptor occupancy in treatment-responsive patients and suggested that sustained D_2 occupancy at or above the accepted threshold (for acute treatment) may not be necessary to maintain response[27]

 Adverse Effects

- The differential percentage of blockade of different receptors, by the antipsychotic, as well as the rate of dissociation from receptors account for many observed adverse effects (e.g., in general, the faster an antipsychotic dissociates from the D_2 receptor, the lesser the risk of EPS and possibly tardive dyskinesia)
- See detailed discussion of adverse effects associated with SGAs (pp. 91–98), TGA (p. 109), FGAs (pp. 116–121) and related charts (pp. 131–132)
- When determining the need for intervention, consideration should be given to: 1) how bothersome the adverse effect is (e.g., is nonadherence a concern?), 2) what (if any) attempts have been tried to resolve the adverse effect and what was the outcome?, 3) the expected duration of treatment with the antipsychotic, 4) the benefits (e.g., therapeutic alliance, better adherence, etc.) vs. risks (relapse, added cost, etc.) associated with any potential interventions. Potential interventions may include : a) do nothing – wait for tolerance to develop and reassure patient, b) alter the administration schedule as appropriate (e.g., divide up daily dose, give sedating drug at bedtime, etc.), c) lower dose of antipsychotic, d) switch to an alternative antipsychotic, e) add a nonpharmacological or pharmacological agent to treat the adverse effect

 Lab Tests/Monitoring

- Initial evaluation – perform complete medical, substance use, smoking, and family history; obtain results of most recent physical examination including laboratory results and ECG
- Body mass index, waist circumference, and weight at treatment initiation, then monthly for first 3 months, thereafter every 3 months while on a stable antipsychotic dose; a waist circumference, measured at the umbilicus, of 35 inches or more in females and 40 inches or more in males is associated with increased cardiovascular risk. Since weight loss is difficult to achieve, health professionals should focus on prevention
- Monitor patients for the onset of symptoms of diabetes (polydipsia, polyuria, polyphagia with weight loss, etc.) regularly. See also Laboratory Tests below

Antipsychotics (cont.)

- Blood pressure and pulse at baseline and during dosage titration with clozapine, risperidone, quetiapine, chlorpromazine, thioridazine and ziprasidone. Regular BP assessments indicated in individuals with cardiovascular risk factors such as smoking, weight gain, dyslipidemias or diabetes
- ECG: prior to prescribing thioridazine, pimozide, and ziprasidone (to rule out contraindications to use), and periodically during course of therapy. When administering a medication that is associated with QT prolongation, a number of risk factors must be considered (e.g., pre-existing conduction abnormalities, heart disease (especially heart failure or recent MI), familial history of early sudden cardiac death, congenital long QT syndrome, electrolyte disturbances, concomitant treatment with medications associated with QT prolongation, etc.) – refer to individual product monographs for specific contraindications[9]
- Evaluate vital signs prior to IM olanzapine administration and monitor for oversedation and cardiorespiratory depression especially if benzodiazepines are co-prescribed. Use caution if benzodiazepine combined with clozapine (see Interactions p. 100)
- EEG: if seizures or myoclonus occurs
- Symptoms related to prolactin elevation (decreased libido, erectile or ejaculatory dysfunction, menstrual changes, galactorrhea) monthly for 3 months after starting an antipsychotic, then yearly. Order prolactin level if symptomatic
- Evaluate patients at baseline for EPS, TD, and other abnormal involuntary movements. Reassess at regular intervals

Laboratory Tests

- Laboratory tests are indicated as follows:
  - Fasting blood glucose (including HbA1c), at baseline, 3 months after initiation or change of the antipsychotic, and annually thereafter (recommended every 3–6 months in patients with obesity, a family history of diabetes, who gain > 5% of their body weight while on medication or experience a rapid increase in waist circumference)
  - Fasting lipid profile at baseline, after 3 months and at least every 2 years (more frequently if LDL exceeds target or if other cardiovascular risk factors are present)
  - Electrolytes, renal function tests, liver function tests, and thyroid function tests at baseline and as clinically indicated
  - CBC at baseline and as clinically indicated
  - Monitor white blood cell count and CPK with fever, rigidity and diaphoresis/autonomic instability (rule out neuroleptic malignant syndrome)
  - Liver function tests if pruritus or signs of jaundice occur
  - Prolactin level if symptomatic (see Patient Monitoring, above)
- ☞ **Clozapine monitoring:**
  - Normal WBC* and differential count required at baseline prior to commencing clozapine treatment. (WBC $\geq 3.5 \times 10^9$/L and ANC** $\geq 2 \times 10^9$/L)
  - Monitor WBC and differential/ANC weekly for the first 26 weeks of treatment; then
  - If WBC $\geq 3.5 \times 10^9$/L and ANC $\geq 2 \times 10^9$/L during first 26 weeks, monitor WBC and differential/ANC every 2 weeks for the next 26 weeks; then
  - If WBC $\geq 3.5 \times 10^9$/L and ANC $\geq 2 \times 10^9$/L during next 26 weeks, monitor WBC and differential/ANC every 4 weeks thereafter
  - Important considerations:
    - If clozapine therapy is stopped for more than 3 days and then restarted, resume weekly hematological monitoring for 6 weeks. If therapy is interrupted for 4 weeks or more, weekly monitoring is required for an additional 26 weeks
    - If at any time WBC 2–3.5×10^9/L or ANC 1.5–2×10^9/L, or patient develops flu-like symptoms, order hematological testing two times per week
    - If at any time, WBC $< 2.0 \times 10^9$/L or ANC $< 1.5 \times 10^9$/L, stop clozapine treatment immediately and monitor patient closely
    - If at any time, WBC $< 1 \times 10^9$/L or ANC $< 0.5 \times 10^9$/L, stop clozapine treatment, consult hematologist, place in protective isolation and monitor closely for signs of infection
    - After discontinuation of clozapine, weekly hematological monitoring must be performed for 4 weeks

* WBC = white blood count

** ANC = absolute neutrophil count

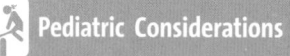 **Pediatric Considerations**

- For detailed information on the use of antipsychotics in this population, please see the *Clinical Handbook of Psychotropic Drugs for Children and Adolescents* (2007)
- SGAs are often preferred in children and adolescents, though few comparative studies available. Likely due to a perceived more tolerable adverse effect profile re EPS and TD. FGAs, like loxapine, are sometimes used on a PRN or short-term basis for hostility or aggression or in those who do not respond or cannot tolerate SGAs[14]

- Antipsychotics may have a number of off-label uses in this population, including psychosis, mood disorders, aggression, agitation, pervasive developmental disorders (e.g., autism), conduct disorder, intermittent explosive disorder, tic disorders; they are often utilized to reduce target symptoms of aggression, temper tantrums, psychomotor excitement, stereotypies, and severe hyperactivity
- Children and adolescents appear to be more sensitive to the effects of antipsychotics; initiate treatment with low doses and increase slowly; reassess dose and need for continued use regularly; monitor closely for adverse effects and potentially developing TD

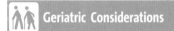 **Geriatric Considerations**

- There are a number of confounders which may alter the response to antipsychotic medication in the elderly and influence how these medications are employed and monitored:
- Pharmacokinetic and pharmacodynamic alterations associated with aging (decreased cardiac output, renal and hepatic blood flow, GFR, lean body mass, and hepatic metabolism – e.g., CYP3A4, etc.) may contribute to a marked sensitivity to the effects of antipsychotics
- Higher incidence of comorbid medical conditions often translates into use of multiple medications, thereby increasing the potential for adverse drug reactions, drug interactions, and adherence issues
- Age-related sensory deficits and cognitive impairment may also adversely impact adherence
- As a general rule, start with lower doses (e.g., 1/4–1/2 usual starting dose, and divide doses where possible) and titrate gradually. Assess tolerability following each dosage increase[3]
- Frequently reported adverse effects of antipsychotic medications in the elderly include neurological effects, orthostatic hypotension, sedation, and anticholinergic adverse effects[3]
- **Neurological Effects**
  - The elderly are more sensitive to extrapyramidal reactions (akathisia, pseudoparkinsonism), which can be persistent and create difficulties in moving, eating, and sleeping, and contribute to falls. These effects are typically dose-related and are more common with high-potency FGAs. Exercise caution if opting to treat by adding on anticholinergic agents or benzodiazepines, as these agents may exacerbate other conditions (e.g., constipation, memory impairment, falls, etc.)
- The risk of TD is cumulative over 1 (25%), 2 (34%), and 3 years (53%), and is higher with FGAs
- **Orthostatic Hypotension**
  - As most antipsychotics can cause orthostatic hypotension, use caution during dosage titration and when other hypotensive agents are prescribed – may result in falls
- **Sedation**
  - Tends to last longer in the elderly and can impair arousal levels during the day. May lead to confusion, disorientation, delirium, and increase risk of falls. Typically a dose-related effect; more common with low-potency FGAs, clozapine, quetiapine, and olanzapine. Caution when combining with other CNS depressants
- **Anticholinergic Effects**
  - The elderly are more sensitive to anticholinergic effects; can result in physical as well as mental adverse effects (e.g., tachycardia, constipation, dry mouth and eyes, blurry vision, difficulty urinating, impairment in concentration and memory, delirium, etc.). Most common with low-potency FGAs, clozapine, and olanzapine
- **Cognitive Effects**
  - Data contradictory as to cognitive decline secondary to use of antipsychotics for behavior disturbances in patients with Alzheimer's disease[24]
- **Use in Dementia**
  - Individuals with dementia often develop neuropsychiatric symptoms such as agitation, aggression, and delusions over the course of illness. Many of these are challenging to control via nonpharmacological interventions, frequently resulting in the prescription of antipsychotic medication, especially SGAs. In 2005, both the FDA and Health Canada issued advisories concerning a small but significant increase in overall mortality in elderly patients with dementia receiving treatment with SGAs and aripiprazole. "Black box" warnings describing this risk were added to the labeling of these agents. The warnings were based primarily on the results of a meta-analysis of 15 smaller studies comparing various SGAs and aripiprazole vs. placebo in elderly patients with dementia. The increased risk reached statistical significance only when the results were pooled in the meta-analysis, potentially due to the low event rate and small sample sizes in the individual trials. The increased risk was evident early on, as the studies involved patients treated over the course of 8–12 weeks. The number needed to harm was reported as 100 or 1 death per 100 patients treated with SGAs over 10–12 weeks. Deaths were primarily from cardiac-related events and pneumonias. Subsequent studies have suggested a similar risk with FGAs. It is currently unknown if this risk extends beyond the early treatment period. Consider individual's risk-benefit ratio when prescribing these agents in dementia patients. It has been suggested to limit use to situations in which there is significant

Antipsychotics (cont.)

risk of harm to self or others or when symptoms are causing significant distress despite implementation of alternative treatments. Reassess the need for continued treatment regularly[24,29]

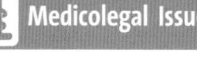 **Medicolegal Issues**

- Antipsychotic therapy has been a source of litigation
- One-on-one medication information sessions, patient and family medication groups, and printed materials can all be used to reinforce and complement psychoeducation
- Keep educating and re-educating patients about their illness and their medication as levels of retention of material are low
- No antipsychotic is perfectly safe. There are pros and cons to every medication. Generally speaking, FGAs are associated with a higher incidence of extrapyramidal adverse effects and tardive dyskinesia, while SGAs may be more likely to result in metabolic-type adverse effects.

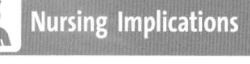 **Nursing Implications**

- Careful observation, data collection, and documentation of patient behavior patterns prior to drug administration, as well as during therapy, are essential nursing measures
- Care is essential in minimizing adverse effects; patients should be educated and reassured about adverse effects to promote positive attitudes toward taking medication; allow patient to ventilate fears about medication. Unrecognized and untreated adverse effects (e.g., akathisia, sexual dysfunction) may play a major role in nonadherence to treatment
- PRN antiparkinsonian agents may be required liberally during first few weeks of treatment with first-generation antipsychotics; patient should take antiparkinsonian agents (e.g., benztropine, procyclidine) only for the extrapyramidal (EPS) adverse effects of antipsychotics; excess use of these agents may precipitate an anticholinergic delirium. Prophylactic antiparkinsonian agents may be required on a temporary basis, by young males, or by individuals with a history of EPS even when prescribed low doses of FGAs
- Blurred vision usually transient; only near vision affected; if severe, pilocarpine eye drops may be prescribed
- A gain in weight may occur in some patients receiving antipsychotics (especially second-generation agents); proper diet, exercise and avoidance of calorie-laden beverages is important; monitor weight, waist circumference, and body mass index during course of treatment
- Monitor patient's intake and output; urinary retention can occur, especially in the elderly; bethanechol (Urecholine) can reverse this
- Anticholinergics reduce peristalsis and decrease intestinal secretions leading to constipation; increasing fluids and bulk (e.g., bran, salads), as well as fruit in the diet is beneficial; increasing exercise may help; if necessary, bulk laxatives (e.g., Metamucil, Prodiem) or a stool softener (e.g., Colace, Surfak) can be used; lactulose is effective in chronic constipation
- Be aware akathisia can be misdiagnosed as anxiety or psychotic agitation and the incorrect treatment prescribed
- Excessive use of caffeine (colas, coffee, tea, chocolate) may worsen anxiety and agitation and counteract the beneficial effects of antipsychotics
- Hold dose and notify physician if patient develops acute dystonia, severe persistent extrapyramidal reactions (longer than a few hours), or has symptoms of jaundice or blood dyscrasias (fever, sore throat, infection, cellulitis, weakness)
- Monitor patients for symptoms that may be associated with QT prolongation (e.g., dizziness, fainting spells, palpitation, nausea and vomiting). Symptomatic patients will require an ECG
- Recommend patient visit family physician yearly for a physical examination, including ophthalmological and neurological examination
- As with all parenteral drug products, injections should be inspected visually for clarity, particulate matter, precipitate, discoloration and leakage prior to administration, whenever solution and container permit. Solution showing haziness, particulate matter, precipitate, discoloration or leakage should not be used
- Store risperidone long-acting injection dose pack in the refrigerator; the powder and solvent should be allowed to come to room temperature prior to reconstitution; it should then be used as soon as possible (see directions in package). Do not combine/mix two different dose strengths of Risperdal Consta. To minimize pain on injection use alternate buttocks as injection sites. Use only supplied teflon-coated needles; use of a higher gauge needles may impede passage of microspheres
- Check patients on depot injections for indurations; Z-track technique is recommended for most depot injections
- "Older" multi-punctured vials of fluphenazine decanoate may contain hydrolyzed ("free") fluphenazine, which can result in higher peak plasma levels within 24 h of injection – monitor for EPS
- Screen for symptoms suggesting obstructive sleep apnea in overweight patients

- Avoid photosensitivity reactions by providing sunscreen agents with UVA protection and suggest protective clothing be worn until response to sun has been determined; patients should wear UVA-protective sunglasses in bright sunlight
- Patients should avoid exposure to extreme heat and humidity as antipsychotics affect the body's ability to regulate temperature
- Because antipsychotics can cause sedation, caution patient not to perform activities requiring alertness until response to the drug has been determined
- For agent-specific administration instructions, see pp. 90–91 (SGAs), p. 108 (TGA), p. 115 (FGAs)

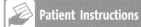 **Patient Instructions**

- For detailed patient instructions on antipsychotics, see the Patient Information Sheets on pp. 337 and 340

Clinical Handbook of Psychotropic Drugs, 18th Edition, © 2009 Hogrefe & Huber Publishers   87   **Antipsychotics**

"Second-Generation" Antipsychotics/SGAs

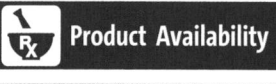
Product Availability

Chemical Class	Generic Name	Trade Name[A]	Dosage Forms and Strengths
Benzisoxazole	Risperidone	Risperdal	Tablets: 0.25 mg, 0.5 mg, 1 mg, 2 mg, 3 mg, 4 mg, 5 mg[C] Oral solution: 1 mg/ml
		Risperdal M-tab	Oral disintegrating tablets: 0.5 mg, 1 mg, 2 mg, 3 mg, 4 mg
		Risperdal Consta	Long-acting injection: 12.5 mg/vial, 25 mg/vial, 37.5 mg/vial, 50 mg/vial
	Paliperidone	Invega	Tablets (extended-release): 3 mg, 6 mg, 9 mg, 12 mg[B]
Dibenzodiazepine	Clozapine	Clozaril FazaClo ODT[B]	Tablets: 12.5 mg[B], 25 mg, 50 mg, 100 mg, 200 mg Oral disintegrating tablets[B]: 12.5 mg, 25 mg, 50 mg, 100 mg
Thienobenzodiazepine	Olanzapine	Zyprexa Zyprexa Zydis Zyprexa Intramuscular	Tablets: 2.5 mg, 5 mg, 7.5 mg, 10 mg, 15 mg, 20 mg Oral disintegrating tablets: 5 mg, 10 mg, 15 mg, 20 mg Short-acting injection: 10 mg/vial
Dibenzothiazepine	Quetiapine	Seroquel Seroquel XR	Tablets: 25 mg, 50 mg[B], 100 mg, 200 mg, 300 mg, 400 mg[B] Tablets (extended-release): 50 mg, 200 mg, 300 mg, 400 mg
Benzothiazolylpiperazine	Ziprasidone	Geodon[B], Seldox[C]	Capsules (ziprasidone hydrochloride): 20 mg, 40 mg, 60 mg, 80 mg Oral suspension (ziprasidone hydrochloride)[B]: 10 mg/ml Short-acting injection (ziprasidone mesylate)[B]: 20 mg/ml

[A] Generic preparations may be available, [B] Not marketed in Canada, [C] Not marketed in USA

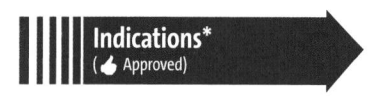
Indications*
(👍 Approved)

Schizophrenia & Psychotic Disorders

- 👍 Acute treatment of schizophrenia and related psychotic disorders (risperidone, olanzapine)
- 👍 Maintenance treatment of schizophrenia and related psychotic disorders (risperidone, olanzapine)
- 👍 Treatment of schizophrenia (paliperidone, quetiapine) and related psychotic disorders (ziprasidone)
- 👍 Treatment-resistant schizophrenia (clozapine)
- 👍 Treatment of schizophrenia in adolescents aged 13–17 years (risperidone – USA)
- 👍 Reducing the risk of recurrent suicidal behavior in patients with schizophrenia or schizoaffective disorder who are judged to be at chronic risk for re-experiencing suicidal behaviour (clozapine – USA)
- • Psychosis associated with depression, Parkinson's disease, psychostimulant use
- • Co-therapy with an antidepressant for psychotic symptoms associated with PTSD
- • Delusions of parasitosis (risperidone – anecdotal reports)
- • Treatment of postpartum psychosis

Bipolar

- 👍 Monotherapy for the acute management of manic episodes associated with bipolar I disorder (risperidone)/bipolar disorder (quetiapine)
- 👍 Monotherapy or co-therapy for the acute treatment of manic or mixed episodes in bipolar I disorder (olanzapine)

* = adult population unless otherwise stated

- 💪 Monotherapy or co-therapy with lithium or valproate for the acute treatment of manic or mixed episodes in bipolar I disorder (risperidone – USA, olanzapine – USA)
- 💪 Monotherapy for the acute treatment of manic or mixed episodes in bipolar I disorder in children and adolescents aged 10–17 years (risperidone – USA)
- 💪 Treatment of acute manic or mixed episodes associated with bipolar disorder, with or without psychotic features (ziprasidone – USA)
- 💪 Monotherapy maintenance treatment in bipolar patients with manic or mixed episodes who responded to acute treatment with olanzapine (olanzapine)
- 💪 Treatment of depressive episodes associated with bipolar disorder (Symbyax – USA, quetiapine – USA)
- Refractory and rapid-cycling bipolar disorder (clozapine; early data)

| Dementia |
- 💪 In severe dementia, for the short-term symptomatic management of inappropriate behavior due to aggression and/or psychosis. The risks and benefits in this population should be considered (risperidone)
- Management of Lewy-body dementia, including reducing visual hallucinations refractory to donezepil without worsening motor effects (quetiapine)

| Autistic Disorder |
- 💪 Treatment of irritability, including symptoms of aggression towards others, deliberate self-injuriousness, temper tantrums and quickly changing moods associated with autistic disorder in children and adolescents aged 5–16 years (risperidone – USA)

| Acute Agitation and Delirium |
- 💪 Rapid control of agitation in patients with schizophrenia and related psychotic disorders, and bipolar mania (olanzapine IM)
- 💪 Treatment of acute agitation in schizophrenic patients for rapid control of agitation (ziprasidone IM – USA)
- Treatment of delirium (olanzapine, quetiapine, risperidone; early data – see Cochrane review[16])

| Depression |
- Adjunct therapy for major depressive disorder (olanzapine, quetiapine, risperidone, ziprasidone)
- Monotherapy for major depressive disorder (olanzapine, quetiapine, risperidone, ziprasidone)
- Monotherapy for combined depression and anxiety (low-dose quetiapine, low-dose risperidone)

| Movement Disorders |
- Levodopa-induced dyskinesias (clozapine, early data with ziprasidone)
- Tardive dyskinesia; improved symptoms (clozapine; case reports – olanzapine, risperidone)
- Movement disorders; decreased motor symptoms in disorders such as tremor, dyskinesia and bradykinesia of Parkinson's disease, essential tremor, akinetic disorders, Huntington's chorea, blepharospasm, and Meige syndrome

| Other |
- Augmentation in treatment-resistant obsessive-compulsive disorder (risperidone, olanzapine, quetiapine); occasional reports of worsening of OCD symptoms, usually in individuals with primary psychotic disorders
- Treatment-resistant PTSD; some improvement in flashbacks, hyperarousal, and intrusive symptoms (clozapine, olanzapine, quetiapine, risperidone; early data)
- Management of pervasive developmental disorders (clozapine, quetiapine, risperidone)
- Tic disorders, Tourette's syndrome, and trichotillomania (olanzapine, quetiapine, risperidone, ziprasidone)
- In dual diagnosis individuals, decrease in addictive behaviors (e.g., smoking, alcoholism, drug abuse)
- Reduced withdrawal symptoms from opiates (clozapine, quetiapine)
- Treatment of cocaine dependence (olanzapine, risperidone; limited data – see Cochrane review[1])
- Treatment of anorexia nervosa (olanzapine; early data – see Cochrane review[8])
- Management of borderline personality disorder (olanzapine, quetiapine, risperidone; early data)
- Moderate nausea related to advanced cancer and associated pain (olanzapine; early data)

💬 General Comments
- Comparable efficacy to FGAs in treatment of positive symptoms; may be advantageous over FGAs in treatment of negative and cognitive symptoms of schizophrenia; may also reduce affective symptomatology in schizophrenia, bipolar disorder, and treatment-resistant depression
- Clozapine has consistently demonstrated superiority over other antipsychotic agents and is a treatment of choice for treating resistant schizophrenia[11]

"Second-Generation" Antipsychotics/SGAs (cont.)

- Lower incidence of extrapyramidal side effects, tardive dyskinesia, and (with the exception of risperidone) minimal to no effect on prolactin elevation
- Unwanted metabolic effects may include weight gain, dyslipidemias, glucose intolerance, and diabetes. The risk appears greatest with olanzapine and clozapine. Individuals who develop a number of these conditions may also meet the criteria for metabolic syndrome
- No evidence of switching to mania when used in patients with bipolar depression; do not induce cycling

 Pharmacology

- See p. 83
- There is significant variation in the receptor profiles of the SGAs (see p. 129 for relative affinities). As a class, they are distinguished by (a) greater 5-HT$_2$ versus D$_2$ blockade, (b) fast dissociation from the D$_2$ receptor, and (c) potentially greater affinity for the mesolimbic tract
- In addition, Ziprasidone is a 5-HT$_{1A}$ agonist (implicated in improving cognition and mood), a 5-HT$_{1D}$ antagonist (causing increased serotonin release), and a moderate inhibitor of 5-HT, DA, and NE transporters (i.e., reuptake) (postulated to contribute to efficacy for affective symptoms)

 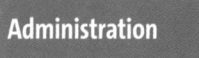 **Dosing**

- See table pp. 133–134 for dosing of individual agents
- In general, lower doses are recommended in the elderly, in children, and in patients with compromised liver or renal function
- Lower doses shown to be effective as augmentation therapy of acute mania
- Initial doses should be lower, and titration slower in patients with mental retardation
- Dosage requirements of clozapine and olanzapine may be higher in smokers due to hepatic enzyme induction by nicotine and polycyclic hydrocarbons
- Prescribing restrictions apply for clozapine – dependent on results of WBC and granulocyte counts (see p. 84 for details): weekly for 26 weeks, then every 2nd week for 26 weeks, monthly thereafter

Administration

Oral

- Paliperidone, olanzapine tablets, quetiapine, risperidone tablets, and risperdone M-tabs may be taken with or without meals
- Ziprasidone should be taken with food. Food increases ziprasidone's bioavailability 2-fold
- AVOID grapefruit juice with clozapine, quetiapine, and ziprasidone (see Drug Interactions pp. 100–106)
- Risperidone solution is compatible with water, coffee, orange juice, and low-fat milk. It is NOT compatible with cola or tea
- Olanzapine Zydis is compatible with water, milk, coffee, orange juice, and apple juice. The mixture should be consumed promptly after mixing
- Risperdone M-tabs and olanzapine zydis disintegrate rapidly in saliva and can be taken with or without liquid
- Risperidone M-tabs and olanzapine zydis break easily. Do NOT push tablet through foil backing as this could damage tablet. Use dry hands to remove tablet and immediately place tablet on tongue
- If half tablets of olanzapine zydis are required, break tablet carefully and wash hands after the procedure. Avoid exposure to powder as dermatitis, eye irritation, and allergic reactions reported. Store broken tablet in tight, light-resistant container (tablet discolors) and use within 7 days
- Paliperidone and quetiapine XR must not be chewed, divided or crushed
- Use liquid (risperidone) or quick-disintegrating tablets (clozapine ODT – USA, olanzapine, risperidone) if patient has difficulty swallowing or is suspected of nonadherence

Short-acting IM

- Olanzapine IM and ziprasidone IM (USA) are powders for reconstitution
- Olanzapine IM is reconstituted using the provided 2.1 ml of sterile water for injection. Use within 1 h of mixing. Inject slowly, deep into the muscle mass
- Concomitant administration of olanzapine IM and parenteral benzodiazepine is NOT RECOMMENDED (see Drug Interactions pp. 100–106)
- Prior to olanzapine IM administration, evaluation of vital signs is recommended. Post-injection monitor for oversedation and cardiorespiratory depression

- Ziprasidone IM (USA) is reconstituted using the provided 1.2 ml of sterile water for injection. Shake vial vigorously until all the drug is dissolved
- Following reconstitution, ziprasidone IM (USA) can be stored, when protected from light, for up to 24 h at 15–30 °C. Since no preservative or bacteriostatic agent is present in this product, any unused portion should be discarded after 24 h
- Ziprasidone IM (USA) may be used with a benzodiazepine. They should NOT be mixed in the same syringe

Long-acting IM

- Risperidone long-acting is a powder for reconstitution; recommended dose pack be allowed to come to room temperature before reconstitution and injection. Reconstitute with diluent provided. Should be used as soon as possible – shelf life is 6 h (nursing administration instructions are provided with the drug); some clinicians recommend a test oral dose of 1–2 mg/day for 2 days if the patient has never taken risperidone
- Shake the preparation vigorously for at least 10 seconds within 2 min before administering; give deep IM into gluteal muscle; rotate sites and specify in charting; only use needles supplied with the kit as use of a higher gauge may impede the passage of microspheres
- DO NOT massage injection site

Pharmacokinetics

- See table pp. 133–134 for kinetics of individual agents

Oral

- Most agents are highly bound to plasma proteins
- Most SGAs are metabolized extensively in the liver; specific agents inhibit cytochrome P-450 metabolizing enzymes (see pp. 133–134)
- Food increases the bioavailability of ziprasidone 2-fold
- Once-daily dosing is appropriate for most drugs because of long elimination half-life; recommended doses of clozapine above 200–300 mg be divided due to seizure risk; manufacturer recommends quetiapine (regular release) and ziprasidone be given twice daily (due to short half-life); despite ziprasidone's short half-life of 6.6 h, PET binding studies show D2 receptor occupancy for 18–24 h and a small double-blind study supports once-daily dosing
- Clozapine exhibits considerable interindividual variability in plasma levels in patients taking similar doses
- Differences in plasma concentration between males and females demonstrated with clozapine (18–50% increase in females) and with olanzapine (30% increase in females)
- Olanzapine and clozapine are eliminated faster in smokers and slower in the elderly
- Studies suggest Asians require lower doses than Caucasians due to pharmacokinetic differences
- Paliperidone is the major active metabolite of risperidone
- Risperidone and metabolite elimination is decreased by 60% in patients with moderate to severe renal disease (See dosing p. 90, pp. 133–134)
- On discontinuation, clozapine and quetiapine are rapidly eliminated from the plasma and brain – may result in rapid re-emergence of symptoms

Disintegrating Tablets

- Supralingual preparations of olanzapine (Zydis) and risperidone (M-Tab) dissolve in saliva within 15 s (can be swallowed with or without liquid) – bioequivalent to oral tablet

Short-acting IM

- Ziprasidone peak plasma level reached within 60 min and is dose-related
- C_{max} occurs in 15–45 min with olanzapine IM compared to 5–8 h with oral form. Half-life for IM and oral forms is similar

Long-acting IM

- See table on p. 139
- Long-acting antipsychotics provide improved bioavailability and more consistent blood levels without the peaks and troughs observed with short-acting oral therapy
- Risperidone long-acting IM is comprised of prolonged-release microspheres. After a single injection, there is a small initial release of drug (< 1%), followed by a lag time of 3 weeks. The main drug release starts from week 3 onward and is maintained from 4–6 weeks. Oral antipsychotic supplementation should be given during the first 3 weeks to maintain therapeutic levels until the main release from the injection site has begun. When administering q 2 weeks, steady-state plasma concentrations are reached after 4 injections and maintained for 4–6 weeks after the last injection. Complete elimination occurs approximately 7–8 weeks after the last injection

Adverse Effects

- See chart on p. 132 for incidence of adverse effects
- Some adverse effects may be preventable by employing simple strategies (e.g., slow upwards titration, dosing a sedating drug at bedtime, etc.)
- Many adverse effects may be transient in nature and require no intervention other than reassurance and follow-up to ensure they resolve

"Second-Generation" Antipsychotics/SGAs (cont.)

- Persistent or bothersome adverse effects typically require intervention. Altering the dosage schedule or dose, adding a nonpharmacological or pharmacological treatment for the adverse effect, or switching to a different antipsychotic may be options to consider
- Certain adverse effects may be more common and/or problematic in females, e.g., weight gain, metabolic syndrome, hyperprolactenemia

CNS Effects

- Activation, insomnia, disturbed sleep, nightmares, vivid dreams – Activation reported with lower doses of ziprasidone, may subside with dosage increase.[25] Insomnia has been reported with clozapine (may be more common following withdrawal), olanzapine, paliperidone, risperidone. Disturbed sleep, nightmares, or vivid dreams occasionally reported for some of these agents (clozapine, olanzapine, quetiapine, risperidone)
- Confusion, disturbed concentration, disorientation (more common with high doses or in the elderly); toxic delirium reported with clozapine. Concomitant anticholinergic agents may exacerbate
- Extrapyramidal – acute onset: A result of antagonism at dopamine D_2 receptors (extrapyramidal reactions correlated with D_2 binding above 80%).
  - Includes acute dystonias, akathisia, pseudoparkinsonism, Pisa syndrome, rabbit syndrome (see p. 142 for onset, symptoms, and treatment options, and pp. 150–157 for detailed treatment options)
  - Extrapyramidal reactions less common with SGAs vs. FGAs (see pp. 142–143 to compare incidence of EPS associated with these agents)
- Extrapyramidal – late onset or tardive movement disorders (TD)
  - Includes tardive akathisia, tardive dyskinesia, and tardive dystonia (see p. 142 for onset, symptoms and therapeutic management options)
  - Late onset movement disorders usually develop after months or years of treatment
  - May be irreversible, so prevention is key – use lowest doses for shortest possible time period and assess for signs of movement disorders regularly. Symptoms are not alleviated and may be exacerbated by antiparkinsonian medications[7]
  - Annual risk of TD with FGAs estimated to be 4–5% with a cumulative risk of up to 50%.[7] Risk of TD lower with SGA and TGA antipsychotics
  - Clozapine has lowest TD risk and has demonstrated a significant reduction in existing TD (especially tardive dystonia), often within 1–4 weeks (sometimes up to 12 weeks)
- Headache – reported with clozapine, olanzapine, paliperidone, quetiapine, and risperidone at an incidence between 5–15% (see product monographs)
- Neuroleptic malignant syndrome (NMS) – rare disorder characterized by autonomic dysfunction (e.g., tachycardia and hypertension), hyperthermia, altered consciousness, and muscle rigidity with an increase in creatine kinase (CK) and myoglobinuria
  - Can occur with any class of antipsychotic agent, at any dose, and at any time (although usually occurs early in the course of treatment). Risk factors may include dehydration, young age, male sex, organic brain syndromes, exhaustion, agitation, and rapid or parenteral antipsychotic administration[7]
  - NMS with clozapine and other SGAs may present with less muscle rigidity, a lower rise in CK and increased autonomic effects; reported incidence with clozapine is 0.2%
  - Potentially fatal (in estimated 5–20%) unless recognized early and medication stopped. Supportive therapy (e.g., maintain hydration, correct electrolyte imbalances, control fever) must be instituted as soon as possible. Additional treatment with dopamine agonists such as dantrolene, amantadine, and bromocriptine may be helpful (controversial – may reduce muscle rigidity without an effect on overall outcome); ECT has also been used successfully to improve symptoms. Treatment with an antipsychotic agent may be recommended several weeks post recovery
  - Case reports of asymptomatic elevation of serum CK with olanzapine; rare cases of rhabdomyolysis with risperidone. Benign elevations of CK also reported with clozapine. Case reports of myalgias (including CK elevations in the absence of NMS) occurring with quetiapine
- Paresthesias – paresthesias or "burning sensations" reported with risperidone
- Sedation, somnolence, and fatigue – common, especially following treatment initiation and dosage increases. Usually transient, but some individuals may complain of persistent effects. May be most bothersome with clozapine and to a lesser extent with quetiapine, and olanzapine.[25] [Management: Prescribe bulk of dose at bedtime; minimize use of concomitant CNS depressants, if possible]
- Seizures – all agents may lower seizure threshold resulting in seizures ranging from myoclonus to grand mal type. May occur if dose increased rapidly or may also be secondary to hyponatremia associated with syndrome of inappropriate antidiuretic hormone secretion (SIADH). Use with caution in patients with a history of seizures. Risk of seizures is greatest with clozapine and is dose-related: 1% (doses below 300 mg), 2.7% (300–599 mg), and 4.4% (above 600 mg); may be preceded by myoclonus (Management: valproate or topiramate in therapeutic doses – recommended as prophylaxis in patients on doses of clozapine over 550 mg daily)

- Stroke – higher incidence of transient ischemic attacks and stroke reported in placebo-controlled trials of elderly patients with dementia treated with risperidone or olanzapine. The relationship, if any, between antipsychotic medication and these events is uncertain[5]

Anticholinergic Effects

- A result of antagonism at muscarinic receptors (ACh)
- More common with clozapine, olanzapine, and quetiapine. See p. 132 for a comparison of the anticholinergic effects of SGAs
- Many of these adverse effects are often dose-related and may also resolve over time without treatment. Treatment options may include reducing the dose of the SGA or switching to another antipsychotic with less potential to cause anticholinergic effects or employing a specific drug or non-drug strategy to treat the adverse effect (see below for suggestions). Many other medications have anticholinergic effects, review patient profiles for their presence and reevaluate the need for their continued use
- Blurred vision [Management: use adequate lighting when reading; pilocarpine 0.5% eye drops]
- Constipation – [Management/prevention: increase dietary fibre and fluid intake, increase exercise, or use a fecal softener (e.g., docusate), or bulk laxative (e.g., Prodiem, Metamucil)] Occasionally associated with olanzapine and quetiapine. Clozapine has been associated with varying degrees of impairment of peristalsis ranging from constipation to intestinal obstruction, fecal impaction, and paralytic ileus (potentially fatal if undetected)
- Delirium – characterized by agitation, confusion, disorientation, visual hallucinations, tachycardia, etc. May result with use of high doses or combination anticholinergic medication. Drugs with high anticholinergic activity have also been associated with slowed cognition and selective impairments of memory and recall
- Dry eyes [Management: artificial tears, wetting solutions]
- Dry mouth/mucous membranes – if severe or persistent, may predispose patient to candida infection [Management: sugar-free gum and candy, oral lubricants (e.g., MoiStir, OraCare D), pilocarpine mouth wash – see p. 39]
- Urinary retention – may be more problematic for older patients especially males with benign prostatic hypertrophy [Management: bethanechol]

Cardiovascular Effects

- Many result from antagonism at α_1-adrenergic and muscarinic receptors
- Arrhythmias and ECG changes:
  - Bradycardia reported with IM olanzapine, often accompanied by decreased resting BP or an orthostatic drop. Caution in patients who have received other medications associated with hypotensive or bradycardic effects
  - ECG changes (e.g., T-wave inversion, ST segment depression, QTc lengthening – may increase risk of arrhythmias) reported with many antipsychotic medications, the clinical significance of which is unclear for many. A QTc of more than 500 ms is associated with an increased risk for torsade de pointes, ventricular fibrillation, and sudden cardiac death. Prominent risk factors for QTc prolongation include congenital long QT syndrome, elderly age, female sex, heart failure, myocardial infarction (MI), and concomitant use of medications that prolong the QT interval (see Drug Interactions pp. 100–106). Other risk factors may include altered nutritional status (e.g., eating disorders, alcoholism), bradycardia, cerebrovascular disease, diabetes, electrolyte imbalances (hypokalemia, hypomagnesemia, hypocalcemia), hypertension, hypothyroidism, and obesity. Clozapine, paliperidone, quetiapine, risperidone, and ziprasidone have been associated with QT interval prolongation.[9] Ziprasidone is contraindicated in patients with prominent risk factors [known history of QT prolongation (including congenital), recent acute MI, uncompensated heart failure, drugs known to prolong QT]. It is recommended to avoid paliperidone in patients with history of cardiac arrhythmia, congenital long QT, drugs that are known to prolong QT. Risperidone, quetiapine, and olanzapine are recommended to be used with caution in cardiovascular disease. Clozapine is contraindicated in severe cardiac disease (e.g., myocarditis)
  - Tachycardia reported with clozapine, olanzapine, quetiapine, risperidone, and ziprasidone. Tachycardia may occur as a compensatory mechanism to orthostatic hypotension caused by α-adrenergic antagonism. Persistent tachycardia at rest accompanied by other signs of heart failure requires cardiology consultation. Tachycardia due to anticholinergic effects in the absence of above conditions may be treated with low-dose peripherally-acting β-blocker[3]
  - Collapse/respiratory/cardiac arrest reported with clozapine alone and in combination with benzodiazepines and other psychotropics
- Cardiomyopathy, pericarditis, myocardial effusion, heart failure, myocardial infarction, mitral valve insufficiency, and myocarditis reported with clozapine. Deaths have been reported. The risk of myocarditis appears greatest in the first month of therapy. DO NOT USE in patients with severe cardiac disease. Investigate patients who develop persistent tachycardia at rest, accompanied by symptoms of heart failure (chest pain, shortness of breath or arrhythmia), and/or fatigue, flu-like symptoms, hypotension, and unexplained fever. Drug should be discontinued and not rechallenged. Rare reports of arrhythmias, myocardial infarction with olanzapine
- Death/dementia – individuals with dementia often develop neuropsychiatric symptoms such as agitation, aggression, and delusions over the course of the illness. Many of these are challenging to control via nonpharmacological interventions, frequently resulting in the prescription of antipsychotic medication, especially SGAs. In 2005, both the FDA and Health Canada issued advisories concerning a small but significant increase

"Second-Generation" Antipsychotics/SGAs (cont.)

in overall mortality in elderly patients with dementia receiving treatment with SGAs and aripiprazole. "Black box" warnings describing this risk were added to the labeling of these agents. The warnings were based primarily on the results of a meta-analysis of 15 smaller studies comparing various SGAs and aripiprazole vs. placebo in elderly patients with dementia. The increased risk reached statistical significance only when the results were pooled in the meta-analysis, potentially due to the low event rate and small sample sizes in the individual trials. The increased risk was evident early on, as the studies involved patients treated over the course of 8–12 weeks. The number needed to harm was reported as 100 or 1 death per 100 patients treated with SGAs over 10–12 weeks. Deaths were primarily related to cardiac-related events and pneumonias. Subsequent studies have suggested a similar risk with FGAs. It is currently unknown if this risk extends beyond the early treatment period. Consider individual's risk-benefit ratio when prescribing these agents in dementia patients. It has been suggested to limit use to situations in which there is significant risk of harm to self or others or when symptoms are causing significant distress despite implementation of alternate treatments. Reassess the need for continued treatment regularly[24]

- Edema – reports of peripheral edema with all SGAs. Tongue and facial edema reported with ziprasidone
- Orthostatic hypotension/compensatory tachycardia/dizziness syncope – may occur as a result of alpha-adrenergic antagonism. Reported with all SGAs. DO NOT USE EPINEPHRINE, as it may further lower the blood pressure (see Drug Interactions). Risperidone, quetiapine or clozapine dosing increases should be gradual to minimize hypotension as well as sinus and reflex tachycardia – may result in falls in the elderly. [Management: rise slowly, divide the daily dose, increase fluid and salt intake, use support hose; treatment with fluid retaining corticosteroid – fludrocortisone]
- Thromboembolism – case reports of pulmonary and/or venous thromboembolism with clozapine, olanzapine, and quetiapine
- Cardiovascular disease (CVD) is the leading cause of death in individuals with schizophrenia. There may be a number of contributing factors to CVD in this population including smoking, sedentary lifestyles, poverty, poor nutrition, reduced access to health care, and a number of metabolic abnormalities including weight gain, dyslipidemias, and glucose intolerance, and hypertension. Please see Endocrine and Metabolic Effects for more details on these effects and their role in CVD

Endocrine & Metabolic Effects

- Antidiuretic hormone dysfunction:
  - Disturbances in antidiuretic hormone function: PIP (polydipsia, intermittent hyponatremia, and psychosis syndrome); prevalence in schizophrenia estimated at 6–20% – can range from mild cognitive deficits to seizures, coma, and death; increased risk in the elderly, smokers, and alcoholics. Monitor sodium levels in chronically treated patients (especially with clozapine) to help identify patients at risk for seizure [Management: fluid restriction, demeclocycline up to 1200 mg/day, captopril 12.5 mg/day, propranolol 30–120 mg/day; replace electrolytes]
- Dyslipidemia:
  - Lipid abnormalities (increases in fasting total cholesterol, LDL cholesterol, and triglycerides) have been associated with certain SGAs. Overall the risk appears greatest with clozapine and olanzapine; moderate with quetiapine; lowest with risperidone and ziprasidone
  - This risk appears to be associated with, but not dependent on, weight gain
  - A 10% increase in cholesterol levels is associated with a 20–30% increase in the overall risk of coronary heart disease. Conversely, lowering cholesterol by 10% decreases the risk by 20–30%[18]
  - See p. 83 for suggested monitoring guidelines
  - Treatment options may include lifestyle and dietary modifications; switching to another antipsychotic associated with a lower potential for lipid dysregulation; add cholersterol lowering medication (e.g., statins, fibrates, salmon oil, etc.)
- Glucose intolerance/insulin resistance/hyperglycemia/type 2 diabetes mellitus (DM):
  - Treatment with SGAs has been associated with an increased risk for insulin resistance, hyperglycemia, and type 2 diabetes (new onset, exacerbation of existing DM, ketoacidosis). A diagnosis of schizophrenia is also a risk factor for developing diabetes
  - Overall the risk of developing disturbances in glucose metabolism appear greatest with clozapine and olanzapine; moderate with quetiapine; lowest with risperidone and ziprasidone[11]
  - Effects tend to occur within 6 months of starting the medication and are often (but not always) associated with substantial weight gain and seem not to be dose dependent
  - See p. 83 for suggested monitoring guidelines
  - Treatment options may include lifestyle and dietary modifications; switching to another antipsychotic associated with a lower potential for glucose dysregulation; adding hypoglycemic agent

- Hyperprolactinemia:
  - Prolactin level may be elevated (related to 50–75% occupancy primarily of peripheral pituitary D_2 receptors) – increases occur several hours after dosing and normalize by 12–24 h with clozapine, olanzapine, quetiapine, and ziprasidone; elevation persists during chronic administration with risperidone (incidence > 30% – less with long-acting IM risperidone) and paliperidone; increased plasma prolactin level related to dose of olanzapine (higher if > 20 mg/day).
  - More common in women than men despite similar doses. Adolescents and children may be at higher risk
  - *Clinical consequences* of elevated prolactin levels may include short-term risks such as galactorrhea, gynecomastia, menstrual irregularities, and sexual dysfunction, and potential long-term risks such as osteoporosis (as a result of decreased bone density secondary to chronic hypogonadism), pituitary tumors, and breast cancer (data conflicting)
  - *Effects in women:* Breast engorgement and lactation (may be more common in women who have previously been pregnant), amenorrhea (with risk of infertility), menstrual irregularities, changes in libido, hirsutism (due to increased testosterone), and possibly osteoporosis (due to decreased estrogen). Recommended that women with hyperprolactinemia or amenorrhea for > 12 months have a bone mineral density evaluation
  - *Effects in men:* Gynecomastia, rarely galactorrhea, decreased libido, and erectile or ejaculatory dysfunction
  - *Monitoring/Investigation:* Recent guidelines suggest routine assessments for the presence of symptoms associated with prolactin elevation. In the event of a positive finding, a prolactin level should be ordered and an attempt made to rule out nonpharmacologic causes.[7,18] The fasting morning serum prolactin level is recommended as it is least variable and best correlated with disease states. In cases where an antipsychotic medication is strongly suspected as the cause, discontinuing the suspected agent (or switching to another antipsychotic agent with less potential for prolactin elevation) for a short period of time (e.g., 3–4 days) if clinically feasible and follow-up monitoring to determine if prolactin levels have fallen, may be a simple means to confirm suspicions and avoid MRI or CT of the hypothalamic/pituitary region[19]
  - *Treatment options:* Assuming discontinuation of antipsychotic therapy is not an option, the preferred treatment is to switch to another antipsychotic agent with a reduced risk of hyperprolactinemia – weighing the potential risk for relapse associated with this action. Other treatment options may include lowering the dose or adding a medication to treat the condition. Use of a dopamine agonist such as bromocriptine (1.25–2.5 mg bid) or cabergoline (0.25–2 mg/week) may be considered but has the potential to exacerbate the underlying illness
- Metabolic syndrome:
  - Metabolic syndrome (also called insulin resistance syndrome, syndrome X, or dysmetabolic syndrome) is an interrelated cluster of cardiovascular disease (CVD) risk factors which include abdominal obesity, dyslipidemia, hypertension, and impaired glucose tolerance. For diagnosis, three of the following five characteristics must be present:
    1. Abdominal Obesity – waist circumference: Men > 102 cm (40 in)/Women > 88 cm (35 in)
    2. Triglycerides: ≥ 1.7 mmol/L (150 mg/dL)
    3. HDL cholesterol: Men < 1.0 mmol/L (40 mg/dL)/Women < 1.3 mmol/L (50 mg/dL)
    4. Blood pressure: ≥ 130/85 mmHg
    5. Fasting glucose: 5.7–7 mmol/L (102–125 mg/dL)
  - Shown to be an important risk factor in the development of type 2 diabetes and CVD. Summary of prospective studies in patients with metabolic syndrome estimates risk of diabetes is 30–52% and risk of CVD is 12–17%; associated with increased risk for coronary artery disease (angina pectoris), myocardial infarction, sudden death, stroke, and congestive heart failure
- Thyroid hormone effects – dose-dependent decrease in total T4 and free T4 concentrations reported with quetiapine; clinical significance unknown
- Weight gain:
  - Reported in up to 50% of patients receiving treatment with antipsychotics. Approximately 50% patients gain an average of 20% of their weight (primarily fat)
  - The mechanism by which antipsychotics may influence weight gain is unknown (may be a result of multiple systems including $5-HT_{1B}$-, $5-HT_{2C}$-, α_1-, and H_1-blockade, prolactinemia, gonadal and adrenal steroid imbalance, and increase in circulating leptin; may also be due to sedation and inactivity, carbohydrate craving, and excessive intake of high-calorie beverages to alleviate drug-induced thirst and dry mouth)
  - Weight gain may contribute to or have deleterious effects on a number of conditions including dyslipidemia, glucose dysregulation and type 2 diabetes, hypertension, coronary artery disease, stroke, osteoarthritis, sleep apnea, and self-image
  - Overall clozapine and olanzapine have been associated with the greatest weight gain potential; quetiapine and risperidone are probably intermediate, ziprasidone is associated with the lowest risk[20]
  - See p. 83 for suggested monitoring guidelines
  - Treatment options: Since it is often challenging to lose weight, preventative strategies which focus on healthy lifestyles (diet and exercise) are recommended. Treatment options may include healthy lifestyle strategies; switching from an antipsychotic with higher weight gain liability to one of lower liability (may result in significant reductions in body weight)[20]; or use of medications to promote weight loss. Treatment with the

"Second-Generation" Antipsychotics/SGAs (cont.)

following agents has been tried with varying degrees of success based on case reports and randomized controlled trials: amantadine (100–300 mg/day), bromocriptine (2.5 mg/day), sibutramine (10 mg/day), famotidine (40 mg/day), topiramate (up to 200 mg/day), nizatidine (300 mg bid), orlistat (120 mg tid)

GI Effects	

- Constipation – see Anticholinergic Effects p. 93
- Dysphagia – dysphagia (difficulty swallowing) and aspiration have been reported with antipsychotic use. Use all agents cautiously in individuals at risk for developing aspiration pneumonia (e.g., advanced Alzheimer's)
- Dry mouth – see Anticholinergic Effects
- GI obstructions – the tablet formulation of paliperidone consists of paliperidone within a nonabsorbable slow-release shell – do not administer to patients with pre-existing severe GI narrowing (e.g., esophageal motility disorders, small bowel inflammatory disease, short gut syndrome, etc.). Clozapine associated with varying degrees of impairment of intestinal peristalsis including bowel obstruction, ischemia, perforation, and aspiration; 102 cases of suspected life-threatening hypomotility disorder reviewed, resulting in mortality rate of 27.5% and considerable morbidity, largely due to bowel resection[21] – see Anticholinergic Effects p. 93
- Parotitis reported with clozapine
- Reflux esophagitis (approximately 11% incidence reported with clozapine)
- Sialorrhea, with difficulty swallowing/gagging which is most profound during sleep; dose related – may lead to aspiration pneumonia – (with clozapine up to 80%). May be due to stimulation of M4 muscarinic or α_2 receptors in salivary glands. [Management: chew sugarless gum, cover pillow with towels, reduce dose. Preliminary evidence suggests benefit with: anticholinergics {amitriptyline (25–100 mg), benztropine (1–4 mg) or trihexyphenidyl (5–15 mg per day)} – caution: additive anticholinergic effects; pirenzepine (25–100 mg); clonidine (0.05–0.4 mg once daily orally or transdermal patch 0.1–0.2 mg applied weekly) – caution: additive hypotension; terazosin (2 mg daily); scopolamine patch (1.5 mg/2.5 cm^2 patch applied every 72 h); atropine "eye" drops (1 drop sublingually 1–2 times a day); ipratropium nasal (given as 2 sprays under the tongue tid)]

Urogenital and Sexual Effects	

- Sexual effects may result from altered dopamine (D_2), serotonergic, ACh, α_1, or H_1 activity; hyperprolactinemia is the main cause of sexual dysfunction in women
- Identify and develop strategies to deal with other co-prescribed medications (e.g., antidepressants especially TCAs and SSRIs, β-blockers, calcium-channel blockers, cimetidine, digoxin diuretics, methyldopa, illicit substances – e.g., cocaine, opioids, etc.) and conditions (e.g., age, alcohol, diabetes, hypertension, smoking, etc.) that may be associated with sexual dysfunction
- Treatment options may include: 1) dosage reduction, 2) waiting 1–3 months to see if tolerance develops, 3) switching antipsychotics, or 4) adding a medication to treat the problem. (See below for treatment suggestions regarding specific types of dysfunction; evidence for their use based primarily on open-label studies and case reports)
- *Anorgasmia* [Management: bethanechol (10 mg tid or 10–25 mg prn before intercourse), neostigmine (7.5–15 mg prn), cyproheptadine (4–16 mg/day), amantadine (100–300 mg/day)]
- *Ejaculation dysfunction* (including inhibition of ejaculation, abnormal ejaculation, retrograde ejaculation – especially risperidone) [Management suggestions for retrograde ejaculation: imipramine (25–50 mg hs), yohimbine (5.4 mg 1–3 × daily, 1–4 h prior to intercourse), or cyproheptadine (4–16 mg/day)]
- *Erectile dysfunction (ED)*, impotence – ED is reported to occur in 23–54% of males on FGAs. The incidence with SGAs is unclear but appears to be lower especially in agents other than risperidone [Management suggestions: bethanechol (10 mg tid or 10–50 mg prn before intercourse), yohimbine (5.4 mg 1–3 × daily, 1–4 h prior to intercourse), sildenafil (25–100 mg prn), amantadine (100–300 mg/day)]
- *Libido* – decreased libido [Management: neostigmine (7.5–15 mg prn) or cyproheptadine (4–16 mg prn) 30 minutes before intercourse]
- Priapism – rare case reports of priapism occurring in patients on all SGAs except paliperidone. As antagonism of α-adrenergic receptors is believed to play a role in this effect, the potential for paliperidone to be associated with priapism cannot be ruled out, as this agent is relatively new to market and the incidence of priapism is rare
- Renal dysfunction – rare reports of interstitial nephritis and acute renal failure with clozapine.

- Urinary incontinence (overflow incontinence); enuresis reported with clozapine (up to 42%); case reports with olanzapine and risperidone [Desmopressin or DDAVP 10 mg nasal spray or 0.2 mg tablets, oxybutynin 5–15 mg, ephedrine 25–150 mg/day, pseudoephedrine 60 mg or tolterodine 1–4 mg/day may be useful.]
- Urinary retention – see Anticholinergic Effects p. 93

Ocular Effects

- Blurred vision/dry eyes: see Anticholingeric Effects p. 93
- Cataracts/lens changes: Development of cataracts reported in association with chronic use of high dose quetiapine in dogs. Lens changes have also been noted (incidence 0.005%) in patients on long-term quetiapine – relationship to medication unknown. Eye examination (e.g., slit lamp exam) recommended at baseline and 6-month intervals thereafter (controversial)
- Esotropia: Case report of esotropia (form of strabismus) with olanzapine
- Palinopsia: Case report of palinopsia with risperidone

Hematological Effects

- Blood dyscrasias, including those affecting erythropoesis, granulopoesis, and thrombopoesis, have been reported with most antipsychotic medications
- Clinically significant hematological abnormalities with antipsychotic medications are, with the exception of clozapine, rare. Accordingly, the development of any blood abnormalities in individuals on antipsychotic medication, especially other than clozapine, should undergo rigorous medical assessment to determine the underlying cause
- Aplastic anemia – reported with risperidone and clozapine
- **Anemia** – reported with clozapine, ziprasidone
- **Eosinophilia** – not typically of clinical significance unless severe. Transient elevations in eosinophil counts without clinical sequalae reported with olanzapine, quetiapine, and ziprasidone. Eosinophilia reported with clozapine frequently between weeks 3 and 5 of treatment; higher incidence in females. Neutropenia can occur concurrently. In most case reports, withdrawal of the drug resulted in normalization of the hematological profile
- **Leukopenia** [defined as WBC $< 4 \times 10^9$/L] and **Neutropenia/Agranulocytosis** [Neutropenia (defined as absolute neutrophil count (ANC) less than 1.5×10^9/L) may be subclassified as mild (ANC = 1–1.5×10^9/L), moderate (ANC = 0.5–1×10^9/L) or severe (also termed agranulocytosis – defined as ANC $< 0.5 \times 10^9$/L or sometimes as ANC $< 0.2 \times 10^9$/L)]
  - Mild neutropenia may be transient (returning to normal without a change in medication/dose), or progressive (continuing to drop, leading to agranulocytosis)
  - Cases of leukopenia and/or neutropenia reported with clozapine, olanzapine, quetiapine, and ziprasidone
  - Transient neutropenia occurring only in the morning (with an afternoon ANC count returning to normal) has been reported with clozapine.
  - Recurrence of previous clozapine-induced neutropenia reported after olanzapine started
  - Agranulocytosis can occur with all antipsychotics but is generally rare (incidence less than 0.1%) except with clozapine (occurs in approximately 1% of patients; 0.38% risk with monitoring). The rate of occurrence is highest in the first 26 weeks of clozapine therapy. Fatalities typically resulting from infections due to compromised immune status have been reported. Patients treated with clozapine must consent to routine hematological monitoring (see p. 84 for guidelines). Risk factors include older age, female gender and certain ethnic groups (i.e., Ashkenazi Jews). Do not use clozapine in patients with myeloproliferative disorders, granulocytopenia or WBC count less than 3.5×10^9/L and/or ANC less than 2×10^9/L. Monitor for, and advise patients to immediately report, any signs of infection or flu-like symptoms (e.g., fever, sore throat, chills, malaise, etc.). Individuals on clozapine may develop transient, benign fever especially during the first few weeks of treatment. Fever due to underlying blood dyscrasia/infection, neuroleptic malignant syndrome or myocarditis must be ruled out. Avoid concomitant use of other medications associated with blood dyscrasias (see Drug Interactions pp. 100–106)
- **Leukocytosis** – 41% risk of transient leukocytosis reported with clozapine. Leukocytosis also reported with ziprasidone
- **Pancytopenia** – case report with quetiapine, hematological profile normalized within 7 days of discontinuing drug
- **Thrombocytopenia** – platelet abnormalities reported infrequently. Case reports of thrombocytopenia with clozapine, olanzapine, risperidone, quetiapine, and ziprasidone; cases of thrombocytosis with clozapine. In most cases, withdrawal of the medication resulted in normalization of platelet counts

Hepatic Effects

- Cholestatic jaundice (reversible if drug stopped). Occurs in less than 0.1% of patients on antipsychotics within first 4 weeks of treatment. Signs include yellow skin, dark urine, pruritus

"Second-Generation" Antipsychotics/SGAs (cont.)

- Hepatomegaly/steatohepatitis – case reports of nonalcoholic steatohepatitis (fatty liver with inflammation, necrosis, and hepatomegaly, with mild to moderate increase in ALT/SGPT and/or AST/SGOT) reported with olanzapine and risperidone; risk factors include weight gain, hyperlipidemia, type 2 diabetes mellitus, and polypharmacy – usually benign but can progress to cirrhosis
- Pancreatitis – reports of pancreatitis with risperidone, olanzapine, quetiapine, and clozapine; generally occurred within first 6 months of therapy (possibly associated with hyperglycemia or hypertriglyceridemia); hyperamylasemia reported with risperidone
- Transaminase elevations – elevations in ALT, AST and/or gamma-GT have been reported with transaminase elevations reported with all SGAs. May be asymptomatic and transient in nature with rare/very rare reports of hepatitis/hepatic failure
- Monitor LFTs at baseline, periodically thereafter, and when clinical signs suggestive of hepatic dysfunction are present

Hypersensitivity Reactions	- Usually appear within the first few months of therapy (but may occur after the drug is discontinued)

- Usually appear within the first few months of therapy (but may occur after the drug is discontinued)
- Photosensitivity and photoallergy reactions including sunburn-like erythematous eruptions which may be accompanied by blistering
- Skin reactions, rashes, rarely abnormal skin pigmentation (risperidone); Rash (5%) and urticaria reported with ziprasidone; potentially dose related; improved with antihistamine/steroid administration and/or discontinuation of ziprasidone in most cases
- Rarely, asthma, laryngeal, angioneurotic or peripheral edema, and anaphylactic reactions occur

Temperature Regulation

- Altered ability of body to regulate response to changes in temperature and humidity; may become hyperthermic or hypothermic; more likely in temperature extremes due to inhibition of the hypothalamic control area
- Transient temperature elevation can occur with clozapine in up to 55% of patients, usually within the first three weeks of treatment and lasting several days; not correlated with dose; older individuals at higher risk; may be accompanied by respiratory and gastrointestinal symptoms, mild creatine kinase elevation, and an elevation in WBC

Other Adverse Effects

- Mild elevations in uric acid (olanzapine)
- Epistaxis (risperidone)
- Rhinitis (risperidone 15%; olanzapine 12%; also with clozapine) – incidence higher with risperidone in children
- Case reports of exacerbation of bulimia nervosa with risperidone and clozapine
- Case report of hyperventilation with quetiapine and olanzapine
- Flu-like symptoms reported with long-acting IM risperidone

D/C Discontinuation Syndrome

- Abrupt discontinuation of an antipsychotic is primarily indicated in situations involving a sudden/severe adverse reaction to a drug (e.g., agranulocytosis with clozapine). Patients may also choose to become nonadherent by stopping their antipsychotic medication abruptly.
- Abrupt discontinuation (or in some cases a large dose reduction) of an antipsychotic may be associated with a number of potential risks including:
  1. Discontinuation syndromes – typically characterized by development of a number of symptoms including nausea, vomiting, diarrhea, diaphoresis, cold sweats, muscles aches and pains, insomnia, anxiety, and confusion. Often the result of cholinergic rebound. Usually appear within days of discontinuation. [Mild cases may only require comfort and reassurance; for more severe symptoms consider restarting the antipsychotic followed by slow taper if possible; or if rebound cholinergic effects present, consider adding an anticholinergic agent short term.]
  2. Psychosis – exacerbation or precipitation of psychosis including a severe, rapid onset or supersensitivity psychosis, most notable with clozapine. Most likely to occur within the first 2–3 weeks of discontinuation or sooner. [Restart antipsychotic.]
  3. Movement disorders – withdrawal dyskinesias noted to appear usually around 2–4 weeks post abrupt withdrawal. [Restart antipsychotic and taper slowly.] Rebound dystonia, parkinsonism, and akathisia also reported to occur usually within days to the first week post discontinuation. [Restart antipsychotic and taper or treat with appropriate anti-EPS medication.]
- Abrupt cessation of a long-acting or depot antipsychotic is of less concern, as plasma concentrations decline slowly (i.e., drug tapers itself)
- Note re: re-initiating clozapine – if restarting clozapine following 2 or more days post last dose, it has been recommended to initiate treatment with 12.5 mg once or twice daily on the first day with potential for more rapid dosage increases thereafter than recommended during initial treatment.
- ☞ **THEREFORE, AFTER PROLONGED USE, THESE MEDICATIONS SHOULD BE WITHDRAWN GRADUALLY.** If switching to another antipsychotic, see pp. 144–145 for specific recommendations.

Precautions

- Use with caution in the elderly, in the presence of cardiovascular disease, chronic respiratory disorder, hypoglycemia, convulsive disorders. Increased mortality reported in elderly patients with dementia mainly due to cardiovascular and infectious causes (deaths increased 220% with quetiapine, 210% with olanzapine, and 50% with risperidine (see Geriatic Considerations p. 85)
- Caution in prescribing to patients with known or suspected hepatic disorder; monitor clinically and measure transaminase level (ALT/SGPT), periodically
- Should be used very cautiously in patients with narrow angle glaucoma or prostatic hypertrophy
- Monitor if QT interval exceeds 420 ms and discontinue drug if patients symptomatic or if QT interval exceeds 500 ms. DO NOT USE ziprasidone or paliperidone in patients with a history of QTc prolongation, recent myocardial infarction or uncompensated heart failure or in combination with drugs known to prolong the QT interval. Patients with hypokalemia or hypomagnesia may also be at risk
- Evaluate clinical status and vital signs prior to IM olanzapine administration and monitor for oversedation and cardiorespiratory depression. DO NOT ADMINISTER together with an IM benzodiazepine (see Interactions p. 100)
- Do not use clozapine in patients with severe cardiac disease; perform a thorough cardiac evaluation prior to starting therapy in all patients
- Cigarette smoking is reported to induce the metabolism and decrease the plasma level of most antipsychotics
- Rapid elimination of clozapine and quetiapine from plasma and brain following abrupt discontinuation may result in early and severe relapse
- Allergic cross-reactivity (rash) between chlorpromazine and clozapine reported
- Quetiapine can be used as a street drug for its sedative and anxiolytic effects – called "quell" or "baby heroin"

Toxicity

- In general, signs and symptoms of toxicity present as exaggerations of known adverse effects
- Mild intoxication may include anticholinergic effects [such as decreased/absent sweating, dry mouth (hypersalivation with clozapine), urinary retention, and tachycardia), sedation, miosis, and orthostatic hypotension
- Major toxicity manifests primarily in the cardiovascular and central nervous systems
- Symptoms of more severe intoxication include coma, seizures, QTc interval prolongation, respiratory arrest, and hypo- or hyperthermia
- Dystonic reactions and other extrapyramidal adverse effects as well as neuroleptic malignant syndrome (NMS) may also occur
- Convulsions appear late, except with clozapine; symptoms may persist as drug elimination may be prolonged following intoxication
- Aspiration pneumonia reported with clozapine at doses above 2,000 mg

Management

- No specific antidotes; provide supportive treatment – establish/maintain airway, ensure adequate oxygenation/ventilation, monitor vital organ functions. Monitor vital signs and ECG for at least 6 h and admit the patient for at least 24 h if significant intoxication apparent. Agents with extended-release technologies such as paliperidone may require longer supervision/monitoring
- Hypotension and circulatory collapse treated with IV fluids and/or sympathomimetic agents. (Caution – use of epinephrine or dopamine or other agents with beta-agonist activity may worsen hypotension in the presence of antipsychotic-induced α blockade; see Drug Interactions pp. 100–106)
- Gastric lavage and/or activated charcoal may be considered, depending on the time elapsed since overdose
- Hemoperfusion/hemodialysis not recommended due to large volumes of distribution and high plasma protein binding profiles of antipsychotics
- Avoid drugs that produce additive QT prolongation (see Drug Interactions pp. 100–106)

Lab Tests/Monitoring

- See p. 83
- Specific guidelines apply to clozapine (p. 84)
- Threshold plasma level suggested for response to clozapine (in the range of 350–550 ng/ml or 1050–1650 nmol/L). Plasma concentration in males is 69% that of females' levels after adjusting for weight. Smokers achieve 82% of plasma concentration of nonsmokers
- Threshold plasma level may be important for response to olanzapine in acutely ill schizophrenic patients (9 ng/ml or 27 nmol/L)
- Recommend clinical status and vital signs be evaluated prior to olanzapine IM administration; monitor for oversedation and cardiorespiratory depression

Use in Pregnancy

- Available data suggest most antipsychotics do not increase the risk of teratogenic effects in humans (risk category C). However, human data for SGAs is limited and ziprasidone has shown possible teratogenic effects in animal studies. The greatest risk of fetal malformations is associated with use during the first trimester.

"Second-Generation" Antipsychotics/SGAs (cont.)

- Early data suggests in utero exposure to SGAs may increase infant birth weight and risk of large size for gestational age. There may be increased weight gain and risk of gestational diabetes (irrespective of the amount of weight gain) in pregnant women taking clozapine, quetiapine or olanzapine during gestation. Some suggest folic acid (4 mg/day) for pregnant women taking SGAs, as they may be at a higher risk of neural tube defects due to inadequate folate intake and obesity.
- Consider the potential for effects on delivery and withdrawal effects in the newborn if used during the third trimester. Third trimester antipsychotic use has been associated with reversible EPS in the newborn.
- Long-term effects on neurodevelopment are largely unknown.
- The benefits of treating the mother's disease may outweigh the unknown risks of SGAs on the fetus. Use lowest effective dose.
- Clozapine is FDA pregnancy risk category B (i.e., limited human data and animal data suggest low risk). However, a case report suggests the concentration of clozapine in the plasma of the fetus exceeds (2-fold) that in the mother and potential adverse effects have had reported (floppy infant syndrome, neonatal seizures, and rare cases of congenital malformations). Monitor WBC of newborn infants if mother on clozapine.
- Animal data suggest olanzapine, quetiapine, and risperidone are not teratogens, but the number of exposures in humans is too low to assess fetal risk. All are risk category C.
- Only animal studies available with paliperidone. As paliperidone is the active metabolite of risperidone, consult risperidone information.
- Ziprasidone is risk category C. However, there is no human data, animal data suggest risk and there is more data with other antipsychotics. Avoid in pregnancy if possible.

Breast Milk

- Antipsychotics have been detected in breast milk. Long-term effects on neurodevelopment are largely unknown. The American Academy of Pediatrics (2001) classifies antipsychotics as drugs "whose effect in the nursing infant is unknown but may be of concern."[2]
- If used while breastfeeding, use lowest effective dose and monitor infant's progress
- In a case report, clozapine concentrations in breast milk exceeded that in the mother's plasma. There are reports of exposed infants developing agranulocytosis, lethargy, and delayed speech acquisition. Suggest those on clozapine do not breastfeed. If the mother does breastfeed, recommend WBC of infant be monitored regularly
- Reports suggest low levels of olanzapine (0.1–1.8% of mother's plasma level) and quetiapine (0.09–6%) pass into breast milk. Case reports with olanzapine of breastfed infants developing diarrhea, sedation, lethargy, sleep disorder, shaking, jaundice, and temporary motor development delay. Case reports of mild neurodevelopmental delay with quetiapine but the infants were also exposed to quetiapine and paroxetine *in utero*
- Low levels of risperidone and its active metabolite (i.e., paliperidone) pass into breast milk (0.84–4.7% of mother's plasma level). Only animal studies available with paliperidone alone
- No human data on ziprasidone during breastfeeding

 Drug Interactions

- Clinically significant interactions are listed below

Class of Drug	Example	Interaction Effects
Acetylcholinesterase inhibitor (central)	Donepezil	May enhance neurotoxicity of antipsychotics, presumably due to a relative acetylcholine/dopamine imbalance (i.e., increased acetylcholine in the presence of dopamine receptor blockade) in the CNS. Case reports of severe EPS (e.g., generalized rigidity, shuffling gait, facial grimacing) in elderly patients within a few days of starting an antipsychotic (risperidone or haloperidol) and an acetylcholinesterase inhibitor (donepezil or tacrine). Symptoms resolved after discontinuing the antipsychotic agent, the acetylcholinesterase inhibitor, or both. Use lowest effective dose of antipsychotic
Adsorbent	Activated charcoal, cholestyramine, attapulgite (kaolin-pectin)	Oral absorption decreased significantly when used simultaneously; give at least 1 h before or 2 h after the antipsychotic

Class of Drug	Example	Interaction Effects
Antiarrhythmic	Amiodarone, Quinidine, Sotalol	With amiodarone and quinidine, increased plasma levels of clozapine (case report with amiodarone) and risperidone likely, due to inhibited metabolism via CYP2D6
		DO NOT COMBINE with paliperidone or ziprasidone. CAUTION with other SGAs. Possible additive prolongation of QT interval and associated life-threatening cardiac arrhythmias. A study suggests ziprasidone causes less QT prolongation than thioridazine but about twice that of quetiapine, risperidone, haloperidol, and olanzapine. Factors which further increase the risk include anorexia, bradycardia, hypokalemia, and hypomagnesemia
Antibiotic Quinolone	Ciprofloxacin, gatifloxacin, levofloxacin, moxifloxacin	With ciprofloxacin, increased clozapine (29–80%) and olanzapine level, due to inhibited metabolism via CYP1A2. Similar interaction likely with norfloxacin. Monitor for increased antipsychotic adverse effects (e.g., sedation, orthostatic hypotension) when starting and antipsychotic efficacy when stopping ciprofloxacin or norfloxacin. Adjust antipsychotic dose as needed
		DO NOT COMBINE with paliperidone or ziprasidone. CAUTION with other SGAs. Possible additive prolongation of QT interval and associated life-threatening cardiac arrhythmias. A study suggests ziprasidone causes less QT prolongation than thioridazine but about twice that of quetiapine, risperidone, haloperidol, and olanzapine. Factors which further increase the risk include anorexia, bradycardia, hypokalemia, and hypomagnesemia. Ciprofloxacin is thought to have less potential for QT prolongation but there are isolated cases of increased QT; also, resistance is high in some areas and ciprofloxacin has limited Gram + coverage in comparison to other quinolones
		CAUTION. Potential to exacerbate psychiatric conditions, as quinolone-induced psychosis has been reported
Macrolide	Erythromycin, clarithromycin	With erythromycin, decreased clearance of clozapine (by 33–54%) and quetiapine (by 52%) due to inhibition of metabolism via CYP3A4. Similar interaction with clarithromycin and telithromycin likely. Change to azithromycin (which does not affect CYP34A) or monitor for increased antipsychotic adverse effects (e.g., sedation, orthostatic hypotension) when starting, and antipsychotic efficacy when stopping clarithromycin/erythromycin/telithromycin. Adjust antipsychotic dose as needed
		DO NOT COMBINE with paliperidone or ziprasidone. CAUTION with other antipsychotics. Possible additive prolongation of QT interval and associated life-threatening cardiac arrhythmias. See above (under quinolones) for further discussion
Anticholinergic	Antiparkinsonian drugs, antidepressants, antihistamines	The concomitant use of two or more drugs that have anticholinergic activity is often clinically appropriate. However, such use increases the risk of anticholinergic adverse effects (e.g., dry mouth, urinary retention, inhibition of sweating, blurred vision, constipation, paralytic ileus, confusion, toxic psychosis). The elderly are particularly vulnerable to these effects – AVOID highly anticholinergic drugs if possible
		Variable effects seen on metabolism, plasma level, and efficacy of antipsychotic
Anticoagulant	Warfarin	Case report of increased INR within 2 weeks of starting quetiapine. Monitor INR at least weekly for 2 weeks when starting, stopping or changing the dose of quetiapine
Anticonvulsant	Carbamazepine	Decreased antipsychotic plasma levels via induction of CYP3A4, CYP1A2, and/or CYP2D6
		Clozapine levels reduced by 50%. AVOID due to potential additive risk for agranulocytosis. Case report of fatal pancytopenia
		Quetiapine C_{max} reduced by 80% and clinically significant carbamazepine level increases have been observed
		Oxcarbazepine is less likely to interact
		Olanzapine levels reduced by 25%. Risperidone reduced by 50%. 9-hydroxyrisperidone (i.e., paliperidone) reduced up to 77% in studies with risperidone. Ziprasidone AUC reduced by 36%. Clinical relevance uncertain. Monitor for antipsychotic response when starting and increased antipsychotic adverse effects when stopping carbamazepine. Adjust antipsychotic dose as needed
	Lamotrigine	Plasma level changes not seen in pharmacokinetic studies, but case reports of clinically significant increased levels of clozapine and risperidone. With concurrent clozapine, monitor blood work as both drugs can depress bone marrow function
	Phenytoin, phenobarbital	Decreased plasma level of antipsychotic due to induction of metabolism; for phenytoin via CYP2C9 and CYP3A4; for phenobarbital primarily via CYP1A2, CYP2C9, and CYP3A4
		With phenytoin, clozapine level decreased by 65–85%; quetiapine clearance increased 5-fold; no data with risperidone or ziprasidine but interaction likely. With phenobarbital, clozapine level decreased by 35%; no data with olanzapine, quetiapine, risperidone or ziprasidine but interaction likely. Changes likely clinically significant. Monitor for antipsychotic response when starting and increased antipsychotic adverse effects when stopping phenytoin or phenobarbital. Adjust antipsychotic dose as needed

"Second-Generation" Antipsychotics/SGAs (cont.)

Class of Drug	Example	Interaction Effects
Anticonvulsant (cont.)	Valproate (divalproex, valproic acid)	Monitor for antipsychotic response and increased antipsychotic adverse effects (e.g., sedation, EPS) when starting, stopping or changing the dose of valproate. Adjust antipsychotic dose as needed
		With clozapine, conflicting information. Both increased and decreased clozapine levels reported. Case report of hepatic encephalopathy. Reports suggest a greater risk of agranulocytosis with concurrent valproate and clozapine than with either alone. Valproate sometimes added to high-dose clozapine to prevent seizures
		With olanzapine, a small study suggests olanzapine levels may decrease by 32–79%. Further study needed to confirm. Incidence of hepatic enzyme elevations may be increased, increasing the risk of hepatic adverse effects. Monitor LFTs q 3–4 months for the first year and q 6 months thereafter
		With quetiapine, case report of severe cervical dystonia with the addition of valproic acid possibly due to increased quetiapine levels
		With risperidone, conflicting information. A single case report of elevated and another of reduced valproate level; two case reports of generalized edema and two cases in children of hyperammonemia. Monitoring of ammonia levels may be warranted if new or increased manic behavior occurs
		With clozapine, olanzapine or risperidone, potential for a high rate of weight gain
Antidepressant		Potential for serotonin syndrome between antidepressant classes that increase serotonin and SGAs. Monitor for symptoms (e.g., myoclonus, tremor). Case reports with clomipiramine and olanzapine; after withdrawal of clozapine in a patient taking clomipramine; with SSRIs and quetiapine, risperidone or ziprasidone; with nefazadone and olanzapine; and with mirtazapine, tramadol and olanzapine
Cyclic	Amitriptyline, clomipramine, maprotiline, trimipramine	DO NOT COMBINE with paliperidone or ziprasidone. CAUTION with other SGAs. Possible additive prolongation of QT interval and associated life-threatening cardiac arrhythmias. A study suggests ziprasidone causes less QT prolongation than thioridazine but about twice that of quetiapine, risperidone, haloperidol, and olanzapine. Factors which further increase the risk include anorexia, bradycardia, hypokalemia, and hypomagnesemia
		Additive sedation, hypotension, and anticholinergic effects
		Case report of increased clomipramine levels and myoclonic jerks followed by seizures with olanzapine possibly due to competitive inhibition for CYP1A2 and/or CYP2D6. Suggest using lowest doses possible if olanzapine and clomipramine used concurrently
		Increased maprotiline levels (up to 60%) with risperidone, possibly due to competitive inhibition of CYP2D6
NDRI	Bupropion	Probable increased plasma levels of risperidone due to competitive inhibition of CYP2D6. Initiate at the lower end of the dosing range
SARI	Nefazodone	Increased plasma levels of clozapine and quetiapine due to inhibited metabolism via CYP3A4. May only be clinically significant when the dose of nefazodone is > 200 mg/day and/or when higher antipsychotic doses are used
SNRI	Venlafaxine	Increased levels of both clozapine and venlafaxine possible due to competitive inhibition of CYP2D6. A study with venlafaxine doses of 150 mg/day or less suggests no clinically significant interaction

Class of Drug	Example	Interaction Effects
SSRI	Citalopram, escitalopram, fluoxetine, fluvoxamine, paroxetine, sertraline	Case report of NMS with fluvoxamine and quetiapine. Monitor for symptoms (e.g., fever, myoclonus, tremor)
		CAUTION with paliperidone and ziprasidone; possible additive prolongation of QT interval and associated life-threatening cardiac arrhythmias. Factors which further increase the risk include anorexia, bradycardia, hypokalemia, and hypomagnesemia
		Increased plasma level of antipsychotic due to inhibition of metabolism of CYP1A2 (potent – fluvoxamine), 2D6 (potent – fluoxetine and paroxetine) and/or 3A4 (fluvoxamine). Monitor for increased antipsychotic adverse effects (e.g., sedation, orthostatic hypotension) when starting and antipsychotic efficacy when stopping SSRI. Adjust antipsychotic dose as needed. Alternatively, consider using a SSRI with no or weak effects on CYPs such as citalopram, escitalopram, and sertraline (at doses of 100 mg/day or less) or use a SSRI that does not affect the specific CYP enzyme which metabolizes the specific SGA
		Clozapine levels: With citalopram, no change to increased. With fluoxetine, 41–76% higher levels plus 38–45% higher norclozapine levels; one fatality reported. With fluvoxamine, 3–11-fold higher levels. With paroxetine, no change to 41% increase plus 45% norclozapine increase. With sertraline, 41% increase plus 45% norclozapine increase; one fatal arrhythmia reported but causality unclear
		Olanzapine levels: With fluoxetine, 15% increase in peak concentration; of little clinical significance. With fluvoxamine, 12–112% increased; cases of increased olanzapine adverse effects
		Risperidone levels: With fluoxetine, *367%* increased levels. With paroxetine *453%* higher; cases of EPS and serotonin syndrome
Irrev. MAOI, RIMA	Tranylcypromine, moclobemide	Additive hypotension
Amylinomimetic	Pramlintide	Pramlintide slows the rate of gastric emptying. Antipsychotics with significant anticholinergic effects can further reduce GI motility. Use drugs with minimal anticholinergic effects at the lowest effective dose
Antidiarrheal	Loperamide	Case report of fatal gastroenteritis with clozapine. Potentially the anticholinergic effects of clozapine added to the antimotility effects of loperamide, leading to toxic megacolon
Antifungal	Ketoconazole, fluconazole, itraconazole, voriconazole	Increased plasma levels of antipsychotics due to inhibition of metabolism via CYP3A4. Increased level/AUC of paliperidone (clinical significance uncertain), quetiapine (level by 335% with ketoconazole), risperidone (level by ~80% with itraconazole), and ziprasidone (AUC by 35–40% with ketoconazole). Consider using fluconazole or voriconazole (less potent inhibitors of CYP3A4 then itraconazole and ketoconazole) or terbinafine. Monitor for increased antipsychotic adverse effects (e.g., sedation, orthostatic hypotension) when starting and antipsychotic efficacy when stopping antifungals. Adjust antipsychotic dose as needed
		CAUTION – possible additive prolongation of QT interval and associated life-threatening cardiac arrhythmias with antipsychotics. Factors which further increase the risk include anorexia, bradycardia, hypokalemia, and hypomagnesemia. Fluconazole has the lowest potential for QT prolongation. One study of the addition of ketoconazole to ziprasidone found no additional QT prolongation
	Terbinafine	Increased plasma level of risperidone possible due to inhibited metabolism via CYP2D6. Consider changing to fluconazole (see above), reducing dose of risperidone or monitoring for an increase in risperidone adverse effects
Antihypertensive	Methyldopa, enalapril, clonidine, guanethidine	Additive hypotensive effect possible
	Lisinopril	Case report of increased plasma level of clozapine
Antiparkinsonian agent	Levodopa, pramipexole, ropinirole	Potential for reduced antiparkinson efficiency. Antipsychotics reduce dopamine while antiparkinson agents increase dopamine in the CNS. If a SGA is necessary, consider using clozapine or quetiapine, which have been reported to be less likely to cause worsening control of movement disorders than other antipsychotics
Antipsychotic combination		Increased risk of EPS and elevated prolactin level with concurrent use of a first-generation antipsychotic (FGA) and a SGA or with concurrent use of two SGAs. Monitor for EPS (e.g., cogwheeling rigidity, unstable gait) and hyperprolactinemia (e.g., galactorrhea)
		CAUTION – possible additive prolongation of QT interval and associated life-threatening cardiac arrhythmias. DO NOT COMBINE with ziprasidone. A study suggests ziprasidone causes less QT prolongation than thioridazine but about twice that of quetiapine, risperidone, haloperidol, and olanzapine. Factors which further increase the risk include anorexia, bradycardia, hypokalemia, and hypomagnesemia

"Second-Generation" Antipsychotics/SGAs (cont.)

Class of Drug	Example	Interaction Effects
Antipsychotic combination (cont.)	Clozapine + risperidone	Isolated case reports suggest increased clozapine and risperidone levels with concurrent use. However, a small study found no effects on levels. Discrepancy potentially due to genetic variability in CYP2D6. Most common adverse effects with concurrent use are EPS, sedation, and hypersalivation. Case report of NMS with combination
	Haloperidol + SGAs	With clozapine, a case of elevated haloperidol levels and a case of NMS
		With olanzapine, a case of extreme parkinsonism potentially due to competitive inhibition of CYP2D6 and/or additive adverse effects
	Paliperidone + risperidone	DO NOT COMBINE. Paliperidone (i.e., 9-hydroxyrisperidone) is the major active metabolite of risperidone, thus no additive benefit of combining but would increase the risk of adverse effects
	Phenothiazines (e.g., chlorpromazine) + SGAs	Possible additive QT prolongation (see above). DO NOT COMBINE with paliperidone or ziprasidone
	Pimozide + SGAs	Possible additive QT prolongation (see above). DO NOT COMBINE with paliperidone or ziprasidone
	Thioridazine + SGAs	Possible additive QT prolongation (see above). DO NOT COMBINE with paliperidone or ziprasidone
		Increased clearance (i.e., decreased plasma levels) of quetiapine by 65%. Possible increased plasma levels of clozapine and risperidone due to inhibition of metabolism via CYP2D6. Increased SGA levels have the potential to further increase the risk of QT prolongation
	Quetiapine + ziprasidone	Case report of increased QTc prolongation possibly due to increased plasma level of either drug as a result of competitive inhibition via CYP3A4
Antitubercular drug	Rifampin, rifabutin, rifapentine	Decreased plasma levels of clozapine (6-fold), quetiapine, risperidone (up to 50%), and 9-hydroxyrisperdine (i.e., paliperidone; 46%) due to induction via CYP3A4 and/or P-glycoprotein with rifampin. Monitor antipsychotic efficacy when starting and antipsychotic adverse effects when stopping rifampin. Suggest monitoring clozapine levels when rifampin therapy is added, changed, or discontinued. Adjust antipsychotic dose as needed
Anxiolytic Benzodiazepines	Clonazepam, diazepam, flurazepam, lorazepam	Increased incidence of dizziness, hypotension, sedation, excessive salivation, and ataxia when combined with clozapine; cases of ECG changes, delirium and cardiovascular or respiratory arrest reported – more likely to occur early in treatment when clozapine added to benzodiazepine regimen (estimated risk 0.36 to 7.7%). Monitor for respiratory depression and hypotension, especially in the first few weeks of therapy and after dose increases
		Concomitant administration of IM olanzapine and parenteral benzodiazepine and/or other drugs with CNS depressant activity has been associated with serious adverse events, including fatalities; thus it is NOT RECOMMENDED. If use of IM olanzapine in combination with parenteral benzodiazepines is considered necessary, careful evaluation of clinical status for excessive sedation and cardiorespiratory depression, and spacing the medications at least 1 h apart is recommended
	Buspirone	Case report of GI bleeding and hyperglycemia with clozapine
Belladonna alkaloid		Additive anticholinergic effects. Because belladonna is typically available as a homeopathic preparation, the clinical significance of the interaction is unknown. Caution is advised
Calcium-channel blocker	Diltiazem, verapamil	Increased plasma level of quetiapine, risperidone (1.8-fold), and 9-hydroxyrisperidone (i.e., paliperidone) with verapamil due to inhibited metabolism via CYP3A4 and/or inhibition of P-glycoprotein

Class of Drug	Example	Interaction Effects
Caffeine	Coffee, tea, cola, guarana or mate containing products	Increased akathisia/agitation Increased plasma levels of clozapine due to competition for metabolism via CYP1A2 More likely to be clinically relevant in those consuming >400 mg of caffeine/day (e.g., >4 cups of caffeinated coffee/day). Variations in caffeine intake should be considered when clozapine concentrations fluctuate Risperidone solution is incompatible with cola or tea (see administration section)
CNS depressant	Alcohol, antihistamines, hypnotics	Increased CNS effects (e.g., sedation, fatigue, impaired cognition). Additive CNS effects and orthostatic hypotension. Alcohol may worsen EPS
Disulfiram		Decreased metabolism and increased plasma level of clozapine
Ginkgo biloba		Potential for increased risperidone levels due to inhibition of metabolism of CYP3A4. Case report of priapism with recent addition of ginkgo to long-standing risperidone
Glucocorticoid	Betamethasone, hydrocortisone, prednisone	Glucocorticoids can induce metabolism via CYP34A. Higher doses of antipsychotics metabolized via CYP3A4 (e.g., quetiapine or ziprasidone) may be needed CAUTION. Potential to exacerbate psychiatric conditions as glucocorticoid-induced psychiatric disorders such as psychosis can occur
Grapefruit		Increased plasma level of quetiapine and ziprasidone possible due to inhibition of metabolism via CYP3A4. Data with clozapine is contradictory but suggests 500 ml or less of grapefruit juice daily may not result in clinical changes Pertinent to avoid or minimize grapefruit and grapefruit juice until more information is available
H₂ antagonist	Cimetidine	Increased plasma levels of clozapine, olanzapine, quetiapine, and risperidone (increased bioavailability by 64%) due to inhibited metabolism via CYP1A2, 2D6, and/or 3A4
	Nizatidine	Higher doses of nizatidine reported to increase plasma level of quetiapine (used in combination with paroxetine) resulting in akathisia, bradykinesia, mild rigidity and bilateral tremor in upper extremities
	Ranitidine	Increased AUC of risperidone (26%) and 9-hydroxyrisperidone (i.e., paliperidone; 20%). May not be clinically significant
Hormone	Oral contraceptive	Estrogen potentiates hyperprolactinemic effect of antipsychotics. Case report of increased plasma level of clozapine with an oral contraceptive (ethinyl estradiol [35 micrograms]/norethindrone [0.5 mg])
Lithium		Important to avoid toxic plasma levels of lithium when it is used concurrently with ziprasidone, since both ziprasidone and toxic lithium levels are associated with QT prolongation Although studies indicate lithium and SGAs can be safely used together, there are rare cases of severe adverse effects; NMS with aripiprazole and olanzapine; diabetic ketoacidosis with clozapine. Potential for increased risk of agranulocytosis and seizures with clozapine. Monitor patients closely, particularly during the first 3 weeks; monitor lithium levels Use the lowest effective doses; consider maintaining lithium in the lower end of the therapeutic range
Metoclopramide		Increased risk of EPS
Modafinil		Case of clozapine toxicity – increased plasma level of clozapine due to inhibited metabolism via CYP2C19
Narcotic	Tramadol	CAUTION. Potential increased risk of seizures with clozapine. Potential for serotonin syndrome; case report with mirtazapine, tramadol, and olanzapine
Protease inhibitor	Ritonavir, indinavir	Increased plasma level of clozapine possible due to inhibition of CYP3A4. AVOID due to potential for clozapine toxicity and additive effects on cardiac conduction Increased plasma level of risperidone reported and associated adverse effects including reversible comatose state. Caution with concurrent use. Monitor for antipsychotic adverse effects (e.g., EPS) when starting and antipsychotic response when stopping a protease inhibitor. Adjust antipsychotic dose as needed Decreased level of olanzapine due to enzyme induction via CYP1A2 or glucuronide conjugation. Peak level reduced by 40% and half-life reduced by 50%. Monitor for antipsychotic response when starting and increased antipsychotic adverse effects when stopping a protease inhibitor. Adjust antipsychotic dose as needed

"Second-Generation" Antipsychotics/SGAs (cont.)

Class of Drug	Example	Interaction Effects
Proton pump inhibitor	Omeprazole	Decreased plasma level of clozapine (by ~40%) likely due to induction of metabolism via CYP1A2 and/or CYP3A4
QT-prolonging agent	Antimalarials (e.g., chloroquine, mefloquine), antiprotozoals (e.g., pentamidine), contrast agents (e.g., gadobutrol), dolasetron, droperidol, methadone, ranolazine, tacrolimus	DO NOT COMBINE with paliperidone or ziprasidine. CAUTION with other SGAs. Possible additive prolongation of QT interval and associated life-threatening cardiac arrhythmias. A study suggests ziprasidone causes less QT prolongation than thioridazine but about twice that of quetiapine, risperidone, haloperidol, and olanzapine. Factors which further increase the risk include anorexia, bradycardia, hypokalemia, and hypomagnesemia
Smoking (tobacco)		Decreased plasma level of clozapine and olanzapine due to induction of metabolism via CYP1A2. Dosage modifications not routinely recommended but smokers may require higher doses for efficacy. Caution when patient stops smoking as level of antipsychotic will increase (case report of serious clozapine toxicity following smoking cessation; serum increases of 72–261% reported); monitor clozapine levels and reduce antipsychotic dose as necessary
Statin	Lovastatin	Case report of prolonged QT_C interval with quetiapine, possibly due to competitive inhibition of CYP3A4
	Simvastatin	Two case reports of rhabdomyolysis with simvastatin plus risperidone. Possibly due to competitive inhibition of CYP3A4
Stimulant	Amphetamine	Antipsychotics can counteract many signs of stimulant toxicity
	Methylphenidate	Case reports of worsening of tardive movement disorder and prolongation or exacerbation of withdrawal dyskinesia following antipsychotic discontinuation
		Antipsychotic agents may impair the stimulatory effect of amphetamines. Concurrent use not recommended. If used, monitor effectiveness of amphetamine therapy when starting, stopping or changing the dose of an antipsychotic
		CAUTION. Potential to exacerbate psychiatric conditions as stimulant-induced psychosis can occur
St. John's Wort		Decreased plasma levels of clozapine and olanzapine possible due to induction of metabolism via CYP1A2. Monitor for antipsychotic response when starting and increased antipsychotic adverse effects when stopping St. John's wort Adjust antipsychotic dose as needed
Sympathomimetic	Epinephrine, norepinephrine	May result in paradoxical fall in blood pressure (due to α-adrenergic block produced by antipsychotics); benefits may outweigh risk in anaphylaxis; phenylephrine is a safe substitute for hypotension

Product Availability

Chemical Class	Generic Name	Trade Name	Dosage Forms and Strengths
Dihydrocarbostyril	Aripiprazole[B]	Abilify	Tablets: 2mg, 5mg, 10 mg, 15 mg, 20 mg, 30 mg Oral solution: 1 mg/ml Injection: 9.75 mg/1.3 ml (7.5 mg/ml)
		Abilify Discmelt	Oral disintegrating tablets: 10 mg, 15 mg, 20 mg, 30 mg

[B] Not available in Canada (available only through Special Access Program)

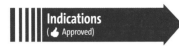 **Indications**
(👍 Approved)

- 👍 Treatment of schizophrenia in adults and adolescents aged 13–17 years (USA)
- 👍 Treatment of acute manic or mixed episodes associated with bipolar I disorder in adults and pediatric patients aged 10–17 years (USA)
- 👍 Adjunctive treatment of major depressive disorder in adults (USA)
- 👍 As an injection for treatment of adults with agitation associated with schizophrenia or bipolar I disorder, manic or mixed (USA)
- Schizoaffective disorder (controlled studies)
- Hostility in schizophrenia and schizoaffective disorder (double-blind studies)
- Psychosis associated with Alzheimer's disease, but potential for increased mortality in the elderly
- Psychosis associated with Parkinson's disease (early data)
- Obsessive-compulsive disorder (early data)
- Decrease in motor and vocal tic frequency in individuals with Tourette's syndrome (early data)
- Reduced craving for cocaine and alcohol in individuals with concurrent schizophrenia (early data)
- Anxiety disorders (early data)

 General Comments

- Decreases both positive and negative symptoms of schizophrenia without producing motor adverse effects
- Comparable efficacy to other antipsychotic agents in the treatment of positive symptoms. May also have potential beneficial effects on cognitive, negative, and affective symptoms
- Appears not to be associated with many of the metabolic adverse effects seen with some SGAs such as weight gain, dyslipidemias, and glucose intolerance/diabetes mellitus
- Not typically sedating; tends to be more activating as the dose increases
- Not typically associated with hyperprolactinemia

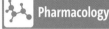 **Pharmacology**

- Aripiprazole has a unique pharmacological profile. It acts as a partial agonist at pre- and post-synaptic D_2 receptors and serotonin (5 HT_{1A}) receptors, and as an antagonist at 5 HT_{2A} receptors
- As a partial dopamine agonist, the intensity of aripiprazole's interaction with the dopamine receptor (intrinsic activity estimated at 25–30%) is less than that of endogenous dopamine (intrinsic activity = 100%). Accordingly, the net effect of dopamine partial agonism depends on whether a hypo- or hyperdopaminergic state exits. In areas of hypodopaminergic activity, partial D_2 agonism results in an increase in overall dopaminergic function (postulated as an explanation for benefit in negative symptoms and affective symptoms, and less EPS). Conversely, in areas of hyperdopaminergic activity, partial D_2 agonism results in a net decrease in dopaminergic function (postulated as explanation for improvement of positive symptoms)
- Partial agonism of the 5 HT_{1A} receptor has been postulated to be associated with anxiolytic action

"Third-Generation" Antipsychotic / TGA (cont.)

- Antagonism of $5\,HT_{2A}$ receptors in the mesocortical tract is believed to enhance dopamine release and thereby alleviate negative symptoms which are postulated to stem from a hypodopaminergic state. $5\,HT_{2A}$ antagonism has also been speculated to produce beneficial effects on anxiety, affective symptoms, and cognition, in addition to negative symptoms
- Partial agonism of D_2 receptors and/or antagonism of $5\,HT_{2A}$ receptors in the tuberinfundibular tract could explain a lack of significant elevations in prolactin level
- Aripiprazole demonstrates low activity at histamine H_1 receptors and sedation is not commonly reported. One of the theories concerning weight gain potential is a combination of antagonism at both H_1 and $5\,HT_{2C}$ receptors (as both olanzapine and clozapine share these affinities). Aripiprazole has low affinity as a partial agonist at the $5\,HT_{2C}$ receptor and is not associated with weight gain

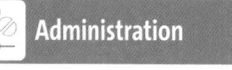 **Dosing**

- See table p. 134 for more information on dosing
- Begin at 10–15 mg once daily; can increase gradually after 2 weeks, up to 30 mg/day (dosing not affected by food); effective dose range: 10–30 mg/day
- Dose adjustment not required in smokers, the elderly or those with renal or hepatic impairment. However, renal and hepatic impairment recommendation is only based on single-dose studies

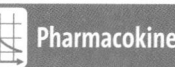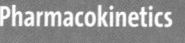 **Administration**

Oral

- Aripiprazole may be taken with or without meals
- AVOID grapefruit juice (see Drug Interactions pp. 110–111)
- Aripiprazole Discmelt disintegrate rapidly in saliva; recommended to be taken without liquid, however, if needed can be taken with liquid
- Aripiprazole Discmelt break easily. Do NOT push the tablet through the foil backing as this could damage the tablet. Use dry hands to remove the tablet and immediately place tablet on the tongue
- Opened bottles of aripiprazole oral solution can be used for up to 6 months after opening, but not beyond the expiration date on the bottle

Short-acting IM

- Aripiprazole IM is a ready-to-use solution for injection. Inject slowly, deep into the muscle mass

Pharmacokinetics

- See p. 134
- Protein binding of parent drug and metabolite is > 99%
- Metabolite dehydroaripiprazole is active, represents 40% of parent drug exposure in plasma, and has similar affinity for D_2 receptors
- The mean half-lives are about 75 h and 94 h for aripiprazole and dehydro-aripiprazole, respectively. Steady-state concentrations are attained within 14 days of dosing for both active moieties
- Metabolized primarily by CYP3A4 and 2D6; Half-life influenced by capacity to metabolize CYP2D6 substrates. In extensive CYP2D6 metabolizers, half-life = 75 h vs. poor metabolizers = 146 h

Oral

- Can be taken with or without food; oral bioavailability is 87%; peak plasma concentration in 3–5 h when taken on an empty stomach, and up to 6 h if taken with meals
- At equivalent doses, the plasma concentrations of aripiprazole from the solution were higher than that from the tablet formulation

Disintegrating Tablets

- Aripiprazole disintegrating tablets (Discmelt) are bioequivalent to oral tablet. Dissolves in saliva within 15 seconds. Recommended to be taken without liquid, but can be given with liquid if needed

Short-acting IM

- Bioavailability of IM aripiprazole slightly greater (100%) vs. oral form (87%). C_{max} occurs in 1–3 h with IM rather than 3–5 h with oral form

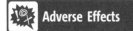 **Adverse Effects**

- See p. 132
- Most adverse effects are dose related

CNS Effects

- Activation – tends to be more activating than sedating; starting at a lower dose or lowering dose my help alleviate this effect
- Commonly reported adverse effects include: headache (> 20%), agitation (> 15%), anxiety (> 25%), insomnia (> 15%), nervousness, lightheadedness, and dizziness (> 10%), somnolence (> 10%), and asthenia. Many of these develop during the first week of treatment and resolve. No dose–response relationship noted, except for somnolence
- EPS – low risk of extrapyramidal adverse effects, though dystonia, akathisia reported; tremor (mostly described as mild intensity, limited duration) reported (> 2%); case report of exacerbation of Parkinson's disease and 2 case reports of rabbit syndrome; reports of tardive dystonia and tardive dyskinesia[22,26]
- Neuroleptic malignant syndrome – a few cases reported with aripiprazole
- Seizures (0.1%) – use cautiously in individuals with a history of seizures, poorly controlled seizures, or medications and/or conditions known to lower the seizure threshold
- Stroke – an increase in cerebrovascular events (i.e., stroke, TIAs) noted in small number of studies of aripiprazole vs. placebo in elderly demented patients; aripiprazole is not recommended for the treatment of dementia-related psychosis

Cardiovascular Effects

- Arrhythmias – no clinically significant increases in QTc interval noted; in some patients QTc interval was shortened.
- Death/dementia – individuals with dementia often develop neuropsychiatric symptoms such as agitation, aggression, and delusions over the course of illness. Many of these are challenging to control via nonpharmacological interventions, frequently resulting in the prescription of anti-psychotic medication, especially SGAs. In 2005 both the FDA and Health Canada issued advisories concerning a small but significant increase in overall mortality in elderly patients with dementia receiving treatment with SGAs and aripiprazole. "Black box" warnings describing this risk were added to the labeling of these agents. The warnings were based primarily on the results of a meta-analysis of 15 smaller studies comparing various SGAs and aripiprazole versus placebo in elderly patients with dementia. The increased risk reached statistical significance only when the results were pooled in the meta-analysis, potentially due to the low event rate and small sample sizes in the individual trials. The increased risk was evident early on, as the studies involved patients treated over the course of 8–12 weeks. The number needed to harm was reported as 100 or 1 death per 100 patients treated with SGAs over 10–12 weeks. Deaths were primarily related to cardiac-related events and pneumonias. It is currently unknown if this risk extends beyond the early treatment period. Consider individual's risk–benefit ratio when prescribing these agents in dementia patients. It has been suggested to limit use to situations in which there is significant risk of harm to self or others or when symptoms are causing significant distress despite implementation of alternate treatments. Reassess the need for continued treatment regularly[24,29]
- Antagonism of α-1-adrenergic receptors may result in postural hypotension, dizziness, and reflex tachycardia
- Orthostatic hypotension reported – more likely to occur during initial dosing or following dosing increases

Endocrine & Metabolic Effects

- Dyslipidemias – risk appears low; monitoring still suggested – see p. 83 for guidelines
- Glucose dysregulation, ketoacidosis, type 2 diabetes mellitus, though association with diabetes is unclear; case reports of hyperglycemia and one report of diabetic ketoacidosis, so monitoring still suggested – see p. 83 for suggested guidelines
- Hyperprolactinemia – appears to have minimal effect on prolactin, although 2 case reports of galactorrhea; assess for signs and symptoms routinely
- Metabolic syndrome – rate and incidence reported in 2 trials to be comparable to placebo[15]
- Weight gain – appears to have minimal effect on weight gain; may be less frequent and/or less significant than with SGAs

GI Effects

- Constipation (> 10%)
- Dysphagia and aspiration reported with antipsychotic use; use all agents cautiously in individuals at risk for developing aspiration pneumonia (e.g., advanced Alzheimer disease).
- Nausea and vomiting (> 10%) seen at start of therapy; higher with increased doses

Urogenital and Sexual Effects

- Priapism – case report of recurrent priapism which started about 6 h following a first dose, successfully treated with intracavernosal phenyleprine and/or cavernal irrigation[17]

"Third-Generation" Antipsychotic / TGA (cont.)

Other Adverse Effects	• Aripiprazole's low affinity for cholinergic M_1 receptors predicts little in the way of anticholinergic adverse effects • Blurred vision (2.5%) • Rhinitis and pharyngitis
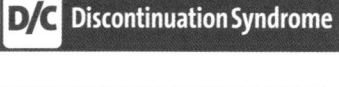 **Discontinuation Syndrome**	• Withdrawal symptoms reported (some studies were in monkeys following abrupt cessation). See p. 98 SGA Abrupt withdrawal/Discontinuation syndromes for a general discussion. Similar to those seen with other classes of antipsychotics
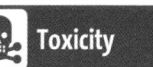 **Precautions**	• Caution in patients with known cardiovascular disease, cerebrovascular disease, seizure disorders or conditions that predispose patients to hypotension or aspiration pneumonia
Toxicity	• Acute ingestions of up to 1080 mg aripiprazole reported with no fatalities • Common adverse effects include emesis, somnolence, and tremor. Other potentially serious effects have been reported in large overdoses including acidosis, electrolyte imbalances, liver function abnormalities, arrhythmias (atrial fibrillation, bradycardia, tachycardia, and QT prolongation), irregular blood pressure, aggression, confusion, loss of consciousness, seizures, coma, and respiratory arrest
Management	• No specific antidote is available. Management relies on close medical supervision and monitoring of vital signs and functions including cardiac function. Supportive therapy to maintain airways and oxygenation and manage symptoms is required. Early administration of charcoal may help in partially preventing absorption. Hemodialysis is not deemed likely to be of benefit due to aripiprazole's high plasma protein binding
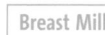 **Use in Pregnancy**	• Aripiprazole is FDA pregnancy risk category C. Animal data suggest a risk of developmental toxicity and possible teratogenicity. Human data limited to two cases; both infants were healthy but one was in fetal distress, including tachycardia, at term. Avoid in pregnancy if possible
Breast Milk	• One case study found a high concentration of aripiprazole in human breast milk (~20% of the maternal plasma level). One case report of failure to lactate post delivery
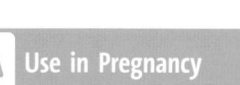 **Drug Interactions**	• Clinically significant interactions are listed below

Class of Drug	Example	Interaction Effects
Acetylcholinesterase inhibitor (central)	Donepezil	May enhance neurotoxicity of antipsychotics presumably due to a relative acetylcholine/dopamine imbalance (i.e., increased acetylcholine in the presence of dopamine receptor blockade) in the CNS. Case reports of severe EPS (e.g., generalized rigidity, shuffling gait, facial grimacing) in elderly patients within a few days of starting an antipsychotic (risperidone or haloperidol) and a acetylcholinesterase inhibitor (donepezil or tacrine). Symptoms resolved after discontinuing the antipsychotic agent, the acetylcholinesterase inhibitor, or both. Use lowest effective dose of antipsychotic
Antiarrhythmic	Quinidine	Increased AUC of aripiprazole by 112% due to decreased metabolism via CYP2D6; AUC of active metabolite decreased by 35%; due to aripiprazole's long half-life, interaction effects may be delayed for up to 10–14 days. Reduce aripiprazole dose by 50%
	Amiodarone, propafenone	Increased plasma level of aripiprazole possible due to inhibited metabolism via CYP2D6
Antibiotic	Clarithromycin, erythromycin	Increased plasma level of aripiprazole due to inhibited metabolism via CYP3A4 likely to occur. Effects may be delayed due to aripiprazole's long half-life. Monitor for aripiprazole adverse effects when antibiotic is added. Adjust aripiprazole dose as needed
Anticonvulsant	Carbamazepine, oxcarbazepine	Decreased plasma level of aripiprazole due to increased metabolism via CYP3A4; C_{max} and AUC of aripiprazole and metabolite decreased by about 70% – doubling the aripiprazole dose may be required
	Valproate (divalproex, valproic acid)	C_{max} and AUC of aripiprazole decreased by 25%; of low clinical significance

Class of Drug	Example	Interaction Effects
Antidepressant SNRI	Venlafaxine	Increased rates of akathisia and fatigue
SSRI	Fluoxetine, paroxetine	Increased plasma level of aripiprazole possible due to inhibited metabolism via CYP2D6 and/or CYP3A4. Case report of NMS with fluoxetine and aripiprazole. Monitor for increased aripiprazole adverse effects when starting and efficacy when stopping a SSRI. Adjust antipsychotic dose as needed. Alternatively, consider using a SSRI with no or weak effects on CYPs such as citalopram, escitalopram, and sertraline (at doses of 100 mg/day or less)
Antifungal	Ketoconazole, itraconazole, fluconazole, voriconazole	Increased plasma levels of aripiprazole due to decreased metabolism via CYP3A4; AUC of aripiprazole and metabolite increased by 63% and 77% with ketoconazole and 48% and 39% with itraconazole, respectively. Reduce the dose of aripiprazole by 50%. Similar interaction may occur with fluconazole and voriconazole
	Terbinafine	Increased plasma level of aripiprazole possible due to inhibited metabolism via CYP2D6
Antiparkinsonian agent	Levodopa, pramipexole, ropinirole	Potential for reduced antiparkinson efficiency. Antipsychotics reduce dopamine while antiparkinson agents increase dopamine in the CNS. If an antipsychotic is necessary, consider using clozapine or quetiapine, which have been reported to be less likely to cause worsening control of movement disorders than other antipsychotics
Cardiac	Ranolazine	DO NOT COMBINE. Increased plasma level of aripiprazole possible due to inhibited metabolism via CYP2D6. Potential additive effects on QT prolongation
CNS depressant	e. g., hypnotics, opioids	Potentiation of CNS effects
Glucocorticoid	Betamethasone, hydrocortisone, prednisone	Glucocorticoids can induce metabolism via CYP3A4. In theory, higher doses of aripiprazole may be needed CAUTION. Potential to exacerbate psychiatric conditions, as glucocorticoid-induced psychiatric disorders such as psychosis can occur
H$_2$ antagonist	Famotidine	Decreased rate (C_{max}) and extent of absorption (AUC) of aripiprazole and its active metabolite; of low clinical significance
	Cimetidine	Increased plasma level of aripiprazole possible due to inhibited metabolism via CYP2D6 and CYP3A4
Lithium		No pharmacokinetic interaction (i.e., drug levels not effected). Increased rates of akathisia and tremor. Case report of NMS
Stimulant	Amphetamine, methylphenidate	Antipsychotics can counteract many signs of stimulant toxicity Antipsychotic agents may impair the stimulatory effect of amphetamines. Concurrent use not recommended. If used, monitor effectiveness of amphetamine therapy when starting, stopping or changing the dose of an antipsychotic CAUTION. Potential to exacerbate psychiatric conditions as stimulant-induced psychosis can occur

"First-Generation" Antipsychotics / FGAs

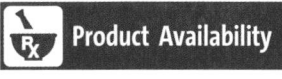 **Product Availability**

Chemical Class	Generic Name	Trade Name[A]	Dosage Forms and Strengths
Butyrophenone	Haloperidol	Haldol	Tablets: 0.5 mg, 1 mg, 2 mg, 5 mg, 10 mg, 20 mg Oral solution[B]: 1 mg/ml Short-acting injection: 5 mg/ml
		Haldol Decanoate	Long-acting injection (depot): 50 mg/ml, 100 mg/ml
Dibenzoxazepine	Loxapine	Loxapac[C], Loxitane[B]	Tablets[C]: 2.5 mg, 5 mg, 10 mg, 25 mg, 50 mg Extended-release Capsules[B]: 5 mg, 10 mg, 25 mg, 50 mg Short-acting injection[C]: 50 mg/ml
Dihydroindolone	Molindone[B]	Moban	Tablets: 5 mg, 10 mg, 25 mg, 50 mg
Diphenylbutylpiperidine	Pimozide	Orap	Tablets: 1 mg[B], 2 mg, 4 mg[C]
Aliphatic phenothiazine	Chlorpromazine	Largactil[C], Thorazine[B]	Tablets: 10 mg[C], 25 mg, 50 mg, 100 mg, 200 mg[B] Oral solution[B]: 30mg/ml, 100 mg/ml Oral syrup[B]: 10 mg/5 ml Short-acting injection: 25 mg/ml
	Methotrimeprazine[C]	Nozinan	Tablets: 2 mg, 5 mg, 25 mg, 50 mg Short-acting injection: 25 mg/ml
Piperazine phenothiazine	Fluphenazine	Moditen[C], Prolixin[B]	Tablets: 1 mg, 2 mg[C], 2.5 mg[B], 5 mg, 10 mg[B] Oral elixir[B]: 2.5 mg/5 ml Oral liquid concentrate[B]: 5 mg/ml Short-acting injection: 2.5 mg/ml[B]
		Modecate[C], Prolixin decanoate[B]	Long-acting injection (depot): 25 mg/ml, 100 mg/ml[C]
	Perphenazine	Trilafon	Tablets: 2 mg, 4 mg, 8 mg, 16 mg Oral liquid concentrate: 16 mg/5ml
	Thioproperazine[C]	Majeptil	Tablets: 10 mg
	Trifluoperazine	Stelazine	Tablets: 1 mg, 2 mg, 5 mg, 10 mg, 20 mg[C] Oral solution: 10 mg/ml
Piperidine phenothiazine	Pericyazine[C]	Neuleptil	Capsules: 5 mg, 10 mg, 20 mg Oral solution: 10 mg/ml
	Pipotiazine[C]	Piportil L4	Long-acting injection (depot): 25 mg/ml, 50 mg/ml
	Thioridazine[B] [D]		Tablets: 10 mg, 15 mg, 25 mg, 50 mg, 100 mg, 150 mg, 200 mg Oral solution: 30 mg/ml, 100 mg/ml

Chemical Class	Generic Name	Trade Name[(A)]	Dosage Forms and Strengths
Thioxanthene	Flupenthixol[(C)]	Fluanxol	Tablets: 0.5 mg, 3 mg
		Fluanxol Depot	Long-acting injection (depot): 20 mg/ml, 100 mg/ml
	Thiothixene	Navane	Capsules: 1 mg[(B)], 2 mg, 5 mg, 10 mg, 20 mg[(B)]
			Oral solution[(B)]: 5 mg/ml
			Short-acting injection[(B)]: 5 mg/ml
	Zuclopenthixol[(C)]	Clopixol	Tablets: 10 mg, 25 mg
		Clopixol Acuphase	Short-acting injection (depot): 50 mg/ml
		Clopixol Depot	Long-acting injection (depot): 200 mg/ml

[(A)] Generic preparations may be available, [(B)] Not marketed in Canada, [(C)] Not marketed in USA, [(D)] Restricted to treatment-refractory schizophrenia in adults

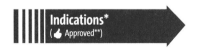

Indications*
(👍 Approved**)

Schizophrenia and Psychotic Disorders

- 👍 Management of the manifestations of schizophrenia
- 👍 Management of the manifestations of chronic schizophrenia in which the main manifestations do not include excitement, agitation or hyperactivity (pimozide, pipotiazine, flupenthixol)
- 👍 Rapid control of acute manifestations of schizophrenia (haloperidol IM, thiothixene IM) and acute psychotic episodes (zuclopenthixol – Acuphase)
- • Management of refractory schizophrenia (flupenthixol, 👍 thioridazine – USA)
- 👍 Management of psychotic disorders
- 👍 As adjunctive medication in some psychotic patients for the control of residual prevailing hostility, impulsivity, and aggressiveness (pericyazine)
- • Management of psychotic depression (loxapine: early data; loxapine metabolized to the antidepressant amoxapine)
- • Management of phencyclidine-induced psychosis (pimozide: early data)
- • Management of monosymptomanic hypochondriacal psychosis, including delusions of parasitosis (pimozide; early data)

Bipolar

- 👍 Rapid control of acute manifestations of manic states (haloperidol IM)
- 👍 Management of psychosis associated with manic-depressive syndromes (methotrimeprazine)
- 👍 Management of manic syndromes (haloperidol, thioproperazine)
- 👍 Symptomatic management of manic phase of bipolar disorder (chlorpromazine – USA, trifluoperazine)

Acute Agitation, Delirium, and Dementia

- 👍 Management of aggressive and agitated behavior in patients with chronic brain syndrome and mental retardation (haloperidol)
- 👍 Management of senile psychoses (methotrimeprazine)
- • Anxiety, tension, and agitation which occur in neuroses (chlorpromazine: early data)
- • Treatment of delirium (chlorpromazine, haloperidol); haloperidol considered drug of choice for most patients

Anxiety

- 👍 Short-term management of nonpsychotic generalized anxiety disorder (trifluoperazine); trifluoperazine is not drug of choice
- 👍 Management of conditions associated with anxiety and tension: Autonomic disturbances, personality disturbances, emotional troubles secondary to such physical conditions as resistant pruritus, etc. (methotrimeprazine)
- 👍 Relief of restlessness and apprehension before surgery (chlorpromazine – USA)

Movement Disorders

- • Management of various dyskinesias, including Huntington's chorea (fluphenazine, pimozide: early data), Sydenham's chorea (chlorpromazine: early data), tardive dyskinesia, and tardive dystonia (pimozide); usefulness is questionable; pimozide tends to worsen levodopa-induced dyskinesias

Mental Health – Other

- 👍 Symptomatic control of tics and vocal utterances of Tourette's syndrome in adults (haloperidol, pimozide – USA) and children (haloperidol – USA, pimozide – USA); haloperidol generally considered the drug of choice

* Canadian approved indications unless otherwise stated

** Adult population unless otherwise stated

"First-Generation" Antipsychotics / FGAs (cont.)

- 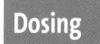 Treatment of severe behavioral problems in children marked by combativeness and/or explosive hyperexcitable behavior (chlorpromazine – USA, haloperidol – USA, thioridazine – USA); the potential risks of these agents should be considered
- 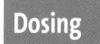 Short-term treatment of hyperactive children who exhibit excessive motor activity with accompanying conduct disorders that are manifested as impulsive behavior, difficulty sustaining attention, aggression, mood lability, and/or poor frustration tolerance (chlorpromazine – USA, haloperidol – USA, thioridazine – USA); generally not considered a first-line option
- 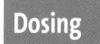 Management of insomnia (methotrimeprazine)
- Management of tic disorders (e.g., Tourette's syndrome) in children with comorbid attention deficit hyperactivity disorder in whom stimulants alone cannot control tics (haloperidol, pimozide)
- Treatment of depression (flupenthixol: short-term studies)
- Management of personality disorders (e.g., paranoid, schizoid, compulsive) (pimozide: early data)
- Management of trichotillomania (haloperidol, pimozide: early data)
- Management of erotomania (pimozide: early data)
- Management of drug withdrawal; alcohol (haloperidol: early data); cocaine (flupenthixol: early data)

Other

- Prevention and control of nausea and vomiting ($\clubsuit$ chlorpromazine – USA, haloperidol, $\clubsuit$ methotrimeprazine, $\clubsuit$ perphenazine, $\clubsuit$ trifluoperazine)
- $\clubsuit$ Management of nausea, vomiting and restlessness/anxiety associated with attacks of acute intermittent porphyria (chlorpromazine – USA)
- $\clubsuit$ Analgesia in pain due to cancer, zona (i.e., herpes zoster/shingles), trigeminal neuralgia, and neurocostal neuralgia, and in phantom limb pains and muscular discomforts (methotrimeprazine)
- $\clubsuit$ Potentiator of anesthetics; in general anesthesia, can be used as both a pre- and post-sedative and analgesic (methotrimeprazine)
- $\clubsuit$ Adjunct in the treatment of tetanus (chlorpromazine – USA)
- Treatment of intractable hiccoughs ($\clubsuit$ chlorpromazine – USA, haloperidol)

Pharmacology

- See p. 83
- All first-generation (previously called typical or conventional) antipsychotics antagonize postsynaptic dopamine-2 (D_2) receptors as their main pharmacological activity. They may be further subclassified as low (e.g., chlorpromazine), moderate (e.g., perphenazine, loxapine, zuclopenthixol), or high (e.g., haloperidol) potency agents according to their affinity for the D_2 receptor
- Antagonism of D_2 receptors in the various dopaminergic pathways is thought responsible for the efficacy and also for some of the adverse effects associated with these agents. D_2 receptor antagonism in the mesolimbic pathway relieves positive symptoms of psychosis; D_2 antagonism in the mesocortical pathway may worsen negative symptoms or cognition; D_2 antagonism in the nigrostriatal pathway may result in EPS (short-term) and TD (long-term); D_2 antagonism in the tuberoinfundibular tract may lead to hyperprolactinemia
- FGAs also have varying abilities to antagonize three other main receptors – alpha-1-adrenergic (a_1), histamine-1 (H_1), and muscarinic-cholinergic (M_1) receptors. Generally, their affinities for these three receptors are the inverse of their affinities for the D_2 receptor. For example, haloperidol has high affinity for D_2, but low affinity for a_1, H_1, and M_1. Based on haloperidol's pharmacological profile, it could be predicted that EPS and hyperprolactinemia would be more common; whereas adverse effects related to a_1 (e.g., postural hypotension), H_1 (e.g., sedation), and M_1 (e.g., constipation) antagonism would be less common

Dosing

- See Table pp. 135–138
- Current opinion suggests use of lower doses (i.e., haloperidol 2–10 mg daily, or equivalent); clinical efficacy of FGAs is correlated with D_2 binding above 60%, while hyperprolactinemia and EPS are associated with D_2 occupancies of 50–75% and 78%, respectively (see pp. 116 and 118); outcome studies show that most patients respond similarly to low doses as to high doses, with decreased adverse effects
- Acute patients may require slightly higher doses than chronic patients; manic patients may need even higher doses; maintenance doses for bipolar patients tend to be about half those used in schizophrenia
- Lower doses are recommended in the elderly, in children, and in patients with compromised liver or renal function
- Lower doses are used in first-episode patients

Administration

Oral

- May be taken with or without meals. AVOID grapefruit juice with pimozide (See Drug Interaction section pp. 123–128)
- Oral solutions should be diluted just prior to administration to improve palatability. Not compatible with all beverages. Dilute chlorpromazine solution with tomato or fruit juice, milk, simple syrup, orange syrup, carbonated beverages, coffee, tea, water or semisolid foods (e.g., soups, puddings) as a vehicle. Dilute fluphenazine and perphenazine solution with water, Seven-Up, sodium chloride solution, milk, V-8, or pineapple, apricot, prune, orange, or tomato juice. Dilute thioridazine solution with water or fruit juice
- Protect liquids from light
- Discard markedly discolored solutions; however, a slight yellowing does not affect potency
- Some liquids such as chlorpromazine and methotrimeprazine have local anesthetic effects and should be well diluted to prevent choking
- If patient is suspected of not swallowing tablet medication, liquid medication can be given

Short-acting Injections

- Watch for orthostatic hypotension, especially with parenteral administration of chlorpromazine or methotrimeprazine; keep patient supine or seated for 30 minutes afterwards; monitor BP before and after each injection
- Give IM into upper outer quadrant of buttocks or in the deltoid (deltoid offers faster absorption as it has better blood perfusion); alternate sites, charting (L) or (R); massage slowly after, to prevent sterile abscess formation; tell patient injection may sting
- Prevent contact dermatitis by keeping drug solution off patient's skin and clothing and injector's hands
- Do not let drug stand in syringe for longer than 15 min as plastic may adsorb drug

Long-acting IM

- Use a needle of at least 21 gauge; give deep IM into large muscle (e.g., buttock, using Z-track method); rotate sites and specify in charting
- As with all oily injections, it is important to ensure, by aspiration before injection, that inadvertent intravascular injection does not occur
- Do not let drug stand in syringe for longer than 15 min as plastic may adsorb drug
- DO NOT massage injection site
- "Older" multi-punctured vials of fluphenazine decanoate may contain hydrolyzed ("free") fluphenazine, which can result in higher peak plasma levels within 24 h of injection
- SC administration can be used for fluphenazine decanoate

Intravenous

- Some SHORT-acting injection formulations can be administered intravenously. Long-acting formulations CANNOT be administered via this route.
- IV administration generally occurs in the intensive care or surgical setting
- Haloperidol lactate and chlorpromazine can be given via direct IV injection or IV infusion
- Methotrimeprazine injection diluted with 5% dextrose can be given as a slow infusion (20–40 drops per minute) as a potentiator of anesthetics during surgery.
- Haloperidol administered IV associated with higher rates of sudden death, torsades de pointes, and QT prolongation[10]

Blood Levels

- The usefulness of serum levels is still unclear; it is suggested that a curvilinear relationship is true with some antipsychotics, and they may be effective within a narrow plasma level range (therapeutic window, e.g., haloperidol)

Pharmacokinetics

- See table pp. 135–138 for kinetics of individual agents
- Varies with individual agents

Oral

- Peak plasma levels of oral doses reached 1–4 h after administration
- Highly bound to plasma proteins
- Most phenothiazines and thioxanthenes have active metabolites
- Metabolized extensively by the liver; specific agents inhibit cytochrome P450 metabolizing enzymes (see pp. 107–110)

Short-acting IM

- Generally peak plasma level reached sooner than with oral preparation
- Bioavailability usually greater than with oral drug (loxapine excepted); dosage should be adjusted accordingly

"First-Generation" Antipsychotics / FGAs (cont.)

- With loxapine, single IM doses produce lower concentrations of active metabolite, for first 12–16 h, than does oral therapy – this may result in a different balance between D_2 and 5-HT$_2$ blockade

Long-acting IM	• See chart on pp. 139–140

- Bioavailability is greater than with oral agents (by a factor of at least 2); eliminates bioavailability problems related to absorption and first-pass metabolism and maintains stable plasma concentrations
- Injections can be painful; highest pain reported 5 minutes after administration and tends to decrease gradually over 2–10 days
- Presence of "free" fluphenazine in multi-dose vials of fluphenazine decanoate is responsible for high peak plasma level seen within 24 h of injection – monitor for EPS

Zuclopenthixol Acuphase	• Short-acting depot injection (see p. 135)

- Peak plasma level: 24–48 h; elimination half-life = 48–72 h

---

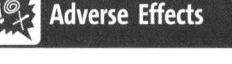 **Adverse Effects**

- See charts on pp. 131–132 for incidence of adverse effects; the incidence may differ between different dosage forms of the same drug (e.g., oral vs long-acting vs short-acting injection)
- Many adverse effects are transient; persistent effects often have remedies, but are generally best dealt with by altering the drug administration schedule or dosage, or a change in drug

CNS Effects

- Confusion, disturbed concentration, disorientation (more common with high doses or in the elderly). Concomitant anticholinergic agents may exacerbate
- Extrapyramidal – acute onset: A result of antagonism at dopamine D_2 receptors (extrapyramidal reactions correlated with D_2 binding above 80%)
  - Includes acute dystonias, akathisia, pseudoparkinsonism, pisa syndrome, rabbit syndrome – see p. 142 for onset, symptoms, and treatment options and pp. 150–157 for detailed treatment options
  - More common with high potency FGAs vs. moderate–low potency agents, also more common with FGAs vs. SGAs/TGA – see pp. 142–143 to compare incidence of EPS associated with these agents
- Extrapyramidal – late onset or tardive movement disorders
  - Includes tardive akathisia, tardive dyskinesia, and tardive dystonia – see p. 142 for onset, symptoms, and therapeutic management options
  - Late onset movement disorders usually develop after months or years of treatment
  - May be irreversible so prevention is key – use lowest doses for shortest possible time period and assess for signs of movement disorders regularly. Symptoms are not alleviated and may be exacerbated by antiparkinsonian medications[7]
  - Annual risk of TD with FGAs estimated to be 4–5% with a cumulative risk of up to 50%.[7] Risk of TD lower with SGA and TGA antipsychotics.
  - Other tardive syndromes may include:
    - Tardive parkinsonism
    - Tardive akathisia (some think this is indistinguishable from early akathisia) (see p. 142)
    - Tardive ballismus
    - Tardive Tourette's syndrome
    - Tardive vomiting (especially in smokers)
    - Tardive hypothalamic syndrome; associated with polydipsia
- Neuroleptic malignant syndrome (NMS) – rare disorder characterized by autonomic dysfunction (e.g., tachycardia and hypertension), hyperthermia, altered consciousness, and muscle rigidity with an increase in creatine kinase and myoglobinuria
  - Can occur with any class of antipsychotic agent, at any dose, and at any time (although usually occurs early in the course of treatment). Risk factors may include dehydration, young age, male sex, organic brain syndromes, exhaustion, agitation, and rapid or parenteral antipsychotic administration[7]
  - Potentially fatal (in estimated 5–20%) unless recognized early and medication stopped. Supportive therapy (e.g., maintain hydration, correct electrolyte imbalances, control fever) must be instituted as soon as possible. Additional treatment with dopamine agonists such as dantrolene, amantadine, and bromocriptine may be helpful (controversial – may reduce muscle rigidity without an effect on overall outcome); ECT has also been used successfully to improve symptoms. Treatment with an antipsychotic agent may be recommended several weeks post recovery

- Sedation – common, especially with low potency agents, following treatment initiation and with dosage increases. Usually transient, but some individuals may complain of persistent effects. [Management: Prescribe bulk of dose at bedtime; minimize use of concomitant CNS depressants, if possible; data regarding treatment with specific agents is lacking – caffeine as well as other psychostimulants including modafinil 200 mg q am (see Drug Interactions p. 123) have been suggested if symptoms persist (controversial)]
- Seizures – all FGAs may lower seizure threshold resulting in seizures ranging from myoclonus to grand mal type. At usual dosage ranges, seizure rates are less than 1% for FGAs. Risk greater with low potency agents and is dose-related. May occur if dose increased rapidly or may also be secondary to hyponatremia associated with syndrome of inappropriate antidiuretic hormone secretion (SIADH). Use with caution in patients with a history of seizures

| Anticholinergic Effects |
- A result of antagonism at muscarinic receptors (ACh)
- More common with low potency FGAs. See p. 131 for a comparison of the anticholinergic effects of FGAs
- Many of these adverse effects are often dose-related and may also resolve over time without treatment. Treatment options may include reducing the dose of the FGA or switching to another antipsychotic with less potential to cause anticholinergic effects or employing a specific drug or non-drug strategy to treat the adverse effect (see below for suggestions). Many medications have anticholinergic effects, review patient profiles for their presence and reevaluate the need for their continued use
- Blurred vision, dry eyes [Management: Use adequate lighting when reading; pilocarpine 0.5% eye drops]
- Constipation [Management/prevention: increase dietary fibre and fluid intake, increase exercise, or use a fecal softener (e.g., docusate) or bulk laxative (e.g., Prodiem, Metamucil)]
- Delirium – characterized by agitation, confusion, disorientation, visual hallucinations, tachycardia, etc. May result with use of high doses or combination anticholinergic medication. Drugs with high anticholinergic activity have also been associated with slowed cognition and selective impairments of memory and recall
- Dry eyes (Management: Artificial tears, wetting solutions)
- Dry mouth/mucous membranes – if severe or persistent, may predispose patient to candida infection [Management: sugar-free gum and candy, oral lubricants (e.g., MoiStir, OraCare D), pilocarpine mouth wash – see p. 39]
- Urinary retention – May be more problematic for older patients, especially males with benign prostatic hypertrophy [Management: bethanechol]

| Cardiovascular Effects |
- Many result from antagonism at α1-adrenergic and muscarinic receptors
- Arrhythmias and ECG changes:
  - ECG changes (e.g., flattened T-waves, ST segment depression, QTc lengthening – may increase risk of arrhythmias) reported with many antipsychotic medications, the clinical significance of which is unclear for many. A QTc of more than 500 ms is associated with an increased risk for torsade de pointes, ventricular fibrillation and sudden cardiac death. Prominent risk factors for QTc prolongation include congenital long QT syndrome, elderly age, female sex, heart failure, myocardial infarction (MI), and concomitant use of medications that prolong the QT interval (see Drug Interactions pp. 123–128). Other risk factors may include altered nutritional status (e.g., eating disorders, alcoholism), bradycardia, cerebrovascular disease, diabetes, electrolyte imbalances (hypokalemia, hypomagnesemia, hypocalcemia), hypertension, hypothyroidism, and obesity. FGAs that have been associated with QT interval prolongation include thioridazine, pimozide, and haloperidol (high dose, IV route)[9]
  - Tachycardia may occur as a compensatory mechanism to orthostatic hypotension caused by α-adrenergic antagonism. Tachycardia due to anticholinergic effects in the absence of above conditions, may be treated with a low dose peripherally-acting β-blocker[3]
- Death/dementia – individuals with dementia often develop neuropsychiatric symptoms such as agitation, aggression, and delusions over the course of illness. Many of these are challenging to control via nonpharmacological interventions, frequently resulting in the prescription of antipsychotic medication. In 2005, both the FDA and Health Canada issued advisories concerning a small but significant increase in overall mortality in elderly patients with dementia receiving treatment with SGAs and aripiprazole. "Black box" warnings describing this risk were added to the labeling of these agents. Deaths were primarily related to cardiac-related events and pneumonias. Subsequent studies have suggested a similar risk with FGAs. It is currently unknown if this risk extends beyond the early treatment period. Consider individual's risk-benefit ratio when prescribing antipsychotics in dementia patients. It has been suggested to limit use to situations in which there is significant risk of harm to self or others or when symptoms are causing significant distress despite implementation of alternate treatments. Reassess the need for continued treatment regularly[24,29]
- Orthostatic hypotension/compensatory tachycardia/dizziness/syncope – may occur as a result of alpha-adrenergic antagonism. More likely to occur with low potency FGAs. DO NOT USE EPINEPHRINE, as it may further lower the blood pressure (see Drug Interactions). When employing antipsychotics that are potent α-adrenergic antagonists, increase doses gradually to minimize hypotension as well as sinus and reflex tachycardia.

"First-Generation" Antipsychotics / FGAs (cont.)

Elderly patients are susceptible to this adverse effect and syncopal episodes may result in falls and fractures. [Management: Rise slowly, divide the daily dose, consider a switch to another agent, increase fluid and salt intake, use support hose; treatment with fluid retaining corticosteroid-fludrocortisone]
- Venous thrombosis – low potency agents may be a risk factor for venous thrombosis in predisposed individuals, case reports of deep vein thrombosis in patients on chlorpromazine – usually occurs in first 3 months of therapy
- Cardiovascular disease (CVD) is the leading cause of death in individuals with schizophrenia. There may be a number of contributing factors to CVD in this population, including smoking, sedentary lifestyles, poverty, poor nutrition, reduced access to health care, and a number of metabolic abnormalities including weight gain, dyslipidemias, glucose intolerance, and hypertension. Please see Endocrine and Metabolic Effects for more details on these effects and their role in CVD

Endocrine & Metabolic Effects
- Antidiuretic hormone dysfunction:
  - Disturbances in antidiuretic hormone function: PIP (polydipsia, intermittent hyponatremia and psychosis syndrome); prevalence in schizophrenia estimated at 6–20%, can range from mild cognitive deficits to seizures, coma, and death; increased risk in the elderly, smokers and alcoholics. Monitor sodium levels in chronically treated patients to help identify risk for seizures [Management: Fluid restriction, demeclocycline up to 1200 mg/day, captopril 12.5 mg/day, propranolol 30–120 mg/day; replace electrolytes]
- Dyslipidemia:
  - Lipid abnormalities (increases in fasting total cholesterol and triglycerides) have been reported in patients on some FGAs. Risk appears to be more often associated with certain SGAs (see p. 94)
  - See p. 83 for suggested monitoring guidelines
  - Treatment options may include lifestyle and dietary modifications; switching to another antipsychotic associated with a lower potential for lipid dysregulation; add cholersterol lowering medication (e.g., statins, fibrates, salmon oil, etc.)
- Hyperglycemia or type 2 diabetes mellitus:
  - Schizophrenia is a risk factor for the development of type 2 diabetes. Certain antipsychotic medications have also been associated with an increased risk for glucose intolerance/diabetes. While the risk appears highest with SGAs (most notably clozapine and olanzapine), there are also reports in the literature of glycosuria, glucose intolerance, hyperglycemia, and diabetes mellitus occurring in association with FGAs.[13] Within FGAs, the risk may be greater with low potency agents[12]
  - See p. 83 for suggested monitoring guidelines
  - Treatment options may include lifestyle and dietary modifications; switching to another antipsychotic associated with a lower potential for glucose dysregulation; adding hypoglycemic agent
- Hyperprolactinemia:
  - Prolactin level may be elevated up to 10-fold from baseline. Develops over first week of treatment and usually remains throughout treatment course
  - More common in women than men despite similar doses. Adolescents and children may be at higher risk
  - *Clinical consequences* of elevated prolactin levels may include short-term risks such as galactorrhea, gynecomastia, menstrual irregularities, and sexual dysfunction, and potential long-term risks such as osteoporosis (as a result of decreased bone density secondary to chronic hypogonadism), pituitary tumors, and breast cancer (data conflicting)
  - *Effects in women:* Breast engorgement and lactation (may be more common in women who have previously been pregnant), amenorrhea (with risk of infertility), menstrual irregularities, changes in libido, hirsutism (due to increased testosterone). Bone mineral density loss may be more intense in females than males and may vary by ethnic group; extent of loss may correlate with duration of hyperprolactinemia. Recommended women with hyperprolactinemia or amenorrhea for > 12 months have a bone mineral density evaluation
  - *Effects in men:* Gynecomastia, rarely galactorrhea, decreased libido, and erectile or ejaculatory dysfunction
  - *Monitoring/investigation:* Recent guidelines suggest routine assessments for the presence of symptoms associated with prolactin elevation. In the event of a positive finding, a prolactin level should be ordered and an attempt made to rule out nonpharmacologic causes.[7,18] The fasting morning serum prolactin level is recommended as least variable and best correlated with disease states. In cases where an antipsychotic medication is strongly suspected as the cause, discontinuing the suspected agent (or switching to another antipsychotic agent with less potential for

prolactin elevation) for a short period of time (e.g., 3–4 days) if clinically feasible and follow-up monitoring to determine if prolactin levels have fallen may be a simple means to confirm suspicions and avoid MRI or CT of the hypothalamic/pituitary region[19]

– *Treatment options:* Assuming discontinuation of antipsychotic therapy is not an option, the preferred treatment is to switch to another antipsychotic agent with a reduced risk of hyperprolactinemia – weighing the potential risk for relapse associated with this action. Other treatment options may include lowering the dose or adding a medication to treat the condition. Use of a dopamine agonist such as bromocriptine (1.25–2.5 mg bid) or cabergoline (0.25–2 mg/week) may be considered but has the potential to exacerbate the underlying illness

- Metabolic syndrome:
  - Metabolic syndrome (also called insulin resistance syndrome, syndrome X, or dysmetabolic syndrome) is an interrelated cluster of cardiovascular disease risk (CVD) factors which include abdominal obesity, dyslipidemia, hypertension, and impaired glucose tolerance. For diagnosis, three of the following five characteristics must be present:
    1. Abdominal obesity – waist circumference: Men > 102 cm (40 in)/Women > 88 cm (35 in)
    2. Triglycerides: ≥ 1.7 mmol/L (150 mg/dL)
    3. HDL cholesterol: Men < 1.0 mmol/L (40 mg/dL)/Women < 1.3 mmol/L (50 mg/dL)
    4. Blood pressure: $\geq 130/85$ mmHg
    5. Fasting glucose: 5.7–7.0 mmol/L (102–125 mg/dL)
  - Experts now pay attention to waist over hip percentage, which should be < 85% in women and < 90% in men
  - Shown to be an important risk factor in the development of type 2 diabetes and CVD. Summary of prospective studies in patients with metabolic syndrome estimates risk of diabetes is 30–52% and risk of CVD is 12–17%; associated with increased risk for coronary artery disease (angina pectoris), myocardial infarction, sudden death, stroke, and congestive heart failure

- Weight gain:
  - Reported in up to 40% of patients receiving treatment with FGAs. More likely to occur early in treatment (e.g., within first 6 months) and the risk appears greater with low potency FGAs[3]
  - The mechanism by which antipsychotics may influence weight gain is unknown (may be a result of multiple systems including $5-HT_{1B}$-, $5-HT_{2C}$-, $\alpha 1$-, and H1-blockade, prolactinemia, gonadal and adrenal steroid imbalance, and increase in circulating leptin; may also be due to sedation and inactivity, carbohydrate craving, and excessive intake of high-calorie beverages to alleviate drug-induced thirst and dry mouth)
  - Weight gain may contribute to or have deleterious effects on a number of conditions, including dyslipidemia, glucose dysregulation, and type 2 diabetes, hypertension, coronary artery disease, stroke, osteoarthritis, sleep apnea, and self-image
  - See p. 83 for suggested monitoring guidelines
  - Treatment options: Since it is often challenging to lose weight, preventative strategies which focus on healthy lifestyles (diet and exercise) are recommended. Treatment options may include healthy lifestyle strategies; switching from an antipsychotic with higher weight gain liability to one of lower liability (may result in significant reductions in body weight)[20] or use of medications to promote weight loss. Treatment with the following agents has been tried with varying degrees of success based on case reports and randomized controlled trials: Amantadine (100–300 mg/day), bromocriptine (2.5 mg/day), sibutramine (10 mg/day), famotidine (40 mg/day), topiramate (up to 200 mg/day), nizatidine (300 mg bid), orlistat (120 mg tid)

| GI Effects | • Constipation – see Anticholinergic Effects p. 93 |

- Dysphagia – dysphagia (difficulty swallowing) and aspiration have been reported with antipsychotic use. Use all agents cautiously in individuals at risk for developing aspiration pneumonia (e.g., advanced Alzheimer's)
- Dry mouth – see Anticholinergic Effects
- Pancreatitis – rare reports of pancreatitis with haloperidol
- Anorexia, dyspepsia, constipation, occasionally diarrhea
- Peculiar taste, glossitis
- Vomiting common after prolonged treatment, especially in smokers
- Sialorrhea, difficulty swallowing, gagging [see p. 96, GI Effects]

| Urogenital and Sexual Effects | • Sexual effects may result from altered dopaminergic (including hyperprolactinemia-main cause of sexual dysfunction in women), serotonergic, ACh, α_1, or H_1 activity |

- An estimated 25–60% of patients on FGAs report sexual dysfunction

"First-Generation" Antipsychotics / FGAs (cont.)

- Identify and develop strategies to deal with other medications (e.g., antidepressants, especially TCAs and SSRIs, β-blockers, calcium channel blockers, cimetidine, digoxin, diuretics, methyldopa, illicit substances – e.g., cocaine, opioids, etc.) and conditions (e.g., age, alcohol, diabetes, hypertension, smoking, etc.) that may be associated with sexual dysfunction
- Treatment options may include: 1) dosage reduction, 2) waiting 1–3 months to see if tolerance develops, 3) switching antipsychotics, or 4) adding a medication to treat the problem (see below for treatment suggestions regarding specific types of dysfunction; evidence for their use is based primarily on open-label studies and case reports)
- *Anorgasmia* [Management: Bethanechol (10 mg tid or 10–25 mg prn before intercourse), neostigmine (7.5–15 mg prn), cyproheptadine (4–16 mg/day), amantadine (100–300 mg/day)]
- *Ejaculation dysfunction* (incl. inhibition of ejaculation, abnormal ejaculation, retrograde ejaculation – especially thioridazine) – reported to be the most common sexual disturbance associated with FGAs [Management suggestions: For retrograde ejaculation – imipramine (25–50 mg hs), yohimbine (5.4 mg 1–3 × daily, 1–4 h prior to intercourse), or cyproheptadine (4–16 mg/day)]
- *Erectile dysfunction*, impotence – ED is reported to occur in 23–54% of males on FGAs [Management suggestions: Bethanechol (10 mg tid or 10–50 mg prn before intercourse), yohimbine (5.4 mg 1–3 × daily, 1–4 h prior to intercourse), sildenafil (25–100 mg prn), amantadine (100–300 mg/day)]
- *Libido* – decreased libido [Management: Neostigmine (7.5–15 mg prn) or cyproheptadine (4–16 mg prn 30 minutes before intercourse)]
- *Priapism* – rare case reports of priapism occurring in patients on FGAs (i.e., chlorpromazine, fluphenazine, mesoridazine, perphenazine, prochlorperazine, thioridazine, thiothixene, and trifluoperazine). Antagonism of α-adrenergic receptors is believed to play a role in this effect
- *Urinary retention* – see Anticholinergic Effects p. 93

Ocular Effects

- Blurred vision/dry eyes: see Anticholingeric Effects p. 93.
- Cataracts/lens changes: Association reported between phenothiazine use and cataract formation. Though eye examination (e.g., slit lamp exam) has been recommended at baseline and 6 month intervals thereafter, this recommendation is controversial
- Lenticular pigmentation
  - Related to long-term use of antipsychotics (primarily chlorpromazine)
  - Presents as glare, halos around lights or hazy vision
  - Granular deposits in eye
  - Vision usually is not impaired; may be reversible if drug stopped
  - Often present in patients with antipsychotic-induced skin pigmentation or photosensitivity reactions
- Pigmentary retinopathy (retinitis pigmentosa)
  - Primarily associated with chronic use of thioridazine or chlorpromazine [annual ophthalmological examination recommended]
  - Reduced visual acuity (may occasionally reverse if drug stopped)
  - Blindness can occur
- With chronic use, chlorpromazine can cause pigmentation of the endothelium and Descemet's membrane of the cornea; it can color the conjunctiva, sclera and eyelids a slate-blue color – may not be reversible when drug stopped

Hematological Effects

- Blood dyscrasias, including those affecting erythropoesis, granulopoesis, and thrombopoesis, have been reported with most antipsychotic medications
- Clinically significant hematological abnormalities with antipsychotic medications are, with the exception of clozapine, rare. Accordingly, the development of any blood abnormalities in individuals on antipsychotic medication, especially other than clozapine, should undergo rigorous medical assessment to determine the underlying cause
- *Aplastic Anemia* – Reported primarily with chlorpromazine and trifluoperazine. Also noted to have occurred in patients treated with fluphenazine, flupenthixol, haloperidol, perphenazine, and thioridazine
- *Eosinophilia* – not typically of clinical significance unless severe. Reported with chlorpromazine and trifluoperazine
- *Leukopenia* [defined as WBC $< 4 \times 10^9$/L] and *Neutropenia/Agranulocytosis* [Neutropenia (defined as absolute neutrophil count (ANC) less than 1.5×10^9/L) may be subclassified as mild (ANC = $1–1.5 \times 10^9$/L), moderate (ANC = $0.5–1 \times 10^9$/L) or severe (also termed agranulocytosis – defined as ANC $< 0.5 \times 10^9$/L or sometimes as ANC $< 0.2 \times 10^9$/L)].

- Mild neutropenia may be transient (returning to normal without a change in medication/dose), or progressive (continuing to drop, leading to agranulocytosis).
- Reported incidence of severe neutropenia in 1 study was (0.02%) with phenothiazines and (0.003%) with butyrophenones
- *Thrombocytopenia* – Reported with a number of FGAs including chlorpromazine, prochlorperazine, and thiordiazine. In most cases withdrawal of the medication was reported to result in normalization of platelet counts

Hepatic Effects	

- Cholestatic jaundice (reversible if drug stopped)
  - Occurs in less than 0.1% of patients within first 4 weeks of treatment, with most antipsychotics
  - Noted to occur in 0.1–0.5% of patients taking chlorpromazine[3]
  - Signs include yellow skin, dark urine, pruritus
- Transient asymptomatic transaminase elevations (ALT 2–3 times the upper limit of normal) reported with haloperidol (up to 16% of patients)

Hypersensitivity Reactions	

- Usually appear within the first few months of therapy (but may occur after the drug is discontinued)
- Photosensitivity and photoallergy reactions including sunburn-like erythematous eruptions which may be accompanied by blistering
- Rarely, asthma, laryngeal, angioneurotic or peripheral edema, and anaphylactic reactions occur
- Hypersensitive reactions at injection site (especially haloperidol decanoate 100 mg/ml); indurations reported with higher doses (see p. 139)
- Cases of systemic lupus erythematosus reported with chlorpromazine

Temperature Regulation	

- Altered ability of body to regulate response to changes in temperature and humidity; may become hyperthermic or hypothermic in temperature extremes due to inhibition of the hypothalamic control area

Other Adverse Effects	

- Low potency antipsychotics associated with increased risk of fatal pulmonary embolism (highest risk with thioridazine)

 Discontinuation Syndrome

- Abrupt discontinuation of an antipsychotic is primarily indicated in situations involving a sudden/severe adverse reaction to a drug (e.g., hepatic insufficiency with chlorpromazine). Patients may also choose to become nonadherent by stopping their antipsychotic medication abruptly
- Abrupt discontinuation (or in some cases a large dose reduction) of an antipsychotic may be associated with a number of potential risks including:
  1. Discontinuation syndromes – typically characterized by development of a number of symptoms including nausea, vomiting, diarrhea, diaphoresis, cold sweats, muscles aches and pains, insomnia, anxiety, and confusion. Often the result of cholinergic rebound. Usually appear within days of discontinuation [Mild cases may only require comfort and reassurance; for more severe symptoms consider restarting the antipsychotic followed by slow taper if possible; or if rebound cholinergic effects present, consider adding an anticholinergic agent short term]
  2. Psychosis – exacerbation or precipitation of psychosis including a severe, rapid onset or supersensitivity psychosis, most notable with clozapine and possibly quetiapine vs. FGAs. Most likely to occur within the first 2–3 weeks post discontinuation or sooner [Restart antipsychotic]
  3. Movement disorders – withdrawal dyskinesias noted to appear usually around 2–4 weeks post abrupt withdrawal [Restart antipsychotic and taper slowly]. Rebound dystonia, parkinsonism, and akathisia also reported to occur usually within days to the first week post discontinuation [Restart antipsychotic and taper or treat with appropriate anti-EPS medication]
- Abrupt cessation of a long-acting or depot antipsychotic is of less concern as plasma concentrations decline slowly (i.e., drug tapers itself)
- ☞ **THEREFORE, AFTER PROLONGED USE, THESE MEDICATIONS SHOULD BE WITHDRAWN GRADUALLY.** If switching to another antipsychotic, see pp. 144–145 for specific recommendations

 Precautions

- Hypotension occurs most frequently with parenteral use, especially with high doses; the patient should be in supine position during short-acting IM administration and remain supine or seated for at least 30 minutes; measure the BP before and following each IM dose
- IM injections should be administered slowly; the deltoid offers faster absorption as it has better blood perfusion
- Use with caution in the elderly, in the presence of cardiovascular disease, chronic respiratory disorder, hypoglycemia, convulsive disorders
- Caution in prescribing to patients with known or suspected hepatic disorder; monitor clinically and measure transaminase level (ALT/SGPT), periodically
- Should be used very cautiously in patients with narrow angle glaucoma or prostatic hypertrophy
- Prior to prescribing thioridazine, or pimozide, a baseline ECG and serum potassium should be done, and monitored periodically during the course of therapy. DO NOT USE these drugs in patients with QT_c interval over 450 ms
- Monitor if QT interval exceeds 420 ms and discontinue drug if exceeds 500 ms; do not exceed 800 mg thioridazine or 20 mg pimozide daily

"First-Generation" Antipsychotics / FGAs (cont.)

- Cigarette smoking is reported to induce the metabolism and decrease the plasma level of some antipsychotics; see drug interaction section
- Allergic cross-reactivity (rash) between chlorpromazine and clozapine reported

Toxicity

- In the majority of cases, overdose is associated with a low mortality and morbidity rate
- Symptoms may include nausea and vomiting, confusion, hallucinations, agitation, drowsiness progressing to coma, hypotension, respiratory depression, electrolyte imbalances, ECG changes and arrhythmias, and/or EPS
- No specific antidotes; provide supportive treatment – establish/maintain airway, ensure adequate oxygenation/ventilation, monitor vital organ functions. Monitor vital signs and ECG for at least 6 h and admit the patient for at least 24 h if significant intoxication apparent
- Hypotension and circulatory collapse treated with IV fluids and/or sympathomimetic agents (CAUTION – use of epinephrine or dopamine or other agents with β-agonist activity may worsen hypotension in the presence of antipsychotic-induced α-blockade; see Drug Interactions pp. 123–128)
- Gastric lavage and/or activated charcoal may be considered depending on the time elapsed since overdose
- Hemoperfusion/hemodialysis not recommended due to large volumes of distribution and high plasma protein binding profiles of antipsychotics
- Avoid drugs that produce additive QT prolongation (see Drug Interactions pp. 123–128)

Management

- Supportive treatment should be given

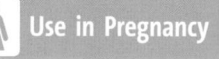

Use in Pregnancy

- Available data suggests most antipsychotics do not increase the risk of teratogenic effects in humans. However, human data for some FGAs is limited and there have been cases of limb defects after first trimester (time of greatest risk for malformations) exposure in humans to haloperidol. If use of haloperidol during pregnancy cannot be avoided, ultrasound with particular attention to limb formation should be considered in first trimester exposures
- Early data suggests *in utero* exposure to FGAs may decrease infant birth weight and increase the risk of small size for gestational age
- Consider the potential effects on delivery (e.g., maternal hypotension with chlorpromazine) and for withdrawal effects in the newborn if used during the third trimester. There are case reports of fetal and neonatal toxicity including NMS, dyskinesia, EPS (manifested by heightened muscle tone and increased rooting and tendon reflexes persisting for several months), neonatal jaundice and postnatal intestinal obstruction
- Long-term effects on neurodevelopment are largely unknown
- The benefits of treating the mother may outweigh the unknown risks of FGAs on the fetus. Use lowest effective dose
- Most FGAs are FDA pregnancy risk category C, yet vary in the amount of information available. Avoid, if possible, FGAs that have no human pregnancy data (e.g., loxapine, pimozide, and zuclopenthixol) or very limited human data (e.g., flupenthixol, molindone, thiothixene)
- High-potency FGAs may yield the best therapeutic benefit with the least anticholinergic and sedative effects, however, comparative safety with other FGAs in pregnancy is unavailable
- Chlorpromazine was initially used for nausea and vomiting of pregnancy. This data suggests chlorpromazine is safe if used in low doses during pregnancy. However, chlorpromazine when given near term in doses of 500 mg or greater may cause an increased incidence of respiratory distress in the neonate, and has been implicated in producing lethargy and EPS in the neonate.

Breast Milk

- Antipsychotics have been detected in breast milk in concentrations of 0.2–11%. The American Academy of Pediatrics (2001) classified antipsychotic drugs as drugs whose "effect in the nursing infant is unknown but may be of concern"[2]
- If used while breastfeeding, use lowest effective dose and monitor infant's progress.
- Very limited data. Single or small numbers of case reports have found no short-term adverse effects of breastfeed infants exposed to flupenthixol, perphenazine, or zuclopenthixol. One report of drowsiness and lethargy with chlorpromazine. Cases of a decline in mental and psychomotor development at age 12–18 months with higher dose haloperidol (20–40 mg/day) and chlorpromazine (200–600 mg/day). Long-term effects on neurodevelopment are largely unknown. A 5-year follow-up study of 7 breastfed infants exposed to chlorpromazine found no developmental deficits

- Clinically significant interactions are listed below

Class of Drug	Example	Interaction Effects
Acetylcholinesterase inhibitor (central)	Donepezil	May enhance neurotoxicity of antipsychotics presumably due to a relative acetylcholine/dopamine imbalance (i.e., increased acetylcholine in the presence of dopamine receptor blockade) in the CNS. Case reports of severe EPS (e.g., generalized rigidity, shuffling gate, facial grimacing) in elderly patients within a few days of starting an antipsychotic (risperidone or haloperidol) and an acetylcholinesterase inhibitor (donepezil or tacrine). Symptoms resolved after discontinuing the antipsychotic agent, the acetylcholinesterase inhibitor, or both. Use lowest effective dose of antipsychotic
Adsorbent	Antacids, activated charcoal, cholestyramine, attapulgite (kaolin-pectin)	Oral absorption decreased significantly when used simultaneously; give at least 1 h before or 2 h after the antipsychotic
Anesthetic	Enflurane	Additive hypotension with chlorpromazine
Amylinomimetic	Pramlintide	Pramlintide slows the rate of gastric emptying. Antipsychotics with significant anticholinergic effects can further reduce GI motility. Use drugs with minimal anticholinergic effects at the lowest effective dose
Antiarrhythmic	Amiodarone, quinidine, sotalol	With quinidine, increased peak plasma level and AUC of haloperidol by ~2-fold due to inhibited metabolism via CYP2D6 and/or displacement from tissue binding. Monitor for haloperidol adverse effects (e.g., EPS). Amiodarone and quinidine likely to increase chlorpromazine, fluphenazine, and thioridazine levels via inhibition of CYP2D6; further increasing risk of QT prolongation
		DO NOT COMBINE with chlorpromazine, fluphenazine, pimozide or thioridazine. NOT recommended with phenothiazines. CAUTION with other FGAs. Possible additive prolongation of QT interval and associated life-threatening cardiac arrhythmias. Factors which further increase the risk include anorexia, bradycardia, hypokalemia, and hypomagnesemia
Antibiotic		
Macrolide	Clarithromycin, erythromycin, telithromycin	With clarithromycin, decreased clearance of pimozide by 46% due to inhibition of metabolism via CYP3A4. May decrease clearance of chlorpromazine and haloperidol. Similar interaction with erythromycin and telithromycin likely. Increased antipsychotic adverse effects including prolonged QT interval possible
		DO NOT COMBINE with pimozide or thioridazine. NOT recommended with phenothiazines. CAUTION with other FGAs. Possible additive prolongation of QT interval and associated life-threatening cardiac arrhythmias. Two reports of deaths occurring within days of adding clarithromycin to pimozide. Azithromycin (which doesn't inhibit CYP3A4) may have a lower risk when used with pimozide, although all macrolides are specifically listed as contraindicated in the pimozide product monograph. Factors which further increase the risk include anorexia, bradycardia, hypokalemia, and hypomagnesemia
Quinolone	Ciprofloxacin, gatifloxacin, levofloxacin, moxifloxacin	With ciprofloxacin, may increase plasma level of trifluorperazine due to inhibition of metabolism via CYP1A2. Clinical significance unknown
		DO NOT COMBINE with pimozide or thioridazine. NOT recommended with phenothiazines. CAUTION with FGAs. Possible additive prolongation of QT interval and associated life-threatening cardiac arrhythmias. Factors which further increase the risk include anorexia, bradycardia, hypokalemia, and hypomagnesemia. Ciprofloxacin is thought to have less potential for QT prolongation but there are isolated cases of increased QT
		CAUTION. Potential to exacerbate psychiatric conditions as quinolone-induced psychosis has been reported

"First-Generation" Antipsychotics / FGAs (cont.)

Class of Drug	Example	Interaction Effects
Anticholinergic	Antiparkinsonian drugs, antidepressants, antihistamines	The concomitant use of two or more drugs that have anticholinergic activity is often clinically appropriate. However, such use increases the risk of anticholinergic adverse effects (e.g., dry mouth, urinary retention, inhibition of sweating, blurred vision, constipation, paralytic ileus, confusion, toxic psychosis). AVOID highly anticholinergic drugs in the elderly who are particularly vulnerable to those effects Variable effects seen on metabolism, plasma level, and efficacy of antipsychotic (see specific classes or individual drugs)
Anticoagulant	Warfarin	Decreased INR possible with chlorpromazine or haloperidol. Monitor INR at least weekly for 2 weeks when starting, stopping or changing the dose of the antipsychotic
Anticonvulsant	Carbamazepine	Decreased antipsychotic plasma levels via induction of CYP3A4, CYP1A2, and/or CYP2D6 With haloperidol, decreased plasma levels of carbamazepine (40%). Conflicting reports on haloperidol levels likely a result of a dose-dependent interaction (i.e., the interaction is more significant with increasing carbamazepine doses). Carbamazepine 100 mg daily reduced haloperidol levels by 15% while carbamazepine 600 mg daily reduced haloperidol levels by 75%. Monitor for antipsychotic efficacy. Adjust dose as needed Likely to decrease levels of chlorpromazine, fluphenazine, flupenthixol, and zuclopenthixol With loxapine, increased plasma levels of carbamazepine epoxide metabolite. Monitor for carbamazepine adverse effects (ataxia, nystagmus, diplopia, headache, vomiting). Adjust carbamazepine as needed
	Lamotrigine	Chlorpromazine may inhibit metabolism of lamotrigine resulting in increased lamotrigine levels. Clinical significance unknown
	Phenytoin, phenobarbital	Decreased plasma level of antipsychotic due to induction of metabolism; for phenytoin via CYP2C9 andCYP3A4; for phenobarbital primarily via CYP1A2, CYP2C9, and CYP3A4 With phenytoin, reduced levels of chlorpromazine, haloperidol, and thioridazine reported. With phenobarbital, reduced levels of chlorpromazine (by 25%) and haloperidol reported. Limited data available; interactions with other FGAs probable. Monitor for antipsychotic response when starting and increased antipsychotic adverse effects when stopping phenytoin or phenobarbital. Adjust antipsychotic dose as needed Loxapine decreased phenytoin levels in one case report
	Valproate (divalproex, valproic acid)	Chlorpromazine inhibits the metabolism of valproate resulting in increased valproate levels. Clinical significance unknown
Antidepressant		DO NOT COMBINE with pimozide or thioridazine and CAUTION with other FGAs applies to the majority of antidepressants, due to possible additive prolongation of QT interval and associated life-threatening cardiac arrhythmias. Factors which further increase the risk include anorexia, bradycardia, hypokalemia, and hypomagnesemia
Cyclic	Amitriptyline, trimipramine	DO NOT COMBINE with pimozide or thioridazine; CAUTION with other FGAs; due to additive prolongation of QT interval Additive sedation, hypotension, and anticholinergic effects Haloperidol and phenothiazines may increase the plasma level of cyclic antidepressants (TCAs). TCAs may increase the plasma level of chlorpromazime. Clinical significance unknown

Class of Drug	Example	Interaction Effects
SSRI	Citalopram, fluoxetine, fluvoxamine, paroxetine, sertraline	DO NOT COMBINE with pimozide or thioridazine; CAUTION with other FGAs; due to additive prolongation of QT interval. Case report of QT prolongation and patient collapsing with concurrent chlorpromazine and fluoxetine Increased EPS and akathasia Increased plasma level of antipsychotic due to inhibition of metabolism of CYP1A2 (potent – fluvoxamine), 2D6 (potent – fluoxetine and paroxetine), and/or 3A4 (fluvoxamine). Monitor for increased antipsychotic adverse effects (e.g., EPS) when starting and antipsychotic efficacy when stopping SSRI. Adjust antipsychotic dose as needed. Alternatively, consider using a SSRI with no or weak effects on CYPs such as citalopram, escitalopram, and sertraline (at doses of 100 mg/day or less) or use a SSRI that does not affect the specific CYP enzyme which metabolizes the specific FGA Haloperidol levels: With fluoxetine, 20–35% higher levels. With fluvoxamine, 23–60% higher. With sertraline, 28% higher Phenothiazine levels: With fluvoxamine, thioridazine levels 3-fold higher. With paroxetine, perphenazine peak levels 2- to 13-fold higher Pimozide levels: With paroxetine, 151% higher AUC and 62% higher peak level. With sertraline, 40% higher peak level
SNRI	Duloxetine, venlafaxine, desvenlafaxine	DO NOT COMBINE with pimozide or thioridazine; CAUTION with other FGAs; due to additive prolongation of QT interval. Increased plasma levels of thioridazine and other phenothiazines possible due to inhibition of CYP2D6 by duloxetine
SARI	Nefazodone	DO NOT COMBINE with pimozide or thioridazine; CAUTION with other FGAs; due to additive prolongation of QT interval. Increased plasma levels of pimozide possible due to inhibition of CYP3A4 by nefazodone Increased AUC (36%) and peak plasma level (13%) of haloperidol. Clinical significance likely minor
Irrev. MAOI, RIMA	Tranylcypromine, moclobemide	Additive hypotension
Antifungal	Ketoconazole, fluconazole, itraconazole, voriconazole	DO NOT COMBINE with pimozide or thioridazine. CAUTION with other FGAs. Possible additive prolongation of QT interval and associated life-threatening cardiac arrhythmias. Factors which further increase the risk include anorexia, bradycardia, hypokalemia, and hypomagnesemia Increased plasma levels of antipsychotics due to inhibition of metabolism via CYP3A4. Increased plasma level of haloperidol (by 30% with itraconazole). Consider using fluconazole or voriconazole (less potent inhibitors of CYP3A4 than itraconazole and ketoconazole) or terbinafine. Monitor for increased antipsychotic adverse effects (e.g., EPS) when starting and antipsychotic efficacy when stopping antifungals. Adjust antipsychotic dose as needed
Antihypertensive	Methyldopa, enalapril, clonidine Guanethidine	Additive hypotensive effect Reversal of antihypertensive effect with chlorpromazine, haloperidol, and thiothixene (not reported with molindone) due to blockade of guanethidine uptake into postsynaptic neurons
Antiparkinsonian	Levodopa, pramipexole, ropinirole	Potential for reduced antiparkinson efficiency. Antipsychotics reduce dopamine while antiparkinson agents increase dopamine in the CNS. If an antipsychotic is necessary, consider using clozapine or quetiapine, which have been reported to be less likely to cause worsening control of movement disorders than other antipsychotics
Antipsychotic combination		Increased risk of anticholinergic effects, EPS, and elevated prolactin level with concurrent use of a second-generation antipsychotic (SGA) and a FGA or with concurrent use of two FGAs. Monitor for anticholinergic effects (e.g., dry mouth, urinary retention), EPS (e.g., cogwheeling rigidity, unstable gait), and hyperprolactinemia (e.g., galactorrhea) CAUTION – possible additive prolongation of QT interval and associated life-threatening cardiac arrhythmias. Factors which further increase the risk include anorexia, bradycardia, hypokalemia, and hypomagnesemia

"First-Generation" Antipsychotics / FGAs (cont.)

Class of Drug	Example	Interaction Effects
	Haloperidol + SGAs	With clozapine, a case of elevated haloperidol levels and a case of NMS
		With olanzapine, a case of extreme parkinsonism potentially due to competitive inhibition of CYP2D6 and/or additive adverse effects
	Haloperidol + phenothiazines	Increased plasma levels of haloperidol due to inhibition of metabolism via CYP2D6 (by 29% with chlorpromazine). Clinical significance unknown. Possible additive QT prolongation (see above)
	Phenothiazines (e.g., chlorpromazine) + SGAs	Possible additive QT prolongation (see above). DO NOT COMBINE with risperidone, paliperidone or ziprasidone
	Pimozide + SGAs	Possible additive QT prolongation (see above). DO NOT COMBINE with risperidone, paliperidone or ziprasidone
	Thioridazine + SGAs	Possible additive QT prolongation (see above). DO NOT COMBINE with risperidone, paliperidone or ziprasidone
		Increased clearance (i.e., decreased plasma levels) of quetiapine by 65%. Possible increased plasma levels of clozapine and risperidone due to inhibition of metabolism via CYP2D6. Increased SGA levels have the potential to further increase the risk of QT prolongation
	Pimozide, thioridazine + FGAs	DO NOT COMBINE. Possible additive QT prolongation (see above)
Antitubercular drug	Isoniazid	Limited data suggests some may experience increased plasma levels of haloperidol. Monitor antipsychotic for antipsychotic adverse effects when starting and antipsychotic efficacy when stopping isoniazid. Adjust antipsychotic dose as needed
	Rifampin, rifabutin, rifapentine	Decreased plasma levels of haloperidol (by 30–63%) due to induction via CYP3A4 and/or P-glycoprotein with rifampin. Monitor antipsychotic efficacy when starting and antipsychotic adverse effects when stopping rifampin. Adjust antipsychotic dose as needed
Anxiolytic Benzodiazepines	Clonazepam, buspirone, diazepam, lorazepam	Increased plasma level of haloperidol (by 19%) Synergistic effect with antipsychotics; used to calm agitated patients May increase extrapyramidal reactions Conflicting information with respect to effects on haloperidol levels from no change to increased levels. Likely no clinically significant interaction
Belladonna alkaloid		Additive anticholinergic effects. Because belladonna is typically available as a homeopathic preparation, the clinical significance of the interaction is unknown. Caution is advised
Beta-blocker	Propranolol	DO NOT COMBINE with thioridazine. Increased plasma level of thioridazine (3- to 5-fold) due to inhibition of metabolism via CYP2D6, thus increasing the risk of cardiotoxicity (QT prolongation, cardiac arrest)
		Increased plasma level of both chlorpromazine (5-fold) and propranolol (decreased clearance by 25–32%). Case report of delirium and seizures. With haloperidol, case report of a severe hypotensive reaction. Start propranolol at a reduced dose. Monitor blood pressure and for antipsychotic adverse effects when starting propranolol
	Pindolol	DO NOT COMBINE with thioridazine. Increased plasma level of thioridazine due to inhibition of metabolism via CYP2D6, thus increasing the risk of cardiotoxicity (QT prolongation, cardiac arrest) and pindolol levels may be increased. Pindolol may increase plasma levels of other phenothiazines
Betel nut		Increased EPS adverse effects due to potent cholinergic effects of the herb
Calcium-channel blocker	Diltiazem, verapamil	DO NOT COMBINE with pimozide or thioridazine. Increased risk of cardiotoxicity (QT prolongation, cardiac arrest) due to possible additive calcium-channel blocking effects and increased plasma levels of pimozide due to inhibition of metabolism via CYP3A4

Class of Drug	Example	Interaction Effects
Caffeine	Coffee, tea, cola, guarana or mate containing products	Increased akathisia/agitation
CNS depressant	Alcohol, hypnotics, antihistamines	Increased CNS effects (e.g., sedation, fatigue, impaired cognition). Additive orthostatic hypotension Alcohol may worsen EPS
Disulfiram		Case report of decreased plasma level of perphenazine, increased level of its metabolite, and clinical decline Potentially due to inhibition of CYP2E1
Evening primrose oil		CAUTION. May lower the seizure threshold. Case reports of seizures with concurrent use of evening primrose oil and phenothiazines
Grapefruit juice		AVOID with pimozide. Increased plasma level of pimozide possible due to inhibition of metabolism via CYP3A4, which increases the risk cardiotoxicity (QT prolongation, cardiac arrest)
H$_2$ antagonist	Cimetidine	Both elevated chlorpromazine plasma levels and decreased absorption of chlorpromazine have been reported. Chlorpromazine absorption may be decreased at higher doses of cimetidine, possibly due to increased gastric pH. Chlorpromazine metabolism may be decreased by inhibition of CYP2D6. May interact with other phenothiazines. Monitor for antipsychotic efficacy and adverse effects. OR switch to a H2-antagonist (e.g., ranitidine or famotidine) that has less potential to alter drug metabolism
Hormone	Oral contraceptive	Estrogen potentiates hyperprolactinemic effect of antipsychotics Case report of increased plasma level of chlorpromazine (6-fold) with an oral contraceptive (ethinyl estradiol [50 micrograms]/norgestrel [0.5 mg])
Lithium		Particular care should be taken to avoid toxic plasma levels of lithium when it is used concurrently with pimozide or thioridazine, since both pimozide/thioridazine and toxic lithium levels are associated with QT prolongation Although numerous studies indicate lithium and FGAs can be safely used together, there are rare cases of severe neurotoxicity (e.g., delirium, seizures, encephalopathy) and EPS with concurrent lithium and haloperidol, loxapine, thiothixene or phenothiazines. In the majority of these cases, lithium was within therapeutic range. Factors that may increase the risk of developing this interaction are the presence of acute mania, pre-existing brain damage, infection, fever, dehydration, a history of EPS and high doses of one or both agents. Monitor patients closely particularly during the first 3 weeks; monitor lithium levels. Use the lowest effective doses; consider maintaining lithium in the lower end of the therapeutic range Decreased plasma levels of chlorpromazine (by 40%) and both increased and decreased lithium levels reported
Narcotic	Codeine	Inhibition of conversion of codeine to its active metabolite, morphine, with haloperidol and phenothiazines. May only be clinically relevant in those with the extensive metabolizer CYP2D6 phenotype. Monitor for efficacy of pain control. Switch to an analgesic which doesn't require CYP2D6 conversion if needed
	Methadone	DO NOT COMBINE with pimozide or thioridazine. CAUTION with other FGAs. Possible additive prolongation of QT interval and associated life-threatening cardiac arrhythmias. Factors which further increase the risk include anorexia, bradycardia, hypokalemia, and hypomagnesemia
	Tramadol	CAUTION. Potential increased risk of seizures with FGAs
Protease inhibitor	Ritonavir, indinavir	AVOID with pimozide and thioridazine. Increased plasma levels of pimozide/thioridazine possible due to inhibition of metabolism via CYP3A4 or CYP2D6, respectively, which increases the risk cardiotoxicity (QT prolongation, cardiac arrest) Increased levels of haloperidol and phenothiazines possible. Clinical significance unknown
QT-prolonging agent	Antimalarials (e.g., chloroquine, mefloquine), antiprotozoals (e.g., pentamidine), contrast agents (e.g., gadobutrol), dolasetron, droperidol, ranolazine, tacrolimus	DO NOT COMBINE with pimozide or thioridazine. CAUTION with other FGAs. Possible additive prolongation of QT interval and associated life-threatening cardiac arrhythmias. A study suggests ziprasidone causes less QT prolongation than thioridazine but about twice that of quetiapine, risperidone, haloperidol, and olanzapine. Factors which further increase the risk include anorexia, bradycardia, hypokalemia, and hypomagnesemia

Clinical Handbook of Psychotropic Drugs, 18th Edition, © 2009 Hogrefe & Huber Publishers

Antipsychotics

"First-Generation" Antipsychotics / FGAs (cont.)

Class of Drug	Example	Interaction Effects
Smoking (tobacco)		Decreased plasma levels of chlorpromazine (by 24%) and thioridazine (by 46%) due to the induction of metabolism via CYP1A2. Similar interaction with other phenothiazines possible. Dosage modifications not routinely recommended but smokers may require higher doses for efficacy. Caution when patient stops smoking as level of antipsychotic will increase; reduce antipsychotic dose as necessary
Stimulant	Amphetamine Methylphenidate	Antipsychotics can counteract many signs of stimulant toxicity Case reports of worsening of tardive movement disorder and prolongation or exacerbation of withdrawal dyskinesia following antipsychotic discontinuation Antipsychotic agents may impair the stimulatory effect of amphetamines. Concurrent use not recommended. If used, monitor effectiveness of amphetamine therapy when starting, stopping or changing the dose of an antipsychotic CAUTION. Potential to exacerbate psychiatric conditions as stimulant-induced psychosis can occur
Sympathomimetic	Epinephrine, norepinephrine	May result in paradoxical fall in blood pressure (due to α-adrenergic block produced by antipsychotics); benefits may outweigh risk in anaphylaxis; phenylephrine is a safe substitute for hypotension

Effects of Antipsychotics on Neurotransmitters/Receptors*

	Chlor-promazine	Methotrime-prazine	Pericyazine	Pipotiazine	Thioridazine	Fluphena-zine	Perphena-zine	Thiopro-perazine	Trifluo-perazine	Haloperidol	Loxapine
D_1 blockade	+++	?	?	?	+++	+++	+++	?	+++	+++	+++
D_2 blockade	++++	+++	++++	+++++	++++	+++++	+++++	+++++	++++	+++++	++++
D_3 blockade	++++	?	?	+++++	++++	+++++	?	++++	?	++++	?
D_4 blockade	+++	?	?	?	+++	++++	?	+++	+++	+++	+++
H_1 blockade	+++	+++++	?	?	+++	+++	++++	?	++	+	+++
M_1 blockade	+++	?	?	?	++++	+	+	?	+	+	++
α_1 blockade	++++	?	?	?	++++	+++	+++	?	+++	+++	+++
α_2 blockade	++	?	+	?	+	+	++	+	+	+	+
$5\text{-}HT_{2A}$ blockade	++++	++++	?	+++	++++	++++	++++	++	++++	+++	++++

	Molindone	Pimozide	Flupenthixol	Thiothixene	Zuclopen-thixol	Clozapine	Risperidone	Olanzapine	Quetiapine	Ziprasidone	Aripiprazole	Paliperidone
D_1 blockade	+	++	++++	++	+++++	+++	+++	+++	++	+++	?	?
D_2 blockade	++++	++++	+++++	+++++	+++++	++	++++	+++	++	++++	+++++[A]	++++
D_3 blockade	?	++++	++++	?	?	++	+++	+++	++	++++	++++	?
D_4 blockade	+	+++	?	?	+++	++++	++++	+++	−	+++	+++	?
H_1 blockade	+/−	+	+++	+++	+++	++++	+++	++++	+++	+++	+++	+++
M_1 blockade	−	+	+++	+	++	++++	+	++++	++	+/−	+/−	+/−
α_1 blockade	+	+++	+++	++	++++	++	++++	+++	++++	+++	+++	++++
α_2 blockade	++	++	++	++	++	++	++++	++	+++	+−	?	+++
$5\text{-}HT_{2A}$ blockade	+	+++	++++	+++	++++	++++	+++++	++++	+++	+++++	++++	+++++

* The ratio of K_i values between various neurotransmitters/receptors determines the pharmacological profile for any one drug.
Key: K_i (nM) > 100,000 = −; 10,000–100,000 = +/−; 1000–10,000 = +; 100–1000 = ++; 10–100 = +++; 1–10 = ++++; 0.1–1 = +++++; $1/K_i$ < 0.001 = −; .001–.01 = +/−; .01–.1 = +; .1–1 = ++; 1–10 = +++; 10–100 = ++++; 100–1000 = +++++;
? = unknown

See p. 130 for Pharmacological Effects on Neurotransmitters. [A] Partial agonist; [B] Agonist

Adapted from: Seeman P. Receptor Tables Vol. 2: Drug Dissociation Constants for Neuroreceptors and Transporters. Toronto: SZ Research, 1993; Leysen JE, Janssen PM, Schotte A, et al. Interaction of antipsychotic drugs with neurotransmitter receptor sites in vitro and in vivo in relation to pharmacological and clinical effects: Role of 5-HT2 receptors. Psychopharmacology (Berl). 1993;112(1 Suppl):S40–S54; Seeman P, Corbett A, Nam D, et al. Dopamine and serotonin receptors: amino acid sequences, and clinical role in neuroleptic parkinsonism. Jpn J Pharmacol. 1996;71(3):187–204.; Richelson E, J Clin Psychiatry. 1996;57(11 Suppl):4–11; Seeman P. Atypical antipsychotics: Mechanism of action. Can J Psychiatry. 2002;47(1):27–38; Brunton LL, Lazo JS, Parker KL. Goodman & Gilman's The pharmacological basis of therapeutics (11th ed.). New York: McGraw Hill, 2006; Buckley PF. Receptor-binding profiles of antipsychotics: Clinical strategies when switching between agents. J Clin Psychiatry. 2007;68(Suppl 6):5-9; Gardner DM, Baldessarini RJ, Waraich P. Modern antipsychotic drugs; a critical overview. CMAJ 2005;172(13):1703–1711; Horacek J, Bubenikova-Valesova V, Kopecek M. Mechanism of action of atypical antipsychotic drugs and the neurobiology of schizophrenia. CNS Drugs 2006;20(5):389–409.

Pharmacological Effects of Antipsychotics on Neurotransmitters/Receptors

Dopamine Blockade	• Additive or synergistic interactions occur between various dopamine receptor subtypes
D_1 Blockade	• May mediate antipsychotic effect; the clinical significance of D_1 receptor antagonism is currently unknown
D_2 Blockade	• In mesolimbic area – antipsychotic effect: correlates with clinical efficacy in controlling positive symptoms of schizophrenia; an inverse relationship exists between D_2 blockade and therapeutic antipsychotic dosage (i.e., potent blockade = low mg dose) • In nigrostriatal tract – adverse effect: extrapyramidal (e.g., tremor, rigidity, etc.) • In tuberinfundibular area – adverse effect: prolactin elevation (e.g., galactorrhea, etc.)
D_3 Blockade	• The clinical significance of D_3 receptor antagonism is currently unknown
D_4 Blockade	• The clinical significance of D_4 receptor antagonism is currently unknown
H_1 Blockade	• Anti-emetic effect • Adverse effects: sedation, drowsiness, postural hypotension, weight gain • Potentiation of effects of other CNS drugs
ACh Blockade	• Mitigation of extrapyramidal adverse effects • Adverse effects: dry mouth, blurred vision, constipation, urinary retention and incontinence, sinus tachycardia, QRS changes, memory disturbances, sedation • Potentiation of effects of drugs with anticholinergic properties
α_1 Blockade	• Adverse effects: postural hypotension, dizziness, reflex tachycardia, sedation, hypersalivation, urinary incontinence • Potentiation of antihypertensives acting via α_1 blockade (e.g., prazosin)
α_2 Blockade	• May lead to increased release of acetylcholine and increased cholinergic activity • Adverse effect: sexual dysfunction • Antagonism of antihypertensives acting via α_2 stimulants (e.g., clonidine)
5-HT$_2$ Blockade	• May correlate with clinical efficacy in decreasing negative symptoms of schizophrenia (data speculative); may modulate (decrease) extrapyramidal effects caused by D_2 blockade • Anxiolytic (5-HT_{2C}); antidepressant, antiaggressive and anti-agitation and antipsychotic effect (5-HT_{2A}) • Adverse effects: hypotension, sedation, weight gain (5-HT_{2C})

Frequency (%) of Adverse Reactions to Antipsychotics at Therapeutic Doses

"FIRST-GENERATION" AGENTS

Reaction	Phenothiazines – Aliphatic		Phenothiazines – Piperidine			Phenothiazines – Piperazine				Haloperidol	Pimozide
	Chlor-promazine	Metho-trimeprazine	Pericyazine	Pipotiazine	Thioridazine	Fluphenazine	Perphenazine	Thiopro-perazine	Trifluo-perazine		
CNS Effects											
Drowsiness, sedation	> 30	> 30	> 30	> 10	> 30	> 2	> 10	> 2	> 2	> 2[c]	> 10
Insomnia, agitation	< 2	< 2	< 2	< 2	< 2	> 2	> 10	> 2	> 2	> 10	> 2
Extrapyramidal Effects											
Parkinsonism	> 10	> 10	> 2	> 30	> 2	> 30	> 10	> 30	> 30	> 30[h]	> 30
Akathisia	> 2	> 2	> 2	> 10	> 2	> 30	> 10	> 30	> 30	> 30	> 10
Dystonic reactions	> 2	< 2	< 2	< 2	< 2	> 10	> 10	> 10	> 10	> 30[h]	> 2
Anticholinergic Effects	> 30	> 30	> 30	> 10	> 30	> 2	> 10	> 2	> 10	> 2	> 2
Cardiovascular Effects											
Orthostatic hypotension	> 30[c]	> 30[b,c]	> 10	> 2	> 30	> 2	> 10	> 2	> 10	> 2	> 2
Tachycardia	> 10	> 10	> 10	< 2	< 2	> 10	> 10	> 10	< 2	< 2	> 2
ECG abnormalities*	> 30[d]	> 10	< 2	< 2	> 30[d]	< 2	> 2	< 2	< 2	< 2	> 2[j]
QTc prolongation (> 450 ms)	> 2[d]	> 2	> 2	> 2	> 10[d]	> 2[d]	< 2	–	> 2	> 2[d]	> 2[j]
Endocrine Effects											
Sexual dysfunction[e]	> 30[f]	> 2[f]	> 10[f]	> 10	> 30[f]	> 30[f]	> 10[f]	> 2	> 30[f]	> 30[f]	> 30
Galactorrhea	> 30	> 30	> 10	> 30	> 30	> 10	> 10	> 10	> 10	< 2	< 2
Weight gain	> 30	> 10	> 10	> 10	> 30	> 30	> 10	> 10	> 10	> 10	> 2[p]
Hyperglycemia	> 30	> 2[s]	> 2[s]	> 2[s]	> 2[s]	> 10	> 10	> 2[s]	> 2	> 10	> 2
Hyperlipidemia	> 30	?	?	?	> 30	?	> 2[s]	?	?	> 2	?
Ocular Effects[a]											
Lenticular pigmentation	> 2	> 2	> 2	> 2	> 2	< 2	< 2	< 2	< 2	< 2	< 2
Pigmentary retinopathy	> 2[a]	> 2[a]	–	–	> 10[a]	–	< 2	< 2	< 2	–	–
Blood dyscrasias	< 2	< 2	< 2	< 2	< 2	< 2	< 2	< 2	< 2	< 2	< 2
Hepatic disorder	< 2	< 2	< 2	< 2	< 2	< 2	< 2	< 2	< 2	< 2	< 2
Seizures[g]	< 2[c]	< 2	< 2	< 2	< 2	< 2	< 2	< 2	< 2	< 2	< 2
Skin Reactions											
Photosensitivity	> 10	> 10	> 2	> 2	> 10[d]	< 2	< 2	< 2	< 2	< 2	–
Rashes	> 10	> 2	> 2	> 2	> 10	< 2	< 2	< 2	< 2	< 2	> 2
Pigmentation[a]	> 30[d]	< 2	–	–	> 2	–	–	–	–	< 2	–

Clinical Handbook of Psychotropic Drugs, 18th Edition, © 2009 Hogrefe & Huber Publishers

Antipsychotics

Frequency (%) of Adverse Reactions to Antipsychotics at Therapeutic Doses (cont.)

| | "FIRST-GENERATION" AGENTS | | | | | "SECOND-GENERATION" AGENTS | | | | | | "3RD GEN." |
| | | | Thioxanthenes | | | | | | | | | |
Reaction	Loxapine	Molindone	Flupenthixol	Thiothixene	Zuclopen-thixol	Clozapine	Paliperidone	Risperidone	Olanzapine	Quetiapine	Ziprasidone	Aripiprazole
CNS Effects												
Drowsiness, sedation	> 30	> 30	> 2	> 10	> 30	> 30	> 2	> 10[b]	> 30	> 30	> 10	> 10
Insomnia, agitation	< 2	> 2	< 2	> 10	> 10	> 2	> 10	> 10	> 10	> 10	> 30	> 10
Extrapyramidal Effects												
Parkinsonism	> 30	> 30	> 30	> 30	> 30	> 2	> 2	> 10[i]	> 2	> 2	> 2	> 2
Akathisia	> 30	< 30	> 30	> 30	> 10	> 10	> 2	> 10[i]	> 10	> 2	> 2	> 10
Dystonic reactions	> 10	> 30	> 10	> 2	> 10[h]	< 2	< 2	< 2[i]	< 2	< 2	> 2	< 2
Anticholinergic Effects	> 10	> 10	> 10	> 2	> 10[k]	> 30[k]	> 2	> 10	> 30	> 30	> 10	> 2
Cardiovascular Effects												
Orthostatic hypotension	> 10	> 2	> 2	> 2	> 2	> 10[b]	> 2	> 10[b]	> 2	> 10	> 10	> 2
Tachycardia	> 10	< 2	> 2	> 2	> 2	> 10[b]	> 2	> 10	< 2[q]	> 2	> 2	> 2
ECG abnormalities*	< 2	< 2	> 2	< 2	< 2	> 30[d]	< 2	> 2	< 2	< 2	> 2[d]	< 2
QTc prolongation (> 450 ms)	–	–	< 2	< 2	< 2	< 2[d]	> 2	< 2	< 2	< 2	< 2[d]	–
Endocrine Effects												
Sexual dysfunction[e]	> 2	< 2[f]	> 30[f]	> 2[f]	> 30[f]	< 2[f]	< 2	> 30[f]	> 30[f]	> 30[f]	< 2[f]	< 2[f]
Galactorrhea	> 2	< 2	–	< 2	–	< 2	< 2	> 10	> 2	–	> 2	< 2
Weight gain	< 2[p]	< 2[p]	> 10	> 10	> 10	> 30	> 10	> 30	> 30	> 10	> 2	> 2[r]
Hyperglycemia	> 2[s]	> 2	> 10	> 2[s]	> 2[s]	> 30	?	> 10	> 30	> 30	> 2	< 2
Hyperlipidemia	> 10	?	?	?	?	> 30	?	> 10	> 30	> 10	< 2	< 2
Ocular Effects[a]												
Lenticular pigmentation	< 2	–	< 2	< 2	< 2	–	?	–	–	< 2	–	–
Pigmentary retinopathy	< 2	–	< 2	< 2	–	–	–	–	–	–	–	–
Blood dyscrasias	< 2	< 2	< 2	< 2	< 2	< 2[n]	?	< 2	< 2	–	< 2	< 2
Hepatic disorder	< 2	> 2	< 2	< 2	< 2	> 2	?	< 2	> 2	> 2	–	< 2
Seizures[g]	< 2	> 2[m]	< 2	< 2	< 2	> 2[o]	< 2	< 2	< 2	< 2	–	< 2
Skin Reactions												
Photosensitivity	< 2	–	< 2	< 2	< 2	> 2	?	> 2	–	–	–	< 2
Rashes	> 2	> 2	> 2	< 2	< 2	> 2	?	< 2	< 2	< 2	> 2	> 2
Pigmentation[a]	–	–	–	> 2	< 2	–	?	< 2	–	–	–	–

Data are pooled from separate studies and are not necessarily comparable

– = None reported in literature perused, *= ECG abnormalities usually without cardiac injury including ST segment depression, flattened T waves, and increased U wave amplitude

[a] Usually seen after prolonged use, [b] May be higher at start of therapy or with rapid dose increase, [c] More frequent with rapid dose increase, [d] Higher doses pose greater risk, [e] Includes impotence, inhibition of ejaculation, anorgasmia, [f] Priapism reported, [g] In nonepileptic patients, [h] Lower incidence with depot preparation, [i] Increased risk with oral doses above 10 mg daily, [j] Pimozide above 20 mg daily poses greater risk, [k] Sialorrhea reported, [m] Doses above 300 mg daily pose greater risk, [n] Risk < 2% with strict monitoring (legal requirement in North America), [o] Risk lower with doses below 300 mg, and increased at higher doses or single doses above 300 mg, [p] Weight loss reported, [q] Bradycardia frequent with IM olanzapine; often accompanied by hypotension [r] Weight loss reported [s] Reported to occur, but no definitive data published as to incidence

Antipsychotic Doses and Pharmacokinetics (Oral and Short-Acting Injections)

SECOND-GENERATION AGENTS (SGAs)											
Drug	CDD (mg)**	ACE in Schizo- phrenia (mg)*	Monograph Doses for Psychosis	Bioavail- ability	Protein Binding	Peak Plasma Level (h) T_{max}	Elimination Half-Life (h)	Metabolizing Enzymes[j] (CYP-450; other)	Enzyme Inhibition[k] (CYP-450; other)	%D2 Receptor Occupancy[o] (dose & plasma level)[b]	%5-HT2A Occupancy (dose)
Benzisoxazole Risperidone (Risperdal)	2–2.5	1.5	Orally: 1–2 mg od to bid to start and increase by 0.5–1 mg q 3–7 days Usual daily dose: 4–6 mg daily Doses above 10 mg/day do not usually produce further im- provement	60–80%	88–90% (parent) 77% (metabolite)	1–1.5 (parent) 3 (metabolite)	3–15 (active metabolite = 20–24) Increased in hepatic or renal disease	**2D6**[p], 3A4; P-gp	2D6, 3A4[w]	60–75% (2–4 mg) 63–85% (2–6 mg; 36–252 nmol/l)	60–90% (1–4 mg)
Paliperidone (active metabolite of risper- idone; Invega)			Orally: 6 mg od If needed, increase by 3 mg q 5 days to a maximum of 12 mg/ day	28–38%	74% (to albu- min and alpha- 1-AGP)	24	23	2D6[w], 3A4[w]	–		
Dibenzodiazepine Clozapine (Clozaril)	200–250? (CDD un- clear)[g]	100	Orally: 12.5 mg od or bid on day 1, 25–50 mg on day 2, then in- crease gradually by 25–50 mg daily increments up to 300– 450 mg daily Doses not to exceed 900 mg daily Prescribing restrictions: see p. 90	40–60%	95–97% (to alpha-1-AGP)	1.5–4.5	6–33 11–105 (active metabolite) Caution in the elderly Reduced in smokers (20–40% shorter)	**1A2**[p], 2D6[w], 3A4, 2C9[w], 2C19[w], 2E1[w]; FMO; UGT1A4; P-gp[w]	1A2[w], 2D6[w], 3A4, 2C9[w], 2C19, 2E1[w]	38–68%[i] (300–900 mg; 600–2500 nmol/l)[g]	85–94% (> 125 mg)
Dibenzothiazepine Quetiapine (Seroquel)	300–400? (CDD un- clear)	200	Orally: 25 mg bid to start; increase by 25–50 mg bid per day, as tolerated, to a target dose of 300 mg per day (given bid) within 4–7 days Usual daily dose: 300–600 mg daily, in divided doses Doses above 800 mg/day not recommended	~73% (rela- tive bioavail- ability; absolute un- known)	83%	0.5–3	6–7 Prolonged in hepatic dis- ease (45% longer; based on a low-, single-dose study in those with mild disease), renal disease (25% longer; based on a low-, single- dose study in those with severe disease), and the elderly (30–50% longer)	**3A4**[p], 2D6[w]; P-gp	1A2[w], 2D6[w], 3A4[w], 2C9[w], 2C19[w]	20–44%[i] (300–700 mg) 13–41% (150–750 mg)	21–80%[i] (150–600 mg) 38–74% (150–750 mg)
(Seroquel XR)			Orally (XR): 300 mg once daily on day 1, 600 mg daily on day 2, then increase to 800 mg daily if needed. Maximum 800 mg/day			~6	~6–7				

Antipsychotic Doses and Pharmacokinetics (Oral and Short-Acting Injections) (cont.)

SECOND-GENERATION AGENTS (SGAs)

Drug	CDD (mg)**	ACE in Schizophrenia (mg)*	Monograph Doses for Psychosis	Bioavailability	Protein Binding	Peak Plasma Level (h) T_{max}	Elimination Half-Life (h)	Metabolizing Enzymes[j] (CYP-450; other)	Enzyme Inhibition[k] (CYP-450; other)	%D2 Receptor Occupancy[a] (dose & plasma level)[b]	%5-HT2A Occupancy (dose)
Thienobenzodiazepine Olanzapine (Zyprexa)	7.5–10	5	Orally: 5–10 mg daily to start; target dose of 10 mg Further dose increases at intervals of not less than 1 week Doses above 20 mg/day not recommended IM: 5–10 mg to start (2.5–5 mg in the elderly) If a third dose is required, give no sooner than 4 h after the second dose. Maximum 20 mg/day with no more than 3 injections in 24 h	57–80%	93% (to albumin and alpha-1-AGP)	5–8 IM: 15–45 min	21–54 (30 mean) No change in hepatic disease (only based on single-dose study) or renal disease Prolonged in the elderly (1.5 times longer) and females (30% longer – clinical significance unclear) Reduced in smokers (40% shorter)	1A2, 2D6[w]; FMO; UGT1A4	1A2[w], 2D6[w], 3A4[w], 2C9[w], 2C19[w]	55–80% (5–20 mg; 59–187 nmol/l) 83–88% (30–40 mg)	80–90% (5–20 mg)
Benzothiazolylpiperazine Ziprasidone (Geodon[c], Zeldox[d])	40–80	40	Orally: 20–40 mg bid to start. If needed, increase q 2 days or longer. Doses above 80 mg bid generally not recommended IM: 10 mg q 2 h or 20 mg q 4 h to a maximum of 40 mg/24 h for up to 3 days	30% (60% with food) IM: 100%	>99% (to albumin and alpha-1-AGP)	6–8 (C_{max} increased 32–72% in mild renal impairment) IM: ~60 min	4–10 dose-dependent (6.6 mean) No change in the elderly or renal disease Prolonged in hepatic disease (mean in hepatic disease = 7.1 vs. 4.8 in control group) IM: 2–5 h IM: Caution in renal disease due to excipient (cyclodextrin)	**3A4**[p], 1A2[w], 2D6, 3C18/19; Aldehyde oxydase[p]	2D6[w], 3A4[w]	45–75% (40–80 mg)	80–90% (40–80 mg)

THIRD-GENERATION AGENT (TGA)

Drug	CDD (mg)**	ACE in Schizophrenia (mg)*	Monograph Doses for Psychosis	Bioavailability	Protein Binding	Peak Plasma Level (h) T_{max}	Elimination Half-Life (h)	Metabolizing Enzymes[j] (CYP-450; other)	Enzyme Inhibition[k] (CYP-450; other)	%D2 Receptor Occupancy[a] (dose & plasma level)[b]	%5-HT2A Occupancy (dose)
Aripiprazole (Abilify)[c]	5–10	10	Orally: Start and usual dose: 10–15 mg od. If needed, increase dose q 2 weeks (up to 30 mg – doses above 15 mg not shown to be more effective)	87% (tablet; slightly higher with solution form) IM: 100%	99% (to albumin)	3–5 IM: 1–3	75–146 (active metabolite = 94) No change in renal or hepatic impairment or in elderly Only based on single-dose studies in those with renal or hepatic impairment	2D6, 3A4	–	40–95% (0.5–30 mg)	?

Drug	CDD (mg)**	ACE in Schizo-phrenia (mg)*	Monograph Doses for Psychosis	Bioavail-ability	Protein Binding	Peak Plasma Level (h) T_{max}	Elimination Half-Life (h)	Metabolizing Enzymes[i] (CYP-450; other)	Enzyme Inhibition[k] (CYP-450; other)	%D2 Receptor Occupancy[a] (dose & plasma level)[b]	%5-HT2A Occupancy (dose)
Butyrophenone Haloperidol (Haldol)	2	4	Orally: Start: 0.5–2 mg bid or tid Usual maximum = 20 mg/day 85–100 mg daily used rarely Short-Acting IM (lactate): 2–5 mg q 4–6h prn; may repeat q 1 h if required	40–80%	92% (to alpha-1-AGP)	0.5–3	12–36	1A2[w], 2D6[w], **3A4**[p]	**2D6**, 3A4; P-gp[w]	75–89% (4–6 mg; 6–13 nmol/l)	?
Dibenzoxazepine Loxapine (Loxapac, Loxitane)	15	40	Orally: Start: 10 mg bid (up to 50 mg daily if needed) Usual = 60–100 mg daily in divided doses 2–4 times daily; higher than 250 mg/day is not recommended	33%	?	?	Oral = 4 h IM = 12 h 8–30 (metabolite)	1A2, 2D6, 3A4; UGT1A4	–	60–80% (15–30 mg)	58–75% (10–30 mg) 75–90% metabolite (> 30 mg)
Dihydroindolone Molindone (Moban)[c]	10	50	Orally: Start: 50–75 mg daily in divided doses; increase by 25 mg q 3–4 days; Maximum = 225 mg/day	?	76%	0.5–2	6.5	2D6	–	?	?
Diphenylbutyl-piperidine Pimozide (Orap)	2	2	Orally: Start: 2–4 mg once daily; increase by 2–4 mg q week; average dose: 6 mg/day Doses above 20 mg/day not recommended[e]	15–50%	97%	8	29–55[f]	1A2[w], **3A4**[p]	**2D6**[p], 3A4; P-gp[p]	77–79% (4–8 mg)	?

Antipsychotic Doses and Pharmacokinetics (Oral and Short-Acting Injections) (cont.)

FIRST-GENERATION AGENTS (FGAs)

Drug	CDD (mg)**	ACE in Schizo-phrenia (mg)*	Monograph Doses for Psychosis	Bioavail-ability	Protein Binding	Peak Plasma Level (h) T_{max}	Elimination Half-Life (h)	Metabolizing Enzymes[i] (CYP-450; other)	Enzyme Inhibition[k] (CYP-450; other)	%D2 Receptor Occupancy[a] (dose & plasma level)[b]	%5-HT2A Occupancy (dose)
Phenothiazines – Aliphatic											
Chlorpromazine (Largactil, Thorazine)	100	100	Orally: Start: 25–75 mg daily in 2–4 divided doses; increase by 20–50 mg twice weekly. Recommended maximum 1 g/day Short-Acting IM: Start: 25 mg followed by 25–50 mg in 1 h if needed. Can increase over several days. Recommended maximum 400 mg q 4–6 h	25–65%	95–99% (to albumin)	0.5–1	16–30	1A2[w], **2D6**[p], 3A4[w]; UGT1A4	1A2, **2D6**[p], 3A4[w], 2C9[w], 2C19, 2E1; P-gp	78–80% (100–200 mg; 10 nmol/l)	?
Methotrimeprazine[d] (Nozinan)	70	Rarely used	Orally (for severe psychosis): Start: 50–200 mg daily divided into 2 or 3 daily doses. Caution if starting with 100 mg or greater/day. Increase up to 1 g or more day if needed. Short-Acting IM: 75–100 mg daily given as 3 or 4 deep IM injections	?	?	1–3	16–78	1A2, 2D6; P-gp	**2D6**[p]; P-gp	?	?
Phenothiazines – Piperazine											
Fluphenazine HCl (Moditen, Prolixin)	2	4	Orally: Start: 2.5–10 mg daily in divided doses q 6–8 h. Doses greater than 20 mg = use with caution Short-Acting IM or SC: Start: 1.25 mg. Doses may range from 2.5 to 10 mg daily in divided doses q 6–8 h. Doses greater than 10 mg = use with caution	1–50%	90–99%	1.5–2	13–58	1A2, 2D6; P-gp	1A2, **2D6**[p], 3A4[w], 2E1 2C8/9; P-gp	?	?
Perphenazine (Trilafon)	10	8	Orally: Start: 8–16 mg bid to qid. Recommended maximum = 64 mg/day	25%	91–92%	1–4	9–21	1A2, **2D6**[p], 3A4, 2C9, 2C19	1A2[w], **2D6**[p], 3A4, 2C9, 2C19; P-gp	79% (4–8 mg)	?

FIRST-GENERATION AGENTS (FGAs)

Drug	CDD (mg)**	ACE in Schizo-phrenia (mg)*	Monograph Doses for Psychosis	Bioavail-ability	Protein Binding	Peak Plasma Level (h) T_{max}	Elimination Half-Life (h)	Metabolizing Enzymes[i] (CYP-450; other)	Enzyme Inhibition[k] (CYP-450; other)	%D2 Receptor Occupancy[a] (dose & plasma level)[b]	%5-HT2A Occupancy[a] (dose)
Thioproperazine (Majeptil)	5	10	Orally: Start: 5 mg in a single dose or divided doses; increase by 5 mg q 2–3 days. Usual dose = 30–40 mg/day. In some cases 90 mg or more daily may be needed	?	?	?	?	?	P-gp	?	?
Trifluoperazine (Stelazine)	5	6	Orally: Start: 2–5 mg bid or tid. Usual = 15–20 mg/day. A few may need 40 mg/day or more. 80 mg/day or more rarely necessary	?	95–99%	?	13	1A2[w]; P-gp; UGT1A4	P-gp	75–80% (5–10 mg)	?
Phenothiazines – Piperidine											
Pericyazine[d] (Neuleptil)	15	Not used	Orally: 5–20 mg in the morning and 10–40 mg in the evening	?	?	?	?	2D6	P-gp	?	?
Thioridazine[c] [l]	100	Not recom-mended	Orally: 150–400 mg daily in outpatients with severe symptoms given in 2–4 divided doses; 200–800 mg daily in hospitalized patients; Recommended maximum 800 mg/day	10–60%	97–99%	1–4	9–30	1A2[w], 2D6[w], 2C19[w]	1A2, **2D6**[p], 2C8/9, 2E1; P-gp; Inducer of 3A4	74–81% (100–400 mg; 620–900 nmol/l)	?
Thioxanthenes											
Flupenthixol (Fluanxol)	5	8	Orally: Start: 1 mg tid; increase by 1 mg q 2–3 days if needed. Usual = 3–6 mg daily in divided doses; up to 12 mg daily used in some patients	30–70%	99%	3–8	26–36	?	2D6[w]	70–74% (5–10 mg; 2–5 nmol/l)	?
Thiothixene (Navane)	5	10	Orally: Start: 5–10 mg daily. Usual = 15–30 mg daily; > 60 mg daily rarely increases response Short-Acting IM: 4 mg bid-qid. Usual = 16–20 mg/day. Range = 6–30 mg/day	50%	90–99%	1–3	34	**1A2**[p]	2D6[w]	?	?

Antipsychotic Doses and Pharmacokinetics (Oral and Short-Acting Injections) (cont.)

FIRST-GENERATION AGENTS (FGAs)

Drug	CDD (mg)**	ACE in Schizo-phrenia (mg)*	Monograph Doses for Psychosis	Bioavail-ability	Protein Binding	Peak Plasma Level (h) T_{max}	Elimination Half-Life (h)	Metabolizing Enzymes[i] (CYP-450; other)	Enzyme Inhibition[k] (CYP-450; other)	%D2 Receptor Occupancy[a] (dose & plasma level)[b]	%5-HT2A Occupancy (dose)
Zuclopenthixol[d] (Clopixol)	12	40	Orally: Start: 10–50 mg daily divided bid-tid; increase by 10–20 mg every 2 to 3 days; usual daily dose: 20–60 mg; doses above 100 mg daily not recommended	44%	98%	2–4	12–28	**2D6**[p]	2D6	?	?
Zuclopenthixol acetate[d] (Clopixol acuphase)	30 mg q 2–3 days	15 mg q 3 days	Usual dose: 50–150 mg IM and repeated every 2–3 days as needed to a maximum cumula-tive dose of 400 mg and maxi-mum of 4 injections (a second injection may need to be given 1–2 days after the first, in some patients)	–	98%	24–48	48–72	**2D6**[p]	2D6	?	?

NOTE: Comparable doses are only approximations. Generally doses used are higher in the acute stage of the illness than in maintenance. Monograph doses are just a guideline, and each patient's medication must be individualized. Plasma levels are available for some antipsychotics but their clinical usefulness is limited. The use of conversion ratios from an oral to a depot preparation is appropriate as a starting point, but wide intra- and interindividual variations in pharma-cokinetic parameters require careful clinical monitoring of the patient. It is recommended that the initially effective dose be reduced, or the injection interval increased, after 4–6 weeks to prevent possible accumulation of the drug as plasma concentrations approach steady-state.

CYP activity data from www.gentest.com/human_p450_database/srchh450.asp (December 2003) and Oesterheld JR, Osser DN. P450 Drug Interactions, http://www.mhc.com/Cytochromes; Flockhart DA. Drug interactions: Cytochrome P450 drug interaction table. Indiana University School of Medicine (2007). http://medicine.iupui.edu/flockhart/table.htm (Accessed July 2008); Product monographs of as July 2008; Lexicomp's Drug Interactions Handbook (2nd ed.) 2004 [Note: data regarding CYP450 profiles may not be consistent among references].

* Views of Dr. Jeffries, based on clinical judgment, ** Based on D_2 affinity and pharmacokinetics.

[a] D_2 receptor occupancy correlates better to plasma level than to dose, and appears to relate to clinical efficacy in controlling positive symptoms of schizophrenia as well as risk of extrapyramidal adverse effects (if > 80%), [b] Approximate conversion: nmol/l = 3 × ng/ml, [c] Not marketed in Canada, [d] Not marketed in USA, [e] Monitor cardiac function in doses above 15 mg/day, [f] Half-life longer (mean 66–111 h) in children and adults with Tourette's syndrome, [g] Threshold plasma level suggested for response in range of 350–500 ng/ml (see p. 99), [i] Cytochrome P-450 isoenzymes involved in drug metabolism, [k] CYP-450 isoenzymes inhibited by drug, [l] Indicated only for patients with schizophrenia who cannot tolerate other antipsychotic drugs or who fail to respond to them, [p] Potent activity, [w] Weak activity

ACE = Apparent Clinical Equivalence; Alpha-1-AGP = alpha-1-acid-glycoprotein; CDD = Comparable Daily Dose; FMO = flavin monooxygenase enzyme involved in N-oxidation reactions; P-gp = p-glycoprotein – a transporter of hydrophobic substances in or out of specific body organs (e.g., block absorption in the gut); UGT = uridine diphosphate glucuronosyl transferase – involved in Phase 2 reactions (conjugation)

Comparison of Long-acting IM Antipsychotics

	Flupenthixol decanoate (Fluanxol)	Fluphenazine decanoate (Modecate; Prolixin)	Haloperidol decanoate (Haldol LA)	Pipotiazine palmitate (Piportil L4)	Zuclopenthixol decanoate (Clopixol Depot)	Risperidone (Risperdal Consta)
Chemical class	Thioxanthene	Piperazine phenothiazine	Butyrophenone	Piperidine phenothiazine	Thioxanthene	Benzisoxazole
Form	Esterified with decanoic acid (a 10-carbon chain fatty acid) and dissolved in vegetable oil; must be hydrolyzed to free flupenthixol; metabolites inactive	Esterified with decanoic acid and dissolved in sesame oil; must be hydrolyzed to free fluphenazine	Esterified with decanoic acid and dissolved in sesame oil; must be hydrolyzed to free haloperidol	Esterified with palmitic acid in sesame oil; must be hydrolyzed to free pipotiazine	Esterified with decanoic acid in coconut oil; must be hydrolyzed to free zuclopenthixol	Encapsulated in a polymer as microspheres in an aqueous base; must be reconstituted just prior to use
Strength supplied	(2%)–20 mg/ml (10%)–100 mg/ml	25 mg/ml 100 mg/ml[B]	50 mg/ml 100 mg/ml	25 mg/ml[B] 50 mg/ml[B]	200 mg/ml[B]	12.5 mg/vial, 25 mg/vial, 37.5 mg/vial, 50 mg/vial
Starting dose	Long-acting IM naive: test dose of 5–20 mg; assess over next 5–10 days Non-naive: 20–40 mg Increase in increments not exceeding 20 mg	IM or SC: 2.5–12.5 mg	10–20 times previous oral dose to a max. of 100 mg	50–100 mg; Increase in increments of 25 mg q 2–3 weeks, if needed	100–200 mg	12.5–25 mg
Usual dose range	20–80 mg	12.5–50 mg	50–200 mg	50–250 mg	150–300 mg	25–50 mg
Maximum dose***	> 80 mg doses generally unnecessary	> 50 mg doses generally unnecessary; doses up to 100 mg have been used in some cases	450 mg/month	250 mg	400 mg q 2 weeks	50 mg q 2 weeks
Usual duration action	2–4 weeks	3–4 weeks	4 weeks	4 weeks	2–4 weeks	2 weeks
Dose comparative to 100 mg CPZ (approx.)	1.8 mg/day (50 mg q 4 weeks)	0.3 mg/day (6.25 mg q 3 weeks)	0.7 mg/day (20 mg q 4 weeks)	0.85 mg/day (24 mg q 4 weeks)	4.3 mg/day (60 mg q 2 weeks)	1.8 mg/day (25 mg q 2 weeks)
Clinical equivalence in schizophrenia[a]	24 mg q 4 weeks	15 mg q 4 weeks	40 mg q 4 weeks	20 mg q 4 weeks	120 mg q 4 weeks	5 mg q 2 weeks
Pharmacokinetics Peak plasma level*	4–7 days	First peak in 8–10 h (due to presence of hydrolyzed "free" fluphenazine); level drops, then peaks again in 8–12 days	3–9 days	12–24 h	3–7 days	see Long-acting p. 91 4–6 weeks
Elimination half-life**	8 days (after single injection), 17 days (multiple dosing)	6.8–9.6 days (single injection), up to 102 days (multiple dosing)	18–21 days	Approx. 15 days	19 days	7–8 weeks, see Long-acting p. 91 Increased in hepatic or renal disease

Comparison of Long-acting IM Antipsychotics (cont.)

	Flupenthixol decanoate (Fluanxol)	Fluphenazine decanoate (Modecate; Prolixin)	Haloperidol decanoate (Haldol LA)	Pipotiazine palmitate (Piportil L4)	Zuclopenthixol decanoate (Clopixol Depot)	Risperidone (Risperdal Consta)
Adverse effects: Generally similar to oral drugs in same class	Flupenthixol (see p. 132)	Fluphenazine (see p. 131)	Haloperidol (see p. 131)	Pipotiazine (see p. 131)	Zuclopenthixol (see p. 132)	Risperidone (see p. 132)
CNS	Both sedating and alerting effect reported; may have energizing effects at low doses	Both drowsiness and insomnia reported	Both drowsiness and insomnia reported	Low sedative potential; excitation reported in approx. 12% of patients	Both drowsiness and insomnia reported (less frequent than with oral zuclopenthixol)	Adverse effects increase with dose > 50 mg q 2 weeks Drowsiness 3–6%, anxiety 25%, insomnia 23%, headache 13%, depression 16%
Extrapyramidal	Frequent	Less frequent than with oral preparation. Increased frequency of dystonia noted with use of "older" multi-punctured multidose vials due to presence of "free" fluphenazine	Frequent, however, reported less often than with oral haloperidol	Frequent, esp. if dose over 100 mg q 4 weeks	Reported in 5–15% of patients	Akathisia and parkinsonism reported in 12.7% Hyperkinesia 12%
Skin and local reactions	Indurations rarely seen (at high doses) Photosensitivity and hyperpigmentation very rare; dermatological reactions seen Pain at injection site	One case of induration seen at a high dose; dermatological reactions have been reported Pain at injection site	Local dermatological reactions; Inflammation and nodules at injection site (may be more common with 100 mg/ml preparation or with higher volumes); Less common if deltoid used One case of photosensitization reported; "tracking" reported Pain at injection site can continue for 2 days after administration	No indurations reported; dermatological changes reported	No indurations but local dermatological reactions reported Pain at injection site	Pain at injection site Redness, swelling or induration > 10% [ensure solution is at room temperature and inject into alternate buttocks]
Laboratory changes	Rarely leukopenia, eosinophilia	One case of jaundice reported; rarely agranulocytosis; ECG changes seen in some patients	Rarely jaundice, leukopenia, agranulocytosis	Transient changes in liver function seen Rarely jaundice, leukopenia	Transient changes in liver function seen Rarely neutropenia, agranulocytosis	Within normal variation

(a) View of Dr Jeffries, based on clinical judgment. (B) = Not marketed in the USA. * Important as indicator when maximum adverse effects will occur; ** Useful for determining dosing interval; steady state will be reached in approximately 5 half-lives; *** Typical maximal doses based on product monographs. Some clinicians may use higher doses if they are effective with minimal adverse effects.

Extrapyramidal Adverse Effects of Antipsychotics

	Acute Extrapyramidal Effects	Tardive Syndromes
Onset	Acute or insidious (up to 30 days)	After months or years of treatment, especially if drug dose decreased or discontinued
Proposed mechanism	Most EPS symptoms are due to dopamine (D$_2$) blockade (if > 80%)	Supersensitivity of postsynaptic dopamine receptors induced by long-term blockade
Treatment	Respond to antiparkinsonian drugs See p. 150 Akathisia may be mediated by different mechanisms and is therefore more responsive to other treatments (e.g., benzodiazepines, β-blockers – see page 155)	Antiparkinsonian drugs are not effective and may exacerbate tardive dyskinesia Most treatments unsatisfactory; some are aimed at balancing dopaminergic and cholinergic systems. Open and controlled studies suggest that branched-chain amino acids (Tarvil, 222 mg/kg tid) can reduce symptoms of tardive dyskinesia in adults and children Can mask symptoms temporarily by further suppressing dopamine with antipsychotics Novel antipsychotics are less likely to induce tardive dyskinesia and may have antidyskinetic properties See p. 142 for treatments

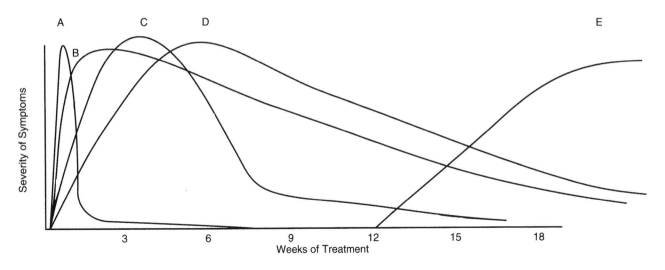

A: Dystonic reactions: uncoordinated spastic movements of muscle groups (e.g., trunk, tongue, face)

B: Akathisia: restlessness, pacing (may result in insomnia)

C: Akinesia: decreased muscular movements
Rigidity: coarse muscular movement; loss of facial expression

D: Tremors: fine movement (shaking) of the extremities ("pill-rolling")
Rabbit syndrome: involuntary movements around the lips
Pisa syndrome: can either be acute or tardive in nature (rare; occurs more commonly in people with brain damage/abnormality)

E: Tardive syndromes: Symptoms of movement disorders that start about 3 months (or later) after therapy is initiated

Extrapyramidal Adverse Effects of Antipsychotics (cont.)

Type	Physical (Motor) Symptoms	Psychological Symptoms	Onset	Possible Risk Factors	Clinical Course	Treatment	Differential Diagnosis
Acute dystonias	Torsions and spasms of muscle groups; muscle spasms, e.g., oculogyric crisis, trismus, laryngospasm, torti/retro/antero-collis tortipelvis, opisthotonus, blepharospasm	Anxiety, fear, panic Dysphoria Repetitive meaningless thoughts	Acute (usually within 24–48 h after the first dose)	Young males, children Antipsychotic naive High potency FGAs; low risk with SGAs and TGA Rapid dose increase Lack of prophylactic antiparkinsonian medication Previous dystonic reaction Hypocalcemia, hyperthyroidism, hypoparathyroidism Recent cocaine use	Acute, painful, spasmodic; oculogyria may be recurrent Acute laryngeal/pharyngeal dystonia may be potentially life-threatening	Sublingual lorazepam, IM benztropine, IM diphenhydramine To prevent recurrence: prophylactic antiparkinsonian agents Reduce dose or change antipsychotic	Seizures Catatonia Hysteria Malingering Hypocalcemia
Acute akathisia	Motor restlessness, fidgeting, pacing, rocking, swinging of leg, trunk rocking forward and backward, repeatedly crossing and uncrossing legs, inability to lie still, shifting from foot to foot Respiratory symptoms: dyspnea or breathing discomfort	Restlessness, irritability Agitation, violent outbursts, dysphoria, feeling "wound-up" or "antsy"; sensation of skin crawling Mental unease Irresistible urge to move	Acute to insidious (within hours to days)	Elderly female, young adults High caffeine intake High potency FGAs; low risk with SGAs and TGA Anxiety Diagnosis of mood disorder Microcytic anemia Low serum ferritin Concurrent use of SSRI	May continue through entire treatment Suggested that may contribute to suicide and/or violence	Antiparkinsonian drugs not very effective Diazepam, clonazepam, lorazepam, β-blockers, cyproheptadine (preliminary reports) Reduce dose or change antipsychotic	Psychotic agitation/decompensation Severe agitation Anxiety Drug-seeking behavior/withdrawal Excess caffeine intake
Acute pseudoparkinsonism	Stiffness, shuffling, mask-like face, "pill-rolling"-type tremor (4–8 cycles per second; greater at rest and bilateral), cogwheel rigidity, stooped posture, postural instability, micrographia, bradykinesia, drooling, loss of arm swing	Slowed thinking Fatigue, anergia Cognitive impairment Depression	Acute to insidious (within 30 days)	Elderly female High potency FGAs; low risk with SGAs and TGA Increased dose Concurrent neurological disorder	May continue through entire treatment	Reduce dose or change antipsychotic Antiparkinsonian drug	Negative symptoms of schizophrenia Idiopathic Parkinson's disease Depression
Pisa syndrome	Leaning to one side		Can be acute or tardive	Elderly patients Compromised brain function, dementia	Often ignored by patients	Antiparkinsonian drug (higher doses)	
Rabbit syndrome	Fine tremor of lower lip		After months of therapy	Elderly patients		Antiparkinsonian drug	

Type	Physical (Motor) Symptoms	Psychological Symptoms	Onset	Possible Risk Factors	Clinical Course	Treatment	Differential Diagnosis
Tardive dyskinesia	Involuntary choreo-athetoid movements of face (e.g., tics, frowning, grimacing), lips (pursing, puckering, smacking), jaw (chewing, clenching), tongue ("fly-catcher," rolling, dysarthria), eyelids (blinking, blepharospasm), limbs (tapping, twitching), trunk (rocking, twisting), neck (nodding), respiratory (dyspnea, gasping, sighing, grunting, forceful breathing) Often coexists with parkinsonism and akathisia. Abnormal movements disappear during sleep	Cognitive impairment, distress (talking, swallowing, eating) and embarrassment	After 3 or more months of therapy in adults and earlier in the elderly Common early sign is "worm-like" movement of the tongue ("fly-catcher tongue")	Elderly female Previous acute persistent EPS Chronic use of high doses of antiparkinsonian drugs Nonpsychotic diagnosis, affective disorder Diabetes Cognitive impairment/brain damage Alcohol/drug abuse may predispose to buccolingual masticatory symptoms May be associated with genetic variation of the D3 receptor gene High homocysteine levels as seen in smokers	Persistent – discontinuation of antipsychotic early increases chance of remission Spontaneous remission in 14–24% after 5 years	Suggestions for treatment include: Switch to a SGA or TGA Pyridoxine up to 400 mg/ day Clonazepam 0.5–6 mg/day Tetrabenazine 25–75 mg/day Clonidine 0.05–0.2 mg/ day Branched-chain amino acids (Tarvil, 222 mg/kg tid)	Spontaneous or withdrawal dyskinesia Stereotypic behavior Tourette's Syndrome Huntington's Chorea or other neurological conditions Movement disorder secondary to co-prescribed drug
Tardive dystonia	Sustained muscle contractions of face, eyes, neck, limbs, back, or trunk (craniocervical area involved most frequently), e.g., blepharospasm, laryngeal dystonia, dysarthria, retroflexed hands		After months or years of therapy	Young male Genetic predisposition (?) Neurological disorder, mental retardation Coexisting tardive dyskinesia Akathisia	Persistent; discontinuation of antipsychotic early increases chance of remission	Switch to a SGA or TGA (clozapine reported to decrease symptoms by at least 50%, including blepharospasm) Suggestions for treatment include: Tetrabenazine 25–75 mg; higher doses of anticholinergics (e.g., trihexyphenidyl 40 mg/ day); Reserpine 0.125–5 mg/day Botulinum toxin 25–50 mg/site (multiple sites used) Benzodiazepines	Myoclonus Motor tics Idiopathic dystonia Meige syndrome
Tardive akathisia	Persistent symptoms of akathisia	As for akathisia	After months of therapy; after drug withdrawal	As for akathisia Coexisting tardive dyskinesia and dystonia	Persistent, discontinuation of antipsychotic early increases chance of remission. Fluctuating course	Switch to a SGA or TGA Suggested treatments include: Clonidine 0.05–0.5 mg/day; Benzodiazepines; β-blockers	As for akathisia

Switching Antipsychotics

Reasons for Considering a Switch	• 1. To enhance efficacy or improve response to treatment: A switch may be considered in cases of nonresponse, partial or less than optimal response, or relapse despite adherence. Motivating factors may include:
	   – Persistent positive symptoms (consider a FGA or a SGA; switching to clozapine may offer additional response in up to a further 50% of patients)
	   – Persistent negative symptoms (consider alternate SGA, lowering dose or aripiprazole)
	   – Persistent cognitive or affective symptoms (consider SGA)
	   – Persistent suicidal ideation or behaviors (consider clozapine)
	   – A request for change from patient or family member
	   – A change in patient's medical or psychiatric condition warranting a change in treatment
	• 2. To relieve or decrease a bothersome adverse effect (e.g., sexual dysfunction, sedation, EPS) or one that may be associated with short- or long-term morbidity (e.g., TD, metabolic effects). These are often major contributors to nonadherence and eventual treatment failure
	• A combination of 1. and 2. – Less than optimal response in the face of bothersome or persistent adverse effects does little to promote confidence in the treatment plan and probably facilitates nonadherent behaviors

Pre-Switch Check List	• Reaffirm diagnosis
	• Address confounding or complicating factors:
	   – Attempt to rule out partial adherence or nonadherence. If present identify and address barriers to adherence if possible (e.g., some adverse effects may be resolved by lowering the dose, changing the administration schedule or waiting for tolerance to develop)
	   – Ensure adequate trial period was employed – adequate dose for adequate duration [at least 4–6 weeks at maximally tolerated dose (longer for clozapine)]
	   – Determine if any drug interactions may be impacting on efficacy or adverse effects
	   – Determine if substance abuse or psychosocial stressors may be confounding response
	   – Give thoughtful consideration to the pros and cons of making a change
	   – Determine if the patient is agreeable to making a change
	   – Establish a thorough plan including how to make the switch and what to expect. How long will it take to work? What unwanted effects might occur and how to monitor for them?
	   – Communicate the plan to the patient

Problems Which May Arise During the Switch	• Two main types of problems that may be anticipated during a switch are:
	   – Withdrawal effects related to discontinuation of the initial antipsychotic
	   – Adverse effects that result from the addition of a new agent
	• These, coupled with a time lag to response, may discourage the patient and negatively impact on adherence unless the patient is educated as to what to expect.

Withdrawal Effects	• Abrupt withdrawal of an antagonist medication opens up a sensitized receptor, leaving it vulnerable to excessive stimulation. This may result in:
	   – Dopaminergic rebound – if a high D_2 affinity medication (e.g., risperidone) is abrupty replaced with a low D_2 affinity medication or a rapid on/off fast dissociating antipsychotic (e.g., quetiapine) or a partial D_2 agonist (e.g., aripiprazole), dopaminergic rebound may result. In the mesolimbic tract, this could lead to supersensitivity psychosis; in the nigrostriatal tract, treatment-emergent EPS and TD may materialize
	   – Cholinergic rebound – if a high affinity cholinergic antagonist (e.g., olanzapine) is abruptly replaced by an antipsychotic with little affinity for blocking cholinergic receptors, cholinergic rebound may ensue, causing the patient to complain of flu-like symptoms such as nausea, vomiting, diarrhea, diaphoresis, and insomnia
	   – Histaminic rebound – abrupt replacement of a high affinity histamine blocker (e.g., clozapine) with a low affinity agent (e.g., aripiprazole) may see improvement in several metabolic parameters such as weight gain, glucose intolerance, and dyslipidemias. Sedation may also improve, but some individuals may experience distressing rebound insomnia which may be interpreted as a sign of relapse
	   – Serotonergic rebound – it has been suggested that abrupt discontinuation of a high affinity serotonin 5-HT_{2A} antagonist may result in serotonin syndrome (agitation, diaphoresis, fever, tremor, confusion, etc.) or NMS-like symptoms
	   – In the absence of any strong scientific evidence, empirical recommendations favor a slow cross-taper method to minimize rebound and the addition/continuation of adjunctive treatments (e.g., anticholinergics for cholinergic rebound or benzodiazepines for insomnia) when necessary

Switching Methods	• Four options (no clear evidence to support one method over another)

• Four options (no clear evidence to support one method over another)
1. Washout/start:
   • Withdraw the first drug gradually and begin the second drug following a suitable washout period. May minimize withdrawal-emergent reactions. Not clinically practical when patient is symptomatic. May increase the risk of relapse
2. Stop/start:
   • Abruptly discontinue the first drug, then start the second drug at its usual initial dose; increase the dose to a therapeutic range accordingly. This technique is often used when the patient has a significant/serious adverse reaction to the initial drug (e.g., agranulocytosis, NMS, ketoacidosis). Potential drawbacks include an increased risk of relapse and withdrawal-emergent reactions
3. Cross-taper:
   • Taper the dose of the first medication while simultaneously increasing the dose of the second drug. Commonly used when stable patients are experiencing bothersome adverse effects and require a medication change. The duration of the cross-titration usually lasts between 1 and 4 weeks. Generally the most well accepted or preferred strategy, thought to minimize the potential for withdrawal-emergent effects and relapse. Drawbacks of this strategy include an increased risk of relapse should the patient spend time with subtherapeutic doses of both antipsychotics, an increased risk of polypharmacy should the patient improve during the switch and the practitioner become reluctant to make further changes, and an increased risk of additive or synergistic effects from both drugs
4. Delayed withdrawal:
   • Establishing the patient on a therapeutic dose of the second drug before reducing the existing medication. The strategy may be preferred in situations for which relapse is a significant concern. There is an increased risk for polypharmacy with this method if the change-over is not completed. As well, there is an increased risk of additive or synergistic effects from both drugs during the procedure

• Rate of switching/cross-tapering should be slow in the elderly and in young patients

Antipsychotic Augmentation Strategies

- The addition of another pharmacological agent or treatment to an antipsychotic in an attempt to augment or improve the response to the initial antipsychotic
- The ultimate goal is to combine different mechanisms of action to create a synergistic effect that will enhance efficacy while minimizing the potential for increased adverse effects and drug interactions
- Some published double-blind studies exist that evaluate augmentation strategies, however, the majority of the evidence for augmentation strategies is derived from open-label studies and case reports
- Most of the literature on augmentation strategies includes augmentation of clozapine therapy, the assumption being that monotherapy with clozapine would often be attempted first before less well studied alternatives such as augmentation strategies with other antipsychotics would be employed. There are still circumstances in which augmentation of other antipsychotics may be considered before a clozapine trial. In many of these cases the target symptom is something other than residual psychotic symptoms – e.g., benzodiazepines for agitation and hostility, antidepressants for depressive symptomatology, mood stabilizers for affective lability
- Should a decision to employ an augmentation strategy be made, a detailed plan should be documented that clearly states the agent to be used, the planned dosage strategy, the target symptoms to be evaluated, and the anticipated time to see effect/trial period (e.g., 3–4 months), and how and when to monitor for efficacy and safety. The plan should also include a strategy for discontinuing the augmenting agent should it prove to be ineffective
- In addition to the information provided below, refer to the corresponding drug interaction section

Anticonvulsants

Carbamazepine

- The available evidence does not support the routine use of carbamazepine for augmentation of antipsychotic treatment of schizophrenia. In particular, the combination of carbamazepine with clozapine is discouraged due to concerns over an additive risk for agranulocytosis (see Drug Interactions p. 101)

Lamotrigine

- One randomized, double-blind trial reported benefit on positive symptoms with the addition of lamotrigine to clozapine therapy
- A review from the Cochrane Collaboration[23] concluded that there was evidence of a marginal beneficial effect on some psychotic symptoms with the addition of lamotrigine, but that the current evidence was not sufficient to recommend the routine addition of lamotrigine in treatment-resistant schizophrenia
- Caution – one case report of a tripling in the clozapine level with the addition of lamotrigine, the mechanism of this potential drug interaction is unknown
- Caution – both lamotrigine and clozapine have the potential to depress bone marrow function

Topiramate

- Case reports of augmentation of clozapine with topiramate have not been favorable

Valproic acid

- There is conflicting evidence regarding the use of valproic acid as augmentation agent. Case reports suggest benefit in refractory patients on clozapine. A meta-analysis of five randomized controlled trials examining valproate as an add-on to various antipsychotics did not report beneficial results
- Caution – there are conflicting reports that valproic acid may increase serum clozapine levels and worsen the severity of weight gain

Antidepressants

- TCAs, SSRIs, mirtazapine, and MAOIs reported to decrease negative symptoms, poor social or work functioning in some patients. Benefits may be due to improvements in secondary (vs. primary) negative symptoms
- Much of the literature involves the combination of an SSRI and clozapine with conflicting reports regarding the efficacy of the duo. It has been speculated that any beneficial effects could be due to an increase in clozapine levels as a result of a drug interaction in which the SSRI inhibits clozapine's metabolism

Benzodiazepines	• Used primarily to calm acutely agitated patients early in treatment
	• A review from the Cochrane Collaboration[28] concluded that there was no evidence to support a beneficial effect of benzodiazepines as adjunctive therapy to antipsychotics to alleviate positive symptoms of schizophrenia. The only significant effect noted was short-term sedation
	• Caution – reports of cardiorespiratory collapse, delirium, loss of consciousness, and death with the combination of benzodiazepines and clozapine. In many cases, the incidences occurred shortly after the addition of clozapine to existing benzodiazepine treatment. Also, reports of cardiorespiratory depression with the combination of benzodiazepines and olanzapine IM (see Drug Interactions p. 104).
Combination Antipsychotics	• There are few controlled studies that evaluate the efficacy of combining two antipsychotics and no convincing evidence in favor of this strategy; the risk of adverse effects and drug interactions as well as costs are increased
	• Combining a FGA with a SGA is generally discouraged as the risk of potential adverse effects may be increased with such combinations, subjecting patients to both EPS, TD, and hyperprolactinemia from the FGAs and weight gain and other metabolic disturbances from the SGAs. There is some suggestion that loxapine, while a FGA at higher doses, may behave more like a SGA at lower doses (i.e., less than 50 mg daily), making it a potentially more attractive option as an add-on to a SGA
	• Some data support adjunctive (low-dose) FGA augmentation of clozapine or olanzapine in treatment-refractory patients
	• A small open-label study combining clozapine and aripiprazole demonstrated decreased sedation, weight loss, and reduction in lipids (mainly triglyceride) levels; decreased weight and lipids also reported with clozapine-ziprasidone combination
	• Decreasing the dose of clozapine and adding quetiapine has also been reported to decrease weight and improve glucose regulation
Electroconvulsive Therapy	• Of benefit in acute schizophrenia, especially if catatonia or affective symptoms are present
	• Some reports suggest superiority with bilateral treatment; usually 12–20 treatments required for schizophrenia
	• Meta-analysis of 36 studies of clozapine + ECT showed marked improvement in 67.2% of patients; adverse effects included prolonged seizure duration in 16.6% of patients
	• Symptoms noted to improve included: Delusions, hallucinations, agitation, hostility, and depression
	• Modest evidence of efficacy in treatment-refractory patients and benefits appear short lived
	• Lack of guidelines regarding maintenance ECT in those who have responded
Ethyl Eicosapentanoic Acid (E-EPA)	• Suggested to exert augmenting effect by inhibiting phospholipase-A2, an enzyme found to be overactive in patients with schizophrenia (see p. 308)
	• Review of double-blind studies suggests E-EPA can be of benefit (at a dose of 2 g/day) as an augmenting drug in patients refractory to clozapine
	• May have a beneficial effect on elevated triglyceride levels and on tardive dyskinesia
	• The purity and consistency among products may not be reliable
Lithium	• Caution – reports of increased potential for neurotoxic reactions (e.g., NMS-like syndrome) with the combination of lithium and mainly haloperidol – controversial
	• There are case reports of beneficial effects from a combination of lithium and clozapine in patients with schizophrenia and schizoaffective disorder. A double-blind study reported that the combination of lithium and clozapine was effective in patients with schizoaffective disorder but not in those with schizophrenia.
Selegiline	• A case report and a number of small open-label trials reported improvement in negative symptoms of schizophrenia following the augmentation of antipsychotic therapy with selegiline
	• These findings were not supported by two controlled trials which showed either no benefit or benefit that was not deemed clinically significant. Currently low-dose selegiline cannot be recommended as augmentation treatment for negative symptoms
Stimulants	• E. g., dextroamphetamine, methylphenidate
	• Transient improvement in negative symptoms and cognitive function reported
	• Exacerbation of positive symptoms can occur

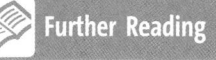 **Further Reading**

References

1 Amato L, Minozzi S, Pani PP, Davoli M. Antipsychotic medications for cocaine dependence. *Cochrane Database of Systematic Reviews* 2007, Issue 3. Art. No.: CD006306. DOI: 10.1002/14651858.CD006306.pub2.

2 American Academy of Pediatrics Committee on Drugs. The transfer of drugs and other chemicals into human milk. Pediatrics. 2001;108(3):776–789.

3 American Psychiatric Association. Practice guideline for the treatment of patients with schizophrenia. Am J Psychiatry. 2004;161(2Suppl.):1–56.

4 Ascher-Svanum H, Faires DE, Zhu B, et al. Medication adherence and long-term functional outcomes in the treatment of schizophrenia in usual care. J Clin Psychiatry. 2006;67(3):453–460.

5 Brodaty H, Ames D, Snowdon J, et al. A randomized placebo controlled trial of risperidone for the treatment of aggression, agitation, and psychosis of dementia. J Clin Psychiatry 2003;64:134–143.

6 Burton, SCF. Strategies for improving adherence to second-generation antipsychotics in patients with schizophrenia by increasing ease of use. J Psychiatr Pract. 2005;11(6):369–378.

7 Canadian Psychiatric Association Working Group. Clinical practice guidelines: Treatment of schizophrenia. Can J Psychiatry. 2005;50(13Suppl.1):S1–S56.

8 Claudino AM, Hay PJ, Lima MS, Schmidt U, Bacaltchuk J, Treasure JL. Antipsychotic drugs for anorexia nervosa. (Protocol) *Cochrane Database of Systematic Reviews* 2007, Issue 4. Art. No.: CD006816. DOI: 10.1002/14651858.CD006816.

9 Crouch MA, Limon L, Cassano AT. Clinical relevance and management of drug-related QT interval prolongation. Pharmacotherapy. 2003;23(7):881–908.

10 Federal Drug Administration. Information for Healthcare Professionals: Haloperidol. 2007, September 17. Available from www.fda.gov/cder/drug/InfoSheets/HCP/haloperidol.htm (Accessed November 24, 2008).

11 Gardner DM, Baldessarini RJ, Waraich P. Modern antipsychotic drugs: A critical overview. CMAJ. 2005;172(13):1703–1711.

12 Gianfrancesco FD, Grogg AL, Mahmoud RA, et al. Differential effects of risperidone, olanzapine, clozapine, and conventional antipsychotics on type 2 diabetes: Findings from a large health plan database. J Clin Psychiatry. 2003;63:920–930.

13 Haddad PM. Antipsychotics and diabetes: A review of non-prospective data. Br J Psychiatry. 2004;184(Suppl.47):S80–S86.

14 Kumar S, Oberstar JV, Sikich L, et al. Efficacy and tolerability of second-generation antipsychotics in children and adolescents with schizophrenia. Schizophr Bull. 2008;34(1):60–71.

15 L'Italien GJ, Casey DE, Kan HJ, Carson WH, Marcus RN. Comparison of metabolic syndrome incidence among schizophrenia patients treated with aripiprazole versus olanzapine or placebo. J Clin Psychiatry. 2007;68(10):1510–1516.

16 Lonergan E, Britton AM, Luxenberg J. Antipsychotics for delirium. *Cochrane Database of Systematic Reviews* 2007, Issue 2. Art. No.: CD005594. DOI: 10.1002/14651858.CD005594.pub2.

17 Mago R, Anolik R, Johnson RA, Kunkel EJ. Recurrent priapism associated with use of aripiprazole. J Clin Psychiatry. 2006;67(9):1471–1472.

18 Marder SR, Essock SM, Miller AL, et al. The Mount Sinai conference on the health monitoring of patients with schizophrenia. Am J Psychiatry. 2004;161(8):1334–1349.

19 Molitch ME. Medication-induced hyperprolactinemia. Mayo Clin Proc. 2005;80(8):1050–1057.

20 Newcomer J. Metabolic considerations in antipsychotic medications. J Clin Psychiatry. 2007;68(Suppl.1):S20–S27.

21 Palmer SE, McLean RM, Ellis PM, et al. Life-threatening clozapine-induced gastrointestinal hypomotility: An analysis of 102 cases. J Clin Psychiatry 2008;69(5):759–768.

22 Pinninti NR, Mago R, Adityanjee. Tardive dystonia-associated prescription of aripiprazole. J Neuropsychiatry Clin Neurosci. 2006;18(3):426–427.

23 Premkumar TS, Pick J. Lamotrigine for schizophrenia. Cochrane Database of Systematic Reviews 2006, Issue 4. Art. No.: CD005962. DOI: 10.1002/14651858.CD005962.pub2.

24 Schneider LS, Dagerman KS, Insel P. Risk of death with atypical antipsychotic drug treatment for dementia. JAMA. 2005;294(15):1934–1943.

25 Stahl SM. Essential Psychopharmacology: The Prescriber's Guide. Cambridge, UK: Cambridge University Press, 2006.

26 Swainston Harrison T, Perry CM. Aripiprazole: a review of its use in schizophrenia and schizoaffective disorder. Drugs. 2004;64:1715–1736.

27 Uchida H, Mamo DC, Kapur S, et al. Monthly administration of long-acting injectable risperidone and striatal dopamine D2 receptor occupancy for the management of schizophrenia. J Clin Psychiatry. 2008;69(8):1281–1286.

28 Volz A, Khorsand V, Gillies D, et al. Benzodiazepines for schizophrenia. Cochrane Database of Systematic Reviews 2007, Issue 1. Art. No.: CD006391. DOI: 10.1002/14651858.CD006391.

29 Wang PS, Schneeweiss S, Avorn J, et al. Risk of death in elderly users of conventional vs. atypical antipsychotic medications. N Engl J Med. 2005;353(22):2335–2341.

Additional Suggested Reading

• Aichhorn W, Whitworth AB, Weiss EM, et al. Second-generation antipsychotics: Is there evidence for sex differences in pharmacokinetics and adverse effect profiles? Drug Saf. 2006;29(7):581–598.

• Alexopoulos GS, Streim J, Carpenter D, et al. The Expert Consensus Guideline Series: Using antipsychotic agents in older patients. J Clin Psychiatry. 2004;65 Suppl 2:S1–S105.

• Altamura AC, Sassella F, Santini A, et al. Intramuscular preparations of antipsychotics. Drugs. 2003;63(5):493–512.

• American Diabetes Association, American Psychiatric Association, American Association of Clinical Endocrinologists, North American Association for the Study of Obesity. Consensus development conference on antipsychotic drugs and obesity and diabetes. J Clin Psychiatry. 2004;65(2):267–272.

• Ananth J, Parameswaran S, Gunatilake S, et al. Neuroleptic malignant syndrome and atypical antipsychotic drugs. J Clin Psychiatry. 2004;65(4):464–470.

• Argo TR, Carnahan RM, Perry PJ. Aripiprazole, a novel atypical antipsychotic drug. Pharmacotherapy. 2004;24(2):212–228.

• Basan A, Kissling W, Leucht S. Valproate as an adjunct to antipsychotics for schizophrenia: A systematic review of randomized trials. Schizophr Res. 2004;70(1):33–37.

• Bergman RN, Ader M. Atypical antipsychotics and glucose homeostasis. J Clin Psychiatry. 2005;66(4):504–514.

• Brunton L, Lazo J, Parker K. Goodman & Gillman's the pharmacological basis of therapeutics (11th ed.) New York, NY: McGraw-Hill, 2006.

• Buckley PF, Correll CU. Strategies for dosing and switching antipsychotics for optimal clinical management. J Clin Psychiatry. 2008;69(Suppl 1):4–17.

• Buckley PF. Receptor-binding profiles of antipsychotics: Clinical strategies when switching between agents. J Clin Psychiatry. 2007 68(Suppl.6):S5–S9.

• Buckley PF. Treating movement disorders and akathisia as side effects of antipsychotic pharmacotherapy. J Clin Psychiatry. 2008;69(5):e14.

- Casey DE. Dyslipidemia and atypical antipsychotic drugs. J Clin Psychiatry. 2004;65 (Suppl 18):S27–S35.
- Chouinard G, Chouinard VA. Atypical antipsychotics: CATIE study, drug-induced movement disorder and resulting iatrogenic psychiatric-like symptoms, supersensitivity rebound psychosis and withdrawal discontinuation syndromes. Psychother Psychosom. 2008;77:69–77.
- Czekalla J, Kollack-Walker S, Beasley CM. Cardiac safety parameters of olanzapine: Comparison with other atypical and typical antipsychotics. J Clin Psychiatry. 2001;62 Suppl 2:S35–S40.
- Davis JM, Chen N. Dose response and dose equivalence of antipsychotics. J Clin Psychopharmacol. 2004;24(2):192–208.
- Duggal HS, Singh I. Psychotropic drug-induced neutropenia. Drugs Today. 2005;41(8):517–526.
- Fink M. NMS: Effective recognition and treatment. Int Drug Ther Newsl. 2003;38(3):17–21.
- Fohey KD. The role of selegiline in the treatment of negative symptoms associated with schizophrenia. Ann Pharmacother. 2007;41:851–856.
- Gareri P, De Fazio P, Stilo M, et al. Conventional and atypical antipsychotics in the elderly. A review. Clin Drug Investig. 2003;23(5):287–322.
- Gentile S. Clinical utilization of atypical antipsychotics in pregnancy and lactation. Ann Pharmacother. 2004;38:1265–1271.
- Haddad PM, Sharma SG. Adverse effects of atypical antipsychotics: Differential risk and clinical implications. CNS Drugs. 2007;21(11):911–936.
- Hall RL, Smith AG, Edwards JG. Haematological safety of antipsychotic drugs. Expert Opin Drug Saf. 2003;2(4):395–399.
- Harvey PD, Green MF, Keefe RSE, et al. Cognitive functioning in schizophrenia: A consensus statement on its role in the definition and evaluation of effective treatment for the illness. J Clin Psychiatry. 2004;65(3):361–372.
- Henderson DC, Nguyen DD, Copeland PM, et al. Clozapine, diabetes mellitus, hyperlipidemia, and cardiovascular risks and mortality: Results of a 10-year naturalistic study. J Clin Psychiatry. 2005;66(9):1116–1121.
- Horacek J, Bubenikova-Valesova V, Kopecek M. Mechanism of action of atypical antipsychotic drugs and the neurobiology of schizophrenia. CNS Drugs 2006;20(5):389–409.
- Iraqi A. A case report of pancytopenia with quetiapine use. Am J Geriatr Psychiatry. 2003;11(6):694.
- Kane SM, Leucht S, Carpenter D, et al. Optimizing pharmacologic treatment of psychotic disorders: The Expert Consensus Guideline Series. J Clin Psychiatry. 2003;64(Suppl 12):S1–S100.
- Kane SM. Tardive dyskinesia rates with atypical antipsychotics in adults: Prevalence and incidence. J Clin Psychiatry. 2004;65(Suppl 9):S16–S20.
- Kirshner SJ, Lander A, Kjernisted M, et al. Do antipsychotics ameliorate or exacerbate obsessive compulsive disorder symptoms? A systematic review. J Affect Disord. 2004;82(2):167–174.
- Kontaxakis UP, Ferentinos PP, Havaki-Kontaxakis BJ, et al. Randomized controlled augmentation trials in clozapineresistant schizophrenic patients: A critical review. European Psychiatry. 2005;20:409–415.
- Lieberman JA, Stroup TS, McEvoy JP, et al. Effectiveness of antipsychotic drugs in patients with chronic schizophrenia. N Engl J Med. 2005;353(12): 1209–1223.
- Marder SR, Essock SM, Miller AL, et al. Physical health monitoring of patients with schizophrenia. Am J Psychiatry. 2004;161(8):1334–1349.
- Marder SR. A review of agitation in mental illness: Treatment guidelines and current therapies. J Clin Psychiatry. 2006;67(Suppl 10):13–21.
- Miller AL, Hall CS, Buchanan RW, et al. The Texas medication algorithm project, antipsychotic algorithm for schizophrenia: 2003 update. J Clin Psychiatry. 2004;65(4):500–508.
- Minzenberg MJ, Poole JH, Benton C, et al. Association of anticholinergic load with impairment of complex attention and memory in schizophrenia. Am J Psychiatry. 2004;161:116–124.
- Moller HS. Management of the negative symptoms of schizophrenia: New treatment options. CNS Drugs. 2003;17(11):793–823.
- Moncrieff J. Does antipsychotic withdrawal provoke psychosis? Acta Psychiatr Scand. 2006;114:3–13.
- Nasrallah HA. Atypical antipsychotic-induced metabolic side effects: Insights from receptor-binding profiles. Mol Psychiatry. 2008;13(1):27–35.
- Newcomer JW. Abnormalities of glucose metabolism associated with atypical antipsychotic drugs. J Clin Psychiatry. 2004;65(Suppl 18):S36–S46.
- Praharaj SK, Arora M, Gandotra S. Clozapine-induced sialorrhea: Pathophysiology and management strategies. Psychopharmacol (Berl). 2006;185:265–273.
- Remington G, Saha A, Chong SA, et al. Augmentation strategies in clozapine-resistent schizophrenia. CNS Drugs. 2005;19(10):1–30,843–872.
- Sacks FM. Metabolic syndrome: Epidemiology and consequences. J Clin Psychiatry. 2004;65(Suppl 18):S3–S12.
- Saha S, Chant D, McGrath J. A systematic review of mortality in schizophrenia. Arch Gen Psychiatry 2007;64(10):1123–1131.
- Simpson GM. The treatment of tardive dyskinesia and tardive dystonia. J Clin Psychiatry. 2000;61(Suppl 4):S39–S44.
- Stahl SM, Grady MM. A critical review of atypical antipsychotic utilization: Comparing monotherapy with polypharmacy and augmentation. Curr Med Chem. 2004;11:313–327.
- Tandon R. Comparative effectiveness of antipsychotics in the treatment of schizophrenia: What CATIE (phase 1) tells us – Part 1. Intern Drug Ther Newsl. 2006;41(7):51–58.
- Wirshing DA. Schizophrenia and obesity: Impact of antipsychotic medications. J Clin Psychiatry. 2004;65(Suppl 18):S13–S26.
- Woods SW. Chlorpromazine equivalent doses for the newer atypical antipsychotics. J Clin Psychiatry. 2003;64(6):663–667.
- Zemrak WR, Kenna GA. Association of antipsychotic and antidepressant drugs with Q-T interval prolongation. Am J Health Syst Pharm. 2008;65(11):1029–1038.
- Ziegenbein M, Steinbrecher A, Garlipp P. Clozapine-induced aplastic anemia in a patient with Parkinson's disease. Can J Psychiatry. 2003;48(5):352.

AGENTS FOR TREATING EXTRAPYRAMIDAL SIDE EFFECTS

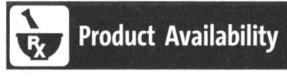 **Product Availability**

Chemical Class	Generic Name	Trade Name[A]	Dosage Forms and Strengths
Dopamine agonist[D]	Amantadine	Symmetrel	Capsules: 100 mg; Tablets 100mg Syrup: 50 mg/5 ml
Antihistamine[D]	Cyproheptadine	Periactin	Tablets: 4 mg Syrup: 2 mg/5 ml
	Diphenhydramine	Benadryl	Caplets/Capsules/Liquigels/Tablets: 25 mg, 50 mg Chewable tablets: 12.5 mg Lozenge (thin strips): 12.5 mg[B], 19 mg[C], 25 mg[B] Elixir: 12.5 mg/5 ml Solution: 6.25 mg/5 ml[C], 12.5 mg/5 ml Injection: 10 mg/ml[B], 50 mg/ml
	Orphenadrine	Norflex	Extended-release tablets: 100 mg Injection: 30 mg/ml
β-blocker	Propranolol	Inderal	Tablets: 10 mg, 20 mg, 40 mg, 60 mg[B], 80 mg, 90 mg[B], 120 mg[C] Solution[B]: 4 mg/ml, 8 mg/ml Injection: 1 mg/ml
		Inderal LA	Sustained-release capsules: 60 mg, 80 mg, 120 mg, 160 mg
Benzodiazepine	Clonazepam	Rivotril[C], Klonopin[B]	Oral concentrated solution[B]: 2.5 mg/ml Tablets: 0.25 mg[C], 0.5 mg, 1 mg, 2 mg Oral disintegrating tablets[B]: 0.125 mg, 0.25 mg, 0.5 mg, 1 mg, 2 mg Injection[B]: 1 mg/ml
	Diazepam	Valium	Tablets: 2 mg, 5 mg, 10 mg Oral solution: 1 mg/ml Injection: 5 mg/ml
		Diazepam Intensol[B]	Oral concentrate[B]: 5 mg/ml Injection: 5 mg/ml
		Diastat	Rectal gel: 5 mg/ml
		Diazemuls[C], Dizac[B]	Emulsion injection (IM/IV): 5 mg/ml
	Lorazepam	Ativan	Tablets: 0.5 mg, 1 mg, 2 mg Sublingual tablets[C]: 0.5 mg, 1 mg, 2 mg Oral solution: 0.5 mg/5 ml Injection: 2 mg/ml[B], 4 mg/ml
		Lorazepam Intensol[B]	Solution[B]: 2 mg/ml

Chemical Class	Generic Name	Trade Name[A]	Dosage Forms and Strengths
Anticholinergic agent[D]	Benztropine	Cogentin	Tablets: 0.5 mg, 1 mg, 2 mg Oral solution[C]: 0.4 mg/ml Injection: 1 mg/ml
	Biperiden[B]	Akineton	Tablets: 2 mg
	Ethopropazine[C]	Parsitan	Tablets: 50 mg
	Procyclidine	Kemadrin	Tablets: 2.5 mg[C], 5 mg Elixir[C]: 2.5 mg/5 ml
	Trihexyphenidyl	Artane	Tablets: 2 mg, 5 mg Elixir[B]: 2 mg/5 ml

[A] Generic preparations may be available, [B] Not marketed in Canada, [C] Not marketed in USA, [D] Antiparkinsonian agents

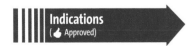

Indications
(👍 Approved)

To relieve the neurological (muscular) side effects induced by antipsychotics (see p. 155 for comparison of drugs):
- 👍 Acute dyskinesias, dystonias
- 👍 Pseudoparkinsonian effects (tremor, rigidity, shuffling)
- 👍 Akathisia (restlessness)
- 👍 Akinesia (decreased muscle movement)
- 👍 "Rabbit syndrome," "Pisa syndrome"
- Antipsychotic-induced sexual dysfunction (amantadine, cyproheptadine); galactorrhea (amantadine)
- Treatment of cocaine withdrawal and use (amantadine – limited evidence, propranolol)

General Comments

- No clear evidence that one drug is more efficacious than another; individual patients may respond better, or tolerate one drug over another
- Controversy exists whether antiparkinsonian agents should be given prophylactically to patients at risk of developing EPS with FGA drugs, or whether they should only be started when EPS develops
- There is a wide variance (e.g., 2–50%) in the reported incidence of drug-induced parkinsonian effects. Rates are higher in the elderly and in females and are dose related
- Consider dosage reduction or discontinuation of the offending antipsychotic agent (if appropriate) or switching to a newer generation antipsychotic as potential treatment options

Pharmacology

- Centrally-active anticholinergic drugs cross the blood-brain barrier, block excitatory cholinergic pathways in the basal ganglia, and restore the dopamine/acetylcholine balance disrupted by neuroleptic drugs, thus treating EPS
- Muscarinic receptors are subclassified into M_1 (predominate in the striatum) and M_2 (predominate in cardiac ventricles) subtypes. Antiparkinsonian drugs show a range of selectivity on M_1 vs M_2 as follows: biperiden > procyclidine > trihexyphenidyl > benztropine. M_1 selectivity predicts lower peripheral side effects
- Anticholinergic drugs also block presynaptic reuptake of dopamine (primarily benztropine), norepinephrine (primarily diphenhydramine), and serotonin (weakly)
- Amantadine and ethopropazine have moderate NMDA (n-methyl-D-aspartate) receptor blocking properties; amantadine exerts its activity by increasing dopamine at the receptor

Dosing

- See chart pp. 156–157
- Dosage increases must be balanced against the risk of evoking anticholinergic adverse effects
- Plasma-level monitoring is not currently advocated

* 👍 Approved indications in psychiatric disorders

Agents for Treating Extrapyramidal Side Effects (cont.)

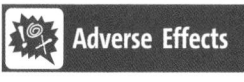 **Adverse Effects**

CNS Effects	• CNS effects: seen primarily in the elderly and at high doses; include stimulation, disorientation, confusion, hallucinations, restlessness, weakness, incoherence, headache; cognitive impairment including decreased memory and distractibility • Excess use/abuse of these drugs may lead to an anticholinergic (toxic) psychosis with symptoms of disorientation, confusion, euphoria (see Toxicity p. 152), in addition to physical signs such as dry mouth, blurred vision, dilated pupils, dry flushed skin • Dopamine-agonist activity of amantadine can occasionally cause worsening of psychotic symptoms, nightmares, insomnia, and mood disturbances
Anticholinergic Effects	• Related to anticholinergic potency: atropine > trihexyphenidyl > benztropine > biperiden > procyclidine > orphenadrine > diphenhydramine • Common: dry mouth, blurred vision, constipation, dry eyes, flushed skin • Occasional: delayed micturition, urinary retention, sexual dysfunction • Excess doses can suppress sweating, resulting in hyperthermia
Cardiovascular Effects	• Palpitations, tachycardia; high doses can cause arrhythmias
GI Effects	• Nausea, vomiting

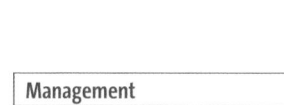 **Precautions**

• Use cautiously in patients with conditions in which excess anticholinergic activity could be harmful, e.g., prostatic hypertrophy, urinary retention, narrow-angle glaucoma, myasthenia gravis
• May decrease sweating; educate and monitor patients on these medications in hot weather to prevent hyperthermia
• Monitor breathing patterns in patients with respiratory difficulties since antiparkinsonian medications can dry bronchial secretions and make breathing difficult
• Caution when using amantadine in patients with peripheral edema or history of congestive heart failure
• If withdrawn abruptly, antiparkinsonian drugs may cause restlessness, anxiety, dyskinesia, dysphoria, sweating and diarrhea
• Euphorigenic and hallucinogenic properties may lead to abuse of anticholinergic agents
• Use of antiparkinsonian agents in patients with existing TD can exacerbate the movement disorder and may unmask latent TD

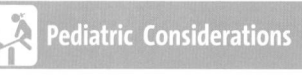 **Toxicity**

• Can occur following excessive doses, with combination therapy, in the elderly, or with drug abuse
• Autonomic signs: dilated pupils, dry flushed skin, thirst, tachycardia, urinary retention, constipation, paralytic ileus, anorexia, staggering gait
• Mental signs: clouded sensorium, dazed, perplexed or fearful countenance, insomnia, euphoria, irritability, excitation, disorientation in time and space, difficulties in thinking and concentration, exacerbation of psychotic behavior, visual hallucinations (grasping at air), and tactile hallucinations (picking objects from skin)

Management	• If toxicity is suspected, stop all drugs with anticholinergic activity; symptoms should abate within 24–48 h • Physostigmine 1–3 mg IM has been used to reverse both central and peripheral effects; use of this drug is not currently recommended as it can cause seizures, cardiac effects, and excessive cholinergic effects

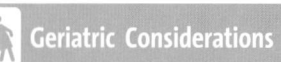 **Pediatric Considerations**

• For detailed information on the use of antiparkinsonian agents in this population, please see the *Clinical Handbook of Psychotropic Drugs for Children and Adolescents* (2007)
• Doses up to 80 mg trihexyphenidyl have been employed in the treatment of dystonic movements in children; these were well tolerated with few side effects

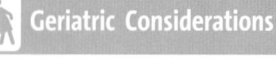 **Geriatric Considerations**

• The elderly are very sensitive to anticholinergic drugs. Monitor for constipation, urinary retention as well as increased confusion, memory loss, and disorientation. Avoid drugs with potent central or peripheral anticholinergic activity (biperiden may be most appropriate agent)
• Caution when using two or more drugs with anticholinergic properties

Use in Pregnancy

- Greatest risk of malformation during first trimester use
- Consider potential for withdrawal or other effects (e.g., metabolism) in newborn and effects on delivery during third trimester
- Limited human data with many of these agents
- Amantadine – contraindicated during first trimester
- Propranolol – use in second/third trimester associated with decreased fetal and placental weight
- Diazepam and lorazepam – effects on human embryo/fetus controversial. Neonatal withdrawal is a concern if used close to delivery
- Clonazepam – limited human data
- Diphenhydramine – data suggest it is safe for use in pregnancy

Breast Milk

- No specific data available; however, infants are sensitive to anticholinergic effects of drugs, therefore breastfeeding is discouraged
- Anticholinergic properties may inhibit lactation

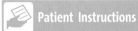 **Nursing Implications**

- Antiparkinsonian drugs should be given only to relieve extrapyramidal side effects of antipsychotics; excess use or abuse can precipitate a toxic psychosis
- Some adverse effects of these drugs (i.e., anticholinergic) are additive to those of antipsychotics; observe patient for signs of side effects or toxicity
- Monitor patient's intake and output. Urinary retention can occur, especially in the elderly; bethanechol (Urecholine) can be used to reverse this problem
- To help prevent gastric irritation, administer drug after meals
- Relieve dry mouth by giving patient cool drinks, ice chips, sugarless chewing gum, or hard, sour candy. Suggest frequent rinsing of the mouth, and teeth should be brushed regularly. Patients should avoid calorie-laden beverages and sweet candy as they not only increase the likelihood of dental caries, but will also promote weight gain. Formerly well-fitting dentures may become ill-fitting, and can cause rubbing and/or ulceration of the gums. May predispose patient to monilial infections. Products that promote or replace salivation (e.g., MoiStir, Saliment) may be of benefit
- Blurring of near vision is due to paresis of the ciliary muscle. This can be helped by wearing suitable glasses, reading by a bright light or, if severe, by the use of Pilocarpine eye drops 0.5%
- Dry eyes may be of particular difficulty to the elderly or those wearing contact lenses. Artificial tears or contact lens wetting solutions may be of benefit in dealing with this problem
- Anticholinergics reduce peristalsis and decrease intestinal secretions, leading to constipation. Increasing fluids and bulk (e.g., bran, salads) as well as fruit in the diet is beneficial. If necessary, bulk laxatives (e.g., Metamucil, Prodiem) or a stool softener (e.g., docusate) can be used; lactulose may be used for chronic constipation
- Warn the patient not to drive a car or operate machinery until response to the drug has been determined
- Appropriate patient education regarding medication and side effects is necessary prior to discharge
- If akathisia does not respond to standard antiparkinsonian agents, diphenhydramine, propranolol, lorazepam, clonazepam, or diazepam can be tried

Patient Instructions

- For detailed patient instructions on antiparkinsonian agents for treating extrapyramidal side effects, see the Patient Information Sheet on p. 341

Agents for Treating Extrapyramidal Side Effects (cont.)

→← Drug Interactions

• Only clinically significant interactions are listed below

Class of Drug	Example	Interaction Effects
Adsorbent	Activated charcoal, antacids, kaolin-pectin (attapulgite), cholestyramine	Oral absorption decreased when used simultaneously
Anticholinergic	Antidepressants, antihistamines, FGAs (low potency)	Increased atropine-like effects causing dry mouth, blurred vision, constipation, etc. May produce inhibition of sweating and may lead to paralytic ileus High doses can bring on a toxic psychosis
Antidepressant SSRI NDRI	 Paroxetine, fluoxetine Bupropion	 Case reports of reversal of antidepressant and antibulimic effects of fluoxetine and paroxetine with cyproheptadine Increased plasma level of procyclidine (by 40%) with paroxetine Case reports of neurotoxicity in elderly patients, in combination with amantadine
Antihypertensive	Hydrochlorothiazide, triamterene	Reduced renal clearance of amantadine resulting in drug accumulation and possible toxicity
Antipsychotic	Haloperidol, trifluoperazine Thioridazine	Antiparkinsonian drugs may aggravate tardive dyskinesia or unmask latent TD May decrease plasma level of the antipsychotic Propranolol may significantly increase thioridazine levels or cause arrhythmias Potential for additive hypotensive effects with propranolol
Caffeine		May offset beneficial effects by increasing tremor and akathisia
Co-trimoxazole (Trimethoprim/Sulfamethoxazole)		Competition for renal clearance resulting in elevated plasma level of amantadine
Digoxin		Increased bioavailability of digoxin tablets (not capsules or liquids) Increased plasma level of digoxin due to decreased gastric motility
Quinidine		Inhibited renal clearance of amantadine (in males) – may be of low clinical significance
Quinine		Increased plasma level of amantadine due to inhibited renal clearance (by 27% in males)

Effects on Extrapyramidal Symptoms

Agent	Tremor	Rigidity	Dystonia	Akinesia	Akathisia
Amantadine (Symmetrel)	++	++	+	+++	++
Benztropine (Cogentin)	++	+++	+++	++	++
Biperiden (Akineton)	++	++	++	+++	++
β-Blockers (e.g., propranolol, nadolol)	+	–	–	–	+++
Clonazepam (Rivotril, Klonopin)	–	+	+	–	+++
Cyproheptadine (Periactin)	–	–	–	–	+++
Diazepam (Valium)	+	++	++	+	+++
Diphenhydramine (Benadryl)	++	+	+++	–	+++
Ethopropazine (Parsitan)	+++	++	+	+	++
Lorazepam (Ativan)	+	+	+++	–	+++
Orphenadrine (Norflex)	++	++	–	++	+
Procyclidine (Kemadrin)	++	++	++	++	++
Trihexyphenidyl (Artane)	++	++	++	+++	++

Based on literature and clinical observations: – effect not established, + some effect (20% response), ++ moderate effect (20–50% response), +++ good effect (> 50% response)

Comparison of Agents for Treating Extrapyramidal Side Effects

Agents	Therapeutic Effects	Adverse Effects	Dose in Adults	CYP-450/UGT Metabolizing Enzymes[A]	CYP-450 Inhibition[B]
Amantadine (Symmetrel)	An NMDA-receptor antagonist May improve akathisia, akinesia, rigidity, acute dystonia, parkinsonism, and tardive dyskinesia; may enhance the effects of other antiparkinsonian agents Tolerance to fixed dose may develop after 1–8 weeks May be useful in levodopa-induced movement disorder Used to treat antipsychotic- and SSRI-induced sexual dysfunction Early data suggest a possible role in ADHD, conduct disorder and in treating cocaine craving and use	Common: indigestion, excitement, difficulty in concentration, dizziness Less often: peripheral edema, skin rash, livido reticularis (mottled skin discoloration), tremors, slurred speech, ataxia, depression, insomnia, and lethargy (these are dose-related and disappear on drug withdrawal) Confusion, hallucinations and seizures reported in the elderly and in patients with renal insufficiency Less anticholinergic than other agents	Orally: 100–400 mg daily Dose must be decreased in patients with renal insufficiency Cocaine withdrawal: 100 mg bid to tid	–[C]	–[C]
Antihistamines **Cyproheptadine** (Periactin)	Useful for akathisia Sedative and anticholinergic effects Has been used to increase appetite May help ameliorate drug-induced sexual dysfunction	Drowsiness, confusion, weight gain	Initial: 4 mg tid up to 32 mg/day	?	?
Diphenhydramine (Benadryl)	Has effect on tremor Sedative effect may benefit tension and excitation; may enhance the effects of other antiparkinsonian agents Some effect on rigidity	Somnolence, confusion, and dizziness, especially in the elderly; delirium reported	IM/IV: 25–50 mg for dystonia Orally: 25–50 mg tid to qid	2D6; UGT1A3	2D6
Orphenadrine (Disipal, Norflex)	Modest effect on sialorrhea Mild stimulant Beneficial effects tend to wear off in 2–6 months	Slight dryness of mouth, sedation, dizziness, mild central excitation	Orally: 50 mg tid up to 400 mg/day	2D6, 2B6 3A4, 1A2	1A2, 2A6, 2D6, 2B6, 3A4, 2C8/9, 2C19, 2E1
β-Blockers Propranolol (Inderal)	Very useful for akathisia and tremor	Monitor pulse and blood pressure; do not stop high dose abruptly due to rebound tachycardia	Orally: 10 mg tid to 120 mg daily	**1A2**[P], **2D6**[P], **2C19**[P], 3A4[W]	1A2[W], 3A4, 2D6[W]
Benzodiazepines **Diazepam** (Valium, etc.)	Beneficial effect on akathisia and acute dystonia Muscle relaxant	Drowsiness, lethargy (see p. 161–162)	Orally: up to 5 mg qid IV: 10 mg for acute dystonia by slow direct IV push (rate of 5 mg (1 ml)/ min)	3A4, 2C9, 2C19, 2B6	
Lorazepam (Ativan)	Beneficial effect on akathisia Excellent for acute dyskinesia (sublingual works quickest)	Drowsiness, lethargy (see p. 161–162)	Orally: up to 2 mg qid Sublingual: 1–2 mg up to tid IM: 1–2 mg for dystonia	–	–
Clonazepam (Rivotril, Klonopin)	Useful for akathisia	Drowsiness, lethargy (see p. 161–162)	Orally: 1–4 mg/day in divided doses	2B4, 2E1, 3A4	2B4
Benztropine (Cogentin)	Beneficial effect on rigidity Relieves sialorrhea and drooling Powerful muscle relaxant; sedative action Cumulative and long-acting; once-daily dosing can be used (preferably in the morning) IM/IV: dramatic effect on dystonic symptoms	Dry mouth, blurred vision, urinary retention, constipation Increases intraocular pressure Toxic psychosis when abused or overused	Orally: 1–2 mg bid up to 4 mg bid if needed IM/IV: 1–2 mg; may repeat in 30 min	2D6	

Agents	Therapeutic Effects	Adverse Effects	Dose in Adults	CYP-450/UGT Metabolizing Enzymes[A]	CYP-450 Inhibition[B]
Biperiden (Akineton)	Has effect against rigidity and akinesia	Has higher affinity for muscarinic receptors in the CNS, and is less likely to cause peripheral anticholinergic effects May cause euphoria, sedation, confusion, and increased tremor	Orally: 2 mg tid to qid	?	?
Ethopropazine (Parsitan, Parsidol)	Has effect against rigidity; improves posture, gait, and speech Specific for tremor	Dry mouth, postural dizziness, somnolence, and confusion can occur Low anticholinergic activity; safe to use in moderate doses in patients with glaucoma	Starting oral dose: 50 mg tid up to 400 mg per day; for severe symptoms up to 600 mg/day	?	?
Procyclidine (Kemadrin)	Similar to trihexyphenidyl Milder and questionable effect on tremor Useful agent to use in combination when muscle rigidity is severe	Less pronounced side effects than with trihexyphenidyl; slight blurring of vision Stimulation and giddiness in some patients Can be abused	Starting oral dose: 2.5 mg bid to tid; increase by 2.5 mg/day if required May need up to 30mg/day	2D6	2D6
Trihexyphenidyl (Artane)	Mild to moderate effect against rigidity and spasm (occasionally get dramatic results) Tremor alleviated to a lesser degree; as a result of relaxing muscle spasm, more tremor activity may be noted Stimulating – can be used during the day for sluggish, lethargic, and akinetic patients	Dry mouth, blurred vision, GI distress Less sedating potential Severe and persistent mental confusion, cognitive impairment may occur, esp. in the elderly; must recognize this as a toxic state At toxic doses get restlessness, delirium, hallucinations; these disappear when the drug is discontinued (most anticholinergic of the antiparkinsonian agents – liable to be abused as a euphoriant)	Orally: 4–15 mg daily, up to 30 mg tolerated in younger patients	?	?

[A] Cytochrome P-450 isoenzymes involved in liver metabolism of drug (data not consistent among references), [B] CYP-450 isoenzymes inhibited by drug, [C] Undergoes little metabolism; 90% of dose recovered unchanged in the urine; does not affect the metabolism of other drugs

P-gp = p-glycoprotein – a transporter of hydrophobic substances in or out of specific body organs (e.g., block absorption in the gut); UGT = uridine diphosphate glucuronosyl transferase – involved in Phase 2 reactions (conjugation)

Extrapyramidal

ANXIOLYTIC (ANTIANXIETY) AGENTS

Classification

- Anxiolytic agents can be classified as follows:

Chemical Class	Agent	Page

Antidepressants
  SSRI
  SNRI
  Tricyclic Antidepressant (TCA)
	Examples: Paroxetine, sertraline, escitalopram
	Example: Venlafaxine
	Example: Clomipramine
		See p. 3
		See p. 21
		See p. 37

Antihistamine[A]	Example: Hydroxyzine[A] (Atarax, Vistaril)	See below[A] and p. 174
Azaspirodecanedione (Azaspirone)	Example: Buspirone	See p. 170
Barbiturates[B]	Examples: Phenobarbital[C] (Luminal)	See below[B] [C]
Benzodiazepines	See below for examples	

[A] CNS depressant; used primarily for pruritus of psychogenic origin. Dose: 10–400 mg/day. Double-blind studies suggest benefit for GAD in adults; onset of anxiolytic action takes 4–6 weeks, but efficacy maintained long-term; [B] Act as CNS depressants; seldom used as anxiolytics, because they are habit-forming, causing physical dependence; they can have severe withdrawal symptoms; tolerance develops quickly, requiring increased dosage; they have a low margin of safety (therapeutic dose close to toxic dose); they are involved in many drug interactions (induce metabolizing enzymes); they can evoke behavioral complications including hyperactivity and conduct disorders in children, and depression in adults; [C] Phenobarbital has been used as an anxiolytic for those unable to benefit from benzodiazepines or buspirone (dose: 30–90 mg/day)

Benzodiazepines

General Comments

- Benzodiazepines can be categorized as follows:

		Anxiolytic	Sedative/Hypnotic	Anticonvulsant	Potency
Short-acting	Midazolam (Versed)[A]	+	+++	–	
	Triazolam (Halcion)	+	+++	high	
Intermediate	Alprazolam (Xanax)	++	+	+	high
	Bromazepam (Lectopam)[C]	++	+		high
	Estazolam (ProSom)[B]	+	+++	+	
	Lorazepam (Ativan)	+++	++	++	high
	Oxazepam (Serax)	++	+		low
	Temazepam (Restoril)	+	+++	+	low
Long-acting	Chlordiazepoxide (Librium)	++			low
	Clobazam[D]			+++	high
	Clonazepam (Rivotril, Klonopin)	++	+	+++	high
	Clorazepate (Tranxene, Tranxilene)	++			medium
	Diazepam (Valium)	+++	++	++	medium
	Flurazepam (Dalmane)	+	+++		medium
	Nitrazepam (Mogadon)(C)	+	+++	++	high
	Quazepam (Doral)[B]	+	+++	+	medium

Activity: + weak, ++ moderate, +++ strong, [A] Acute use only, [B] Not marketed in Canada, [C] Not marketed in the USA, [D] Not used in anxiety and not reviewed in this chapter.

Chemical Class	Generic Name	Trade Name[A]	Dosage Forms and Strengths
Benzodiazepine	Alprazolam	Xanax Xanax TS[C] Xanax XR[B] Niravam[B]	Tablets: 0.25 mg, 0.5 mg, 1 mg, 2 mg[B] Oral concentrate: 1 mg/ml Triscored tablets: 2 mg Extended-release tablets[B]: 0.5 mg, 1 mg, 2 mg, 3 mg Oral disintegrating tablet: 0.25 mg, 0.5 mg, 1 mg, 2 mg
	Bromazepam[C]	Lectopam	Tablets: 1.5 mg, 3 mg, 6 mg
	Chlordiazepoxide	Librium Libritabs[B]	Capsules: 5 mg, 10 mg, 25 mg Tablets: 5 mg, 25 mg
	Clonazepam	Rivotril[C], Klonopin[B]	Tablets: 0.25 mg, 0.5 mg, 1 mg, 2 mg Oral disintegrating tablets[B]: 0.125 mg, 0.25 mg, 0.5 mg, 1 mg, 2 mg Oral concentrated solution[B]: 2.5 mg/ml Injection[B]: 1 mg/ml
	Clorazepate	Tranxene[C], Tranxilene[B] Tranxene SD[B]	Tablets: 3.75 mg, 7.5 mg, 15 mg Tablets: 11.25 mg, 22.5 mg
	Diazepam	Valium Diazepam Intensol[B] Diastat Diazemuls[C], Dizac[B]	Tablets: 2 mg, 5 mg, 10 mg Oral solution: 5 mg/5 ml Injection: 5 mg/ml Oral concentrate[B]: 5 mg/ml Injection: 5 mg/ml Rectal gel: 5 mg/ml Emulsion injection (IM/IV): 5 mg/ml
	Estazolam[B]	ProSom	Tablets: 1 mg, 2 mg
	Flurazepam	Dalmane	Capsules: 15 mg, 30 mg
	Lorazepam	Ativan Lorazepam Intensol[B]	Tablets: 0.5 mg, 1 mg, 2 mg Sublingual tablets[C]: 0.5 mg, 1 mg, 2 mg Oral solution[B]: 0.5 mg/5 ml Injection: 2 mg/ml[B], 4 mg/ml Solution[B]: 2 mg/ml
	Midazolam	Versed	Syrup[B]: 2 mg/ml Injection: 1 mg/ml, 5 mg/ml
	Nitrazepam[C]	Mogadon	Tablets: 5 mg, 10 mg
	Oxazepam	Serax	Tablets: 10 mg[C], 15 mg, 30 mg[C] Capsules[B]: 10 mg, 15 mg, 30 mg
	Quazepam[B]	Doral	Tablets: 15 mg
	Temazepam	Restoril	Capsules: 7.5 mg[B], 15 mg, 22.5 mg, 30 mg
	Triazolam	Halcion	Tablets: 0.125 mg, 0.25 mg

[A] Generic preparations may be available, [B] Not marketed in Canada, [C] Not marketed in USA

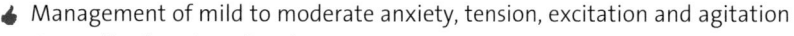

Benzodiazepines (cont.)

Indications (👍 Approved)	👍 Management of mild to moderate anxiety, tension, excitation and agitation 👍 Generalized anxiety disorder 👍 Management of acute and chronic alcohol withdrawal syndromes 👍 Tetanus (diazepam) 👍 Convulsions: status epilepticus, absence seizures, infantile spasms, simple-partial and complex-partial seizures 👍 Insomnia 👍 Panic disorder with or without agoraphobia (alprazolam, clorazepate) 👍 Muscle spasms, dystonia, "restless legs" syndrome 👍 Other: cardioversion, endoscopy and bronchoscopy, enhancement of analgesia during labor and delivery, preoperative sedation • Akathisia due to antipsychotic agents • May reduce abnormal movements associated with tardive dyskinesia (clonazepam) • Sedation in severe agitation (IV) • In mania used concomitantly with antipsychotic or lithium to control agitation; may potentiate antipsychotics and decrease dosage requirements • Depression (alprazolam) • Mania • In schizophrenia used with antipsychotic to control agitation; diazepam used alone in high doses suggested to improve paranoia • Social phobia (alprazolam, clonazepam, diazepam, lorazepam) • Catatonia (parenteral and sublingual lorazepam, diazepam, clonazepam) • Myoclonus, restless legs syndrome, Tourette's syndrome (clonazepam) • Acute dystonia (SL or IM lorazepam) • Delirium (lorazepam); delirium tremens (diazepam) • Neuralgic pain (clonazepam) • Premenstrual dysphoric disorder (alprazolam) • Control of violent outbursts, assaultive behavior (clonazepam, lorazepam) reduce agitation and behavioral problems associated with severe over-arousal or anxiety; used also in combination with mood stabilizers, antipsychotic, or β-blocker
General Comments	• The potency of a benzodiazepine is the affinity of the parent drug, or its active metabolites, for benzodiazepine receptors, in vivo • Benzodiazepines are suggested to relieve behavioral and somatic manifestations of anxiety, but have little effect on psychic or cognitive symptoms (e.g., worry, anger, interpersonal sensitivity, and obsessionality); may be most helpful during the beginning phase of treatment not recommended long-term
Pharmacology	• Depress the CNS at the levels of the limbic system, the brain-stem reticular formation, and the cortex Benzodiazepines bind to the "benzodiazepine"-GABA-chloride receptor complex, facilitating the action of GABA (an inhibitory neurotransmitter) on CNS excitability. Intensity of action depends on degree of receptor occupancy • Clonazepam has 5-HT potentiating properties
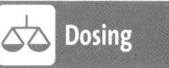 **Dosing**	• See pp. 166–169 for individual agents • Although the majority of indications for benzodiazepines are for short-term (less than 2 months) treatment, many patients are prescribed these agents for extended periods of time (>3 months). Clinicians should discuss the risks and benefits of long-term use with patients early on in therapy • Following IV administration of diazepam, local pain and thrombophlebitis may occur due to precipitation of the drug, or due to an irritant effect of propylene glycol; IV diazepam emulsion (Diazemuls) is less likely to cause this problem

- IM use is discouraged with diazepam as absorption is slow, erratic, and possibly incomplete; local pain often occurs. Lorazepam IM is adequately absorbed (though absorption can be erratic by this method)
- When switching from immediate-release (divided dose) to XR (single dose), alprazolam, 0.5 mg tid = alprazolam XR 1.5 mg od. Alprazolam XR administered once daily, preferably in the morning; should not be chewed, crushed, or broken. Dosage titration recommended of no more than 1 mg/day every 3–4 days. Slower absorption rate results in a relatively constant concentration that is maintained for 5–11 h after dosing. Dose reductions should be in increments of 0.5 mg q 3 days, or less

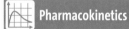

Pharmacokinetics

- See pp. 166–169 for individual agents
- Marked interindividual variation (up to 10-fold) is found in all pharmacokinetic parameters. Age, smoking, liver disease, physical disorders, as well as concurrent use of other drugs may influence parameters by changing the volume of distribution and elimination half-life of these drugs
- Well absorbed from GI tract after oral administration; food can delay the rate, but not the extent of absorption; onset of action is determined by rate of absorption and lipid solubility
- Lipid solubility denotes speed of entry into (lipid) brain tissue, followed by extensive redistribution to adipose tissue. Benzodiazepines have a high volume of distribution (i.e., the tissue drug concentration is much higher than the blood drug concentration)
- The duration of action is determined mainly by the distribution and not by elimination half-life (except for ultra-short half-life drugs like midazolam and triazolam)
- Differences in pharmacokinetics between the various benzodiazepines have been presumed to indicate clinical differences as well – this is not necessarily so. However, present rationale for selection of a benzodiazepine remains the difference in pharmacokinetic profile. Generally, short-acting agents can be used as hypnotics and for acute problems relating to anxiety, while long-acting agents can be used for chronic conditions where a continuous drug effect is needed
- It is suggested that the longer the half-life of a benzodiazepine, the greater the likelihood that the compound will have an adverse effect on daytime functioning (e.g., hangover). However, with shorter half-life benzodiazepines, withdrawal and anxiety between doses (rebound) and anterograde amnesia are seen more often
- The major pathways of metabolism are hepatic microsomal oxidation and demethylation. Conjugation to more polar (water-soluble) glucuronide derivatives allows for excretion. Biotransformation by oxidation can be impaired by disease states (e.g., hepatic cirrhosis), by age or by drugs that impair the metabolism. Drugs undergoing conjugation only (e.g., oxazepam) are not so affected

Onset & Duration of Action

- Benzodiazepines that undergo conjugation (e.g., temazepam, oxazepam) have longer elimination half-lives in women than in men

Adverse Effects

- Are few, and often disappear with adjustment of dosage

CNS Effects

- Most common are extensions of the generalized sedative effect, e.g., fatigue, drowsiness; alprazolam XR may prolong daytime sedation
- Impaired mental speed, central cognitive processing ability, memory and perceptomotor performance (related to dose, high lipid solubility – see table pp. 166–169, and to peak plasma level of benzodiazepine)
- Tolerance to acute short-term memory impairment does not develop with time
- Anterograde amnesia (more likely with high potency agents or higher doses); sexual dysmnesia (midazolam)
- Chronic use: impaired visuospacial and visuomotor abilities, e.g., decreased motor coordination, psychomotor speed and response time, decreased concentration, speed of information processing and verbal learning; patients may underestimate their memory deficits. Data suggests that cognitive function may improve gradually after drug discontinuation
- Behavior dyscontrol with irritability and impulsivity; paradoxical agitation – insomnia, hallucinations, nightmares, euphoria, rage, and violent behavior; most likely in patients with a history of aggressive behavior or unstable emotional behavior, e.g., borderline personality disorder (less likely with oxazepam)
- Confusion and disorientation – primarily in the elderly. Periods of blackouts or amnesia have been reported
- Treatment-emergent depression (13% incidence with clonazepam)
- Excessive doses (parenterally) can result in respiratory depression and apnea

Benzodiazepines (cont.)

- Dysarthria, muscle weakness, incoordination, ataxia (up to 22% with clonazepam at doses above 2 mg/day), nystagmus
- Headache

Other Adverse Effects

- Anticholinergic effects, e.g., blurred vision (mild), dry mouth
- Sexual dysfunction including decreased libido, erectile dysfunction, anorgasmia, ejaculatory disturbance and gynecomastia; abnormal size and shape of sperm reported
- Dizziness (up to 12% with higher doses of clonazepam)
- Increased salivation (clonazepam)
- Rare reports of purpura and thrombocytopenia with diazepam
- Few documented allergies to benzodiazepines; rarely reported skin reactions include rashes, fixed drug eruption, photosensitivity reactions, pigmentation, alopecia, bullous reactions, exfoliative dermatitis, vasculitis, erythema nodosum

D/C Discontinuation Syndrome

- Benzodiazepines present different risks of physiological dependence at therapeutic doses, depending on the individual as well as the drug's potency and its elimination half-life. Up to 30% of patients suggested to experience withdrawal after 8 weeks of benzodiazepine treatment
- Discontinuation of a benzodiazepine can produce:
  - Withdrawal: occurs 1–2 days (shortacting) to 5–10 days (longacting) following any drug discontinuation. Common symptoms include insomnia, agitation, anxiety, perceptual changes, dysphoria, headache, muscle aches, twitches, tremors, loss of appetite and GI distress. Catatonia and depression have also been reported. Severe reactions can occur such as grand mal or petit mal seizures, coma, and psychotic states
  - Rebound: occurs hours to days after drug withdrawal; symptoms (of anxiety) are similar but more intense than those reported originally
  - Relapse: symptoms occur weeks to months after drug withdrawal, are similar to original symptoms of anxiety, and get progressively worse until treated
- Pseudo withdrawal is a psychological withdrawal as a result of the patient's apprehension about discontinuing the drug – consists of anxiety symptoms unaccompanied by true withdrawal symptoms

Management

- To withdraw a patient from a benzodiazepine, an equivalent dose of diazepam should be substituted (see pp. 166–169) and withdrawal done according to one of the following protocols depending on patient history and psychological issues regarding benzodiazepine use
  1. Reduce diazepam by 10 mg daily until a total daily dose of 20 mg is reached – then reduce by 5 mg daily to an end point of total abstinence; propranolol may aid in the withdrawal process; or
  2. Reduce diazepan at a rate of 25% per week; or
  3. For patients with long-standing benzadiazepine use, reduce the first 50% of the dose over 4–8 weeks, then taper the final 50% more gradually, as tolerated by the patient
  ☞ **This protocol should not be used for alprazolam, which must be decreased by 0.5 mg weekly; quicker withdrawal may result in delirium and seizures**
  - Carbamazepine (in therapeutic doses) may aid in the withdrawal process
  - Alternatively, alprazolam may be substituted with an equal dose of clonazepam (in divided doses), then decreased by 1 mg daily

⚠ Precautions

- Do not use in patients with sleep apnea
- Administer with caution to elderly or debilitated patients, those with liver disease, and to patients performing hazardous tasks requiring mental alertness or physical coordination
- Benzodiazepines may diminish the therapeutic efficacy of electroconvulsive therapy (ECT) by raising the seizure threshold
- Anxiolytics lower the tolerance to alcohol, and high doses may produce mental confusion similar to alcohol intoxication
- Can cause physical and psychological dependence, tolerance, and withdrawal symptoms – correlated to dose and duration of use
- Benzodiazepines are at risk of being abused by susceptible individuals (e.g., habitual polydrug users); they prefer agents with rapid peak drug effects (e.g., diazepam, lorazepam, alprazolam). Methadone users may take a benzodiazepine a few hours after their methadone dose to augment a 'high'. Users of opiates use benzodiazepines to self-medicate symptoms of withdrawal. Benzodiazepines also used to treat adverse effects of cocaine or alcohol

- Withdrawal symptoms resemble those of alcohol and barbiturates, e.g., tremor, agitation, headache, nausea, delirium, hallucinations, metallic taste. Abrupt withdrawal following prolonged use of high doses can produce grandmal seizures (especially with alprazolam)

Toxicity
- Rarely if ever fatal when taken alone; may be lethal when taken in combination with other drugs, such as alcohol and barbiturates
- Symptoms of overdose include hypotension, depressed respiration, and coma

Management
- Flumazenil injection (a benzodiazepine antagonist) reverses the hypnotic-sedative effects of benzodiazepines. Repeated doses may be required due to the short duration of action of flumazenil

Pediatric Considerations
- For detailed information on the use of anxiolytics in this population, please see the *Clinical Handbook of Psychotropic Drugs for Children and Adolescents* (2007)
- Probable indications for anxiolytics include seizure disorder, generalized anxiety disorder, adjustment disorder, insomnia, night terrors, and somnambulism
- High potency benzodiazepines (clonazepam) useful for panic disorder/agoraphobia, social phobia and separation anxiety disorder
- Benzodiazepines are metabolized faster in children than in adults; may require small divided doses to maintain blood level
- Adverse effec include sedation, cognitive, and motor effects; disinhibition with irritability and agitation reported in up to 30% of children – primarily in younger impulsive patients with mental retardation

Geriatric Considerations
- Caution when using drugs that are metabolized by oxidation (e.g., diazepam, estazolam) as they can accumulate in the elderly or in persons wih liver disease
- Caution when combining with other drugs with CNS effects; excessive sedation can cause confusion, disorientation
- Elderly are more vulnerable to adverse CNS effects, specifically as to balance, gait, memory, cognition, behavior – longterm use should be discouraged
- Data indicates that benzodiazepine use increases risk of falls 3-fold, leading to femur fractures; risk increased with dose and in females
- Higher risk of motor vehicle accidents documented in elderly taking long-acting benzodiazepines

Use in Pregnancy
- Benzodiazepines and metabolites freely cross the placenta and accumulate in fetal circulation
- Some studies suggest an association between benzodiazepine use in the first trimester and teratogenicity; data contradictory; absolute risk of cleft palate increased by 0.01% (level B evidence)[1] – suggest ultrasound screening of fetus
- High doses or prolonged use by mother in third trimester may precipitate fetal benzodiazepine syndrome (level A evidence)[1]: including floppy infant syndrome, impaired temperature regulation and withdrawal symptoms in newborn

Breast Milk
- Benzodiazepines are excreted into breast milk in levels sufficient to produce effects in the newborn, including sedation, lethargy, and poor temperature regulation, e.g., infant can receive up to 13% of maternal dose of diazepam and 7% of lorazepam dose
- Metabolism of benzodiazepines in infants is slower, especially during the first 6 weeks; long-acting agents can accumulate
- American Academy of Pediatrics considers benzodiazepines as drugs "whose effect on nursing infants is unknown but may be of concern"

Nursing Implications
- Assess the anxiety level of patients on these drugs to determine if anxiety control has been accomplished or if oversedation has occurred
- The dose should be maintained as prescribed; caution patient not to increase or decrease the dose without consulting the physician
- Inform patients that activities requiring mental alertness should not be performed after taking drug; advise the patient to report any memory lapses or amnesia to the physician immediately
- Caution patients not to use other CNS depressant drugs including over-the-counter drugs (e.g., antihistamines or alcohol) without consulting the doctor
- Excessive consumption of caffeinated beverages will counteract the effects of anxiolytics
- Tolerance and physical addiction can occur; caution patient that withdrawal symptoms can occur with abrupt discontinuation after prolonged use
- Alprazolam XR should be administered at a consistent time of day, once daily (preferably in the morning); a highfat meal prior to drug administration can affect the plasma level of this drug. Alprazolam XR should not be broken, crushed, or chewed, but should be swallowed whole
- Advise patient to avoid ingestion of grapefruit juice while on alprazolam and triazolam as blood levels of these drugs can be elevated

Benzodiazepines (cont.)

Patient Instructions

- For detailed patient instructions on anxiolytic drugs, see the Patient Information Sheet on p. 342

Drug Interactions

- Many interactions; only clinically significant ones are listed below

Class of Drug	Example	Interaction Effects
Allopurinol		Decreased metabolism and increased half-life of benzodiazepines that are metabolized by oxidation (see charts pp. 166–169), leading to increased drug effect
Anesthetics	Ketamine	Prolonged recovery with diazepam due to decreased metabolism
	Volatile (e.g., halothane)	Decreased protein binding of diazepam resulting in increased pharmacological effects
Antiarrhythmic	Amiodarone	Reduced metabolism and increased plasma level of midazolam
Antibiotic	Erythromycin, clarithromycin, troleandomycin	Decreased metabolism and increased plasma levels of benzodiazepines metabolized by CYP3A4, including midazolam (by 54%), triazolam (by 52%), alprazolam (by 60%), estazolam, and diazepam; no interaction with azithromycin
	Chloramphenicol	Decreased metabolism of benzodiazepines that are metabolized by oxidation
	Quinolones: ciprofloxacin, enoxacin	Decreased metabolism of diazepam
	Quinupristin/dalfopristin	Decreased metabolism of midazolam and diazepam via CYP3A4
Anticoagulant	Warfarin	Decreased PT ratio or INR response with chlordiazepoxide
Anticonvulsant	Carbamazepine, barbiturates	Increased metabolism and decreased plasma level of benzodiazepines metabolized by CYP3A4, including alprazolam (> 50%) and clonazepam (19–37%), diazepam Additive CNS effects
	Phenytoin	Decreased phenytoin plasma level reported with clonazepam Increased phenytoin level and toxicity reported with diazepam and chlordiazepoxide Increased metabolism and decreased plasma level of benzodiazepines metabolized by CYP3A4
	Valproate	Displacement by diazepam from proteinbinding resulting in increased plasma level Decreased metabolism and increased pharmacological effects of clonazepam and lorazepam

Antidepressant
  Cyclic
  SSRI
 	
  SARI
	Desipramine, imipramine
	Fluoxetine, fluvoxamine, sertraline
	
	Nefazodone
		Increased plasma levels of desipramine and imipramine with alprazolam (by 20% and 31%, respectively)
		Decreased metabolism and increased plasma level of benzodiazepines metabolized by CYP3A4, including alprazolam (by 100% with fluvoxamine and 46% with fluoxetine) and diazepam (13% decrease with sertraline)
		Increased plasma levels of alprazolam (by 200%) and triazolam (by 500%) due to inhibited metabolism via CYP3A4

Antifungal	Itraconazole, ketoconazole, fluconazole	Decreased metabolism and increased half-life of chlordiazepoxide and midazolam; decreased metabolism of triazolam (6-7 fold); reduce dose by 50–75%; AUC of alprazolam increased up to 4 fold
Antipsychotic	Clozapine	Marked sedation, increased salivation, hypotension (collapse), delirium, and respiratory arrest reported; more likely to occur early in treatment when clozapine is added to benzodiazepine regimen
	Olanzapine	Synergistic increase in somnolence when lorazepam given with IM olanzapine. Recommend lorazepam be given at least 1 h after IM olanzapine
Antituberculosis therapy	Isoniazid Rifampin	Decreased metabolism of benzodiazepines that are metabolized by oxidation (triazolam clearance decreased by 75%) Increased metabolism of benzodiazepines that aremetabolized by oxidation due to enzyme induction of CYP3A4 (diazepam by 300%, midazolam by 83%, estazolam)

Class of Drug	Example	Interaction Effects
β-Blocker	Propranolol	Increased half-life and decreased clearance of diazepam and bromazepam (no interaction with alprazolam, lorazepam, or oxazepam)
Caffeine		May counteract sedation and anxiolytic effects and increase insomnia
Ca-channel Blocker	Diltiazem	Decreased metabolism and increased plasma level of drugs metabolized by CYP3A4 including triazolam (by 100%), and of midazolam (by 105%)
	Verapamil	Increased plasma level of midazolam by 97% due to inhibited metabolism via CYP3A4
CNS depressant	Barbiturates, antihistamines Alcohol	Increased CNS depression; with high doses coma and respiratory depression can occur Alprazolam reported to increase aggression in moderate alcohol drinkers Brain concentrations of various benzodiazepines altered by ethanol: triazolam and estazolam concentrations decreased, diazepam concentration increased, no change with chlordiazepoxide
Digoxin		Decreased metabolism and elimination of digoxin reported with alprazolam
Disulfiram		Decreased metabolism of benzodiazepines that are metabolized by oxidation
Grapefruit juice		Increased absorption of diazepam and triazolam due to inhibition of CYP3A4 in the gut by grapefruit juice Decreased metabolism of alprazolam, midazolam, diazepam, and triazolam via CYP3A4 resulting in increased peak concentration and bioavailability
H$_2$ antagonist	Cimetidine	Decreased metabolism of benzodiazepines that are metabolized by oxidation (no effect with ranitidine, famotidine or nizatidine); peak plasma concentration of alprazolam increased by 86%
Hormone	Estrogen, oral contraceptives	Decreased metabolism of benzodiazepines that are metabolized by oxidation, e.g., diazepam, chlordiazepoxide, nitrazepam; increased half-life of alprazolam by 29% Clearance of combined oral contraceptives may be reduced with diazepam due to inhibited metabolism
Immunosuppressant	Cyclosporin	Decreased metabolism of cyclosporin with midazolam via CYP3A4
Kava Kava		May potentiate CNS effects causing increased side effects and toxicity
Lithium		Increased incidence of sexual dysfunction (up to 49%) when combined with clonazepam
L-Dopa		Benzodiazepines can reduce the efficacy of L-dopa secondary to the GABA agonist effect
Pomegranate juice		May decrease the metabolism of benzodiazepines that are metabolized via CYP3A4 (e.g., triazolam, alprazolam)
Probenecid		Decreased clearance of lorazepam (by 50%)
Propoxyphene		Increased half-life of alprazolam (by 58%) due to inhibited hydroxylation
Protease inhibitor	Ritonavir, indinavir	Increased plasma level of benzodiazepines that are metabolized by oxidation via CYP3A4 (e.g., triazolam, alprazolam)
Proton pump inhibitor	Omeprazole	Increased ataxia and sedation due to decreased metabolism of benzodiazepines metabolized by oxidation (no effect with lansoprazole)
Smoking – cigarettes		Increased clearance of diazepam and chlordiazepoxide due to enzyme induction Alprazolam concentration reduced by up to 50%
St. John's Wort		Decreased AUC of alprazolam by 40%, half-life by 24%, and increased C_{max} by 15% due to induced metabolism via CYP3A4 Increased oral clearance of midazolam by 108%, decreased oral bioavailability by 39% and AUC by 10% due to induced metabolism via CYP3A4[3]

Comparison of the Benzodiazepines

Drug	Compara-tive Dose (mg)**	Peak Plasma Level PO (C_{max})	Lipid Solubil-ity[c]	Elimination Half-life	Metabolites*** (m = main metabolite)	Comments	Use in Renal and Hepatic Disorders	Clinical Considerations
Alprazolam	0.5	Oral tablet = 1–2 h XR = 5–11 h (a high-fat meal increases C_{max} by 25% and decreases T_{max} by about 30%) Asians reported to reach higher C_{max}	moderate	Oral tablet = 6–27 h XR = 11–16 h Half-life increased in obese patients and in Asians.	Metabolized by oxidation: 29 metabolites; principal ones are: α-hydroxyalprazolam[m] desmethylalprazolam 4-hydroxyalprazolam Metabolized by CYP3A4[p] and 1A2	Rapidly and completely absorbed. Absorption rate for XR preparation differs significantly depending on time of day administered. 80% protein bound Well absorbed sublingually Plasma level of alprazolam may correlate with efficacy in panic disorder Plasma level decreased in smokers by up to 50% Clearance in elderly only 50–80% that of young adults	*Renal* – increased plasma level of free (unbound) alprazolam and possible decreased clearance *Hepatic* – half-life increased	Use: – anxiolytic – alcohol withdrawal – depression characterized by anxiety – panic attack prophylaxis – adjunct in depression tid dosing recommended Increases stage 2, and decreases stages 1 and 4 and REM sleep; caution on withdrawal (see p. 162) Low degree of sedation Case reports of behavioral side effects including mania XR preparation may prolong side effects such as sedation
Bromaze-pam[b]	3.0	0.5–4 h (2–12 h in elderly)	low	8–30 h	Metabolized by oxidation: 3-hydroxybromazepam Metabolized by CYP3A4	Metabolite reported to have anxiolytic activity; does not accumulate on chronic dosing In elderly C_{max} and half-life increased	?	Use: – anxiolytic
Chlordiazep-oxide	25.0	1–4 h	moderate	4–29 h (parent drug) 28–100 h (metabolites)	Metabolized by oxidation: desmethylchlordiazepoxide[m] oxazepam desmethyldiazepam	Onset of activity may be delayed; parent compound less potent than metabolites Metabolites accumulate on chronic dosing	*Renal* – decrease dose by 50% in patients with creatinine clearance < 10 ml/min *Hepatic* – half-life increased (2–3-fold) in patients with cirrhosis	Use: – anxiolytic – alcohol withdrawal Antacids* delay absorption in GI tract, but do not influence completeness of absorption Moderate degree of sedation
Clonazepam	0.25	1–4 h	low	19–60 h	Metabolized by oxidation: no active metabolite Metabolized primarily by CYP2B4, 2E1 and 3A4	Quickly and completely absorbed; slow onset of activity Dosage varies depending on usage Anxiety: 0.5–8 mg/day Panic disorder/agoraphobia: 2–8 mg/day Acute mania: 4–24mg/day Aggression: 1–3 mg/day Adjunct in psychotic states: 2–10 mg/day	*Renal* – no change *Hepatic* – increase in free (unbound) clonazepam in patients with cirrhosis	Use: – anticonvulsant – anxiolytic – panic attack prophylaxis – prophylaxis of BD – manic episode of BD – akathisia – restless legs syndrome – aggressive behavior Moderate degree of sedation

Drug	Comparative Dose (mg)**	Peak Plasma Level PO (C_{max})	Lipid Solubility[c]	Elimination Half-life	Metabolites*** (m = main metabolite)	Comments	Use in Renal and Hepatic Disorders	Clinical Considerations
Clorazepate Dipotassium	10.0	0.5–2 h	high	1.3–120 h (metabolites)	Metabolized by oxidation: N-desmethyldiazepam	Hydrolyzed in the stomach to active metabolite (parent compound inactive) Rate of hydrolysis depends on gastric acidity, therefore absorption is unreliable (one study disputes this) Metabolite accumulates on chronic dosing	*Renal* – clearance of metabolite impaired *Hepatic* – ?	Use: – anxiolytic – alcohol withdrawal Antacids and sodium bicarbonate reduce the rate and extent of appearance of active metabolite in the blood Fast onset of action Moderate degree of sedation
Diazepam	5	1–2 h	high	14–80 h (parent drug) 30–200 h (metabolites) Males have a shorter half-life and higher clearance rate than females	Metabolized by oxidation: N-desmethyldiazepam[m] oxazepam 3-hydroxydiazepam temazepam Metabolized by CYP3A4, 2C9, 2C19 and 2B6 Inhibitor of UGT2B7	Less protein bound in elderly, therefore attains higher serum levels Rapid onset of action followed by a redistribution into adipose tissue; accumulation on chronic dosing IM drug erratically absorbed Smoking: associated with higher diazepam clearance especially in the young	*Renal* – increased plasma level of free (unbound) diazepam and decreased clearance *Hepatic* – 2- to 3-fold increase in half-life in patients with cirrhosis	Use: – anxiolytic – anticonvulsant (status epilepticus) – alcohol withdrawal – akathisia – muscle relaxant – preoperative sedation Increases stage 2, and decreases stages 1 and 4 and REM sleep Fast onset of action High degree of sedation
Estazolam[a]	1	0.5–6 h	low	8–24 h	Metabolized by oxidation: 4-hydroxyestazolam 1-oxoestazolam Metabolized by CYP3A4	Metabolites inactive Metabolism impaired in the elderly and in hepatic disease	*Renal* – ? *Hepatic* – metabolism impaired	Use: – hypnotic Caution on withdrawal High doses can cause respiratory depression
Flurazepam	15	0.5–1 h	high	0.3–3 h (parent drug) 40–250 h (metabolites)	Metabolized by oxidation: N-desalkylflurazepam[m] OH-ethylflurazepam flurazepam aldehyde Metabolized by CYP2C and 2D6	Rapidly metabolized to active metabolite Elderly males accumulate metabolite more than young males on chronic dosing	*Renal* – ? *Hepatic* – metabolism impaired	Use: – hypnotic Decreases stage 1 and increases stage 2 sleep; no effect on REM Increase in daytime sedation over time; hangover Fast onset of action

Comparison of the Benzodiazepines (cont.)

Drug	Compara-tive Dose (mg)**	Peak Plasma Level PO (C_{max})	Lipid Solubil-ity[c]	Elimination Half-life	Metabolites*** (m = main metabolite)	Comments	Use in Renal and Hepatic Disorders	Clinical Considerations
Lorazepam	1	Oral: 1–6 h IM: 45–75 min IV: 5–10 min SL: 60 min	mode-rate	8–24 h	Conjugated to form loraze-pam glucuronide by UGT2B7	Metabolite not pharmacologically active Slow onset of action Give at least twice daily to maintain steady state levels Well absorbed sublingually Clearance reduced in elderly by 22% (one study) Not involved in metabolic interactions via CYP enzymes	*Renal* – half-life of metabolite increased *Hepatic* – half-life and Vd doubled in patients with cirrhosis	Use: – anxiolytic – hypnotic – preoperative sedation – muscle relaxant – catatonia – manic phase of BD – akathisia – acute dystonia Produces anterograde amnesia Blood levels fall quickly on discontinuation; withdrawal symptoms appear sooner than with long-acting drugs Decreases stage 1 and REM
Midazolam	Acute use only	0.5–1 min	high	1–4 h (parent) 1–20 h (metabolites)	Metabolized by oxidation: 1-OH-methylmidazolam 4-OH-midazolam Metabolized primarily by CYP3A4 Inhibitor of P-gp	Metabolites active	*Renal* – decrease dose by 50% in patients with creatinine clearance < 10 ml/min *Hepatic* – metabolism significantly impaired in patients with cirrhosis	Use: – preoperative – sedative – anxiolytic – IV induction of anesthesia (in 30–60 s) – post-ECT agitation IV dose: 1–2.5 mg over at least 2 min May lower blood pressure Fast onset of action Produces anterograde amnesia; may induce false sexual beliefs
Nitrazepam[b]	2.5	0.5–7 h	low	15–48 h	Metabolized by nitroreduction by CYP2E1 No active metabolites	Excreted as amino and acetamide analogs Metabolism impaired in elderly Accumulates with chronic use	*Renal* – ? *Hepatic* – metabolism impaired	Use: – hypnotic Decreases REM sleep
Oxazepam	15	1–4 h	low	3–25 h	Conjugated to oxazepam glucuronide by UGT2B7	Metabolites not pharmacologically active Half-life and plasma clearance not affected much by age or sex Slow onset of action Give at least twice daily to maintain steady state No metabolic interactions	*Renal* – prolonged half-life *Hepatic* – no effect	Use: – anxiolytic – hypnotic – alcohol withdrawal – muscle relaxant Can lower aggression levels in patients with a history of belligerence and assault without releasing paradoxical rage responses Low sedative potential

Drug	Compara-tive Dose (mg)**	Peak Plasma Level PO (C_{max})	Lipid Solubil-ity[c]	Elimination Half-life	Metabolites*** (m = main metabolite)	Comments	Use in Renal and Hepatic Disorders	Clinical Considerations
Quazepam[a]	7.5	1.5 h	high	15–40 h (parent) 39–120 h (metabolites)	Metabolized by oxidation: 2-oxoquazepam Desalkylflurazepam Metabolized primarily by CYP2D6	Rapidly absorbed and metabolized Accumulation on chronic dosing – not associated with marked residual effects	?	Use: – hypnotic – anxiolytic Suppresses REM sleep, prolongs REM latency, increases stage 2 and decreases stages 1, 3, and 4 Rebound effects, anterograde amnesia and impaired performance not reported
Temazepam	10	2.5 h mean	moderate	3–25 h	Conjugated by UGT2B7	Hard gelatin capsule; variable rate of absorption depending on formulation; 5% excreted as oxazepam in the urine; plasma concentration too low to detect No accumulation with chronic use; no metabolic interactions	*Renal* – ? *Hepatic* – no effect	Use: – anxiolytic – hypnotic On doses of 30 mg/day or more, may cause hangover, morning nausea, headache, drowsiness, and vivid dreaming Decreases sleep stages 3 & 4 Rebound insomnia has been reported
Triazolam	0.25	1–2 h	moderate	1.5–5 h	Metabolized by oxidation: 7-α-hydroxyderivative Metabolized by CYP3A4[p]	Well absorbed sublingually Metabolite inactive; negligible accumulation of drug due to high hepatic clearance (dependent on hepatic blood flow and microsomal oxidizing capacity) Although half-life is short, clinical effects have been observed up to 16 h after a single dose Clearance in elderly only 50–80% that of young adults	*Renal* – no change *Hepatic* – reduced clearance	Use: – hypnotic Decreases stage 1, and increases stage 2 sleep; significantly increases latency to REM compared with baseline Rebound insomnia and anxiety reported Dose-related anterograde amnesia reported, especially in doses above 0.5 mg daily Reports of rage, automatism Report of hypothermia when combined with desipramine (neither drug causes this effect alone); potentiates anorexic effect of desipramine

* Apply to all benzodiazepines except where noted, ** Doses are approximate (alprazolam and clonazepam are relatively less potent, when dealing with anxiety, relatively more when dealing with panic); the doses used are substitute doses when switching among various benzodiazepines (they are approximately equal to phenobarbital 30 mg or pentobarbital 100 mg), *** See comments under Pharmacokinetics p. 161

[a] Not marketed in Canada, [b] Not marketed in USA, [c] High lipid solubility denotes fast entry into (lipid) brain tissue, rapid onset and increased risk of memory impairment,
[p] Primary route of metabolism, where known

P-gp = p-glycoprotein – a transporter of hydrophobic substances in or out of specific body organs (e.g., block absorption in the gut); UGT = uridine diphosphate glucuronosyl transferase – involved in Phase 2 reactions (conjugation)

Buspirone

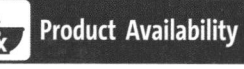 **Product Availability**

Chemical Class	Generic Name	Trade Name[A]	Dosage Forms and Strengths
Azaspirone	Buspirone	Buspar	Tablets: 5 mg, 7.5 mg[B], 10 mg, 15 mg[B], 30 mg[B]

[A] Generic preparations may be available, [B] Not marketed in Canada

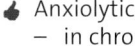 **Indications**
(👍 Approved)

- 👍 Anxiolytic, useful:
  - – in chronic anxiety
  - – as an alternative to benzodiazepines in situations where sedation or psychomotor impairment may be dangerous
  - – in patients with a history of substance abuse or alcohol abuse
- Treatment of obsessive compulsive disorder; may potentiate antiobsessional effects of SSRIs or clomipramine – data contradictory
- Double-blind, randomized clinical trials have demonstrated some benefits for the treatment of generalized anxiety disorder
- Antidepressant effects reported in doses of 40–90 mg/day; useful in patients with concomitant anxiety; may augment effect of antidepressants in treatment refractory depression; 30% of patients in step 2 of STAR*D trial reached remission when given buspirone plus citalopram (n = 286)[2]
- Contradictory evidence as to efficacy in social phobia; may be useful as an augmenting agent in partial responders to SSRIs
- Premenstrual dysphoric disorder
- Preliminary reports show some efficacy in posttraumatic stress disorder and body dysmorphic disorder
- Preliminary reports show buspirone may aid in smoking cessation and alcohol withdrawal (primarily in patients with concomitant anxiety) studies show mixed results on alcohol consumption
- Treatment of agitation, aggression/antisocial behavior, sexual preference disorders
- Preliminary data suggest efficacy in the treatment of anxiety and irritability in pervasive developmental disorders and ADHD
- Treatment of antipsychotic-induced akathisia
- May be useful in alleviating sexual side effects (data contradictory) and bruxism caused by SSRI antidepressants

General Comments

- Buspirone (Buspar) is a selective anxiolytic of the azaspirone class; unlike the benzodiazepines, it has no anticonvulsant or muscle-relaxant properties
- Tolerance to effects of buspirone has not been reported
- Has a low potential for abuse or addiction
- Lack of effect on respiration may make it useful in patients with pulmonary disease or sleep apnea; may actually stimulate respiration
- Minimal effect on cognition, memory or driving performance
- May have a preferential effect for symptoms of anxiety, irritability and aggression with little effect on behavioral manifestations

Pharmacology

- Unlike the benzodiazepines, buspirone does not bind to the GABA"benzodiazepine" receptor complex, but has a marked effect on serotonin transmission and affects nonadrenergic and dopaminergic activity
- A partial 5-HT$_{1A}$ agonist; chronic administration causes downregulation of 5-HT$_2$ receptors; a major metabolite (1-(2-pyrimidinyl)-piperazine) enhances norepinephrine release
- Low doses (< 15 mg/day) have effects on PRE-synaptic 5-HT$_{1A}$ receptors; higher doses (> 15 mg/day) have agonistic effects on POST-synaptic 5-HT$_{1A}$ receptors

Dosing

- 5–30 mg daily in divided doses
- A lag time of 1–2 weeks may be needed for the anxiolytic effect to occur; rarely doses up to 60 mg daily are required
- ☞ **Not effective on a prn basis**
- Decrease dose by 25–50% in patients with creatinine clearance < 10 ml/min

Pharmacokinetics	• Absorption is virtually complete; firstpass effect reduces bioavailability to about 4%
	• Food may reduce rate of absorption (95%), decrease extent of firstpass effect and therefore increase oral bioavailability, C_{max} increased up to 116%
	• Highly bound to plasma proteins
	• Peak plasma level: 0.7–1.5 h. Onset of action takes days to weeks; maximum effect seen in 34 weeks
	• Elimination half-life: 1–11 h. Metabolite: 1-(2-pyrimidinyl) piperazine (active); parent drug metabolized by CYP3A4 and 2C19; metabolite metabolized by 2D6
	• Clearance reduced in renal and hepatic impairment

Adverse Effects	• Causes little sedation; does not impair psychomotor or cognitive functions
	• headache (up to 6%), dizziness (up to 12%), lightheadedness (3%), nervousness (5%), excitement (2%), fatigue, paresthesia, numbness and GI upset seen in less than 10% of patients
	• Due to its effect on dopamine, the possible risk of neurological effects has been a concern; however, buspirone does not lead to postsynaptic dopamine receptor hypersensitivity since it binds only to presynaptic dopamine autoreceptors; when combined with antipsychotic, increases in extrapyramidal reactions (including dyskinesias) have been reported
	• Can precipitate hypomania or mania (primarily in elderly); high doses may worsen psychosis
	• Dose-dependent increase in prolactin and growth hormone levels reported
	• Cases of priapism reported

D/C Discontinuation Syndrome	• Withdrawal effects have not been reported

Precautions	• Has no crosstolerance with benzodiazepines and will not alleviate benzodiazepine withdrawal; when switching, taper benzodiazepine dose while adding buspirone to the regimen
	• Caution in patients with seizure disorder as drug has no anticonvulsant activity

Toxicity	• No deaths have been reported
	• Excessive doses produce extension of pharmacological effects including dizziness, nausea, and vomiting; monitor respiration, BP, and pulse, and give symptomatic and supportive therapy

Pediatric Considerations	• For detailed information on the use of buspirone in this population, please see the *Clinical Handbook of Psychotropic Drugs for Children and Adolescents* (2007)
	• Buspirone used in ADHD, aggression, autism, and to augment SSRIs in obsessive-compulsive disorder (10–30 mg/day)
	• Dizziness, behavior activation, euphoria, increased aggression and psychosis reported

Geriatric Considerations	• Buspirone does not cause sedation, cognitive impairment, disinhibition or motor impairment in the elderly
	• Used in behavior disturbances of dementia at doses of 20–45 mg/day
	• Dosage should be decreased in patients with reduced hepatic or renal function

Use in Pregnancy	• Safety in pregnancy has not yet been determined; no teratogenicity in animal studies
Breast Milk	• Buspirone and metabolites are excreted in human milk; no data on safety

Buspirone (cont.)

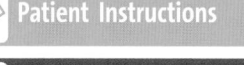 **Nursing Implications**

- The effect of buspirone is gradual; improvement may be seen 7–10 days after starting therapy
- When switching from a benzodiazepine to buspirone, it is important to gradually taper the benzodiazepine to avoid precipitating a withdrawal reaction
- Buspirone should be taken consistently, not on a prn basis

Patient Instructions

- For detailed patient instructions on buspirone, see the Patient Information Sheet on p. 343

Drug Interactions

- Clinically significant interactions are listed below

Class of Drug	Example	Interaction Effect
Antibiotic	Erythromycin	Increased plasma level of buspirone (5-fold) due to inhibited metabolism via CYP3A4
Antidepressant SARI Irreversible MAOI SSRI	Trazodone Phenelzine, tranylcypromine Fluoxetine, fluvoxamine	Case of serotonin syndrome with high dose of trazodone Elevated blood pressure reported May potentiate antiobsessional effects of the antidepressants Increased plasma level of buspirone (3-fold) with fluvoxamine Case reports of serotonin syndrome, euphoria, seizures or dystonia with combination
Antifungal	Itraconazole	Increased plasma level of buspirone (13-fold) due to inhibited metabolism via CYP3A4
Antipsychotic	Haloperidol	Increased plasma level of haloperidol by 26% due to inhibited metabolism
Antitubercular drug	Rifampin	Decreased peak plasma concentration and half-life of buspirone due to induced metabolism via CYP3A4
Benzodiazepine	Diazepam	Increased serum level of benzodiazepine
Ca-channel blocker	Verapamil, diltiazem	Increased peak plasma level of buspirone (3- to 4-fold) due to inhibited metabolism via CYP3A4
Digoxin		Effects of digoxin may be increased
Grapefruit juice		Increased peak plasma level of buspirone (up to 15-fold), AUC (up to 20-fold) and half-life (1.5-fold) due to inhibited metabolism via CYP3A4
Immunosuppressant	Cyclosporin A	Increased serum level of cyclosporin A with possible renal adverse effects
St. John's Wort		Case report of possible serotonin syndrome

Further Reading

References

1 ACOG Committee on Practice Bulletins – Obstetrics. ACOG Practice Bulletin: Clinical management guidelines for obstetrician-gynecologists number 92, April 2008. Use of psychiatric medications during pregnancy and lactation. Obstet Gynecol. 2008;111(4):1001–1020.
2 Trivedi MH, Rush AJ, Wisniewski SR, et al. Evaluation of outcomes with citalopram for depression using measurement-based care in STAR*D: Implications for clinical practice. Am J Psychiatry 2006;163(1):28–40.
3 Zhou SF, Zhou ZW, Li CG, et al. Identification of drugs that interact with herbs in drug development. Drug Discov Today. 2007;12(15–16):664–673.

Additional Suggested Reading

- American Psychiatric Association. Practice guideline for the treatment of patients with obsessive-compulsive disorder. Arlington, VA: American Psychiatric Association, 2007. Available from http://www.psychiatryonline.com/pracGuide/loadGuidelinePdf.aspx?file=OCDPracticeGuidelineFinal05-04-07 (Accessed March 16, 2009).

- American Psychiatric Association. Practice guideline for the treatment of patients with panic disorder (2nd ed). Arlington, VA: American Psychiatric Association, 2008. Available from http://www.psychiatryonline.com/pracGuide/loadGuidelinePdf.aspx?file=PanicDisorder_2e_PracticeGuideline (Accessed March 16, 2009).
- Baldwin DS, Anderson IM, Nutt DJ, et al. Evidence-based guidelines for the pharmacological treatment of anxiety disorders: Recommendations from the British Association for Psychopharmacology. J Psychopharmacol. 2005;19(6):567–596. Available from http://www.bap.org.uk/consensus/Anxiety_Disorder_Guidelines.pdf (Accessed March 16, 2009).
- Culpepper L. Use of algorithms to treat anxiety in primary care. J Clin Psychiatry. 2003;64 Suppl 2:S30–S33.
- Fricchione G. Clinical practice. Generalized anxiety disorder. N Engl J Med. 2004;351(7):675–682.
- Goodman WK. Selecting pharmacotherapy for generalized anxiety disorder. J Clin Psychiatry. 2004;65 Suppl 13:S8–S13.
- Gorman JM. Treating generalized anxiety disorder. J Clin Psychiatry. 2003;64 Suppl 2:S24–S29.
- Jenike MA. Clinical practice. Obsessive-compulsive disorder. N Engl J Med. 2004;350(3):259–265.
- Katon WJ. Clinical practice. Panic disorder. N Engl J Med. 2006;354(22):2360–2367.
- Labellarte MJ, Ginsburg GS, Walkup JT, et al. The treatment of anxiety disorders in children and adolescents. Biol Psychiatry. 1999;46(11):1567–1578.
- Mancuso CE, Tanzi MG, Gabay M. Paradoxical reactions to benzodiazepines: Literature review and treatment options. Pharmacotherapy. 2004;24(9):1177–1185.
- Monnier J, Labbate LA, Wolitzky K, et al. Pharmacotherapy for generalized anxiety disorder. Int Drug Ther Newsl. 2004;39(12):89–96.
- Muller JE, Keon L, Seedat S, et al. Social anxiety disorder, current treatment recommendations. CNS Drugs. 2005;19(5):377–391.
- National Institute for Health and Clinical Excellence. Post-traumatic stress disorder (PTSD): The management of PTSD in adults and children in primary and secondary care [Clinical Guideline 26]. London: NICE; 2005. Available from http://www.nice.org.uk/nicemedia/pdf/CG026NICEguideline.pdf (Accessed March 16, 2009).
- Nelson J, Chouinard G. Guidelines for the clinical use of benzodiazepines: Pharmacokinetics, dependency, rebound and withdrawal. Can J Clin Pharmacol. 1999;6(2):69–83.
- Nemeroff CB. Anxiolytics: Past, present and future agents. J Clin Psychiatry. 2003;64 Suppl 3:S3–S6.
- O'Brien CP. Benzodiazepine use, abuse, and dependence. J Clin Psychiatry. 2005;66 Suppl 2:S28–S33.
- Pallanti S, Hollander E, Goodman WK. A qualitative analysis of nonresponse: Management of treatment-refractory obsessive-compulsive disorder. J Clin Psychiatry. 2004;65(Suppl 14):6–10.
- Petrovic M, Mariman A, Warie H, et al. Is there a rationale for prescription of benzodiazepines in the elderly? Review of the literature. Acta Clin Belg. 2003;58(1):27–36.
- Steward SA. The effects of benzodiazepines on cognition. J Clin Psychiatry. 2005;66 Suppl 2:S9–S13.

HYPNOTICS/SEDATIVES

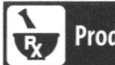 **Product Availability**

Chemical Class	Generic Name	Trade Name[A]	Dosage Forms and Strengths
Antihistamines	Hydroxyzine	Atarax, Vistaril[B]	Capsules: 10 mg, 25 mg, 50 mg, 100 mg[B] Oral syrup: 10 mg/5 ml, 25 mg/5 ml[B] Injection: 25 mg/ml[B], 50 mg/ml
	Diphenhydramine	Benadryl	Capsules: 25 mg, 50 mg Chewable tablets: 12.5 mg Oral solution: 6.25 mg/5 ml, 10 mg/5 ml[B], 12.5 mg/5 ml Injection: 10 mg/ml[B], 50 mg/ml
	Doxylamine[B]	Unisom	Tablets: 25 mg
	Promethazine	Phenergan	Tablets: 12.5 mg[B], 25 mg, 50 mg Oral Solution: 6.25 mg/5ml[B], 10 mg/5ml[C], 25 mg/5ml[B] Suppositories[B]: 12.5 mg, 25 mg, 50 mg Injection 25 mg/5 ml
Barbiturate*	Pentobarbital	Nembutal	Capsules: 100 mg Injection: 50 mg/ml
	Secobarbital	Seconal	Capsules: 50 mg[B], 100 mg
Benzodiazepines			see pp. 158–165
Chloral derivative	Chloral hydrate	Noctec, Aquachloral[B]	Capsules: 500 mg Oral solution: 500 mg/5 ml
Acetaldehyde polymer	Paraldehyde[C]	Paral	Injection: (100%) 5 ml
Amino acid	L-Tryptophan[C]	Tryptan	Tablets: 500 mg, 1 g Capsules: 500 mg
Cyclopyrrolone	Zopiclone[C]	Imovane	Tablets: 5 mg, 7.5 mg
	Eszopiclone[B][D]	Lunesta	Tablets: 1 mg, 2 mg, 3 mg
Imidazopyridine derivative	Zolpidem[B]	Ambien Ambien CR[B]	Tablets: 5 mg, 10 mg Tablets[B]: 6.25 mg, 12.5 mg
Pyrazolopyrimidine	Zaleplon	Sonata[B], Starnoc[C]	Capsules: 5 mg, 10 mg
Selective melatonin agonist	Ramelteon[B]	Rozerem	Tablets: 8 mg (see pp. 307–308)

[A] Generic preparations may be available, [B] Not marketed in Canada, [C] Not marketed in USA, [D] S-isomer of zopiclone

* Many of these drugs are no longer recommended for use as hypnotics because of their low therapeutic index and high addiction liability.

Indications
(👍 Approved)
- 👍 Nocturnal sedation; short-term management of insomnia
- 👍 Preoperative sedation
- 👍 Chronic insomnia (ramelteon)
- 👍 Long-term management of insomnia (eszopiclone – USA)

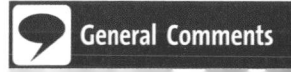 **General Comments**
- Prior to treatment of insomnia, determine if sleep disturbance is
  - Due to a primary sleep disorder (e.g., sleep apnea, restless legs syndrome, narcolepsy)

- – Due to psychiatric disorder (e.g., depression, mania)
- – Drug-induced (e.g., theophylline, sympathomimetics)
- – Due to medical disorder (e.g., thyroid, peptic ulcer, pain)
- – Due to use of excessive caffeine, alcohol
- Treat the primary cause, wherever possible
- Use of hypnotics is recommended for limited time periods; long-term, continuous treatment is not recommended (except L-tryptophan and ramelteon)
- One small (n = 46) randomized clinical trial found that cognitive-behavioral therapy was as effective (or more) as zopiclone for chronic primary insomnia (in older adults) after 6 weeks of treatment and more effective than zopiclone at 6-month follow-up

 Pharmacology

- Hypnotics suppress the reticular formation of the midbrain to various degrees resulting in sedation, sleep, or anesthesia
- Benzodiazepines bind to the "benzodiazepine"-GABA-chloride receptor complex in the brain; they act nonselectively at two central receptor sites: omega 1 receptors which modulate sedative effects, and omega 2 receptors responsible for memory and cognitive functions
- Zolpidem, zopiclone, eszopiclone, and zaleplon bind selectively to $GABA_{A1}$ (omega 1) receptors
- Ramelteon has high binding affinity for MT_1 and MT_2 melatonin receptors and enhances the effect of endogenous melatonin – not a CNS depressant; has no anxiolytic or muscle relaxant properties, and no tolerance or abuse potential

 Dosing

- See pp. 182–185 for individual agents
- Dosage should be adjusted in the elderly and in patients with hepatic impairment

 Pharmacokinetics

- See pp. 182–185
- Zaleplon: absorption and peak plasma level decreased with high fat meal (C_{max} and T_{max} decreased by 35%). Japanese patients showed increased C_{max} and AUC by 37% and 64%, respectively
- Zolpidem: peak plasma level increased (by more than 50%) and half-life increased in female elderly patients and in cirrhosis. CR preparation formulated with an immediate-release layer and a slow-release layer; C_{max} occurs later and is higher than with regular release product
- Zopiclone: half life doubled in elderly patients
- Eszopiclone: T_{max} delayed after high-fat meal; increased AUC by 41% and $T_{1/2}$ to 9 h in elderly; AUC increased 2-fold in moderate to severe liver impairment
- Ramelteon: high inter-patient variability in C_{max} and AUC; absorption affected by food, especially high fat meals. Drug exposure increased 4-fold in mild hepatic impairment; 4 active metabolites; 84% of drug is eliminated in urine

 Onset & Duration of Action

- See pp. 182–185
- Tolerance to effects of many hypnotics occurs after 2–4 weeks of continuous use

Adverse Effects

- See chart pp. 183–185
- Day-time sedation and impairment; dependent on drug dosage, half-life, and patient tolerance
- Anterograde amnesia is dependent on drug potency and dose
- Rebound insomnia is dependent on drug dose, half-life, and duration of use
- High dose can impair respiration and decrease blood pressure
- Ramelteon has been associated with an effect on reproductive hormones (decreased testosterone and increased prolactin) in adults; long-term effects unknown
- Priapism reported with hydroxyzine

D/C Discontinuation Syndrome

- Can occur with chronic use of all hypnotics except L-tryptophan and ramelteon
- Discontinuation of hypnotics can produce:
  - – Withdrawal: occurs within 1–2 days (short-acting) to 3–7 days (long-acting) following discontinuation of regular use of most hypnotics (for more than 2 weeks); suggested to occur less frequently with zopiclone and zolpidem. Common symptoms include insomnia, agitation, dizziness,

 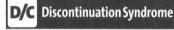

Hypnotics/Sedatives (cont.)

nausea/vomiting, anxiety, perceptual disturbances (e.g., photophobia), malaise and anorexia. Abrupt withdrawal of high doses may result in twitching, hyperthermia, tremors, seizures and/or psychosis and possibly death
- Rebound: occurs hours to days after drug withdrawal; described as worsening of insomnia beyond pretreatment levels. More likely to occur with short-acting agents
- Relapse: recurrence of the insomnia, to pretreatment levels, when the hypnotic is discontinued

Management
- Withdrawal of a hypnotic (after chronic use) should be tailored to each patient; consider switching medications (if on a short-acting agent) to a comparable dose of a long-acting agent and gradually tapering the dose over several weeks. For benzodiazepines examples, see p. 162

 **Precautions**
- Abrupt withdrawal of hypnotics (excluding antihistamines, zopiclone, ramelteon, and L-tryptophan) may produce a significant discontinuation syndrome. See preceding section for symptoms and consequences of abrupt discontinuation
- Caution re drug interactions
- Long-term use (for years) of hypnotics occurs as patients report unsuccessful efforts to decrease use (due to withdrawal effects); can result in memory impairment or falls (in the elderly)
- Long-term administration of barbiturates has been associated with osteomalacia in adults, because of altered vitamin D metabolism
- Recreational abuse can occur (especially with benzodiazepines) to achieve a "high"; avoid use in addiction-prone individuals (except L-tryptophan and ramelteon)
- Abuse may result in clouding of consciousness and visual hallucinations
- Use in individuals with sleep apnea is contraindicated
- CR zolpidem reported to cause incidents of sleepwalking, driving while "asleep" and food binging while "asleep"

 **Toxicity**
- Symptoms of overdose include: excitement, restlessness, delirium, nystagmus, ataxia, and stupor (does not apply to L-tryptophan); hypothermia has been reported with barbiturates
- Lethal dose of chloral hydrate is approximately 10 times the therapeutic dose (5–10 g)
- Onset of CNS symptoms occurs rapidly with zolpidem following overdose

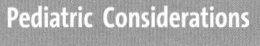 **Pediatric Considerations**
- For detailed information on the use of hypnotics in this population, please see the *Clinical Handbook of Psychotropic Drugs for Children and Adolescents* (2007)
- Barbiturates:
  - Chronic use has been associated with hyperkinetic states with symptoms such as reduced attention span, and destructive or aggressive reactions; developmental delays reported with mental slowing
  - Long-term administration associated with rickets due to altered vitamin D metabolism
- Chloral hydrate:
  - Dosage: 50 mg/kg body weight, to a maximum of 1000 mg per single dose; high doses can depress respiration and blood pressure
  - Used as a sedative for non-invasive procedures (e.g., EEG, CT scan) and for sedation of neonates, infants, and children (under age of 6)
- Antihistamines:
  - Paradoxical CNS excitation can occur

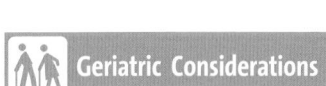 **Geriatric Considerations**
- Lowest effective dose should be utilized in the elderly for the least amount of time (preferably less than 2 months)
- Caution when using drugs that are metabolized by oxidation (e.g., flurazepam), as they can accumulate in the elderly or in persons with liver disease
- Caution when combined with other drugs with CNS properties; additive effects can cause confusion, disorientation
- Anterograde amnesia reported with higher doses
- Diphenhydramine reported to decrease disturbed behavior in patients with dementia, however, elderly more sensitive to CNS and anticholinergic effects; can increase risk of falls
- Ramelteon: AUC and C_{max} increased 97% and 86%, respectively, and half-life increased in elderly subjects

Use in Pregnancy

- See pp. 183–185 for individual agents. For benzodiazepines, see p. 162

Breast Milk

- The American Academy of Pediatrics considers many hypnotics/sedatives compatible with breastfeeding – See table pp. 183–185

Nursing Implications

- Assess personal sleep habits to determine causes or factors contributing to insomnia (e.g., alcohol, caffeine, etc.)
- Counsel patient regarding chronic use of hypnotic and loss of efficacy of drug over time (tolerance) (with the exception of ramelteon, L-tryptophan, zopiclone, and zolpidem). Increasing the dose may not increase efficacy but may result in adverse or toxic effects
- Patients on ramelteon should avoid taking the drug with or after a high-fat meal
- Suggest that abrupt withdrawal after chronic use of most hypnotics may result in serious side effects and rebound symptoms (see Discontinuation Syndrome, p. 175); drugs should be tapered over time
- Suggest alternative methods of treating insomnia (e.g., cognitive-behavioral therapy, relaxation exercises, regular sleep/wake cycle 7 days/week, avoiding daytime naps, and avoiding caffeine after midday), stop offending medications/substances (nicotine, stimulants, alcohol)
- Patients taking CR zolpidem should not split, crush or chew the tablet

Patient Instructions

- For detailed patient instructions on hypnotics/sedatives, see the Patient Information Sheet on p. 344

Drug Interactions

- Only clinically significant interactions are listed below

Class of Drug	Example	Interaction Effects
Antibiotic/Antiinfective	Ciprofloxacin Clarithromycin Doxycycline Erythromycin Linezolid	*Ramelteon:* Increased plasma level of ramelteon possible due to inhibited metabolism via CYP1A2 *Eszopiclone:* increased plasma level of eszopiclone due to inhibited metabolism via CYP3A4 *Zopiclone, zaleplon,* and *zolpidem* increased plasma level of hypnotic due to decreased clearance *Diphenhydramine:* case report of acute delirium
Anticoagulant	Dicumarol, warfarin	*Chloral hydrate* will displace drugs that are protein-bound and temporarily enhance hypoprothrombinemic response; increased or decreased PT ratio or INR response *Paraldehyde:* decreased PT ratio or INR response
Anticonvulsant	Carbamazepine, phenytoin Valproate	*Zopiclone:* decreased plasma level of zopiclone due to induced metabolism via CYP3A4 *Zolpidem:* case of somnambulism
Antidepressant SSRI, RIMA, MAOI SSRI SSRI/NDRI SNRI Tricyclics	Fluoxetine, moclobemide, phenelzine, tranylcypromine Fluoxetine, fluvoxamine Fluvoxamine Sertraline, bupropion Venlafaxine Imipramine Desipramine Amitriptyline, clomipramine, desipramine, imipramine	*L-Tryptophan* combination may produce increased serotonin activity resulting in twitching, agitation ("serotonin syndrome") Additive antidepressant effect in treatment-resistant patients Increased sedation and side effects of *chloral hydrate* due to inhibited metabolism *Ramelteon:* DO NOT COMBINE; increased C_{max} (90-fold) and AUC (190-fold) of ramelteon due to inhibited metabolism via CYP1A2 *Zolpidem:* case reports of hallucinations and delirium with sertraline, fluoxetine, paroxetine, and bupropion *Zolpidem:* case report of hallucinations and delirium *Diphenhydramine:* decreased metabolism of venlafaxine via CYP2D6 *Zolpidem:* in one study 5/8 patients on combination experienced anterograde amnesia *Zolpidem:* case report of visual hallucinations with combination *Diphenhydramine:* increased plasma level of antidepressants metabolized primarily by CYP2D6 due to inhibited metabolism

Hypnotics/Sedatives (cont.)

Class of Drug	Example	Interaction Effects
Antifungal	Ketoconazole, itraconazole	*Eszopiclone*: increase C_{max} and $T_{1/2}$ of eszopiclone (1.4- and 1.3-fold, respectively with ketoconazole) due to decreased metabolism via CYP3A4 *Zolpidem*: decreased clearance of zolpidem by 41%; half-life increased by 26% with ketoconazole *Zopiclone*: increased AUC and elimination half-life of zopiclone due to decreased metabolism *Zaleplon*: increased plasma level of zaleplon due to decreased metabolism Barbiturates induce the metaboilsm and reduce the efficacy of griseofulvin *Ramelteon*: increased C_{max} and AUC (34% and 84% respectively) due to inhibited metabolism by ketoconazole via CYP3A4
	Fluconazole	*Ramelteon*: increased AUC and C_{max} of ramelteon by 150% due to inhibited metabolism via CYP2C9
Antipsychotic	Chlorpromazine, fluphenazine, perphena-zine, thiothixene, risperidone	*Diphenhydramine*: possible increase in plasma level of antipsychotic metabolized via CYP2D6 due to inhibited metabolism Additive CNS depression and psychomotor impairment
Antitubercular drug	Rifampin	*Zolpidem*: decreased peak plasma level of zolpidem by 60% and increased elimination half-life by 36% *Zaleplon*: decreased AUC of zaleplon by 80% due to induced metabolism *Zopiclone*: decreased AUC of zopiclone by 80% due to induced metabolism *Eszopiclone*: decreased AUC of eszopiclone due to induced metabolism *Ramelteon*: decreased C_{max} and AUC of ramelteon by 40–90% due to induced metabolism
Anxiolytic	General	Additive CNS effects
	Lorazepam	*Eszopiclone*: C_{max} of both drugs increased by 22%
Barbiturates		Barbiturates are potent and known inducers of several CYP-450 enzymes (see p. 182). Since these agents are rarely utilized as a hypnotic agent and they are associated with lots of important drug interactions, many of these interactions have been left off this table. Please refer to a drug interaction text for a list of drugs that interact with barbiturates
β-Blocker	Metoprolol	*Diphenhydramine*: decreased clearance of metoprolol 2-fold due to inhibited metabolism
Ca-channel blocker	Diltiazem	*Diphenhydramine*: initial sharp increase seen in diltiazem concentration secondary to displacement from tissue binding sites, followed by an increase in steady-state plasma levels secondary to inhibited metabolism via CYP2D6
Caffeine	Tea, coffee, colas	May counteract sedation and increase insomnia
Cimetidine		*Zaleplon*: increased peak plasma level and AUC of zaleplon by 85% due to inhibited metabolism via CYP3A4 and aldehyde oxidase *Zopiclone* and *zolpidem*: increased plasma level of hypnotic due to inhibited metabolism *Diphenhydramine, zolpidem*: increased AUC and half-life, and decreased clearance of diphenhydramine
CNS depressant	Alcohol	Increased CNS depression and psychomotor impairment; in "high" doses coma and respiratory depression can occur
CNS stimulant	Methylphenidate, dextroamphetamine	May counteract sedation and increase insomnia
Disulfiram		*Paraldehyde*: avoid since it is metabolized to acetaldehyde; an alcohol-like reaction will occur
Flumazenil		*Zolpidem* and *zaleplon*: antagonism of hypnotic effects
Grapefruit juice		*Zaleplon*: increased plasma level of zaleplon due to inhibited metabolism via CYP3A4
Lithium		Increased efficacy and increased plasma level of lithium with *L*-tryptophan
Narcotic	Codeine	*Diphenhydramine*: inhibited conversion of codeine to its active moiety morphine, via CYP2D6, resulting in decreased analgesic efficacy
	Methadone	*Diphenhydramine, zolpidem*: increased plasma levels of methadone possible due to inhibited metabolism via CYP2D6
Oral contraceptive		*Chloral hydrate*: decreased efficacy of the oral contraceptive due to induction of microsomal enzymes
Protease inhibitor	Ritonavir	*Zolpidem* and *eszopiclone*: increased plasma level of hypnotic due to decreased metabolism via CYP3A4

Product Availability

Chemical Class	Generic Name	Trade Name(A)	Dosage Forms and Strengths
Tryptophan	L-Tryptophan(C)	Tryptan	Capsules: 500 mg Tablets: 250 mg, 500 mg, 750 mg, 1 g

(A) Generic preparations may be available, (C) Not marketed in USA

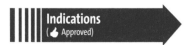 **Indications**
(Approved)

- 👍 Adjunct in the treatment of bipolar disorder (BD); may potentiate the effects of lithium and antipsychotics in acute mania; some efficacy if used alone
- 👍 Potentiates the effects of lithium in prophylaxis
- Sedative; will reduce sleep latency without distorting usual stages of sleep
- Potentiates the effects of antidepressants in depression and obsessive compulsive disorder
- Decrease aggression and antisocial behavior
- Placebo-controlled trial reports benefit for premenstrual dysphoric disorder

 Pharmacology

- An essential amino acid that acts as a precursor for the synthesis of serotonin
- Reported to increase melatonin levels

 Dosing

- Depression: 8–16 g/day
- Mania: 8–12 g/day
- Aggression: up to 16 g/day
- Sedation: up to 5 g at bedtime

 Pharmacokinetics

- Half-life = 15.8 h
- Highly bound to plasma protein (80–90%)
- There is no correlation between dose and plasma level

 Adverse Effects

CNS Effects

- Drowsiness
- Headache
- Euphoria, disinhibition of mood and sexual behavior reported
- Tremors

Anticholinergic Effects

- Constipation
- Dry mouth

Cardiovascular Effects

- Dizziness

GI Effects

- GI upset
- Anorexia

L-Tryptophan (cont.)

⚠️ **Precautions**	• Protein-reduced diets can cause an amino acid imbalance when using L-tryptophan • When used with lithium, lithium dose should be decreased (if level high) and plasma levels monitored for toxicity • Eosinophilia-myalgia syndrome reported (cause traced to impurity in raw material); symptoms include fatigue, myalgia, shortness of breath, rash, swelling of extremities, congestive heart failure, and death • Use with caution in patients with cataracts, as they seem to be related to metabolites of tryptophan (e.g., kynurenine) • Caution in patients with a family history of diabetes as diabetogenic effect reported • Vitamin B_6 (pyridoxine) deficiency can predispose to elevated levels of tryptophan metabolites which have been associated with bladder cancer
🛑 **Contraindications**	• Irritation of urinary bladder (cystitis) • Diabetes • Patients with malabsorption in upper bowel • Achlorhydric states
☠️ **Toxicity**	• High doses cause vomiting and "serotonin" overdrive including shivering, diaphoresis, hypomania, and ataxia
Pediatric Considerations	• No data on use in children
Geriatric Considerations	• Used in agitation, aggression, and behavior problems in elderly demented patients • Sedation is primary side effect
Use in Pregnancy	• Contraindicated • Pregnancy has been associated with the accumulation of L-tryptophan metabolites (e.g., xanthurenic acid, kynurenine) due to inhibited metabolism
Breast Milk	• Unknown
Nursing Implications	• Give drug with meals or snacks to reduce nausea • Protein-reduced diets may affect the efficacy of L-tryptophan • When used with lithium, monitor for signs of toxicity including tremor, ataxia, and confusion; dermatological side effects may be exacerbated
Patient Instructions	• For detailed patient instructions on L-tryptophan, see the Patient Information Sheet on p. 346
Drug Interactions	• Clinically significant interactions are listed below

Class of Drug	Example	Interaction Effects
Antidepressant 　Tricyclic 　MAOI – Irreversible, RIMA, SSRI, SNRI	Amitriptyline Tranylcypromine, moclobemide, fluvoxamine, duloxetine	Additive effects in treatment-resistant patients Additive effects in treatment-resistant patients; monitor for increased serotonergic effects
Hormone	Oral contraceptives, estradiol, diethylstilboestrol	Increased levels of metabolites (xanthurenic acid, kynurenine), due to inhibited metabolism

Class of Drug	Example	Interaction Effects
Lithium		Increased lithium level and possible toxicity Enhanced therapeutic effect for mania and prophylaxis of bipolar affective disorder in treatment-resistant patients
Sibutramine		Increased risk of serotonin syndrome

Comparison of Hypnotics/Sedatives

	Usual Oral Adult Dose	Onset of Action	Bioavailability	Protein Binding	Half-life	Efficacy/ Tolerance	CYP-450 Metabo-lizing Enzyme[c]	CYP-450 Effect[d]	Indications
ANTIHISTAMINE									
Diphenhydramine (Benadryl, Nytol)	25–300 mg	15–60 min	40–60%	80–85%	1–3 h	Antihista-mines lose hypnotic effi-cacy with time	2D6	2D6 inhibitor	Sedation, insomnia, allergic reactions
Hydroxyzine (Atarax)	10–400 mg	15–30 min	?	?	8–20 h (short-er in children)		–	2D6 inhibitor	Anxiety, itching of psycho-genic origin
Doxylamine[a] (Unisom)	25–150 mg	2–3 h	25%	?	10 h		–	–	Insomnia
BARBITURATE									
Pentobarbital (Nembutal)	50–200 mg	15 min	61%	35–45%	21–42 h	Loses effect after 2 weeks	2C, 3A4	2A6, 2B6, 2C9, 3A4 inducer	Insomnia, preoperative seda-tion for anxiety and tension, anesthesia
Secobarbital (Seconal)	50–200 mg	15 min	80%	30–45%	2–3 h	Loses effect after 2 weeks		2A6, 2B6, 2C9, 3A4 inducer	Nocturnal and pre-operative sedation, dental procedures, sleep EEGs, acute convulsive disorders
Chloral hydrate (Noctec)	0.5–2 g	30 min	> 95% (active metabolite tri-chloroethanol)	35–41% (tri-chloroacetic acid metabo-lite = 71–88%)	4–12 h (tri-chloroacetic acid metabo-lite = up to 100 h)	Loses effect after 2 weeks	2B, 2E1	inducer	Nocturnal and pre-operative sedation; alcohol, barbiturate, and narcotic withdrawal; porphyria
Eszopiclone[a] (Lunesta)	2–3 ng (1–2 mg in eld-erly; 1 mg in hepatic impair-ment)	1 h (2 h after high-fat meal)	80%	52–59%	5–7 h (9 h in elderly)	No tolerance after 6 months	3A4, 2EI	–	Insomnia
L-Tryptophan[b] (Trofan, Tryptan)	1–5 g	1.8–3.3 h	48–95%	?	2.2–7.4	No tolerance reported	?	?	Insomnia, mood disorder prophylaxis
Paraldehyde (Paral)	10–30 ml (hypnotic) 5–10 ml (sedative)	10 min	4–8 h	?	?	?	?	?	Drug and alcohol withdrawal, convulsive control in tetany and poisoning
Ramelteon (Rozerem)	8 mg	30 min Peak level 0.5–1.5 h (fasting); 2.6 h in elderly Food delays T_{max} by 45 min	Absolute bio-availability 1.8%; due to extensive first-pass metabo-lism	82%	1–2h (M-II metab = 2–5h)	No tolerance	CYP1A2[p], 2C9, 3A4	–	Insomnia

	Usual Oral Adult Dose	Onset of Action	Bioavailability	Protein Binding	Half-life	Efficacy/ Tolerance	CYP-450 Metabo-lizing Enzyme[c]	CYP-450 Effect[d]	Indications
Zaleplon (Sonata, Starnoc)	5–10 mg (5 mg in elderly)	Rapid Peak level: 0.9–1.5 h (delayed after high-fat meal)	30%	60%	0.9–1.1 h	No tolerance after 4 weeks	3A4, aldehyde-oxidase[p]	CYP3A4 inducer	Insomnia – useful for noctur-nal awakenings due to fast onset and short duration of action
Zolpidem[a] (Ambien)	5–20 mg (5 mg in elderly)	30 min Peak level: 1.6 h CR: 2.5–8 h	70%	92%	1.5–4.5 h CR: 2.8	No tolerance after 50 weeks	1A2, 2D6, 3A4[p]	CYP3A4 inhibitor	Insomnia Early data suggest possible efficacy in rigidity of Parkin-son's disease Adjunctive therapy for spas-ticity, including progressive supranuclear palsy
Zopiclone[b] (Imovane)	3.75–15 mg	30 min Peak level: 90 min	> 75% (increased in elderly)	45%	3.8–6.5 h (5–10 h in elderly)	No tolerance after 17 weeks	1A2, 2C9	?	Insomnia

[a] Not marketed in Canada, [b] Not marketed in USA, [c] Cytochrome P-450 isoenzymes involved in drug metabolism, [d] Effect of drug on cytochrome enzymes, [p] primary route of metabolism

	Effect on Sleep Architecture	Pregnancy/Lactation	Precautions	Main Side Effects
Antihistamine		In animals, teratogenicity seen in high doses; case reports in humans, but correla-tion not proven Excreted into human milk; newborn have increased sensitivity to antihistamines Doxylamine is safe to use in pregnancy (Category A) and is a component of the drug Diclectin, which is used for morning sickness associated with pregnancy	Elderly patients more susceptible to adverse effects including increased sedation, cognitive impairment, and increased risk of falls May precipitate seizures in patients with focal lesions Diphenhydramine is a potent inhibitor of CYP2D6 and may interact with a number of drugs (see pp. 177–178) Low abuse potential	Residual daytime sedation, incoordination; anti-cholinergic effects at high doses (dry mouth, blurred vision, confusion, delirium, urinary reten-tion, etc.); elderly more prone to CNS effects in-cluding inattention, disorganized speech, behavior disturbance, altered consciousness GI disturbances; paradoxical CNS excitation can occur; tolerance to effects occurs within days or weeks
Barbiturate	Suppress REM sleep and delta sleep; REM rebound on with-drawal	Barbiturates cross the placenta; an increase in congenital defects and hemorrhagic dis-ease of newborn reported Prolonged elimination of barbiturate re-ported in fetus Withdrawal symptoms seen in newborn Excreted in breast milk; American Academy of Pediatrics considers secobarbital compati-ble with breast-feeding	**AVOID** barbiturates in: severe hepatic impairment, porphyria, uncontrolled pain (delirium may result) pulmonary insufficiency, confused and restless elderly patients With low doses, patient may become euphoric, ex-cited, restless, or violent; at high doses, can develop acute confusional state and respiratory depression Risk of suicide due to low lethal dose Risk of tolerance; high potential for abuse and dependence	CNS: confusion, hangover, drowsiness, excitement if given to patients in severe pain Can cause severe depression (risk of suicide) Skin rash (1–3%), nausea, vomiting Weight gain
Chloral hydrate	REM sleep decreased in doses over 1 g	Crosses placenta; no reports of congenital defects in newborn Excreted in breast milk; one report of drowsiness in newborn; American Academy of Pediatrics considers drug compatible with breast-feeding	**CAUTION** in hepatic and renal impairment, gastritis, peptic ulcer, and cardiac distress Doses above 2 g can impair respiration and decrease blood pressure Tolerance can occur with chronic use; withdrawal reactions reported	Nausea, vomiting, hangover, skin rash Does not accumulate with chronic use Will induce hepatic enzymes and affect metabo-lism of other drugs; will displace other drugs from protein binding

Comparison of Hypnotics/Sedatives (cont.)

	Effect on Sleep Architecture	Pregnancy/Lactation	Precautions	Main Side Effects
Eszopiclone	Decreased sleep latency, decreased nighttime awakenings, increased total sleep time	Not teratogenic in animals No studies in humans Not known if excreted into breast milk	High doses (> 6 mg) can produce amnesia, euphoria, and hallucinations Caution in respiratory impairment, liver dysfunction, depression, elderly, and in combination with CYP3A4 inhibitors Moderate abuse potential	Unpleasant taste (> 30%), headache (> 10%), dry mouth, dizziness No evidence of tolerance after 12 months of nightly use; withdrawal effects have been reported including rebound insomnia Memory impairment reported in the morning, often only in the first week of treatment
L-Tryptophan	Decreased REM latency and REM sleep; increased non-REM and total sleep time	Contraindicated: AVOID	In combination with other serotonergic drugs can cause twitching or jerking, i.e., "serotonin syndrome" Eosinophilic myalgia reported with certain preparations made from impure raw material Chronic use associated with niacin and pyridoxine deficiency No abuse potential	GI upset: nausea, vomiting, dry mouth, dizziness, and headache
Paraldehyde		Crosses placenta; fetal concentration equals that of maternal blood; respiratory depression seen in neonates	**AVOID** in gastroenteritis, liver damage, bronchopulmonary disease; may produce excitement or delirium in presence of pain Decomposed product should not be used (acetic acid odor) Do not give to persons receiving disulfiram Dissolves plastic; use glass container/syringe; use product immediately after drawing up in syringe	Unpleasant taste, odor imparted into exhaled air; may irritate throat and mucous membranes if administered chronically – dilute liberally Injection can be painful if more than 5 ml injected; give deep IM
Ramelteon	Small decreases in stages 3 and 4	Category C: teratogenic in animal studies; effect in humans unknown	Reported to decrease testosterone and increase prolactin levels CAUTION re drug interactions (see pp. 177–178) No habituation, rebound insomnia, or withdrawal effects. No abuse potential AUC and T_{max} increased 4-fold in mild hepatic impairment No effect in renal impairment	Drowsiness, dizziness, fatigue, headache, nausea Cases of worsening insomnia Cases of respiratory infection Increased serum prolactin (in up to 32%) No behavioral impairment reported
Zaleplon	Sleep latency and short-wave sleep decreased	Safety in pregnancy not established Excreted in breast milk; not recommended for nursing mothers	Due to rapid onset of action, should be taken immediately before bedtime Dependance, withdrawal and rebound insomnia reported after prolonged use Moderate abuse potential Caution in liver dysfunction: 4-fold increase in C_{max} and 7-fold increase in AUC	Drowsiness, headache, GI upset, asthenia, myalgia, paresthesias, dry mouth, hangover, anterograde amnesia; cases of non-dose-related ECG changes reported Rarely sleepwalking, confusion, hallucination and mania No persistent sedation or cognitive/motor impairment upon awakening

	Effect on Sleep Architecture	Pregnancy/Lactation	Precautions	Main Side Effects
Zolpidem	Decreased sleep latency and increased total sleep time Time spent in REM sleep decreased with higher doses No effect on stages 3 and 4	Not teratogenic in animal studies Total drug excreted in milk does not exceed 0.02% of administered dose Considered compatible with breast-feeding by the American Academy of Pediatrics	**CAUTION** in liver dysfunction, respiratory impairment; elderly more prone to confusion, falls Habituation reported; moderate abuse potential Withdrawal reactions and rebound insomnia reported with CR preparation	Drowsiness, dizziness, ataxia, agitation, nightmares, diarrhea, nausea, headache, hangover, anterograde amnesia, sleep walking, sleep talking, food binging and driving while "asleep" Dysphoria reported at high doses; rarely confusion, delirium, mania and psychosis reported with perceptual distortions and hallucinations (case reports primarily in females) Residual sedation upon awakening reported especially with CR preparation Withdrawal symptoms and rebound insomnia on discontinuation reported after 4 weeks of nightly use
Zopiclone	REM delayed but duration the same; stage 1 shortened; stage 2 increased	Not teratogenic in animal studies Crosses placenta; no congenital abnormalities reported in humans Newborns have significantly lower birth weights and lower gestational age Excreted in breast milk; infant receives approx. 1% of administered dose – effect unknown	**CAUTION** in respiratory impairment, liver dysfunction and depression; elderly are more prone to adverse effects Anticholinergic agents may decrease plasma level Not recommended in children Dependence rare and withdrawal effects are mild; rebound insomnia reported Moderate abuse potential Caution in liver dysfunction: time to peak (T_{max}) and half-life increased	Generally dose-related: metallic taste, dry mouth, GI distress, palpitations, dyspnea, tremor, rash, chills, sweating, agitation, nightmares Severe drowsiness, confusion, and incoordination are signs of drug intolerance or excessive dosage Rarely hallucinations and behavioral disturbances

Further Reading

- Ancoli-Israel S. Sleep and aging: Prevalence of disturbed sleep and treatment considerations in older adults. J Clin Pychiatry. 2005;66 Suppl 9:S24–S30.
- Doghramji, PP. Trends in the pharmacologic management of insomnia. J Clin Psychiatry. 2006;6(Suppl 13):5–8.
- Erman MK. Therapeutic options in the treatment of insomnia. J Clin Psychiatry. 2005;66 Suppl 9:S18–S23.
- Griffiths RR, Johnson MW. Relative abuse liability of hypnotic drugs: A conceptual framework and algorithm for differentiating among compounds. J Clin Psychiatry. 2005;66 Suppl 9:S31–S41.
- Morin AK, Jarvis CI, Lynch AM. Therapeutic options for sleep-maintenance and sleep-onset insomnia. Pharmacotherapy. 2007;27(1):89–110.
- Sivertsen B, Omvik S, Pallesen S, et al. Cognitive behavioural therapy vs. zopiclone for treatment of chronic primary insomnia in older adults: A randomized controlled trial. JAMA. 2006;295(24):2851–2858.
- Wang JS, DeVane CL. Pharmacokinetics and drug interactions of the sedative hypnotics. Psychopharmacol Bull. 2003;37(1):10–29.

MOOD STABILIZERS

Classification

- Mood stabilizers can be classified as follows:

Chemical Class	Agent	Page
Lithium	Example: Lithium carbonate	See p. 186
Anticonvulsant	Carbamazepine Gabapentin Topiramate Lamotrigine Oxcarbazepine Valproate Clonazepam	See p. 194

Antipsychotics
   Second-generation
   Third-generation
	Olanzapine, risperidone, quetiapine, ziprasidone, clozapine, paliperidone
	Aripiprazole
		See p. 88
		See p. 107

Antipsychotic/antidepressant combination	Olanzapine/fluoxetine[B] (Symbyax)	

[B] Not marketed in Canada

Lithium

Product Availability

Chemical Class	Generic Name	Trade Name[A]	Dosage Forms and Strengths
Lithium salt	Lithium carbonate	Eskalith[B], Lithonate[B], Lithane[C], Carbolith[C] Eskalith CR, Lithobid SR[B], Duralith[C]	Capsules: 150 mg, 300 mg, 600 mg Tablets: 300 mg Sustained-release tablets: 300 mg, 450 mg[B]
	Lithium citrate	Cibalith-S	Oral solution: 300 mg/5 ml (8 mmol/5 ml)

[A] Generic preparations may be available, [B] Not marketed in Canada, [C] Not marketed in USA

Indications
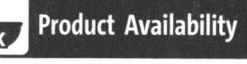
(👍 Approved)

- 👍 Long-term maintenance or prophylaxis of bipolar disorder (BD) I and II
- 👍 Treatment of acute mania, mixed states
- Prevention or diminution of the intensity of subsequent episodes of mania and depression
- Reduces suicidal behavior/risk in BD
- Augments the action of antidepressants in depression and in obsessive-compulsive disorder
- Organic brain syndrome with secondary affective symptoms

- Treatment of chronic aggression/antisocial behavior/impulsivity across a broad range of diagnoses; may be useful in patients with an affective component to symptoms
- May ameliorate restlessness and excitability in up to 50% of patients with schizophrenia
- Migraine, cluster headaches
- Double-blind and open studies suggest that lithium may reduce gambling behavior and affective instability in pathological gamblers
- Anorexia nervosa

General Comments

- "Classic" mania responds best (up to 80%). Other possible predictors of response include: family history of lithium response in first degree relatives, few prior episodes of mania or depression, and complete recovery between episodes
- Considered first-line therapy (in combination with antipsychotic) for the treatment of severe mania
- Less response noted in patients with dysphoric/psychotic mania or mixed states (30–40%), rapid-cycling BD (20–30%), in patients with multiple prior episodes, comorbid medical conditions, in adolescents, in patients with substance abuse and those with high anxiety ratings
- Suggested to be more effective in augmenting antidepressants in bipolar than in unipolar depression
- May be more effective in preventing manic or mixed episodes than depressive episodes especially if mania precedes depression
- As some rapid-cycling may be contributed to by lithium-induced hypothyroidism, it is important to regularly assess thyroid function
- Risk of death from suicide shown to be lower with lithium than with valproate

Pharmacology

- Exact mechanism of action unknown; postulated that lithium may stabilize catecholamine receptors, and may alter calcium-mediated intracellular functions and increase GABA activity. Lithium blocks the ability of neurons to restore normal levels of the second messenger system (phosphatidyl-inositol biphosphate, G-proteins), thereby reducing the responsiveness of neurons to stimuli from muscarinic, cholinergic, and α-adrenergic neurotransmitters
- Research data suggest that chronic lithium use increases N-acetyl-aspartate levels in the brain, and may exert neuroprotective effects
- Lithium therapy requires reaching plasma concentrations that are relatively close to the toxic concentration
- Administration of lithium requires 10–14 days before the complete effect is observed, therefore acute mania is often treated with an antipsychotic; lithium is subsequently added to the treatment regimen

Dosing

- See baseline monitoring recommendations (p. 190)
- Dose is usually guided by plasma level; increase slowly to minimize side effects
  - Acute treatment: 900–2400 mg daily (0.8–1.2 mmol/l)
  - Maintenance: 400–1200 mg daily (0.6–1.0 mmol/l)
- Patients in an acute manic episode appear to have an increased tolerance to lithium; control of mania may require lithium level of 0.9–1.4 mmol/l
- If creatinine clearance is 10–50 ml/min, use 50–75% of the standard dose; if creatinine clearance is < 10 ml/min, use 25–50% of the standard dose. Patients undergoing dialysis should take their dose AFTER each dialysis treatment
- Once patient is stabilized, once-daily dosing is preferable (if patient can tolerate)
- Patients sensitive to side effects that are related to high peak plasma levels, e.g., tremor, urinary frequency, and GI effects (i.e., nausea), may respond to slow release preparations (e.g., Duralith)
- Missed doses or drug interactions may reduce the lithium level and precipitate relapse

Pharmacokinetics

- Lithium is completely absorbed from the GI tract
- Peak plasma level: 1.5–2 h (slow release preparation = 4 h)
- Half-life: 8–35 h; once-daily dosing preferred (improved compliance and decreased urine volume and renal toxicity), half-life increases with duration of therapy (e.g., up to 58 h after 1 year's therapy)
- Excreted primarily (95%) by the kidney; therefore, adequate renal function is essential in order to avoid lithium accumulation and intoxication (see Dosing, above); clearance is significantly correlated with total body weight. Close relationship between level of dehydration and renal clearance
- Monitoring: measure first plasma level 5 days after starting therapy (unless toxicity is suspected). Measure once weekly for the first 2 weeks, thereafter at clinical discretion or whenever a new drug is prescribed or if the dose is increased. Blood levels should be measured at TROUGH, i.e., 9–13 h after last dose
- Lithium is secreted in saliva reaching concentrations 3 times that seen in plasma – saliva composition is altered (see Adverse Effects/GI Effects below)

Lithium (cont.)

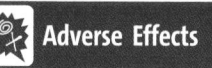 **Adverse Effects**

- See Table p. 214

CNS Effects

- General weakness (up to 33%), fatigue, dysphoria, and restlessness are usually transient and may coincide with peaks in lithium concentration
- Drowsiness, tiredness
- Dizziness and vertigo [Management: administer with food, use slow-release preparation to avoid peak lithium levels, or reduce dosage]
- Cognitive blunting, memory difficulties (up to 28%), decreased speed of information processing, confusion, lack of drive, productivity or creativity [Management: assess lithium plasma level and thyroid function; slow-release preparation, a lower dose, or liothyronine may improve cognitive function]
- Slurred speech, ataxia – evaluate for lithium toxicity
- Neuromuscular: incoordination, muscle weakness, fine tremor/shakiness – up to 65% incidence; more frequent at higher doses and in combination with antidepressant or antipsychotic, with excessive caffeine use, or alcoholism. Frequency of tremor decreases with time [Management: reduce dose, eliminate dietary caffeine; b-blocker (e.g., propranolol or atenolol) may be of benefit]. A coarse tremor may be a sign of lithium toxicity. Cogwheel rigidity and choreoathetosis reported
- Chronic treatment can affect the peripheral nervous system involving motor and sensory function
- Cases of tardive dyskinesia reported in patients on lithium who have not used antipsychotic for at least 6 months
- Seizures rare
- Headaches; rarely, papilledema/elevated intracranial pressure (pseudotumor cerebri) reported
- Cases of somnambulism

Cardiovascular Effects

- Bradycardia
- ECG changes: 20–30% benign T-wave changes (flattening or inversion) and QRS widening at therapeutic doses; use lithium cautiously in patients with pre-existing cardiac disease; arrhythmias and sinus node dysfunction occur less frequently (sinus node dysfunction reported with lithium-carbamazepine combination, with high plasma levels of lithium, in the elderly, and in patients taking other drugs that may affect conduction) [assess patient who has syncopal episode]

Endocrine & Metabolic Effects

- Long-term effects: clinical hypothyroidism occurs in up to 34% of patients, often within the first year – risk greater in women over age 40 and in rapid cyclers – may be more common in regions of high dietary iodine (monitor TSH level – may require levothyroxine therapy). Subclinical hypothyroidism (high TSH and normal free T_4) found in 25% of patients on lithium
- Goiter (not necessarily associated with hypothyroidism) – may be more common in regions of iodine deficiency
- Hyperparathyroidism with hypercalcemia reported in 10–40% of patients on maintenance therapy; may predispose to decreased bone density or to cardiac conduction disturbances; occasional reports of parathyroid adenoma and hyperplasia
- Reports of irregular or prolonged menstrual cycles in up to 15% of females
- Weight gain – up to 60% incidence (25% of patients gain excessive weight); may be related to increased appetite, fluid retention, altered carbohydrate and fat metabolism or to hypothyroidism [Management: reduce caloric intake]. Mean gain is 7.5 kg (range 3–28 kg) on lithium alone (may be higher with drug combinations) and may be related to dose

GI Effects

- Usually coincide with peaks in lithium concentration and are probably due to rapid absorption of the lithium ion; most disappear after a few weeks; if occur late in therapy, evaluate for lithium toxicity
- Nausea – up to 50% incidence, abdominal pain [Management: administer with food, or use slow-release preparation]
- Vomiting – 20% incidence; higher with increased plasma level [Management: use multiple daily dosing, change to a slow-release preparation, or lower dose]
- Diarrhea, loose stools – up to 20% incidence. Slow release preparation may worsen this side effect in some patients [Management: if on a slow-release product, change to a regular lithium preparation; less problems noted with lithium citrate preparations; if all else fails and cannot decrease the lithium dose, loperamide prn]

- Metallic taste: composition of saliva altered (ions and proteins)
- Excessive thirst (up to 36% of incidence), dry mouth, mucosal ulceration (rare), hypersalivation occasionally reported

Renal Effects

- Usually seen after chronic use
- Polyuria and polydipsia – up to 60% risk (dose-related); monitor for fluid and electrolyte imbalance – usually reversible if lithium stopped; however, several cases of persistent diabetes insipidus reported up to 57 months after lithium stopped [potassium-sparing diuretic (amiloride 10–20 mg/day) or DDAVP (10 mg nasal spray or tablets 0.2 mg) may be useful]; sustained-release preparations may cause less impairment of urine concentrating function
- Changes in distal tubular function including impaired urine concentrating ability in about 50% of patients (not always reversible) and chronic focal interstitial nephritis
- Reduced glomerular filtration rates reported with chronic treatment especially in patients who have had one or more episodes of lithium intoxication
- Histological changes include: (a) interstitial fibrosis, tubular atrophy and glomerulosclerosis, seen in 26% patients after treatment beyond two years – primarily those with impaired urine concentrating ability; (b) distal tubular dilatation and macrocyst formation
- Rare cases of nephrotic syndrome with proteinuria, glycosuria and oliguria, edema, and hypoalbuminemia

Dermatological Effects

- Dry skin common
- Skin rash, pruritus, exacerbation or new onset of psoriasis [the latter may respond to inositol up to 6 g/day]
- Acne [may respond to: pyridoxine 50 mg bid, zinc sulfate 110 mg bid, or β-carotene 25,000 IU daily]
- Dryness and thinning of hair – may be related to hypothyroidism; alopecia reported in 12–19% of patients on chronic therapy; changes in color and texture also reported
- Folliculitis (may occur more frequently in the spring) [may respond to antihistamines]
- Case reports of nail pigmentation

Other Adverse Effects

- Blurred vision may be related to peak plasma levels; reduction in retinal light sensitivity, nystagmus
- Changes in sexual function – up to 10% risk; includes decreased libido, erectile dysfunction, priapism and decreased sperm motility; soreness and ulceration of genitalia (rare)
- Edema, swelling of extremities – evaluate for sodium retention [use diuretics with caution – see Drug Interactions – spironolactone may be preferred]
- Anemia, leukocytosis (common), leukopenia, albuminuria; rarely aplastic anemia, agranulocytosis, thrombocytopenia, and thrombocytosis
- Rarely – can induce polyarthritis

 Discontinuation Syndrome

- Rarely anxiety, instability, and emotional lability reported following abrupt withdrawal
- Rapid discontinuation may increase the risk of relapse
- 50% rate of manic or depressive recurrence within 3 to 5 months among previously stable patients reported with abrupt withdrawal

 Precautions

- Good kidney function, adequate salt and fluid intake are essential
- Excessive loss of sodium (due to vomiting, diarrhea, use of diuretics, etc.) causes increased lithium retention, possibly leading to toxicity; lower doses of lithium are necessary if the patient is on a salt-restricted diet (which includes most low-calorie diets)
- Heavy sweating can lead to changes in plasma level of lithium
- Use cautiously and in reduced dosage in the elderly as the ability to excrete lithium decreases with age
- Some researchers suggest that concurrent ECT may increase the possibility of developing cerebral toxicity to lithium; discontinue during courses of ECT, if possible
- Do not rapidly increase lithium and antipsychotic dosage at the same time, due to risk of neurotoxicity

 Contraindications

- Brain damage
- Renal disease
- Cardiovascular disease
- Severe debilitation

Lithium (cont.)

 **Toxicity**

Mild Toxicity	• At lithium levels of 1.5–2 mmol/l; occasionally occurs with levels in the normal range
	• Develops gradually over several days
	• Side effects such as ataxia, coarse tremor, confusion, diarrhea, drowsiness, fasciculation, and slurred speech may occur
Management	• Stop lithium
Moderate/Severe Toxicity	• At lithium levels in excess of 2 mmol/l
	• Acute lithium toxicity can present as acute delirium with disorientation, fluctuating levels of consciousness, hallucinations, and extrapyramidal symptoms; may manifest as a catatonic stupor
	• Severe poisoning may result in coma with hyperreflexia, muscle tremor, hyperextension of the limbs, pulse irregularities, hypertension or hypotension, ECG changes, peripheral circulatory failure, neuroleptic malignant syndrome, and epileptic seizures; acute tubular necrosis (renal failure) can occur
	• In some patients, lithium toxicity causes persistent neurological (cerebellar and basal ganglia) dysfunction
	• At toxic levels lithium may inhibit its own excretion, as can renal dysfunction, sodium depletion, as well as certain drugs (e.g., NSAIDs)
	• Note: The discrepancy between high serum levels and advanced symptoms of toxicity reflects delayed distribution of drug into susceptible tissues; accumulation in the CNS explains persistent symptoms despite falling serum levels
	• Deaths have been reported; when serum lithium level exceeds 4 mmol/l the prognosis is poor
Management	• Symptomatic: Reduce absorption, restore fluid and electrolyte balance, correct sodium depletion and remove drug from the body
	• Blood lithium concentration may be reduced by forced alkaline diuresis or by prolonged peritoneal dialysis or hemodialysis
	• Excretion may be facilitated by IV urea, sodium bicarbonate, acetazolamide, or aminophylline
	• Convulsions may be controlled by a short-acting barbiturate (thiopental sodium)

Lab Tests/Monitoring

At beginning of treatment and at every admission:
1. serum electrolytes
2. Hb, Hct, WBC and differential
3. sensitive TSH, total T4, T4 uptake
4. BUN, creatinine
5. calcium
6. ECG for patients over 45, or with a history of cardiac problems
7. parathormone (recommended by some)

On an outpatient basis, repeat tests (2) + (3) every 6 months; (4) every 12 months; (5) every 2 years; (6) every 5 years. As some rapid cycling may be due to lithium-induced hypothyroidism, it is important to regularly assess thyroid function

• Plasma level monitoring – see Pharmacokinetics p. 187

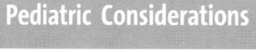 **Pediatric Considerations**

• For detailed information on the use of lithium in this population, please see the *Clinical Handbook of Psychotropic Drugs for Children and Adolescents* (2007)
• Lithium has been used successfully in children with chronic aggressive conduct disorders, in bipolar disorder, in periodic mood and behavior disorders, and pervasive developmental disorder (autism)
• Half-life shorter and clearance is faster than seen in adults

Geriatric Considerations

- Good kidney function, adequate salt and fluid intake are essential; ability to excrete lithium decreases with age, resulting in a longer elimination half-life
- Start therapy at lower doses and monitor serum level
- Incidence of side effects may be greater and occur at lower plasma levels, including tremor, GI disturbances, polyuria, ataxia, myoclonus, and EPS
- Elderly are at increased risk for hyponatremia after an acute illness or if fluid intake is restricted
- Elderly are at higher risk for neurotoxicity and cognitive impairment, even at therapeutic plasma levels
- Slow release preparation may decrease side effects that occur as a result of peak plasma levels

 Use in Pregnancy

- Avoid in pregnancy (esp. first trimester), overall risk of fetal malformations is 4–12%; cardiovascular malformations risk ratio is 1.2–7.7 – level A evidence (e.g., tricuspid valve malformations; 0.05– 0.1% risk of Ebstein's anomaly) – fetal echocardiography may be considered if exposure in first trimester (level C evidence) and high-resolution ultrasound at 16–18 weeks gestation. If necessary, use lithium at the lowest possible divided daily dose to avoid peak concentrations
- A statistically significant association noted between higher doses of lithium in the first trimester and premature deliveries; a higher rate of macrosomia reported in these premature infants
- Monitor drug levels during pregnancy: weekly in first month, then during and immediately after delivery (level C evidence)
- Lithium clearance increased by 50–100% in the third trimester because of increases in plasma volume and greater glomerular filtration rate; rate returns to pre-pregnancy levels after delivery; dose should be decreased, or drug discontinued, 2–3 days prior to delivery
- Use of lithium near term may produce severe toxicity in the newborn, which is usually reversible, including nontoxic goiter, atrial flutter, T-wave inversion, nephrogenic diabetes insipidus, floppy baby syndrome, cyanosis and seizures; can be minimized by withholding maternal lithium 24 h before delivery
- Do neonatal ECG if lithium was used in first trimester; observe infant for lithium toxicity for first 10 days of life

Breast Milk

- Present in breast milk at a concentration of 30–100% of mother's serum (infant's serum concentration is approximately equal to or less than that of the milk). Reported symptoms in infant include lethargy, hypothermia, hypotonia, involuntary movements, dehydration, hypothyroidism, cyanosis, heart murmur, and T-wave changes
- Infant has decreased renal clearance; the American Academy of Pediatrics considers lithium contraindicated during breastfeeding. Avoid until infant is at least 5 months of age due to decreased renal clearance
- If breastfeeding is undertaken, the mother should be educated about signs and symptoms of lithium toxicity and risk of infant dehydration; monitor infant lithium levels and consider periodic thyroid evaluation

Nursing Implications

- Accurate observation and assessment of patient's behavior before and after lithium therapy is initiated is important
- Be alert for, observe, and report any signs of side effects, or symptoms of toxicity; if toxic withhold the dose and call doctor immediately
- Have patient maintain normal salt intake and check fluid intake and output; adjust fluid and salt ingestion to compensate if excessive loss occurs through vomiting or diarrhea
- Expect nausea, thirst, frequent urination, and generalized discomfort during the first few days; therapeutic effects occur gradually and may take up to 3 weeks
- May give lithium with meals to avoid GI disturbances
- Caffeine intake should not be dramatically altered while taking lithium
- Withhold morning dose of lithium until after the blood draw, on mornings when blood is drawn for a lithium level
- The patient and family should be educated regarding the drug's effects and toxicities
- Slow release preparations should not be broken or crushed. They may decrease side effects that occur as a result of high peak plasma levels (i.e., 1–2 h post dose), e.g., tremor
- Because lithium may cause drowsiness, caution patient to avoid activities requiring alertness until response to drug has been determined

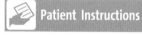 **Patient Instructions**

- For detailed patient instructions on lithium, see the Patient Information Sheet on p. 347

Lithium (cont.)

➡️⬅️ **Drug Interactions**	• Clinically significant interactions are listed below

Class of Drug	Example	Interaction Effects
Alcohol		Increased tremor/shakiness with chronic alcohol use
Anesthetic	Ketamine	Increased lithium toxicity due to sodium depletion
Angiotensin-converting enzyme (ACE) inhibitor ACE-2 inhibitor	Captopril, enalapril, lisinopril Candesartan, losartan, valsartan	Increased lithium toxicity due to sodium depletion; average increase in lithium level of 36% reported Reports of lithium toxicity possibly due to reduced aldosterone levels
Antibiotic/anti-infective	Ampicillin, doxycycline, tetracycline, spectinomycin, levofloxacin, metronidazole	Case reports of increased lithium effect and toxicity due to decreased renal clearance of lithium. Monitor lithium level if combination used
Anticonvulsant	Carbamazepine, phenytoin, valproate	Increased neurotoxicity of both drugs at therapeutic doses Synergistic mood-stabilizing effect with carbamazepine and valproate Valproate may aggravate action tremor
Antidepressant Cyclic, MAOIs, RIMA SSRI/SNRI	Desipramine, tranylcypromine, moclobemide, phenelzine Fluoxetine, fluvoxamine, sertraline, paroxetine, venlafaxine	Synergistic antidepressant effect in treatment-resistant patients May increase lithium tremor Elevated lithium serum level with possible neurotoxicity; serotonin syndrome (see p. 8) reported Synergistic effect in treatment-resistant depression and OCD
Antihypertensive	Amiloride, spironolactone, thiazides, triamterene, methyldopa Acetazolamide, mannitol, urea β-blockers: propranolol, oxprenolol	Increased lithium effects and toxicity due to decreased renal clearance of lithium Increased renal excretion of lithium, decreasing its effect Beneficial effect in treatment of lithium tremor; propranolol lowers glomerular filtration rate and has been associated with a 19% reduction in lithium clearance
Antipsychotic	Molindone Haloperidol, perphenazine, phenothiazines Clozapine	Increased plasma level of molindone reported; variable effects on plasma level of neuroleptics as well as lithium seen Increased neurotoxicity possible at therapeutic doses; may increase EPS; cases of NMS reported Possible increased risk of agranulocytosis with clozapine; two cases of seizures and two cases of diabetic ketoacidosis reported with combination
Antiviral agent	Zidovudine	Reversal of zidovudine-induced neutropenia
Benzodiazepine	Clonazepam	Increased incidence of sexual dysfunction (up to 49%) reported with the combination
Ca-channel blocker	Verapamil, diltiazem	Increased neurotoxicity of both drugs; increased bradycardia and cardiotoxicity with verapamil due to combined calcium blockade
Caffeine		Increased renal excretion of lithium resulting in decreased plasma level May increase lithium tremor
Herbal diuretics	Agrimony, dandelion, juniper, licorice, horsetail, uva ursi Cola nut, guarana, maté	Elevated lithium level possible due to decreased renal clearance Increased excretion and decreased lithium level possible due to high content of caffeine in herbal preparations
Iodide salt	Calcium, potassium iodide	May act synergistically to produce hypothyroidism. AVOID
L-Tryptophan		Increased plasma level and efficacy and/or toxicity of lithium

Class of Drug	Example	Interaction Effects
Metronidazole		Decreased renal clearance of lithium resulting in elevated plasma levels. Monitor lithium level, creatinine and electrolyte levels and osmolality
NSAID	Ibuprofen, ketorolac, diclofenac, indomethacin, mefenamic acid, naproxen, celecoxib, rofecoxib, sulindac (no interaction with ASA)	Increased lithium level and possible toxicity due to decreased renal clearance of lithium (up to 133% increase reported with celecoxib, up to 448% with rofecoxib, up to 300% with mefenamic acid); serum creatinine increased in several reports. Use caution and monitor lithium level every 4–5 days until stable
Neuromuscular blocker	Succinylcholine, pancuronium	Potentiation of muscle relaxation
Psyllium	Metamucil, Prodiem	Decreased lithium level if drugs taken at the same time. Increased water drawn into the colon by the bulk laxatives would increase the amount of ionized lithium, which would remain unabsorbed
Sibutramine		Increased risk of serotonin syndrome
Sodium salt		Increased intake results in decreased lithium plasma level; decreased intake causes increased lithium plasma level
Theophylline	Aminophylline, oxtriphylline, theophylline	Enhanced renal lithium clearance and reduced plasma level (by approx. 20%) May increase lithium tremor
Trimethoprim/Sulfamethoxazole		Case report of lithium toxicity within days of starting antimicrobial
Triptan	Sumatriptan, zolmitriptan	Increased serotonergic effects possible – monitor
Urinary alkalizer	Potassium citrate, sodium bicarbonate	Enhanced renal lithium clearance and reduced plasma level

194

Anticonvulsants

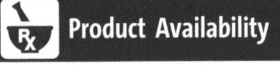 **Product Availability**

Chemical Class	Generic Name	Trade Name[A]	Dosage Forms and Strengths
First-generation	Clonazepam Phenytoin	Rivotril[C], Klonopin[B] Dilantin	See pp. 158–173 See p. 300
Second-generation	Carbamazepine	Tegretol	Tablets: 100 mg[B], 200 mg, 300 mg[B], 400 mg[B] Chewable tablets: 100 mg, 200 mg Oral suspension: 100 mg/5 mg
		Tegretol CR[C]	Controlled-release tablets[C]: 200 mg, 400 mg
		Tegretol XR[B], Equetro[B], Carbatrol[B]	Extended-release capsules[B]: 100 mg, 200 mg, 300 mg, 400 mg
	Divalproex sodium	Depakote sprinkle[B]	Capsules[B]: 125 mg
		Depakote[B]	Delayed-release tablets: 125 mg[B], 250 mg[B], 500 mg
		Depakote ER[B], Epival ER[B]	Extended-release tablets: 250 mg, 500 mg
		Epival (ECT)[C]	Enteric-coated tablets: 125 mg, 250 mg, 500 mg
	Valproic acid	Depakene	Capsules: 250 mg[B], 500 mg[B] Oral syrup: 250 mg/5 ml
	Valproate sodium	Depacon[B]	Injection[B]: 100 mg/ml
Third-generation	Gabapentin	Neurontin	Capsules: 100 mg, 300 mg, 400 mg Tablets: 600 mg, 800 mg Oral solution[B]: 250 mg/5 ml
	Lamotrigine	Lamictal	Tablets: 25 mg, 100 mg, 150 mg, 200 mg[B] Chewable tablets: 2 mg, 5 mg, 25 mg[B]
	Oxcarbazepine	Trileptal	Tablets: 150 mg, 300 mg, 600 mg Oral suspension: 300 mg/5 ml
	Topiramate	Topamax	Tablets: 25 mg, 50 mg[B], 100 mg, 200 mg Sprinkle capsules: 15 mg, 25 mg

[A] Generic preparations may be available, [B] Not marketed in Canada, [C] Not marketed in USA

|||| Indications
(👍 Approved)

	Carbamazepine	Valproate	Gabapentin	Lamotrigine	Topiramate	Oxcarbazepine
Acute mania	👍 +	👍 +	?/–	?/–	?/–	+
Prophylaxis of BD	👍 +	+	?	👍 + (Bipolar I)	–	+/–
Rapid-cycling BD	+/–	+	?/–	+ (Bipolar II)	?/–	–

	Carbamazepine	Valproate	Gabapentin	Lamotrigine	Topiramate	Oxcarbazepine
Mixed states	👍 +	+	?	+	–	+ (preliminary data, adjunctive drug)
Bipolar depression	+ (data contradictory)	+/– (data contradictory)	+/– (open trials)	+ (Bipolar I)*	+ (adjunctive – data contradictory)	+ (preliminary data)
Anticonvulsant	👍 Prophylaxis and treatment of complex partial and limbic region seizures	👍 Absence, simple and complex partial generalized seizures	👍 Adjunctive in refractory epilepsy	👍 Adjunctive or sole therapy in refractory epilepsy	👍 Adjunctive or monotherapy in epilepsy	👍 Partial seizures (sole or adjunctive agent)
Paroxysmal pain syndromes	👍 +	+	👍 + Postherpetic neuralgia + (neuropathic pain)	+ (central pain)	+ (neuropathic pain – preliminay data)	+ (neuropathic pain – open trials)
Migraine headaches	+	👍 +	+ (preliminary data)	+/– (preliminary data)	👍 + (prophylaxis)	–
Behavior disturbances (in dementia, explosive disorder, conduct disorder, mental retardation, brain damage)	+ (alone or in combination with lithium, antipsychotics or β-blockers)	+	+ (preliminary data)	– (preliminary data)	+	+ (preliminary data)
Panic disorder	+	+	+ (severe panic only – preliminary data)	?	–	+ (case report)
Social phobia, generalized anxiety disorder	–	+/– (open trials)	+	?	+ (open trials)	?
Eating disorder; binge eating/ bulimia	?	?	?	?	+	?
Posttraumatic stress disorder	+ (open trials)	+ (open trials)	+ (adjunctive – preliminary data)	+	?	?
Obsessive compulsive disorder	+/– (augmenting drug – preliminary data)	–	+ (adjunctive to SSRIs – preliminary data)	+/– (case report – adjunctive drug)	+ (open trial, adjunctive drug)	+ (case report – adjunctive drug)
Core symptoms of borderline personality disorder	+	+ (preliminary data)	?	+ (preliminary data)	+	+ (preliminary data)
Paranoid ideation, hallucinations and negative symptoms of schizophrenia	+ (adjunctive drug)	+ (adjunctive drug)	–	+ (adjunctive drug – benefit on positive symptoms)	+ (preliminary data – adjunctive drug)	+ (preliminary data – alone or as adjunctive drug)
Movement disorders	Dystonic disorder in children	–	Management of tardive dyskinesia in psychotic patients with mood features (preliminary data)	–	Essential tremor (preliminary data from 3 small RDBCTs)	–

Anticonvulsants (cont.)

	Carbamazepine	Valproate	Gabapentin	Lamotrigine	Topiramate	Oxcarbazepine
Drug dependence	Aid in alcohol or sedative/hypnotic withdrawal; may play a role in cocaine dependence	Aid in alcohol withdrawal (open trials)	May reduce craving for cocaine as well as its usage Adjunct in opioid withdrawal	Aid in alcohol withdrawal (open trials) May reduce craving for cocaine (open trial)	Aid in treating alcohol dependence together with behavior modification (controlled trial) Promotes smoking cessation in alcohol-dependant smokers	–

♦ Approved indication; + = positive data; – = negative data; ? = no data available or data of poor quality to guide therapy; * pivotal trials in acute bipolar depression have been negative; experts recommend lamotrigine as first-line therapy based on other lines of evidence

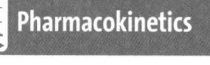 **Pharmacokinetics**

- See table p. 197 for specific agents
- With valproate, pharmacokinetics show significant variation with changes in body weight. Valproate exhibits concentration-dependent protein binding, therefore at high doses and plasma concentrations a larger proportion may exist in unbound (free) form
- The 10,11-epoxide metabolite of carbamazepine can reach up to 50% of the plasma concentration of the parent drug; it is pharmacologically active and is associated with neurological side effects
- Gabapentin shows dose-dependent bioavailability as a result of a saturable transport mechanism (better bioavailability with more frequent dosing; plasma level is proportional to the dose). Elimination is almost entirely by the kidneys, and is reduced in patients with renal dysfunction (see Dosing p. 196)
- Large interindividual variation seen in plasma lamotrigine concentration in patients with renal impairment; half-life is also prolonged in hepatic dysfunction. Age, gender and smoking do not affect pharmacokinetics

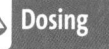 **Dosing**

- See table p. 197 for specific agents
- Plasma level monitoring for carbamazepine and valproate (measured at trough) can help guide dosing
- Slower dosage titration of lamotrigine may decrease risk of rash
- Reduced dosages recommended in the elderly and in hepatic or renal disorders

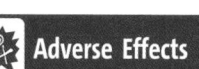 **Adverse Effects**

- See table pp. 197–201 for specific agents
- Many side effects can be minimized with slower dosage titration
- Common (for all anticonvulsants):
  - GI complaints, e.g., nausea [Management: take with food, change to an enteric-coated preparation, use ranitidine 150 mg/day or famotidine 20 mg/day]
  - Dose-related lethargy, sedation, behavior changes/deterioration, reversible dementia/encephalopathy; cognitive effects are more prominent on drug initiation and are minimized with slow dosage increases
  - Dose-related tremor; tends to be rhythmic, rapid, symmetrical and most prominent in upper extremities [reduce dose if possible; responds to propranolol]
  - Ataxia
  - Changes in appetite, weight gain (except topiramate and lamotrigine) – more common in females; may be associated with features of insulin resistance, hyperlipidemia, impaired glucose tolerance, and hyperinsulinemia. Weight increases with duration of treatment. Obesity may increase risk of hyperandrogenism in females [metformin 500 mg tid]
  - Menstrual disturbances (except gabapentin and topiramate), including: prolonged cycles, oligomenorrhea, amenorrhea, polycystic ovaries; elevated testosterone – rates may be higher in females who begin taking valproate before age 20. Clinical features of polycystic ovary syndrome include hirsutism, alopecia, acne, menstrual irregularities, and obesity; lab indices show increased total and free testosterone, decreased FSH, increased serum prolactin and LH, and LH/FSH ratio > 2, incidence most common with valproic acid (10.5%)

- Occasional (for all anticonvulsants):
  - Dysarthria, incoordination
  - Diplopia, nystagmus
- Rare – Anticonvulsant hypersensitivity syndrome with fever, rash and internal organ involvement; cross-sensitivity reported between carbamazepine and lamotrigine

Comparison of Anticonvulsants

	Carbamazepine	Oxcarbazepine	Valproate	Gabapentin	Lamotrigine	Topiramate
General comments	Positive predictors of response include: non-classic or secondary mania, an early age at onset, a negative family history of mood disorder, and patients with neurological abnormalities Less response noted in patients with severe mania, dysphoric mania and rapid cycling disorder	Pharmacological activity is exerted primarily through the 10-monohydroxy metabolite (MHD) of oxcarbazepine Early data suggest similar pharmacological activity as carbamazepine with a lower potential for serious adverse effects	Positive predictors of response include: pure mania, mixed or dysphoric mania and patients with secondary or rapid cycling disorder Good response in adolescents and in mania with comorbid substance use disorder Less response noted in patients with co-morbid personality disorder, severe mania and those previously treated with antidepressants or stimulants May be more effective in treating and preventing manic and mixed episodes	May be effective as an adjunctive medication in both Bipolar I and Bipolar II disorders (evidence of poor quality), especially in the presence of significant anxiety	More effective in Bipolar depression; suggested to have antidepressant properties First-line agent for treatment of bipolar depression in patients with a history of severe refractory manic episodes: does not induce switches to hypomania or mania Prophylaxis of rapid cycling and Bipolar II disorder	May be effective as an adjunct to other mood stabilizers in refractory mania and in ultra-rapid or ultradian cycling disorder (poor quality evidence)
Pharmacology	Anticonvulsant, anti-kindling, and GABA-ergic activity Blocks voltage-dependent sodium channels	MHD metabolite has anticonvulsant, anti-kindling, and GABA-ergic activity Blocks voltage-dependent sodium channels and calcium channels	Anticonvulsant, anti-kindling, and GABA-ergic activity Indirectly blunts excitatory activity of glutaminergic system Blocks Ca channels Indirectly blocks voltage-dependent sodium channels Increases serotonergic function	Anticonvulsant, anti-kindling, and GABA-ergic activity Blocks voltage-dependent sodium channels and calcium channels Inhibits excitatory amino acids (glutamate)	Anticonvulsant and GABA-ergic activity Blocks voltage-dependent sodium channels and calcium channels Inhibits excitatory amino acids (glutamate)	Anticonvulsant, anti-kindling, and GABA-ergic activity Inhibits excitatory amino acids (glutamate) Inhibits carbonic anhydrase and blocks voltage-dependent sodium channels and calcium channels

Comparison of Anticonvulsants (cont.)

	Carbamazepine	Oxcarbazepine	Valproate	Gabapentin	Lamotrigine	Topiramate
Dosing	Begin at 200 mg daily and increase by 100 mg twice weekly, until either side effects limit dose, or reach therapeutic plasma level Extended release: begin at 200 mg bid and increased by 200 mg daily up to a maximum of 1600 mg/day (capsules can be opened and sprinkled on food)	Begin at 150–300 mg/day and increase by 150 mg q 2 weeks When switching from carbamazepine, the equivalent dose is 50% higher	Begin at 250 mg bid and increase dose gradually, until either side effects limit dose, or reach therapeutic plasma level Once daily dosing has been used Loading dose strategy: *Oral:* give stat dose of 20 mg/kg, then 12 h later initiate bid dosing at 10 mg/kg bid *IV:* 1200–1800 mg/day over 3 days	Begin at 300–400 mg/day and increase by 300–400 mg a day BD range 900–4000 mg/day Usual dose: 900–1800 mg/day Anxiety: up to 3600 mg/day	Begin at 25–50 mg/day and increase by 12.5–25 mg a week up to 250 mg bid (lower if co-prescribed with valproate) Antidepressant dose: 200 mg/day	Begin at 25–50 mg/day and increase by 25–50 mg every 4–7 days up to 500 mg/day (a low initial dose and gradual increases minimize cognitive and behavioral side effects)
	Dose range: 300–1600 mg/day in single or divided dose	Dose range: 600–1200 mg/day (divided doses)	Dose range: 750–3000 mg/day in single or divided dose *Max:* 60 mg/kg/day	Dose range: 900–3600 mg/day given as tid dosing	Dose range: 100–500 mg/day given in single or divided dose	Acute dose range: 200–600 mg/day Maintenance range: 50–400 mg/day
Renal impairment	No change	Decrease dose by 50% if creatinine clearance < 30 ml/min	Free valproate level doubles in renal impairment	Decrease dose if creatinine clearance > 60 ml/min (see Precautions, p. 204)	Reduced clearance	Moderate: clearance reduced by 42% Severe: clearance reduced by 54%
Hepatic impairment	Reduced clearance	No effect	See hepatic adverse effects (p. 197) and Precautions (p. 204)	–	Reduce initial and maintenance doses by 50% in mild to moderate impairment and 75% in severe impairment	Reduced clearance
Recommended plasma level	17–54 µmol/L (4–12 micrograms/ml)	15–35 micrograms/ml (MHD metabolite)	350–800 µmol/L (50–115 micrograms/ml)	No correlation	–	–
Pharmacokinetics Bioavailability	75–85%	> 95%	78%	Approx. 60% (dose-dependent; higher with qid dosing)	100%	80%
Peak plasma level	1–6 h	1–3 h (parent) 4–12 h (active MHD metabolite) and 2–4 h at steady state	Oral valproic acid: 1–4 h (may be delayed by food) Divalproex and extended-release: 3–8 h	2–3 h	1–5 h (rate may be reduced by food)	2–3 h (delayed by food)
Protein binding	75–90%	40%	60–95% (concentration dependent); increased by low-fat diets	minimal	55%	13–17%
Half-life	15–35 h (acute use); 10–20 h (chronic use) – stimulates own metabolism	Parent: 1–5 h MHD metabolite: 7–20 h	5–20 h	5–7 h	33 h mean (acute use) 26 h mean (chronic use)	19–23 h

	Carbamazepine	Oxcarbazepine	Valproate	Gabapentin	Lamotrigine	Topiramate
Metabolizing enzymes	CYP1A3, 3A4[M], 2C8, 2C9; P-gp	Rapidly metabolized by cytosolic enzymes to active metabolite MHD	CYP2C9; UGT1A6, 1A9, 2B7	Not metabolized – eliminated by renal excretion	Metabolized primarily by glucuronic acid conjugation; also by UGT1A4, 2B7	P-gp; 70% eliminated unchanged in urine
Metabolism effects	Inducer of CYP1A2, 3A4[P], 2C9, 2B6 and UGT1A4 Induces own metabolism Inhibitor of P-gp	Moderate inducer of CYP3A4 Inhibitor of CYP2C19 and UGT1A4 (does not induce own metabolism)	Inhibitor of CYP2D6[W], 2C9, 2C19; UGT2B7[P], 2B15	–	–	–
Adverse effects CNS	Sedation (11%), cognitive blunting, confusion (higher doses)	Sedation common, lethargy	Sedation (> 10%), lethargy, behavior changes/deterioration, cognitive blunting, encephalopathy	Sedation (19%), fatigue, abnormal thinking, amnesia	Sedation (> 10%), asthenia, cognitive blunting, "spaced-out" feeling	Sedation, lethargy, fatigue common Deficits in word-finding, concentration and memory (dose-dependent) Anxiety, agitation, insomnia
	Agitation, restlessness, irritability, insomnia May exacerbate schizophrenia on withdrawal		Hyperactivity, aggression Case of delirium (following loading-dose strategy) Rare cases of psychosis	Nervousness, anxiety, hostility Rare switches to hypomania/mania Cases of depression	Agitation, activation, irritability, insomnia Switches to hypomania/mania	Increased panic attacks, worsening of depression or psychosis
	Headache Tremors, ataxia (up to 50%), paresthesias (3%), acute dystonic reactions, chronic dyskinesias	Headache Ataxia (> 25%), gait disturbances, tremor	Headache (3%) Tremors (10% adults; 15% children – tend to be rhythmic, rapid, symmetrical and most prominent in the upper extremities), ataxia, dysarthria, incoordination	Tremors (7%), ataxia, incoordination, dysarthria, myalgia	Headache (> 25%) Tremors, ataxia (22%), incoordination, myalgia, arthralgia	Headache Tremors, ataxia; paresthesias common
Anticholinergic	Blurred vision (6%), mydriasis, cycloplegia, ophthalmoplegia, dry mouth, slurred speech Constipation	Blurred vision	–	Dry mouth or throat (2%) Constipation	Blurred vision Constipation Dry mouth (> 5%)	Blurred vision, sweating Acute angle closure reported (glaucoma)
Gastrointestinal	Nausea (4%)	Nausea common, vomiting	Nausea common, vomiting	Nausea	Nausea, vomiting, diarrhea (> 5%) Rarely esophagitis	Nausea (4–13%) Change in taste of carbonated beverages
Cardiovascular	Dizziness Vasculitis	Dizziness, peripheral edema	Rarely dizziness Vasculitis	Dizziness (17%), hypotension Occasionally hypertension Peripheral edema	Breathlessness, dizziness (38%) Conduction changes (prolongation of PR interval)	Dizziness common

Comparison of Anticonvulsants (cont.)

	Carbamazepine	Oxcarbazepine	Valproate	Gabapentin	Lamotrigine	Topiramate
Dermatological	Rash (10–15%) – severe dermatological reactions may signify impending blood dyscrasias Hair loss (6%) Photosensitivity reactions Rarely: fixed drug eruptions, lichenoid-like reactions, bullous reactions, exfoliative dermatitis, vasculitis Hypersensitivity syndrome – rare; with fever, skin eruptions and internal organ involvement	Rash less common than with carbamazepine; 25–30% of patients are cross-sensitive Stevens-Johnson syndrome and toxic epidermal necrolysis reported in adults and children	Rash Hair loss (up to 12% – higher incidence with higher doses); changes in texture or color of hair Case reports of nail pigmentation Rare cases of Stevens-Johnson syndrome (increased risk in combination with lamotrigine), toxic epidermal necrolysis, lupus, vasculitis, erythema multiforme, or skin pigmentation	Pruritus	Rash (up to 10%); in 2–3% require drug discontinuation – risk of severe rash increased with rapid dose titration, in children, and in combination with valproate Stevens-Johnson syndrome in 1–2% of children and 0.1% of adults (usually within first 8 weeks of therapy); increased risk in combination with valproate Rarely, erythema multiforme, hypersensitivity syndrome Photosensitivity reactions	Rash
Hematologic	Transitory leukopenia (10%), persistent leukopenia (2%) Rarely, eosinophilia, aplastic anemia, thrombocytopenia, purpura, and agranulocytosis	Rare	Reversible thrombocytopenia – may be related to high plasma levels; rare episodes of bleeding Macrocytic anemia, coagulopathies Case of pancytopenia (following loading-dose strategy)	Leukopenia (1%), purpura	Neutropenia Rarely, hematemesis, hemolytic anemia, thrombocytopenia, pancytopenia, aplastic anemia	Purpura
Hepatic	Transient enzyme elevation (5–15%) – evaluate for hepatotoxicity if elevation > 3 times normal Rarely, hepatocellular and cholestatic jaundice, granulomatous hepatitis and severe hepatic necrosis	Rare	Asymptomatic hepatic transaminase elevation (44%) Cases of severe liver toxicity (all patients were also taking lamotrigine) Steatosis or nonalcoholic fatty liver disease (a symptom of insulin resistance)	Case reports of abnormal liver function	Rare	Cases of severe liver damage

	Carbamazepine	Oxcarbazepine	Valproate	Gabapentin	Lamotrigine	Topiramate
Endocrine	Menstrual disturbances in females (up to 45%) Decreased libido in males Elevation of total cholesterol (primarily HDL) Can lower thyroxine levels and TSH response to TRH Polycystic ovaries reported in up to 22% of females; hyperandrogenism in up to 17% Weight gain – may be independent of or secondary to peripheral edema/SIADH Occasional weight loss	Hyperthermia	Menstrual disturbances (up to 60%) including prolonged cycles, oligomenorrhea, amenorrhea, polycystic ovaries (up to 67%) – higher incidence in obese women In females: hyperandrogenism (increased testosterone in 33%), android obesity (in up to 53%), hirsutism, hyperinsulinemia Decreased levels of HDL, low HDL/cholesterol ratio, increased triglyceride levels Weight gain (59%) – mean gain of up to 21 kg reported; more common in females and with high plasma levels; may be associated with features of insulin resistance Weight loss (5%)	Weight gain common with higher doses	Menstrual disturbances, dysmenorrhea, vaginitis No weight gain	Decreased sweating, hyperthermia Anorexia; weight loss (4–13%)
Ocular	Diplopia (16%), nystagmus (up to 50%), visual hallucinations, lens abnormalities 2 cases of pigmentary retinopathy	Diplopia, nystagmus	Diplopia, nystagmus, asterixis (spots before the eyes)	Diplopia (6%), nystagmus, amblyopia	Diplopia (28%) nystagmus, amblyopia	Diplopia, nystagmus Cases of acute myopia and secondary angle closure glaucoma
Other	Hyponatremia and water intoxication (4–12%) – more common in the elderly and with higher plasma levels Rarely: acute renal failure, pancreatitis, splenomegaly, lymphadenopathy, systemic lupus erythematosus and serum sickness Can decrease vitamin D levels by increasing its metabolism, resulting in increased bone resorption, osteomalacia, osteoporosis, and fractures [bone density evaluation, supplement with calcium and vitamin D]	Hyponatremia (29% incidence); higher risk in the elderly	Gingival hyperplasia Carnitine deficiency Hyperammonemia (up to 50%); usually asymptomatic, but may cause increased sedation, confusion, stupor and/or coma Increased bone resorption with osteoporosis, osteopenia [bone density evaluation, supplement with calcium and vitamin D] Rarely: osteomalacia, cholecystitis, pancreatitis and serum sickness	Rhinitis, pharyngitis	Rhinitis, pharyngitis Rarely, apnea, pancreatitis	Hyponatremia (up to 25%) Nephrolithiasis (renal stone formation) in up to 1.5% with chronic use Epistaxis Decrease in sodium bicarbonate (up to 30% patients) Metabolic acidosis (may increase risk for nephrolithiasis or nephrocalcinosis and may result in osteomalacia and/or osteoporosis

Comparison of Anticonvulsants (cont.)

	Carbamazepine	Oxcarbazepine	Valproate	Gabapentin	Lamotrigine	Topiramate
Chronic or serious conditions	Bone marrow suppression, ocular effects, SIADH (hyponatremia), hypersensitivity syndrome (0.1%)	Hyponatremia Stevens-Johnson syndrome, toxic epidermal necrolysis	Endocrine (females), thrombocytopenia, leukopenia, hyperammonemia, hepatic toxicity, Stevens-Johnson syndrome, pancreatitis, osteopenia and osteoporosis	None known	Rash, Stevens-Johnson syndrome, toxic epidermal necrolysis, hypersensitivity syndrome (0.1%), PR prolongation	Untreated metabolic acidosis; renal stone formation Acute myopia Hyperthermia
Use in Pregnancy	Avoid in first trimester (level A evidence)[1]. If necessary, use lowest amount possible in divided doses. Monitor drug levels throughout pregnancy, maternal alpha fetoprotein around week 16, and do fetal ultrasound around week 20 Concentration of drug in cord blood equals that in maternal serum Caution: overall incidence of major malformations is 5.7% with lower birth rates reported Risk of spina bifida up to 1%, congenital heart defects 2.9% One prospective study reported craniofacial defects in 11%, fingernail hyperplasia in 26%, and developmental delays in 20% of children exposed prenatally May cause vitamin K deficiency during latter half of gestation resulting in bleeding [vitamin K and folic acid supplementation recommended] Clearance increased 2-fold during pregnancy; dose may need to be increased by 100%	Crosses placenta; teratogenic effects reported in animals; likely to cause teratogenic effects in humans (folic acid supplementation recommended)	AVOID, especially in first trimester (level A evidence)[1]; incidence of malformations is 11.1% – related to dose and drug plasm level. Fetal serum concentrations are 1.4 times that of the mother; half-life prolonged in infant If absolutely necessary, limit use to < 1000 mg/day in 3 or more divided doses. Monitor plasma levels throughout pregnancy, maternal alpha fetoprotein around week 16, and do fetal ultrasound around week 20 Risk of spina bifida 1–2%, neural tube defects up to 5%, neurological dysfunction and developmental deficits seen in up to 71%; musculoskeletal, cardiovascular, pulmonary, craniofacial, genital and skin defects also reported May cause vitamin K deficiency during latter half of gestation resulting in bleeding [vitamin K and folic acid supplementation recommended] Infants may be at higher risk for hypoglycemia Total plasma valproate concentration decreased during pregnancy as a result of increased volume of distribution and clearance; plasma protein binding decreased	Crosses placenta Fetotoxicity reported in animal studies; risk to humans is currently unknown	Crosses placenta; levels comparable to those in maternal plasma; considered a potential maintenance therapy option for pregnant women with mood disorders (level B evidence)[1] Half-life increased in infant 3.2% risk of malformations in first trimester; risk noted to increase to 5.4% when total daily dose > 200 mg Increased risk of cleft lip and/or cleft palate when used in first trimester Decreases fetal folate levels [folic acid supplementation recommended] Lamotrigine metabolism appears to be induced during pregnancy and plasma levels increase rapidly after delivery	Fetotoxicity reported in animal studies. Risk to humans is currently unknown Case reports of hypospadias in male infants [folic acid supplementation recommended]

	Carbamazepine	Oxcarbazepine	Valproate	Gabapentin	Lamotrigine	Topiramate
Breast Milk	American Academy of Pediatrics considers carbamazepine compatible with breastfeeding Breast milk contains 7–95% of maternal drug concentration; infant serum level is 6–65% of mother's Educate mother about signs and symptoms of hepatic dysfunction and CNS effects of drug in the infant Monitor liver enzymes and CBC of infant and mother No long-term cognitive or behavioral effects reported in infant	Excreted into breast milk at levels up to 50% of those in maternal plasma Effects on infant unknown	American Academy of Pediatrics considers valproate compatible with breastfeeding Infant plasma level of valproate is up to 40% of that of mother; half-life in infants is significantly longer than in adults Educate mother about the signs and symptoms of hepatic dysfunction and those of hematological abnormalities in the infant Monitor liver enzymes and CBC of infant and mother No long-term cognitive or behavioral effects reported in infant	Amount of gabapentin in breast milk is approximately equivalent to that in maternal serum No long-term cognitive or behavioral effects reported in infant	Breastfeeding is not recommended Excreted in breast milk; the milk/plasma ratio is about 0.6 Infant serum levels are 25–30% of those of mother Consider risk of life-threatening rash in infant	Breastfeeding is not recommended due to possible psychomotor slowing and somnolence in infant

(m) moderate, (p)potent, (w)weak; P-gp = p-glycoprotein – a transporter of hydrophobic substances in or out of specific body organs (e.g., block absorption in the gut); UGT = uridine diphosphate glucuronosyl transferase – involved in Phase 2 reactions (conjugation)

 D/C Discontinuation Syndrome

- No evidence of psychological or physical dependence to anticonvulsants
- Myoclonic jerks have been reported following the tapering of carbamazepine or valproate
- Case of anhedonia, tremor, tachycardia, and hyperhydrosis reported following rapid discontinuation of lamotrigine
- Abrupt discontinuation (especially in patients with a seizure disorder) may provoke rebound seizures – taper
- Rare reports of psychiatric symptoms on withdrawal, including psychosis (exacerbation of schizophrenia)

⚠ Precautions

- Prior to treatment laboratory investigations should be performed (see p. 206)
- According to the FDA (February 2008), patients receiving antiepileptic drugs have a slightly increased risk of suicidal behavior or ideation (0.43%) compared to patients receiving placebo (0.22%). The increased risk was observed as early as one week and continued through 24 weeks. Patients who were treated for epilepsy, psychiatric disorders, and other conditions were all at increased risk for suicidality but the relative risk for suicidality was higher in the patients with epilepsy than in those with psychiatric or other conditions.

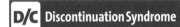
Carbamazepine

- Monitor patients starting drug treatment for behavioral changes that could indicate emergence or worsening of depression, or suicidal thoughts or behaviors
- Carbamazepine induces its own hepatic metabolism; therefore, weekly determinations of serum carbamazepine should be done for the first 2 months, monthly for 6 months, then at clinical discretion (at least every 6 months) or when there is a change in drug regimen
- Carbamazepine induces the metabolism of drugs metabolized by the cytochrome P-450 system (see Interactions pp. 208–210)
- Because of its anticholinergic action, give cautiously to patients with increased intraocular pressure or urinary retention
- Patients of Asian ancestry and with a positive test for HLA-B*1502 are at increased risk of serious skin reactions; they may require lower doses
- Tolerance to effects has been reported; efficacy not improved with dose increase
- Any cutaneous eruption, with fever, should be investigated for internal organ involvement. Check complete blood count (CBC) if patient reports fever, sore throat, petechiae, or bruising. Mild degree of blood cell suppression can occur; stop therapy if WBC levels drop below 3,000 white cells/mm^3; erythrocytes less than 4×10^6/mm^3; platelets less than 100,000/mm^3; hemoglobin less than 11 g/dl; reticulocyte count below 3%; or if serum iron rises above 150 mg/dl
- Patients who develop cutaneous reactions to carbamazepine should avoid the use of amitriptyline (as carbamazepine is a metabolite)
- Do not administer carbamazepine suspension together with any other liquid preparation as formation of an insoluble precipitate can occur

Anticonvulsants (cont.)

- Hypersensitivity syndrome with fever, skin eruptions and internal organ involvement occurs rarely – cross-sensitivity with other anticonvulsants suggested

Oxcarbazepine

- Monitor patients starting drug treatment for behavioral changes that could indicate emergence or worsening of depression, or suicidal thoughts or behaviors
- 25–30% of patients who exhibited hypersensitivity reactions to carbamazepine may also have these reactions with oxcarbazepine
- Monitor sodium levels with chronic use due to risk of hyponatremia
- Hypersensitivity syndrome with fever, skin eruptions and internal organ involvement occurs rarely – cross-sensitivity with other anticonvulsants suggested

Valproate

- Monitor patients starting drug treatment for behavioral changes that could indicate emergence or worsening of depression, or suicidal thoughts or behaviors
- Hepatic toxicity may show no relation to hepatic enzyme levels. Monitor liver function prior to therapy. In high-risk patients, monitor serum fibrinogen and albumin for decreases in concentration, and ammonia for increases secondary to decrease in carnitine levels. Stop drug if hepatic transaminase 2–3 times the upper limit of normal
- In patients with severe abdominal pain, lethargy, and weight loss, rule out pancreatitis – do serum amylase level
- Platelet counts and bleeding time determinations are recommended prior to therapy and at periodic intervals; withdraw if hemorrhage, bruising, or coagulation disorder is detected
- Diabetic patients on valproic acid may show false-positive ketone results
- Due to risk of polycystic ovary syndrome, consider monitoring for bioavailable androgens (free testosterone) as well as prolactin, LH, and TSH in females with menstrual irregularities, obesity, hirsutism, alopecia, and evidence of anovulation
- In patients with decreased or altered protein binding it may be more useful to monitor unbound (free) valproate concentrations rather than total concentrations
- Valproate will inhibit the metabolism of a number of drugs metabolized by cytochrome P-450 (see Drug Interactions pp. 211–212)

Gabapentin

- Monitor patients starting drug treatment for behavioral changes that could indicate emergence or worsening of depression, or suicidal thoughts or behaviors
- Dosing in renal dysfunction: if creatinine clearance (CrCl) 30–59 ml/min, give drug bid to a maximum daily dose of 1400 mg. If CrCl 15–29 ml/min, give drug once daily to a maximum dose of 700 mg/day. If CrCl is 15 ml/min, give drug to a maximum of 300 mg once daily; reduce dose proportionally with decreasing CrCl

Lamotrigine

- Monitor patients starting drug treatment for behavioral changes that could indicate emergence or worsening of depression, or suicidal thoughts or behaviors
- Severe, potentially life-threatening rashes have been reported – higher incidence in children, rapid dosage titration and in combination with valproate. Most occur within first 8 weeks of starting lamotrigine. Patient should be educated to immediately report to the physician any rash or systemic symptoms (fever, malaise, pharyngitis, flu-like symptoms), sores or blisters on soles, palms or mucus membranes. Do not rechallenge
- Use cautiously in patients with renal dysfunction as elimination half-life of lamotrigine is increased
- Due to potential of PR prolongation, lamotrigine should be used cautiously in patients with conduction abnormalities

Topiramate

- Monitor patients starting drug treatment for behavioral changes that could indicate emergence or worsening of depression, or suicidal thoughts or behaviors
- Risk of renal stone (Ca phosphate) formation in males on chronic therapy – ensure adequate fluid intake and avoid excessive antacid use and carbonic anhydrase inhibitors
- Acute myopia secondary to angle closure glaucoma reported; ophthalmological consult recommended for patients who complain of acute visual and/or painful/red eyes

- Decrease in sodium bicarbonate (up to 30% incidence); symptoms include fatigue, anorexia, hyperventilation, cardiac arrhythmia, and stupor. Chronic metabolic acidosis may increase risk for nephrolithiasis or nephrocalcinosis and may result in osteomalacia and/or osteoporosis with an increase in risk of fractures [reduce dose or taper and discontinue drug]
- Cognitive side effects are related to dose

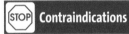 **Contraindications**

- Patients with a history of hepatic or cardiovascular disease or with a blood dyscrasia (gabapentin excluded)
- Hypersensitivity to any tricyclic compound (carbamazepine), and demonstrated hypersensitivity to any of the other agents
- Patients prescribed clozapine due to increased risk of agranulocytosis (carbamazepine)

 Toxicity

Carbamazepine

- Usually occurs with plasma levels above 50 mmol/l; children may be at risk for toxicity at lower serum concentrations due to increased production of toxic epoxide metabolite. Measurement of epoxide level may be beneficial in patients who develop clinical signs of carbamazepine toxicity at therapeutic concentrations of the parent drug
- The maximum plasma concentration may be delayed for up to 70 h after an overdose; onset of symptoms begin 1–3 h after ingestion of extended-release preparation
- Signs:
  - Dizziness, blood pressure changes, sinus tachycardia, ECG changes
  - Drowsiness, stupor, agitation, disorientation, EEG changes, seizures and coma
  - Nausea, vomiting, decreased intestinal motility, urinary retention
  - Tremor, involuntary movements, opisthotonos, abnormal reflexes, myoclonus, ataxia
  - Mydriasis, nystagmus
  - Flushing, respiratory depression, cyanosis
- No known antidote, treat symptomatically

Oxcarbazepine

- No deaths reported following overdose of up to 24,000 mg; no known antidote – treat symptomatically

Valproate

- Maximum plasma concentration may not occur for up to 18 h following an overdose, and serum half-life may be prolonged
- Onset of CNS depression may be rapid (within 3 h); enteric-coated preparations may delay onset of symptoms
- Signs/symptoms: severe dizziness, hypotension, supraventricular tachycardia, bradycardia; severe drowsiness; trembling; irregular, slow or shallow breathing, apnea, and coma; loss of tendon reflexes, generalized myoclonus, seizures; cerebral edema – evident 2 to 3 days after overdose and may last up to 15 days; hematological changes, electrolyte, and metabolic abnormalities; optic nerve damage reported
- Overdose can result in coma and death; naloxone may reverse the CNS depressant effects, and may also reverse anti-epileptic effects
- Supportive treatment [L-carnitine supplementation (50–100 mg/kg/day to a max of 2 g/day) recommended for patients with CNS depression, evidence of hepatic dysfunction, and hyperammonemia]

Gabapentin

- Signs and symptoms: double vision, slurred speech, drowsiness, lethargy and diarrhea – all patients recovered
- Gabapentin can be removed by hemodialysis

Lamotrigine

- Overdose can result in ataxia, nystagmus, delirium, seizures, intraventricular conduction delay, and coma
- No known antidote – treat symptomatically

Topiramate

- Emesis and gastric lavage recommended; topiramate can be removed by hemodialysis
- Treat symptomatically

Anticonvulsants (cont.)

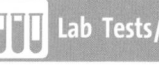 **Lab Tests/Monitoring**

	Carbamazepine	Oxcarbazepine	Valproate	Gabapentin	Lamotrigine	Topiramate
Work-up	1) CBC including platelets and differential 2) Serum electrolytes 3) Liver function 4) ECG (in patients over age 45 or with a cardiac history) 5) Bone density	Serum electrolytes	1) CBC including platelets and differential 2) Liver function 3) Total and HDL cholesterol and triglycerides 4) In females: body weight/BMI 5) Consider serum testosterone level in young females 6) Bone density	BUN and serum creatinine	None required	Baseline serum bicarbonate BUN and serum creatinine
Follow-up	Repeat CBC after the first month, then 2–3 times a year Serum electrolytes every 6 months	Sodium levels periodically and when patient has symptoms of hyponatremia	Repeat test #1 and #2 monthly for 2 months, then 2–3 times a year Test #3 and #4 annually Test #5 if symptoms of hyperandrogenism or menstrual irregularities occur; also test prolactin, LH, and TSH as well as for insulin resistance syndrome and hypertension Ammonia level in event of lethargy, mental status changes	LH and TSH Renal function if suspect toxicity	None required	Periodic serum bicarbonate (to rule out metabolic acidosis) Renal function if suspect toxicity
Plasma level monitoring	Measure drug level 5 days after start of therapy and 5 days after change in dose or addition/deletion of any other drug (see Drug Interactions pp. 208–210)	None required	Measure drug level 5 days after start of therapy and 5 days after change in dose or addition/deletion of any other drug (see Drug Interactions pp. 211–212 and Precautions p. 204)	None required	None required	None required

Pediatric Considerations

- For detailed information on the use of anticonvulsants in this population, please see the *Clinical Handbook of Psychotropic Drugs for Children and Adolescents* (2007)

Carbamazepine
- Used in episodic dyscontrol and assaultive behavior disorder
- Children may be at risk for major toxicities at lower serum concentrations due to increased production of toxic metabolite; case reports of behavior disturbances, mania and worsening of tics
- Common side effects include: unsteadiness, dizziness, diplopia, drowsiness, nausea and vomiting

Oxcarbazepine
- Used in children and adolescents as sole or add-on therapy for partial seizures

Valproate
- Efficacy reported in treatment of bipolar disorder, acute mania, migraine prophylaxis as well as temper/aggressive outbursts in adolescents and young adults
- Children under age 2 with other medical conditions are at risk of developing fatal hepatotoxicity
- Children ages 3–10 taking other anticonvulsants are at high risk for developing fatal hepatotoxicity

- Use in female children and adolescents may result in increased risk of hyperandrogenism and polycystic ovarian syndrome, delayed or prolonged puberty; excessive weight gain, hyperinsulinemia and dyslipidemia; decreased bone mineral density reported (in up to 14%) – may conduce to osteoporosis

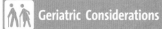

Gabapentin

- Used to reduce anxiety and agitation in children with BD and schizoaffective disorder and to treat neuropathic pain
- Incidence of side effects in children reported to be similar to that in adults. Case reports of behavioral problems including hyperactivity, aggression, irritability

Lamotrigine

- Has been used in adolescents as add-on therapy in refractory bipolar depression. Common side effects included headache, tremor, somnolence, and dizziness
- Risk of severe, life-threatening rash increased in children

Topiramate

- Used as add-on therapy in seizure disorders and prophylaxis of migraine headaches
- Side effects include sedation, cognitive and behavioral problems, and weight loss

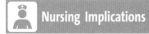

Geriatric Considerations

- Dosing should be instituted more gradually in the elderly and those with liver impairment
- May cause confusion, cognitive impairment, ataxia (may lead to falls)
- Early data suggest efficacy in treating behavior disturbances in dementia
- Caution when combining with other drugs with CNS or anticholinergic properties; additive effects can result in confusion, disorientation, delirium
- Due to reduced protein binding and hepatic oxidation, elderly may have a higher proportion of unbound (free) valproate and a reduced clearance, resulting in elevated levels of unbound valproate (within therapeutic plasma levels of total drug); case report of acute parkinsonism with valproate, in an elderly patient with dementia
- Continuous anticonvulsant use in elderly women is associated with increased rates of bone loss at the calcaneus and hip. It is sufficient to increase the risk of hip fracture by 29% over 5 years among women aged 65 years and older
- May have an increased risk for thrombocytopenia with valproate
- Elderly with pre-existing cardiac disease should have a thorough cardiac evaluation prior to carbamazepine use
- Higher risk of hyponatremia with carbamazepine and oxcarbazepine
- Reduce dose of gabapentin if creatinine clearance < 60 ml/min and of oxcarbazepine if creatinine clearance < 30 ml/min
- Plasma level of lamotrigine increased in elderly patients

Nursing Implications

- Monitor patients starting drug treatment for behavioral changes that could indicate emergence or worsening of depression, or suicidal thoughts or behaviors
- Watch out for signs of fever, sore throat, and bruising or bleeding
- Close clinical and laboratory supervision should be maintained (see Adverse Effects pp. 197–201 and Monitoring p. 183) throughout treatment to detect signs of possible blood dyscrasia or liver involvement
- A rash, especially with carbamazepine or lamotrigine, may signal incipient blood dyscrasia; advise the physician
- Anorexia, nausea, vomiting, edema, malaise and lethargy may signify hepatic toxicity
- Since drowsiness can occur, patients should exercise caution when performing tasks that require alertness; will enhance the effects of alcohol and other CNS drugs
- Check for urinary retention and constipation with carbamazepine; increase fluids to lessen constipation
- Liquid carbamazepine should not be mixed or taken at the same time as any other liquid medication
- Liquid valproate should not be administered with carbonated beverages as mouth irritation can occur
- Patients on topiramate should drink plenty of fluids and avoid the regular use of antacids (e.g., Tums, Maalox, Rolaids, etc.) to reduce risk of renal stone formation
- Enteric-coated or controlled-release tablets should not be broken or crushed but should be swallowed whole; chewing capsules can cause local irritation in the mouth and throat; extended-release capsules can be opened and sprinkled on food
- Grapefruit juice should be avoided as it can elevate the blood level of carbamazepine

Anticonvulsants (cont.)

- In females (particularly on valproate) obtain baseline body weight/BMI, and measure periodically, monitor for menstrual disturbances, hirsutism, obesity, alopecia and infertility – two or more of these symptoms may be associated with polycystic ovaries
- Patients on topiramate should report eye pain or continued visual disturbances to the physician
- To treat occasional pain avoid the use of acetylsalicylic acid (ASA or aspirin) as it can affect the blood level of valproate – acetaminophen or ibuprofen (and related drugs) are safer alternatives
- Monitor patient's height, weight, and body mass index
- In the elderly, monitor for ataxia, confusion and cognitive impairment
- Advise patient to store medication away from heat and humidity as the drug may lose potency

 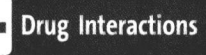 **Patient Instructions**
- For detailed patient instructions on Anticonvulsant Mood Stabilizers, see the Patient Information Sheet on p. 349

Drug Interactions
- Clinically significant interactions are listed below

DRUGS INTERACTING WITH CARBAMAZEPINE

Class of Drug	Example	Interaction Effects
Acetazolamide		Increased plasma level of carbamazepine due to inhibited metabolism
Anesthetic	Halothane	Enzyme induction may result in hepatocellular damage
	Methoxyflurane, isoflurane, sevoflurane	Enzyme induction may result in renal damage
Antibiotic	Erythromycin, troleandomycin, clarithromycin	Increased plasma levels of carbamazepine due to reduced clearance (by 5–41%)
	Doxycycline (no interaction with other tetracyclines)	Decreased serum level and half-life of doxycycline due to enhanced metabolism (Alternatively, tetracycline can be used or doxycycline can be dosed q 12 h)
	Quinupristin/dalfopristin	Increased plasma level of carbamazepine due to inhibited metabolism via CYP3A4
Anticoagulant	Warfarin	Enhanced metabolism of anticoagulant and impaired hypoprothombinemic response; decreased PT ratio or INR response
Anticonvulsant	Felbamate	Decreased carbamazepine level by 50%, but increased level of epoxide metabolite Decreased felbamate level
	Phenytoin, primidone, phenobarbital	Decreased carbamazepine level due to increased metabolism via CYP3A4, but ratio of epoxide metabolite increased Altered plasma level of co-prescribed anticonvulsant
	Clonazepam, clobazam, ethosuximide, topiramate, tiagabine, zonisamide, oxcarbazepine	Clearance of the anticonvulsants is increased by carbamazepine, with possible decrease in efficacy (40% decrease in concentration of topiramate and of oxcarbazepine metabolite)
	Valproate, valproic acid	Increased plasma level of epoxide metabolite of carbamazepine; may result in toxicity even at therapeutic carbamazepine concentrations Decreased valproate level due to increased clearance and displacement from protein binding Effects on carbamazepine levels are variable and inconsistent
	Lamotrigine	Increased plasma level of epoxide metabolite of carbamazepine by 10–45% with resultant increased side effects Increased metabolism of lamotrigine; half-life and plasma level decreased by 30–50%
	Topiramate	Increased plasma level of carbamazepine by 20%

Class of Drug	Example	Interaction Effects
Antidepressant		
SSRI	Fluoxetine, fluvoxamine	Increased plasma level of carbamazepine and its active metabolite with fluoxetine; increased nausea with fluvoxamine
	Sertraline, citalopram	Decreased plasma level of sertraline or citalopram due to enzyme induction via CYP3A4 (case report)
Cyclic (non-selective)	Imipramine, doxepin, amitriptyline, nortriptyline	Decreased plasma level of antidepressant by up to 46% due to enzyme induction
SARI	Trazodone	Decreased plasma level of trazodone
		Increased plasma level of carbamazepine with nefazodone due to decreased metabolism via CYP3A4
MAOI	Phenelzine	Possible decrease in metabolism and increased plasma level of carbamazepine
Antifungal	Ketoconazole, fluconazole	Increased plasma level of carbamazepine with ketoconazole (by 29%) due to inhibited metabolism via CYP3A4; clearance decreased by 50% with fluconazole
	Fluconazole, itraconazole, ketoconazole	Decreased plasma levels of antifungals
Antipsychotic	Phenothiazines, haloperidol, risperidone, thiothixene, olanzapine, zuclopenthixol, flupenthixol, ziprasidone	Decreased plasma level of antipsychotic (up to 100% with haloperidol, 44% with olanzapine)
		Increased akathisia
		Increased neurotoxicity of both antipsychotic and carbamazepine at therapeutic doses
	Clozapine	Avoid combination due to possible potentiation of bone marrow suppression
		Decreased plasma level of clozapine by up to 63%
	Loxapine, haloperidol	Increased plasma level of carbamazepine and metabolite
	Chlorpromazine liquid, thioridazine liquid	Precipitation of a "rubbery mass" when carbamazepine suspension is combined with neuroleptic liquid preparations
Antitubercular drug	Isoniazid	Increased plasma level of carbamazepine; clearance reduced by up to 45%
	Rifampin	Decreased plasma level of carbamazepine
Benzodiazepine	Alprazolam, clonazepam	Decreased plasma level of alprazolam (> 50%) and clonazepam (19–37%) due to enzyme induction
β-Blocker	Propranolol	Decreased plasma level of β-blocker due to enzyme induction
Calcium-channel blocker	Diltiazem, verapamil (no interaction with nifedipine)	Increased plasma levels of carbamazepine due to decreased metabolism (total carbamazepine increased 46%, free carbamazepine increased 33%)
Cimetidine		Transient increase in carbamazepine levels and possible toxicity due to inhibited metabolism (no interaction with ranitidine, famotidine and nizatidine)
Corticosteroids		Decreased plasma level of corticosteroid due to enzyme induction
Danazol		Plasma levels of carbamazepine increased by 50–100%; half-life is doubled and clearance reduced by half
Desmopressin (DDAVP)		Concurrent use may increase antidiuretic effect, resulting in decreased sodium concentration with resultant seizures
Diclofenac		Increased plasma level of carbamazepine due to decreased metabolism
Disopyramide		Increased metabolism and decreased plasma level of disopyramide
Etretinate		Therapeutic failure with etretinate due to decreased plasma level
Folic acid		Decreased plasma level of folic acid
Grapefruit juice		Decreased metabolism of carbamazepine resulting in increased plasma level by up to 40%
Hormone	Oral contraceptive	Increased metabolism of oral contraceptive and increased binding of progestin and ethinyl estradiol to sex hormone binding globulin, may result in decreased contraceptive efficacy

Anticonvulsants (cont.)

Class of Drug	Example	Interaction Effects
Immunosuppressant	Cyclosporin	Decreased plasma level and efficacy of cyclosporin due to enzyme induction via CYP3A4
Influenza vaccine		Decreased elimination and increased half-life of carbamazepine
Isotretinoin		Decreased plasma level of carbamazepine and its metabolite
Lithium		Increased neurotoxicity of both drugs; sinus node dysfunction reported with combination Synergistic mood-stabilizing effect; may potentiate antidepressant or antimanic effect
Modafinil		Decreased plasma level of modafinil due to enhanced metabolism
Metronidazole		Increased plasma level of carbamazepine due to inhibited metabolism
Muscle relaxant (non-depolarizing)	Gallamine, pancuronium	Decreased duration of action and efficacy of muscle relaxant
Narcotic	Methadone	Decreased effect of methadone (up to 60%) due to enhanced metabolism
Propoxyphene		Increased plasma level of carbamazepine due to reduced metabolism
Protease inhibitor	Ritonavir, saquinavir, indinavir, nelfinavir	Increased metabolism and decreased plasma level of ritonavir and saquinavir with possible loss of efficacy Increased plasma level of carbamazepine due to inhibited metabolism via CYP3A4, potentially resulting in toxicity
Proton pump inhibitor	Omeprazole	Increased carbamazepine levels
Quinine		Increased plasma level of carbamazepine (by 37%) and AUC (by 51%) due to inhibited metabolism
Stimulant	Methylphenidate	Decreased plasma level of methylphenidate and its metabolite
Theophylline		Decreased theophylline level due to enzyme induction by carbamazepine; decreased carbamazepine level by up to 50%
Thyroid hormone		Decreased plasma level of thyroid hormone due to enzyme induction

DRUGS INTERACTING WITH OXCARBAZEPINE

Class of Drug	Example	Interaction Effects
Anticonvulsant	Carbamazepine, phenytoin, phenobarbital	Decreased plasma levels of oxcarbazepine MHD metabolite by 40%
	Valproate	Increased level of phenytoin (by 40%) and phenobarbital (by 14%) due to inhibited metabolism via CYP2C19
CNS depressant	Alcohol, hypnotics, narcotics	Increased sedation, disorientation
Diuretic	Furosemide	Increased risk of hyponatremia with oxcarbazepine
Hormone	Oral contraceptives	Increased metabolism of ethinyl estradiol through induction of CYP3A4
Verapamil		Reduced oxcarbazepine MHD metabolite plasma level by about 20% – mechanism unknown

Class of Drug	Example	Interaction Effects
Antibiotic	Erythromycin	Increased valproate plasma level due to decreased metabolism
Anticoagulant	Warfarin	Inhibition of secondary phase of platelet aggregation by valproate, thus affecting coagulation; increased PT ratio or INR response Displacement of protein binding of warfarin (free fraction increased by 33%)
Anticonvulsant	Phenobarbital, primidone	Increased level of anticonvulsant (by 30–50%) due to decreased metabolism caused by valproate
	Carbamazepine	Decreased valproate levels due to increased clearance and displacement for protein binding Effects on carbamazepine levels are variable and inconsistent Synergistic mood-stabilizing effect in treatment-resistant patients
	Phenytoin, mephenytoin	Enhanced anticonvulsant effect due to displacement from protein binding (free fraction increased by 60%) and inhibited clearance (by 25%); toxicity can occur at therapeutic levels Possible decrease in valproate level
	Felbamate	Increased plasma level of valproate (by 31–51%) due to decreased metabolism
	Lamotrigine	Increased lamotrigine plasma level (by up to 200%), half-life (by up to 50%) and decreased clearance (by up to 60%) Both decreases and increases in plasma level of valproate reported. This combination may be dangerous due to high incidence of Stevens-Johnson syndrome and toxic epidermal necrolysis
	Ethosuximide	Increased half-life of ethosuximide (by 25%)
	Topiramate	Case reports of delirium and elevated ammonia levels
Antidepressant Tricyclic SSRI	Amitriptyline, nortriptyline Fluoxetine	Increased plasma level and adverse effects of antidepressant Increased plasma level of valproate (up to 50%)
Antipsychotic	Phenothiazines	Increased neurotoxicity, sedation, and extrapyramidal side effects due to decreased clearance of valproate (by 14%)
	Clozapine	Both increased and decreased clozapine levels reported; changes in clozapine/norclozapine ratio Case report of hepatic encephalopathy
	Haloperidol	Increased plasma level of haloperidol by an average of 32%
	Olanzapine	Combination associated with high incidence of weight gain
Antitubercular drug	Isoniazid	Increased plasma level of valproate due to inhibited metabolism
	Rifampin	Increased clearance of valproate (by 40%)
Antiviral agent	Zidovudine	Increased level of zidovudine (by 38%) due to decreased clearance
	Acyclovir	Decreased level of valproate
Anxiolytic	Clonazepam, chlordiazepoxide, lorazepam	Decreased metabolism and increased pharmacological effects of benzodiazepines resulting in increased sedation, disorientation (lorazepam clearance reduced by 41%)
	Clonazepam	Concomitant use may induce absence status in patients with a history of absence type seizures
	Diazepam	Increased plasma level of diazepam due to displacement from protein binding (free fraction increased by 90%)
Cimetidine		Decreased metabolism and increased half-life of valproate
CNS depressant	Alcohol, hypnotics	Increased sedation, disorientation Valproate displaces alcohol from protein binding and potentiates intoxicating effect
Hypnotic	Zolpidem	Case of somnambulism with combination
Lithium		Synergistic mood-stabilizing effect in treatment-resistant patients Valproate may aggravate action tremor

Anticonvulsants (cont.)

DRUGS INTERACTING WITH VALPROATE (cont.)

Class of Drug	Example	Interaction Effects
Salicylate	Acetylsalicylic acid, bismuth subsalicylate	Displacement of valproate from protein binding and decreased clearance, leading to increased level of free drug (4-fold), with possible toxicity
Sulfonylurea	Tolbutamide	Increase in free fraction of tolbutamide from 20 to 50% due to displacement from protein binding
Thiopental		Displacement of thiopental from protein binding resulting in an increased hypnotic/anesthetic effect

DRUGS INTERACTING WITH GABAPENTIN

Class of Drug	Example	Interaction Effects
Antacid	Al/Mg containing antacids	Co-administration reduces gabapentin bioavailability by up to 24%
CNS depressant	Alcohol, hypnotics	Increased sedation, disorientation
Narcotic	Hydrocodone Morphine	Decreased effectiveness of hydrocodone reported Enhanced analgesic effects

DRUGS INTERACTING WITH LAMOTRIGINE

Class of Drug	Example	Interaction Effects
Anticonvulsant	Carbamazepine, phenytoin, phenobarbital, primidone Valproate Topiramate	Plasma level and half-life of lamotrigine decreased due to increased metabolism (clearance increased 30–50% with carbamazepine; by 125% with phenytoin) Increased plasma level of epoxide metabolite of carbamazepine by 10–45% with resultant increased side effects Increased plasma level of lamotrigine (by up to 200%), half-life (by up to 50%) and decreased clearance (by up to 60%); both decreases and increases in valproate levels reported Increased risk of life-threatening rash with combination (Stevens-Johnson syndrome and toxic epidermal necrolysis) Decreased plasma level of lamotrigine
Antidepressant	Sertraline Fluoxetine	Increased plasma level of lamotrigine (data contradictory) Decreased plasma level of lamotrigine (mechanism unclear)
Antipsychotic	Olanzapine	AUC of lamotrigine decreased by 24%
Antitubercular	Rifampin	Decreased lamotrigine levels and half-life
CNS depressant	Alcohol, hypnotics	Increased sedation, disorientation
Hormones	Oral contraceptive	Decreased plasma level of lamotrigine by 27–64% Reports of breakthrough bleeding and unexpected pregnancies
Lithium		Decreased plasma level of lamotrigine
Protease inhibitor	Lopinavir/ritonavir	Decreased plasma level of lamotrigine by 50% due to increased metabolism

DRUGS INTERACTING WITH TOPIRAMATE

Class of Drug	Example	Interaction Effects
Antacid		Excessive use may increase renal stone (calcium phosphate) formation
Anticonvulsant	Carbamazepine, oxcarbazepine, phenytoin, phenobarbital, primidone Lamotrigine Valproate	Decreased plasma levels of topiramate reported; by 40% with carbamazepine and 48% with phenytoin Increased plasma level of carbamazepine (by 20%) and of phenytoin Decreased plasma level of lamotrigine Case reports of delirium and elevated ammonia levels
Carbonic anhydrase inhibitor	Acetazolamide, zonisamide	Excessive use may increase renal stone (calcium phosphate) formation
CNS depressant	Alcohol, hypnotics, narcotics	Increased sedation, disorientation
Digoxin		Decreased levels of digoxin by 12%
Hormone	Oral contraceptive	Possibly decreased metabolism of oral contraceptive

Comparison of Adverse Reactions to Mood Stabilizers at Therapeutic Doses

Reaction	Lithium	Carbamazepine	Oxcarbazepine	Valproate	Gabapentin	Lamotrigine	Topiramate
CNS							
Drowsiness, sedation	< 2%[f]	>10%	>10%	>10%	>10%	>10%	>10%[d]
Headache	> 2%	> 2%	>30%	>10%	> 2%	>10%	>10%
Cognitive blunting, memory impairment	>10%	> 2%	> 2%	> 2%	< 2%	> 2%	> 2%[d]
Weakness, fatigue	>30%[f]	>10%	>10%	>10%	>10%	> 2%	>10%
Insomnia, agitation	< 2%	< 2%	> 2%	> 2%	> 2%	> 2%	>10%
Neurological							
Incoordination	< 2%[f]	>10%	> 2%	> 2%	< 2%	> 2%	> 2%
Dizziness	–	>10%	> 2%	>10%	>10%	>30%	>10%[d]
Ataxia	< 2%[f]	>10%	> 2%	> 2%	>10%	>10%	> 2%[d]
Tremor	>30%[f]	>30%	>10%	>10%	> 2%	> 2%	> 2%
Paresthesias	–	> 2%	> 2%	> 2%	< 2%	< 2%	>10%
Diplopia	–	>10%	>10%	>10%	> 2%	>10%	> 2%
Anticholinergic							
Blurred vision	> 2%[f]	> 2%	> 2	> 2%	< 2%	>10%	> 2%
Cardiovascular							
ECG changes[a]	>10%	> 2%	< 2	> 2%	–	< 2%	–
Gastrointestinal							
Nausea, vomiting	>30%	>10%	>10%	>10%	> 2%	>10%	> 2%
Diarrhea	>10%[f]	> 2%	> 2%	>10%	–	> 2%	> 2%
Weight gain	>30%	> 2%	> 2%	>30%	>10%[d]	< 2%	–
Weight loss	< 2%	< 2%	< 2%	> 2%	< 2%	> 2%	>10%[d]
Endocrine							
Hair loss, thinning	>10%	> 2%	< 2%	>10%	–	–	< 2%
Menstrual disturbances	>10%	>30%	< 2%	>30%	–	> 2%	–
Polycystic ovary syndrome	–	>10%	?	>30%	–	–	–
Hypothyroidism	>30%	< 2%	?	< 2%	–	< 1%	–
Polyuria, polydipsia	>30%	> 2%	< 2%	–	–	–	–
Skin reactions, Rash	>10%[c]	>10%[e]	> 2%	> 2%	< 2%	>10%[e]	< 2%
Sexual dysfunction	> 2%	< 2%	–	> 2%	< 2%	–	–
Blood dyscrasias							
Transient leukopenia	< 2%	>10%	< 2%	< 2%	< 2%	< 2%	< 2%
Leukocytosis	>10%	< 2%	< 2%	< 2%	–	–	–
Thrombocytopenia	–	> 2%	–	>30%[d]	–	< 2%	–
Hepatic							
Transient enzyme elevation[b]	–	>10%	< 2%	>30%[d]	< 2%	< 2%	–

[a] ECG abnormalities usually without cardiac injury, including ST segment depression, flattened T waves, and increased U wave amplitude; [b] Evaluate for hepatotoxicity if elevation >3 times normal; [c] Worsening of psoriasis reported; [d] Greater with higher doses; [e] May be first sign of impending blood dyscrasia; [f] Higher incidence and more pronounced symptoms with higher serum lithium concentration; may indicate early toxicity – monitor level

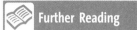**Further Reading**

Reference

[1] ACOG Committee on Practice Bulletins – Obstetrics. ACOG Practice Bulletin: Clinical management guidelines for obstetrician-gynecologists number 92, April 2008 (replaces practice bulletin number 87, November 2007). Use of psychiatric medications during pregnancy and lactation. *Obstet Gynecol* 2008;111(4):1001–1020.

Additional Suggested Reading

- Arnone D. Review of the use of topiramate for treatment of psychiatric disorders. Ann Gen Psychiatry. 2005;4(1):5.
- Aziz R, Lorberg B, Tampi RR. Treatments for late-life bipolar disorder. Am J Geriatr Pharmacother. 2006;4(4):347–364.
- Benazzi F. Bipolar II disorder: Epidemiology, diagnosis and management. CNS Drugs. 2007;21(9):727–740.
- Cohen LS. Treatment of bipolar disorder during pregnancy. J Clin Psychiatry. 2007;68(Suppl 9):4–9.
- Ensrud KE, Walczak, TS. Blackwell T et al. Antiepileptic drug use increases rates of bone loss in older women: A prospective study. Neurology. 2004;62(11):E24–25.
- Ernst CL, Goldberg JF. The reproductive safety profile of mood stabilizers, atypical antipsychotic, and broad-spectrum psychotropics. J Clin Psychiatry. 2002;63(Suppl. 4):42–55.
- Fountoulakis KN, Vieta E. Treatment of bipolar disorder: a systematic review of available data and clinical perspectives. Int J Neuropsychopharmacol. 2008;11(7):999–1029.
- Goodwin FK, Fireman B, Simon GE, et al. Suicide risk in bipolar disorder during treatment with lithium and divalproex. JAMA. 2003;290(11):1467–1473.
- Grunze H. Reevaluating therapies for bipolar depression. J Clin Psychiatry. 2005;66(Suppl 5):17–25.
- Hahn C-G, Gyulai L, Baldassano CF, et al. The current understanding of lamotrigine as a mood stabilizer. J Clin Psychiatry. 2004;65(6):791–804.
- Hebert AA, Ralston JP. Cutaneous reactions to anticonvulsant medications. J Clin Psychiatry. 2001;62 Suppl 14:S22–S26.
- Hirschfeld RMA. Guideline watch: Practice guideline for the treatment of patients with bipolar disorder. Arlington, VA: American Psychiatric Association. Available from http://www.psychiatryonline.com/pracGuide/loadGuidelinePdf.aspx?file=Bipolar.watch (Accessed March 16, 2009).
- Keck PE, McElroy SL. Clinical pharmacodynamics and pharmacokinetics of antimanic and mood-stabilizing medications. J Clin Psychiatry. 2002;63 Suppl 4:S3–S11.
- Ketter TA, Wang PW. Predictors of treatment response in bipolar disorders: Evidence from clinical and brain imaging studies. J Clin Psychiatry. 2002;63 Suppl 3:S21–S25.
- Lepkifker E, Sverdlik A, Iancu I, et al. Renal insufficiency in long-term lithium treatment. J Clin Psychiatry. 2004;65(6):850–856.
- Leucht S, Kissling W, McGrath J. Lithium for schizophrenia revisted: A systematic review and meta-analysis of randomized controlled trials. J Clin Psychiatry. 2004;65(2):177–186.
- McIntyre RS, Konarski JZ. Tolerability profiles of atypical antipsychotics in the treatment of bipolar disorder. J Clin Psychiatry. 2005;66 Suppl 3:S28–S36.
- Perlis RH. The role of pharmacologic treatment guidelines for bipolar disorder. J Clin Psychiatry. 2005;66 Suppl 3:S37–S47.
- Sachs GS. Decision tree for the treatment of bipolar disorder. J Clin Psychiatry. 2003;64 Suppl 8:S35–S40.
- Scottish Intercollegiate Guidelines Network (SIGN). Bipolar affective disorder: A national clinical guideline [Guideline 82]. Edinburgh, UK: SIGN, May 2005. Available from http://www.sign.ac.uk/pdf/sign82.pdf (accessed March 16, 2009). Summary available from http://www.guideline.gov/summary/pdf.aspx?doc_id=7285&stat=1&string=%22electroconvulsive+therapy%22 (accessed March 16, 2009).
- Stahl SM. Psychopharmacology of anticonvulsants: Do all anticonvulsants have the same mechanism of action? J Clin Psychiatry. 2004;65(2):149–150.
- Stowe ZN. The use of mood stabilizers during breastfeeding. J Clin Psychiatry. 2007;68 (Suppl 9):22–28.
- Suppes T, Dennehy EB, Hirschfeld RMA, et al. The Texas implementation of medication algorithms. Update to the algorithms for treatment of Bipolar I Disorder. J Clin Psychiatry. 2005;66(7):870–886.
- Suppes T, Dennehy EB, Swann AC, et al. Report of the Texas Consensus Conference Panel on medication treatment of bipolar disorder 2000. J Clin Psychiatry. 2005;63(4):288–299.
- Yatham LN, Kennedy SH, O'Donovan C, et al. Canadian Network for Mood and Anxiety Treatments (CANMAT) guidelines for the management of patients with bipolar disorder: Update 2007. Bipolar Disord. 2006;8(6):721–739.
- Yatham LN. Newer anticonvulsants in the treatment of bipolar disorder. J Clin Psychiatry. 2004;65(10):28–35.

DRUGS FOR ADHD

Classification

- Drugs for ADHD can be classified as follows:

Chemical Class	Agent[A]	Page
Psychostimulant	🔥 Amphetamine and related drugs (e.g., lisdexamfetamine[B]) 🔥 Methylphenidate, dexmethylphenidate	See p. 216
Selective norepinephrine reuptake inhibitor	🔥 Atomoxetine	See p. 224
Adrenergic agent	Clonidine Guanfacine[B]	See p. 230 See p. 297
Antidepressant	Bupropion Venlafaxine Tricyclic agents	See p. 16 See p. 21 See p. 37
Dopaminergic agent	Modafinil	See p. 299

🔥 Approved indication, [A] Generic preparations may be available, [B] Not available in Canada, [C] Not available in USA

Psychostimulants

Product Availability

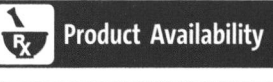

Generic Name	Trade Name[A]	Dosage Forms and Strengths
Dextroamphetamine	Dexedrine, Dextrostat	Tablets: 5 mg, 10 mg[B] Elixir: 5 mg/5 ml
	Dexedrine extended-release	Spansules: 5 mg[B], 10 mg, 15 mg
Lisdexamfetamine[B]	Vyvanse	Capsules: 30 mg, 50 mg, 70 mg
Methamphetamine[B] (desoxyephedrine)	Desoxyn	Tablets: 5 mg
Dextroamphetamine/Amphetamine salts	Adderall[B]	Tablets[B]: 5 mg, 7.5 mg, 10 mg, 12.5 mg, 15 mg, 20 mg, 30 mg
	Adderall XR	Capsules: 5 mg, 10 mg, 15 mg, 20 mg, 25 mg, 30 mg
Methylphenidate	Ritalin Methylin[B]	Tablets: 5 mg, 10 mg, 20 mg Chewable tablets[B]: 2.5mg, 5mg, 10mg Oral solution[B]: 5mg/5ml, 10mg/5ml
	Ritalin SR, Metadate ER[B], Methylin ER[B] Metadate CD[B] Ritalin LA[B] Concerta Biphentin[C]	Sustained-release tablets: 10 mg[B], 20 mg Extended-release capsules[B]: 10 mg, 20 mg, 30 mg, 40 mg, 50 mg, 60 mg Extended-release capsules[B]: 10 mg, 20 mg, 30 mg, 40 mg Osmotic-controlled-release tablets: 18 mg, 27 mg, 36 mg, 54 mg Controlled-release[C]: 10 mg, 15 mg, 20 mg, 30 mg, 40 mg, 50 mg, 60 mg, 80 mg

Generic Name	Trade Name[A]	Dosage Forms and Strengths
Methylphenidate transdermal patch[B]	Daytrana	Transdermal patch: 27.5 mg, 41.3 mg, 55 mg, 82.5 mg
Dexmethylphenidate[B]	Focalin	Tablets: 2.5 mg, 5 mg, 10 mg
	Focalin XR	Extended-release capsules 5mg, 10mg, 20mg

[A] Generic preparations may be available, [B] Not marketed in Canada, [C] Not marketed in USA

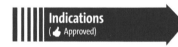

Indications
(👍 Approved)

- 👍 Attention-deficit/hyperactivity disorder (ADHD)
- 👍 Parkinson's disease
- 👍 Narcolepsy
- 👍 Obesity (dextroamphetamine – USA only)
- Treatment-resistant depression
- Major depression in medically or surgically ill patients, or in elderly
- Augmentation of cyclic antidepressants, SSRIs, and RIMA
- Attention-deficit/hyperactivity disorder – in partial remission (ADHD-PR) in adults
- Chronic fatigue syndrome, neurasthenia
- Negative symptoms of schizophrenia; some improvement noted in cognitive deficits, mood, and concentration with low doses of dextroamphetamine
- Improves fatigue and cognition in AIDS-related neuropsychiatric impairment
- Positive results with methylphenidate in decreasing anger, irritability and aggression in brain-injured patients, oppositional defiant disorder, conduct disorder, and ADHD
- Controlled studies suggest methylphenidate has modest efficacy in the treatment of inattention and hyperactivity in autism and mental retardation – adverse effects may be more problematic in this population

General Comments

- All psychostimulants have been found to be equally effective at reducing symptoms of inattention, hyperactivity and impulsivity
- General response occurs within the first week; response seen in approximately 75% of children and 25–78% of adults with ADHD (although individuals may respond better to selective drugs)
- An untreated psychiatric disorder (mood or anxiety disorder) may diminish response to stimulants or may decrease the ability to tolerate the medication
- Psychostimulants suggested to suppress physical and verbal aggression and reduce negative or antisocial interactions
- See Precautions (p. 220) and Contraindications (p. 221) regarding patient risks
- Use with caution and careful monitoring in patients with current abuse of drugs or alcohol due to risk for diversion or abuse
  Stimulant therapy can reduce the risk for substance use disorder in adolescents with ADHD
- Lisdexamfetamine is a prodrug in which d-amphetamine is bonded to l-lysine. It can only be taken orally and therefore has less potential for abuse and diversion than short-acting stimulants

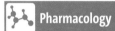

Pharmacology

- Mechanism of action in treating ADHD is not well understood; methylphenidate (MPH) promotes release of stored dopamine from presynaptic vesicles and blocks the return of norepinephrine and dopamine (in a dose-dependant fashion) into presynaptic nerve endings. Amphetamines also block NE and DA reuptake, but appear to promote the release of newly synthesized dopamine more selectively. The combined action of promoting release and blocking reuptake results in a net increase in extracellular dopamine in basal ganglia, cortex, and other brain regions to a lesser extent. Increases in DA are suggested to improve attention, decrease distractibility, and modulate motivation, thus improving performance
- Release of dopamine and norepinephrine in subcortical limbic areas (e.g., nucleus accumbens) may be the mechanism responsible for the abuse potential of these drugs
- See chart p. 230

Psychostimulants (cont.)

Long-acting Formulations

Drug	Drug	Formulation	Duration of Effect	Usual Dosing
Methylphenidate biphasic release	Biphentin	40% immediate-release beads + 60% delayed-release beads in a capsule	10–12h	Once daily; can open and sprinkle on food
	Concerta	22% immediate-release coating + 78% delayed-release osmotic mechanism	10–12h	Once daily
	Metadate CD	30% immediate-release beads + 70% delayed-release beads in a capsule	8h	Once daily
	Ritalin LA	50% immediate-release beads + 50% delayed-release beads in a capsule	6–8h	Once daily; can open and sprinkle on food
Methylphenidate sustained/slow release	Ritalin SR	Provides a slow continual release of drug from a wax matrix	4–6h	Multiple daily dosing
	Methylin ER	Provides a slow continual release of drug due to diffusion and erosion from a hydrophilic polymer	4–8h	Multiple daily dosing
	Metadate ER	Provides a slow continual release of drug from a wax matrix	4–8h	Multiple daily dosing
Methylphenidate transdermal patch	Daytrana	Drug dispersed in an acrylic adhesive which is dispersed in a silicone adhesive. Total dose delivered is dependent on patch size and wear time (see Dosing below)	Depends on length of time patch applied	On in a.m., off after 9h
Dexmethylphenidate extended-release	Focalin XR	50% immediate-release beads + 50% enteric-coated delayed-release beads, in a capsule	10–12h	Once daily; can open and sprinkle on food
Dextroamphetamine/amphetamine salts	Adderall XR	50% immediate-release beads + 50% delayed-release beads in a capsule	10–12h	Once daily; can open and sprinkle on food
Dextroamphetamine	Dexedrine Spansules	Bead system contains both immediate-release and sustained-release drug	4–9h	Multiple daily dosing; can open and sprinkle on food
Lisdexamfetamine	Vyvanse	Lisdexamfetamine is an inactive prodrug of dextroamphetamine and L-lysine. The drug becomes slowly activated as the prodrug molecule is hydrolyzed (cleaving off the amino acid) in the intestines and liver	10–13h	Once daily
Methamphetamine	Desoxyn Gradumet	Slow-release tablet	8h	Once daily

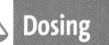 **Dosing**

- See chart p. 227
- Treatment is often started at low doses (e.g., 5–10 mg of methylphenidate) and gradually increased over several days; initial improvement noted may plateau after two to three weeks of continuous use – this does not imply tolerance. Patients should compare the plateau to their baseline
- The effect of stimulants is not always associated with the dose; doses above 1.0 mg/kg/day of methylphenidate often do not result in an increased response, however, side effects can increase. Doses above 1mg/kg/day may be tried in those tolerating the stimulant and have had a moderate response
- To minimize anorexia, give drug with or after meals; food can affect T_{max} and/or C_{max} (see table p. 227)
- Patients who have problems swallowing pills may use one of several medications formulated as beads (Metadate CD, Ritalin LA, Biphentin, Dexedrine Spansules or Adderall XR), by opening the capsule, sprinkling the beads in applesauce, and swallowing the mixture without chewing
- Divided doses required with regular preparations of methylphenidate (dose every 2 to 6 h). Important to document "wear-off" times (changes in behavior attention) and adjust dosing interval accordingly
- Though controversial, as some data suggest continued activation, administration of a small dose (e.g., 5 mg) ½ hour before bedtime can sometimes help to calm the child so as to permit him to go to sleep

- Methylphenidate SR preparation continues to have erratic release in some patients (depending on stomach acidity) and is only slightly longer in duration of action than immediate-release preparations. Compliance may be improved with long-acting formulations
- The extended-release, sustained-release, or controlled-release formulations may decrease inter-dose dysphoria or "wear off" phenomenon (rebound hyperactivity). Supplementation with short-acting preparations may be needed in the morning (to speed up onset) or in the afternoon (to extend duration of action of some preparations)
- Transdermal patch (Daytrana): Total dose delivered is dependent on patch size and wear time. Dose delivered over 9 h: 10 mg for 27.5 mg patch, 15 mg for 41.3 mg patch, 20 mg for 55 mg patch, and 30 mg for 82.5 mg patch. Dose titration recommended on a weekly basis (9 h wear period/day), as required. Patch can be removed earlier than 9 h for shorter duration of effect or if late-day side effects are problematic.

Pharmacokinetics

- See chart p. 227
- Large interindividual variation in absorption and bioavailability; food may affect T_{max} and C_{max} (see table p. 227)
- Extended-release and osmotic-controlled methylphenidate tablets are formulated with different cores which release the active drug at different times, into the body (see Extended-release preparations)
- Transdermal patch releases methylphenidate at a steady rate per hour, related to dose. Absorption and C_{max} may increase with chronic dosing; rate and extent of absorption increase if patch applied to inflamed skin or if heat applied over patch
- Lisdexamfetamine is converted to *d*-amphetamine and L-lysine by enzymatic hydrolysis; peak plasma concentration of *d*-amphetamine after 50 mg dose of lisdexamfetamine = 30 mg of immediate-release *d*-amphetamine. Only a small amount of *d*-amphetamine is released if lisdexamfetamine is administered parenterally

Switching Formulations

- It is generally recommended to start treatment with a low dose of a long-acting preparation and titrate the dose slowly to a therapeutic level.
- Conversion between dosage formulations are always approximations and are dependent on a number of factors:
  - the pharmacokinetics of each preparation, including the duration of action of each product
  - the patient's age and weight (dosing recommendations are usually based on weight)
  - the patient's response may vary between preparations of the same drug.
- It is always important to monitor both response and adverse effects at each dosage level.

Dosage Conversion

Immediate-release Drug	Extended-release Products (Daily Dose)
Methylphenidate	
5 mg bid-tid	Metadate/Methylin ER, Biphentin, or Ritalin LA 10–20 mg, or Metadate CD 10–20 mg, or Concerta 18 mg
10 mg bid-tid	Metadate/Methylin ER, Biphentin, or Ritalin LA 20–30 mg, or Ritalin SR 20 mg, or Metadate CD 30 mg, or Concerta 27–36 mg
15 mg bid-tid	Metadate/Methylin ER, Biphentin, or Ritalin LA 30–40 mg, or Ritalin SR 40 mg or Metadate CD 30-40 mg, or Concerta 36–54 mg
20 mg bid-tid	Metadate/Methylin ER, Biphentin, or Ritalin LA 40–50 mg, or Ritalin SR 40–60 mg, or Concerta 54–72 mg
30 mg bid	Metadate/Methylin ER, Biphentin, or Ritalin LA 50–60 mg, or Ritalin SR 60 mg, or Concerta 72 mg
Dexmethylphenidate Focalin 2.5 mg bid	Focalin XR 5 mg daily
Dextroamphetamine-amphetamine Salts Adderall 5 mg bid	Adderall XR 10 mg daily
Dextroamphetamine 5 mg bid	Dexedrine Spansules 10 mg daily (large inter-patient variance noted in conversion, from 1:1 to about 1:1.5)

Note: Conversion to Daytrana transdermal patch is currently unknown; titration recommended (see Dosing p. 219)

Psychostimulants (cont.)

SUGGESTED DOSE CONVERSIONS BETWEEN DIFFERENT DRUGS USED IN THE TREATMENT OF ADHD, IN ADULTS > 70 KG, ARE AS FOLLOWS:

Methylphenidate immediate-release 35 mg/day given in 2–3 doses	Ritalin LA, Biphentin, or Metadate CD 40 mg once daily, or Ritalin SR, or Metadate/Methylin ER 40 mg/day given in 2 doses	Concerta 36–45 mg given once daily	Dexmethylphenidate immediate-release 15–20 mg/day given in 2–3 doses or Focalin XR 15–20 mg given once daily	Adderall 20 mg/day given in 2 doses or Adderall XR 20 mg given once daily	Dextroamphetamine immediate-release 20 mg/day given in 3 doses or Dextroamphetamine extended-release 20 mg/day given in 2 doses	Dose is variable and dependant on the weight of the individual. Atomoxetine 100 mg given once daily would be appropriate for a 70 kg male

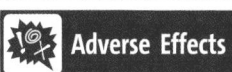

Onset & Duration of Action

- See chart p. 227

Adverse Effects

- See chart pp. 227–229
- Heart rate and blood pressure should be monitored after every dose increase in patients with a history of cardiovascular disease or other risk factors (e.g., hypertension, heart failure, MI or ventricular arrhythmia). Strokes, MI, and sudden death reported with all stimulants in adults and children [Cardiac evaluation recommended if patient exhibits excessive increases in BP or pulse, exertional chest pain or unexplained syncope during treatment]
- Psychostimulants used consistently in children and young teenagers over a period of years have been demonstrated to lead to some growth loss [drug holidays are sometimes used to help mitigate weight and growth loss]
- Common adverse effects include restlessness, irritability, anxiety, insomnia or anorexia; worsening of aggressive behavior or hostility at start of therapy
- Drug-induced insomnia [can be managed by changing the timing of the dose; melatonin (3–6 mg given ½ h before bedtime), L-tryptophan (500–1000 mg), valerian root (450–900 mg extract), antihistamines or trazodone (25–50 mg) at bedtime]. When stimulants wear off at the end of the day, patient may experience rebound, or a period of irritability and return of ADHD symptoms in excess of baseline – this may cause difficulty to fall asleep
- Anorexia common, GI distress and weight loss [can be minimized by taking medication with meals, eating smaller meals more frequently or drinking high-calorie fluids]; if loss of weight exceeds 10% of body weight, consider switching to a shorter-acting agent that allows for return of appetite late in the day, or use of atomoxetine
- Headache most common 2–3 h after a dose (tension-like or 'achy'); tends to decrease over time [accetaminophen as required]
- Hyperactive rebound can occur in the afternoon or evening [an earlier second dose, more frequent dosing, or the use of slow-release preparation can be tried]
- Dysphoria or sadness has been noted to occur on stimulants, both during the day and when they are wearing off; more common with amphetamine-based products
- May exacerbate psychotic symptoms in children with a genetic predisposition or prior history of psychosis; risk of inducing mixed/manic episode in patients with BAD

D/C Discontinuation Syndrome

- Abrupt withdrawal after prolonged use may result in dysphoria, irritability, or a rebound in symptoms of ADHD; increase in sleep and appetite reported
- Case of priapism reported in 16-year-old each time he forgot to take his dose of extended-release methylphenidate (Concerta) 54 mg

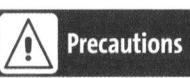

Precautions

- Patients should be screened for cardiovascular risks by history (early cardiac death in the family, family cardiac history, syncope, chest pain on exertion) and given a physical exam. If risk factors are present, an ECG or cardiology consult should be considered according to the judgment of the clinician. In patients with ADHD and cardiac problems, the risks and benefits of using stimulants need to be assessed in conjunction with a cardiologist
- Use cautiously in patients with anxiety, tension, agitation, restlessness
- May lower the seizure threshold (contradictory data)

- May precipitate manic or hypomanic symptoms in a patient with undiagnosed bipolar disorder and exacerbate psychotic symptoms
- Chronic abuse in patients can lead to tolerance and psychic dependence; drug dependence is rare; drug abuse or diversion is a risk, especially in children with comorbid conduct or substance problems. Stimulants can be abused orally, intravenously or nasally
- Use cautiously if there is a positive family history of Tourette's syndrome (tic incidence 20–50% in this population); in patients with Tourette's syndrome there may be an initial worsening of tics; dose may need to be adjusted [clonidine may be effective]
- Some patients become tolerant to stimulant effects; may require an increased dose or a drug holiday
- May exacerbate thought disorder and behavior disturbances in psychotic patients
- Application of external heat (e.g., heating pad, sauna, etc.) over Daytrana patch results in temperature-dependent increase in release of methylphenidate (greater than 2-fold)

 Contraindications

- Patients with structural cardiac abnormalities or cardiovascular disease, tachyarrhythmias, severe angina pectoris, severe hypertension
- Use with caution and with careful monitoring in patients with a recent history of alcohol and/or drug abuse
- Do not use in patients with a history of functional psychosis
- Anorexia nervosa
- Severe anxiety, tension, agitation
- Hyperthyroidism, glaucoma
- Patients taking MAOIs

 Toxicity

- See p. 227

 Lab Tests/Monitoring

- Baseline: height, weight, blood pressure and pulse and repeat regularly throughout treatment. Patients with a prior or family history of cardiac disease should be further evaluated via ECG and echocardiograph. Cardiac evaluation recommended if patient experiences excessive increase in blood pressure or pulse, exertional chest pain, or unexplained syncope

 Pediatric Considerations

- For detailed information on the use of psychostimulants in this population, please see the *Clinical Handbook of Psychotropic Drugs for Children and Adolescents* (2007)
- ADHD is the primary indication in children and adolescents
- Monitor height and weight (children) to ensure children are growing as per usual growth charts; if more than 10% of body weight is lost, consider lowering the dose, using drug holidays or switching treatment
- Tics or dyskinesias can be unmasked in children with ADHD with a genetic predisposition

 Geriatric Considerations

- Useful in the treatment of elderly or medically ill patients with major depression (see precautions and contraindications re cardiac status)
- Dosing before breakfast and lunch may facilitate daytime activity
- Initiate dosage gradually, e.g., 2.5 mg to start, increased by 2.5–5.0 mg every 2–3 days, as tolerated

 Use in Pregnancy

- See p. 227

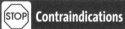 **Nursing Implications**

- While medication has demonstrated superiority, a multimodal approach to treatment of ADHD is necessary in order to increase the probability of a positive outcome for the child; some non-pharmacological approaches include parent training, as well as special education for the child
- Ensure that spansules, sustained-/extended-release, or osmotic-controlled preparations are not chewed, but are swallowed whole
- For patients who have difficulty swallowing pills, Metadate CD, Ritalin LA, Adderall XR, Biphentin or Dexedrine Spansules can be prescribed; capsule can be opened and the beads sprinkled in applesauce and swallowed without chewing
- Monitor therapy by watching for adverse side effects and changes in concentration, mood, and activity level; report any changes in behavior or in sleeping or eating habits
- ADHD: monitor height and weight in children; drug-free periods are advocated

Psychostimulants (cont.)

- In patients with ADHD driving impairment is a common feature of the disorder, and driving is noted to be markedly improved on medication. Patients with a history of driving difficulty should be cautioned about driving while off medication
- Caution patients that abrupt discontinuation may lead to exacerbation of symptoms
- Doses of psychostimulants in latter part of day may cause insomnia
- To minimize anorexia, give drug with or after meals
- Heart rate and blood pressure should be monitored after dose increases
- Patients should be advised that the Concerta tablet shell does not dissolve and may be seen in the stool after a bowel movement
- Daytrana patch should be applied (immediately upon removal of protective pouch) to clean, dry skin on the hip, 2 h before desired effect and taken off about 9 h later; advise patient not to apply patch to inflamed skin, and to avoid exposing area of application to external heat (e.g., electric or heating pads). Dispose patch by folding together the adhesive side – can be flushed down the toilet

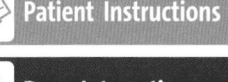 **Patient Instructions**
- For detailed patient instructions on psychostimulants, see the Patient Information Sheet on p. 351

Drug Interactions
- Clinically significant interactions are listed below

DRUGS INTERACTING WITH METHYLPHENIDATE AND DEXMETHYLPHENIDATE

Class of Drug	Example	Interaction Effects
Antibacterial	Linezolid	Linezolid inhibits MAO enzymes – AVOID combination (discontinue stimulant while linezolid used)
Anticoagulant	Warfarin	Decreased metabolism of anticoagulant Increased INR response
Anticonvulsant	Carbamazepine	Decreased plasma level of methylphenidate due to increased metabolism
	Phenytoin, phenobarbital, primidone	Increased level of phenytoin and phenobarbital due to inhibited metabolism by methylphenidate
Antidepressant MAOI (Irreversible)	Phenelzine, tranylcypromine, pargyline	Release of large amount of norepinephrine with hypertensive reaction – AVOID; combination used very RARELY to augment antidepressant therapy with strict monitoring
RIMA	Moclobemide	Increased blood pressure and enhanced effect if used over prolonged period or in high doses
SNRI	Venlafaxine	Case of serotonin syndrome with methylphenidate after one dose of venlafaxine given
SSRI		Additive effects in depression, dysthymia and OCD in patients with ADHD; may improve response in refractory paraphilias and paraphilia-related disorders Plasma level of SSRI antidepressant may be increased
Tricyclic	Amitriptyline, etc.	Used together to augment antidepressant effect Plasma level of tricyclic antidepressant may be increased Cardiovascular effects increased, with combination, in children; monitor blood pressure and ECG Case reports of neurotoxic effects with imipramine, but considered rare; monitor
Antihistamine	Diphenhydramine	Antagonism of sedative effects
Antihypertensive	Clonidine	Additive effect on sleep, hyperactivity, and aggression associated with ADHD – use caution due to case reports of sudden death and monitor ECG
	Guanethidine	Decreased hypotensive effect; may be dose dependent

Class of Drug	Example	Interaction Effects
Antipsychotic		Early data suggest that methylphenidate may exacerbate or prolong withdrawal dyskinesia following antipsychotic discontinuation
Herbal preparations	Ephedra, yohimbine, St. John's Wort Ginkgo biloba	May cause hypertension, arrhythmias and/or CNS stimulation Seizure threshold may be lowered with combination
Theophylline		Reports of increased tachycardia, palpitations, dizziness, weakness and agitation

DRUGS INTERACTING WITH DEXTROAMPHETAMINE AND LISDEXAMFETAMINE

Class of Drug	Example	Interaction Effects
Acidifying agent	Ammonium chloride, fruit juices, ascorbic acid	Decreased absorption, increased elimination and decreased plasma level of dextroamphetamine and lisdexamfetamine
Alkalinizing agent	Potassium citrate, sodium bicarbonate	Increased absorption, prolonged half-life and decreased elimination of amphetamines
Antidepressant MAOI (Irreversible) RIMA SSRIs Tricyclic	 Phenelzine, tranylcypromine Moclobemide Sertraline, paroxetine	 Hypertensive crisis due to increased norepinephrine release; AVOID Slightly enhanced effect if used over prolonged period or in high doses Additive effects in depression, dysthymia and OCD in patients with ADHD Paroxetine may increase plasma level of dextroamphetamine due to inhibited metabolism via CYP2D6 May result in increased level of either the antidepressant or amphetamine
β-Blocker	Propranolol	Increased blood pressure and tachycardia due to unopposed alpha stimulation
Sibutramine		Possible hypertension and tachycardia – use with caution

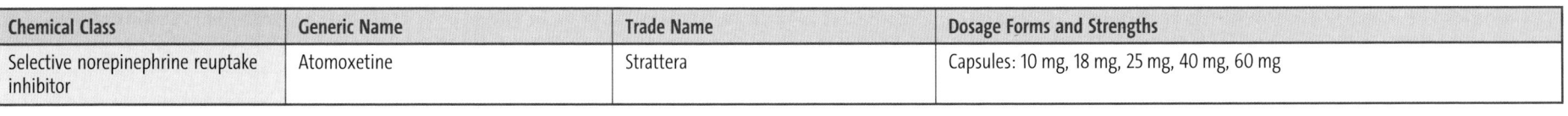

Atomoxetine

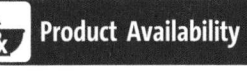 **Product Availability**

Chemical Class	Generic Name	Trade Name	Dosage Forms and Strengths
Selective norepinephrine reuptake inhibitor	Atomoxetine	Strattera	Capsules: 10 mg, 18 mg, 25 mg, 40 mg, 60 mg

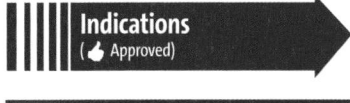 **Indications**
(👍 Approved)

- 👍 Treatment of ADHD in children, adolescents, and adults
- May reduce anxiety symptoms in patients with comorbid anxiety disorder

 **General Comments**

- Some guidelines list atomoxetine as a second line agent, while other guidelines have suggested it for first line use. May be effective for some patients who have not responded to stimulant treatment, who have comorbid anxiety, or individuals who have an active comorbid substance use disorder. Benefits include a lack of euphoria, a lower risk of rebound, and a lower risk of induction of tics or psychosis
- Evidence available indicates that stimulants and atomoxetine have both been found to be superior to placebo for reducing the severity of ADHD symptoms on average in the short term
- Has a slow onset of action and response may take up to 4 weeks – titrate dose gradually. Response is first seen at 4 weeks of full dose and full optimization of drug response requires at least 3 months
- Reduces both the inattentive and hyperactive/impulsive symptoms of ADHD
- Not a controlled substance
- Some head-to-head studies show greater reductions in ADHD symptoms and a greater percentage of responders with stimulants when compared to atomoxetine
- A large head-to-head trial of OROS-MPH vs. atomoxetine in over 600 children demonstrated that 40% of children who do not respond to one drug are responders to the other, indicating selective response

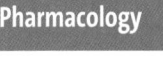 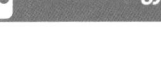 **Pharmacology**

- Selectively blocks the reuptake of norepinephrine; increases dopamine and norepinephrine in the frontal cortex (without increasing dopamine in subcortical areas) – leads to cognitive enhancement without abuse liability; suggested to be important in regulating attention, impulsivity, and activity levels
- No stimulant or euphoriant activity – promising treatment in patients with comorbid substance use disorder

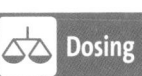 **Dosing**

- Dosing is based on body weight
- Children and adolescents up to 70 kg: see Table p. 227; Do not exceed 1.4 mg/kg or 100 mg/day, whichever is less
- Adults and children over 70 kg: see Table p. 227; maximum of 100 mg/day. Doses > 100 mg/day have not been found to result in additional therapeutic benefit
- In patients with moderate hepatic dysfunction, reduce dose by 50%; in severe hepatic dysfunction reduce dose to 25% of the usual therapeutic range
- No dose adjustment required in renal insufficiency; may exacerbate hypertension in patients with end-stage renal disease
- Lower doses required for those who are poor metabolizers of CYP2D6
- If prescribed in combination with drugs that inhibit CYP2D6 (see Interactions p. 195): initiate dose, as above, but do not increase to the usual target dose unless symptoms fail to improve *after 4 weeks* and the initial dose is well tolerated

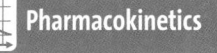 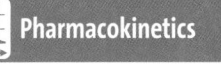 **Pharmacokinetics**

- Rapidly absorbed; may be taken with or without food – high-fat meal decreases rate but not extent of absorption (C_{max} delayed by 3 h and is 37% lower)
- Bioavailability 63%; 94% in poor metabolizers

- Protein binding: 98% atomoxetine and 69% for OH-atomoxetine metabolite
- Peak plasma level reached in 1–2 h; 3–4 h in poor metabolizers
- Half-life = 5 h of atomoxetine and 6–8 h of hydroxyatomoxetine; in poor metabolizers the values are 21.6 h and 34–40 h, respectively; metabolized primarily by CYP2D6, also by CYP2C19
- Hepatic dysfunction: 2-fold increase in AUC in moderate hepatic insufficiency and 4-fold increase in AUC in severe hepatic dysfunction (see dosing)

 Adverse Effects

- See table pp. 227–229
- Common: rhinitis, upper abdominal pain, nausea, vomiting, decreased appetite, weight loss (seen initially, especially if dose titrated too rapidly, but levels off with time), dizziness, headache, fatigue, emotional lability, insomnia
- Less frequent: irritability, sedation, depression, dry mouth, constipation, mydriasis, tremor, pruritus, urinary retention
- Small increases in blood pressure and pulse can occur at start of treatment; usually plateau with time
- Sexual dysfunction (2%) including erectile disturbance, impotence, and abnormal orgasm
- Rare cases of elevated hepatic enzymes and bilirubin; severe hepatic injury reported in at least two individuals (out of 3.4 million) after several months of treatment; injury reversed when atomoxetine withdrawn

 D/C Discontinuation Syndrome

- No evidence, to date, that suggests a drug discontinuation or withdrawal syndrome exists

 Precautions

- Use with caution in patients with cardiovascular disease, including hypertension, arteriosclerosis, and tachyarrhythmias. Do a cardiac history and physical assessment prior to prescribing atomoxetine and evaluate symptoms suggestive of cardiac disease that develop during treatment. DO NOT USE in adults or children with structural cardiac abnormalities – miocardial infarction, stroke, and deaths reported
- Due to risk of hypertension, use cautiously in any condition that may predispose patients to hypertension
- Use caution in patients with liver dysfunction – see dosing, above
- Cases of liver injury reported (rare); discontinue drug in patients with jaundice or laboratory evidence of liver injury – rechallenge not advised
- Has been associated with increased suicidal ideation

 Contraindications

- Patients with structural cardiac abnormalities or cardiovascular disease, tachyarrhythmias, severe hypertension or severe angina
- Should not be administered together with an MAOI or within 2 weeks of discontinuing an MAOI
- Not recommended in patients with narrow angle glaucoma due to increased risk of mydriasis

 Toxicity

- See p. 227
- Symptoms include anxiety, tremulousness, dry mouth; case of seizures and prolonged QTc interval

 Lab Tests/Monitoring

- Liver function test at first symptoms or sign of liver dysfunction

 Pediatric Considerations

- For detailed information on the use of atomoxetine in this population, please see the *Clinical Handbook of Psychotropic Drugs for Children and Adolescents* (2007)
- Safety and efficacy of atomoxetine has not been established in children < 6 years of age
- Pharmacokinetics in children are similar to that in adults

 Geriatric Considerations

- Use with caution in patients with cardiovascular disease or liver dysfunction

 Use in Pregnancy

- Category "C" risk; effect on humans unknown

Breast Milk

- Unknown if atomoxetine is excreted in human milk

Atomoxetine (cont.)

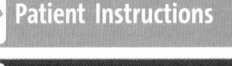 **Nursing Implications**

- Measure pulse and blood pressure at baseline and periodically during treatment
- Monitor for increased irritability, anger, depression, or suicidal ideation
- Monitor growth and weight during treatment
- Monitor for signs of liver toxicity (pruritus, dark urine, jaundice, upper right quadrant tenderness, unexplained flu-like symptoms)
- Capsules of atomoxetine cannot be opened
- Give atomoxetine with or after meals to minimize stomach ache, nausea, and vomiting

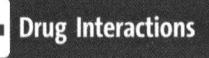 **Patient Instructions**

- For detailed patient instructions on atomoxetine, see the Patient Information Sheet on p. 353

Drug Interactions

- Clinically significant interactions are listed below

Class of Drug	Example	Interaction Effects
Antiarrhythmic	Quinidine	Increased level of atomoxetine due to inhibited metabolism via CYP2D6
Antidepressant SSRI MAOI	Paroxetine, fluoxetine Phenelzine	Increased plasma level and half-life of atomoxetine due to inhibited metabolism via CYP2D6 Do not administer concurrently or within 2 weeks of discontinuing an MAOI
Antiparkinsonian Agent	Pergolide	Increased atomoxetine level due to inhibited metabolism via CYP2D6
Antiviral Agent	Ritonavir, delavirdine	Increased atomoxetine level due to inhibited metabolism via CYP2D6
β-Agonist	Albuterol	Can potentiate cardiovascular effects resulting in increased blood pressure and heart rate
Dextromethorphan (DM)		Competitive inhibition of DM metabolism via CYP2D6, with potential for increased plasma level of either drug
Stimulant	Methylphenidate, amphetamines	Possible potentiation of hypertension and tachycardia

	Methylphenidate	Dexmethylphenidate	Dextroamphetamine/Amphetamine salts/Methamphetamine	Atomoxetine
Pharmacology	Selectively inhibits presynaptic transporters (i.e., reuptake) for dopamine and norepinephrine – dependent on normal neuronal activity Increases levels of synaptic dopamine and NE	Selectively inhibits presynaptic transporters (i.e., reuptake) for dopamine and norepinephrine – dependent on normal neuronal activity Increases levels of synaptic dopamine and NE	Cause release of dopamine, NE and 5-HT into the synapse – occurs independently of normal neuronal activity Inhibit MAO enzyme	Selectively blocks reuptake of NE; increases NE and DA in frontal cortex
Dosing ADHD	Start with 2.5–5 mg bid and increase by 2.5–5 mg weekly Usual dose: 10–60 mg/day or 0.25–1.0 mg/kg body weight (divided doses); up to 3 mg/kg has been used in children Up to 120 mg/day used in adults with ADHD Extended-release: 18–20 mg qam; can increase by 18–20 mg weekly to a maximum of 72 mg/day Transdermal patch: week 1, apply 27.5 mg patch (for 9 h/day); increase dose in weekly intervals as necessary	Over age 6: start with 2.5 mg bid and can increase weekly in 2.5–5 mg increments to a maximum of 20 mg/day (divided dose, given at least q 4 h) Usual dose: 5–20 mg daily given bid When switching from methylphenidate, the starting dose of dexmethylphenidate should be half that of methylphenidate	*Dextroamphetamine*: Age 3–5: start with 2.5 mg and increase by 2.5 mg weekly. Over age 6: start with 5 mg and increase by 5 mg weekly Usual dose: dextroamphetamine: 2.5–40 mg/day or 0.1–0.8 mg/kg (divided doses); Spansules can be sprinkled on food *Adderall*: 2.5–5 mg to start and increase by 2.5–5 mg every 3–7 days up to 30 mg/day (given every 4–7 h). In adults up to 40 mg/day (in divided doses) *Adderall XR*: 10–30 mg qam *Methamphetamine*: start with 5 mg od-bid and increase by 5 mg/week Usual dose: 20–25 mg/day – in divided doses; Gradumet given once daily *Lisdexamfetamine*: Children age 6–12: 30 mg q am and can increase by 20 mg in 7-day increments to a maximum of 70 mg/day	Dosing is based on body weight Children: *Up to 70 kg*: initiate at 0.5 mg/kg/day, and increase after a minimum of 10 days to 0.8 mg/kg/day for 10 days; if clinical response is not achieved, increase to a target dose of 1.2 mg/kg/day, given once daily or bid in the morning and late afternoon. Do not exceed 1.4 mg/kg or 100 mg/day, whichever is less. *Over 70 kg*: initiate at 40 mg/day and increase after a minimum of 10 days to 60 mg/day for 10 days; if clinical response is not achieved, increase to a target dose of 80 mg/day, given once daily or bid in the morning and later afternoon. If response is inadequate after 2–4 weeks, the dose can be increased to a maximum of 100 mg/day *Adults*: see dosing over 70 kg, above
Depression	10–30 mg/day	–	Dextroamphetamine: 5–60 mg/day	–
Narcolepsy	10–60 mg/day (usual dose: 10 mg 2–3 times/day)	–	Dextroamphetamine: 5–60 mg/day	–

Comparison of Drugs for ADHD (cont.)

	Methylphenidate	Dexmethylphenidate	Dextroamphetamine/Amphetamine salts/Methamphetamine	Atomoxetine
Pharmacokinetics				
Bioavailability	> 90%	No change; 22–25%	Dextroamphetamine: > 90% Methamphetamine: 65–70%	63–94%

Peak plasma level	Tabs: 0.3–4 h
	Slow release: 1–8 h
	Metadate CD: 1.5 h first peak and 4.5 h second peak
	Concerta: 1 h first peak and 6.8 h second peak
		1–1.5 h (fasting)	Dextroamphetamine:
			    Tablets 1–4 h,
			    Spansules: 6–10 h
			Adderall:
			    Tablets 1–2 h
			    XR: 7 h
			Lisdexamfetamine: 1 h, d-amphetamine: 3.5 h
				1–2 h
				Poor metabolizers: 3–4 h

Protein binding	8–15%	12–15%	12–15%	98% atomoxetine and 69% OH-atomoxetine metabolite
Onset of effects	0.5–2 h Absorption from GI tract is slow and incomplete	0.5–2 h	0.5–2 h Readily absorbed from the GI tract Adderall: saccharate and aspartate salts have a delayed onset	Delayed up to 4 weeks
Plasma half-life	Regular tabs: 2.9 h mean (range: 2–4 h) SR and Concerta: 3.4 h mean Metadate CD: 6.8 h mean 2.2 h Daytrana: 3–4 h after removal of patch	2.2 h	Dextroamphetamine: 6–8 h in acidic pH, 18.6–33.6 h in alkaline pH Methamphetamine: 6.5–15 h Adderall: 6–8 h Lisdexamfetamine: < 1 h; d-amphetamine: 10–13 h	Atomoxetine = 5 h (poor metabolizers = 21.6 h) OH-atomoxetine = 6–8h (poor metabolizers = 34–40 h

Duration of action	Regular tabs: 3–5 h
	Slow release – theoretically 5–8 h,
	but 3–5 h practically
	Extended release: 8–12 h
		6–7 h	Dextroamphetamine:
			    Tabs 4–5 h, Spansules: 7–8 h
			Adderall:
			    Tabs 5–7 h, XR: 12 h
			Lisdexamfetamine: 10 h
				Approx. 24 h

Metabolism	Metabolized by CYP2D6 Inhibits CYP2D6 and 2C9 enzymes	By de-esterification	Metabolized by CYP2D6	Metabolized primarily by CYP2D6; also by CYP2C19
Hepatic impairment	No change	No change	No change	Moderate: reduce dose by 50% Severe: reduce dose by 75%
Renal impairment		?	Decreased excretion	No adjustment
Effect of food	Metadate CD: delayed T_{max} by 1h Concerta: delayed T_{max} by 1h and C_{max} by 10–30%	–	Decreased extent of absorption Lisdexamfetamine: no change	T_{max} delayed by 3 h
High-fat meal	Ritalin and Ritalin LA: delayed T_{max} Metadate CD: increased C_{max} by 30%	Delayed T_{max}	–	C_{max} 37% lower

	Methylphenidate	Dexmethylphenidate	Dextroamphetamine/Amphetamine salts/Methamphetamine	Atomoxetine
Adverse Effects*				
CNS	Nervousness (16%), anxiety, insomnia (up to 28%), restlessness, activation, irritability (up to 26%), headache (up to 14%), tearfulness, drowsiness (10%), rebound depression, may exacerbate mania or psychosis (See Precautions p. 220) Cases of suicidal thoughts, hallucinations and psychotic or violent behavior reported with Concerta Tourette's syndrome, tics (up to 10% – mostly with higher doses) Social withdrawal, dullness, sadness and irritability reported in children with autism	Drowsiness, headache Fever (5%) Arthralgia, dyskinesias (See Precautions p. 220)	Nervousness, insomnia, activation, restlessness, anxiety, emotional lability, mania (with high doses), dysphoria, irritability, headache, confusion, delusions, rebound depression; may exacerbate mania or psychosis (See Precautions p. 220) Headache Tremor, Tourette's syndrome, tics – usually with higher doses	Insomnia, dizziness, fatigue, headache, emotional inability Less common: drowsiness, irritability, depression, tremor Reports of psychotic/manic symptoms (hallucinations, delusions and mania) in children and adolescents with no prior history of psychotic illness Case reports of tics
GI	Abdominal pain (up to 23%), nausea, vomiting and diarrhea (> 10%), anorexia (up to 41% dose-related)	Abdominal pain (15%), nausea, anorexia (6%)	Abdominal pain common: nausea, vomiting, anorexia	Upper abdominal pain, nausea, vomiting, anorexia
Cardiovascular	Increased heart rate and blood pressure, at start of therapy, dizziness (13%), hypotension, palpitations (See Precautions p. 220)	Increased heart rate and blood pressure at start of therapy (See Precautions p. 220)	Increased heart rate and blood pressure, at start of therapy, dizziness, palpitations (See Precautions p. 220)	Small increases in heart rate and blood pressure at start of treatment (See Precautions p. 225)
Anticholinergic	Dry mouth, blurred vision	Blurred vision	Dry mouth, dysgeusia, blurred vision	Dry mouth, constipation, mydriasis, urinary retention
Endocrine	Growth delay (height and weight), may occur initially but tends to normalize over time (unless high chronic doses used), weight loss	Growth delay, weight loss	Growth delay (height and weight), may occur initially but tends to normalize over time (unless high chronic doses used), weight loss, impotence, changes in libido	Sexual dysfunction, weight loss
Other	Upper respiratory infections: pharyngitis (4%), sinusitis (3%), rhinitis (13%), cough (4%), fever Rash; contact sensitization/dermatitis with Daytrana patch – redness, itching, blistering Leukopenia, blood dyscrasias, anemia, hair loss	Cough, upper respiratory infections	Urticaria, anemia	Cases of liver damage with elevated AST/ALT and bilirubin in adults and children Pruritus, rhinitis
Toxicity	CNS overstimulation with vomiting, agitation, tremors, hyperreflexia, convulsions, confusion, hallucinations, delirium, cardiovascular effects e.g., hypertension, tachycardia; seizures reported Supportive therapy should be given	CNS overstimulation with vomiting, agitation, tremors, hyperreflexia, convulsions, confusion, hallucinations, delirium, cardiovascular effects e.g., hypertension, tachycardia Supportive therapy should be given	Restlessness, dizziness, increased reflexes, tremor, insomnia, irritability, assaultiveness, hallucinations, panic, cardiovascular effects, circulatory collapse, convulsions, and coma Supportive therapy should be given	Anxiety, tremulousness, dry mouth; case of seizures & QT_c prolongation Supportive therapy should be given

Comparison of Drugs for ADHD (cont.)

	Methylphenidate	Dexmethylphenidate	Dextroamphetamine/Amphetamine salts/Methamphetamine	Atomoxetine
Use in Pregnancy	No evidence of teratogenicity reported	Safety not established	High doses have embryotoxic and teratogenic potential; use of amphetamine in pregnant animals has been associated with permanent alterations in the central noradrenergic system of the neonate Increased risk of premature delivery and low birth weight; withdrawal reactions in newborn reported	Category C
Breastfeeding	No data	No data	Excreted into breast milk; recommended not to breastfeed	No data

* Dose related

Clonidine

Product Availability

Chemical Class	Generic Name	Trade Name[(A)]	Dosage Forms and Strengths
Adrenergic agent	Clonidine	Catapres Catapres TTS[(B)]	Tablet: 0.025 mg, 0.1 mg, 0.2 mg, 0.3 mg[(B)] Transdermal patch[(B)]: 0.1 mg/24 h, 0.2 mg/24 h, 0.3 mg/24 h

[(A)] Generic preparations may be available, [(B)] Not available in Canada

Indications
(✚ Approved)

- ADHD: meta-analysis of studies suggests a moderate benefit in children and adolescents; reduced hyperarousal, agitation, aggression, and sleep disturbances; useful in patients with concurrent tic disorders or conduct disorder; minimal benefit on inattentive symptoms
- Some benefit in combining with stimulants; may help ameliorate sleep disturbances caused by psychostimulants (Caution – see Drug Interactions p. 232)
- Improves behavior or impulsivity when used alone or in combination with methylphenidate (Caution – see Interactions p. 232); may reduce hyperarousal behaviors in pervasive developmental disorders
- Reported to be effective for controlling some problematic behaviors in children and adults with autism
- Reported to have synergistic effect with anticonvulsant regimens in controlling aggression and impulsivity
- Of some benefit in generalized anxiety disorder, panic attacks, phobic disorders, and obsessive-compulsive disorders; may augment effects of SSRIs and cyclic antidepressants in social phobia; helpful for symptoms of hyperarousal, hypervigilance, aggression, and irritability of PTSD
- May relieve antipsychotic-induced asthenia and improve symptoms of tardive dyskinesia
- May help decrease clozapine-induced sialorrhea
- Used in heroin and nicotine withdrawal to reduce agitation, tremor, and diaphoresis, and to increase patient comfort. Opioid antagonists (e.g., naltrexone) as well as dicyclomine (for stomach cramps) and cyclobenzaprine (for muscle cramps) often given concomitantly

General Comments	• Reduces the hyperactive/impulsive and aggressive symptoms of ADHD but is less effective for inattention problems; considered generally less effective than psychostimulants, though may be beneficial for some patients who have not responded to stimulant treatment or those with comorbid tic disorder
	• In anxiety disorders, psychological symptoms respond better than somatic symptoms; anxiolytic effects may be short-lived
Pharmacology	• A central and peripheral α-adrenergic agonist; acts on presynaptic neurons and inhibits noradrenergic release and transmission at the synapse
Dosing	• ADHD: 3–10 micrograms/kg body weight per day (0.05–0.4 mg/day) once daily at bedtime, or in divided doses
	• Antisocial behavior/aggression: children – 0.15–0.4 mg/day as tablets or transdermal patch; adults – 0.4–0.6 mg/day
	• Anxiety disorders: 0.15–0.5 mg/day
	• Drug dependence: 0.1–0.3 mg tid to qid for up to 7 days; nicotine withdrawal: 0.1 mg bid to 0.4 mg/day for 3–4 weeks
Pharmacokinetics	• Well absorbed orally and percutaneously (when applied to the arm or chest)
	• Peak plasma level of oral preparation occurs in 3–5 h; therapeutic plasma concentrations of transdermal patch occur within 2–3 days
	• Plasma half-life is 6–20 h; in patients with impaired renal function, half-life ranges from 18–41 h. Elimination half-life is dose-dependent
Onset & Duration of Action	• Oral tablets: onset of effects occurs in 30–60 minutes and lasts about 8 h
	• Transdermal patch: therapeutic plasma concentrations are attained within 2–3 days and effects last for 7 days
Adverse Effects	• Sedation, dizziness, bradycardia, and hypotension common on initiation (monitor BP and heart rate)
	• Less common: anxiety, irritability, decreased memory, headache, dry mouth, and lack of energy
	• Dermatological reactions reported in up to 50% of patients using the transdermal patch
	• May increase agitation and produce depressive symptoms
D/C Discontinuation Syndrome	• Withdrawal reactions occur after abrupt cessation of long-term therapy (over 1–2 months)
	• Taper on drug discontinuation to prevent rebound hypertension and sedation, as well as tic rebound in patients with Tourette's syndrome
	• Cases of rebound psychotic symptoms reported
Precautions	• Use caution in combination with psychostimulants due to case reports of sudden death with combination
	• Use with caution in patients with cerebrovascular disease, chronic renal failure, or a history of depression
Toxicity	• Signs and symptoms of overdose occur within 60 minutes of drug ingestion and may persist for up to 48 h
	• Symptoms include transient hypertension followed by hypotension, bradycardia, weakness, pallor, sedation, vomiting, hypothermia; can progress to CNS depression, diminished or absent reflexes, apnea, respiratory depression, cardiac conduction defects, seizures, and coma
Treatment	• Supportive and symptomatic
Pediatric Considerations	• For detailed information on the use of clonidine in this population, please see the *Clinical Handbook of Psychotropic Drugs for Children and Adolescents* (2007)
	• Children metabolize clonidine faster than adults and may require more frequent dosing (4–6 times/day)
Geriatric Considerations	• Use with caution in patients with cardiovascular disease or chronic renal failure
Use in Pregnancy	• Animal studies suggest teratogenic effects; effects in humans unknown
	• Clonidine crosses the placenta and may lower the heart rate of the fetus
Breast Milk	• Clonidine is distributed into breast milk; effects on infant unknown

Clonidine (cont.)

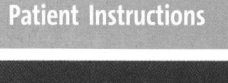 **Nursing Implications**

- Clonidine should not be discontinued suddenly due to risk of rebound hypertension and sedation
- Handle the used transdermal patch carefully (fold in half with sticky sides together)
- Should the transdermal patch begin to loosen from the skin, apply adhesive overlay over the system to ensure good adhesion over the period of application
- Monitor for skin reactions around area when transdermal patch is applied

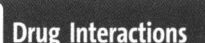 **Patient Instructions**

- For detailed patient instructions on clonidine, see the Patient Information Sheet on p. 354

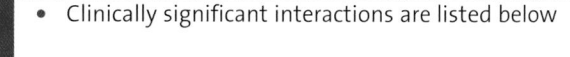 **Drug Interactions**

- Clinically significant interactions are listed below

Class of Drug	Example	Interaction Effects
Antidepressant	Desipramine, bupropion	Clonidine withdrawal may result in excess circulating catecholamines; use caution in combination with noradrenergic or dopaminergic antidepressants
Cyclic	Imipramine, desipramine	Inhibition of antihypertensive effect of clonidine by the antidepressant
Antihypertensives	General	Additive hypotension
β-Blockers	Propranolol	Additive bradycardia
CNS depressants	Antihistamines, alcohol	Additive CNS depressant effects
Stimulants	Methylphenidate	Additive effect on sleep, hyperactivity, and aggression associated with ADHD Use caution due to case reports of sudden death [monitor ECG]

Augmentation Strategies in ADHD

Nonresponse in ADHD	• Ascertain diagnosis is correct • Ascertain if patient is compliant with therapy (speak with caregivers, check with pharmacy for late refills) • Ensure dosage prescribed is therapeutic • Consider trying the alternate stimulant if the first one was ineffective and the patient was adhering to therapy recommendations
Factors Complicating Response	• Concurrent medical or psychiatric condition, e.g., bipolar disorder, conduct disorder, learning disability • Concurrent prescription drugs may interfere with efficacy, e.g., antipsychotics (see Drug Interactions) • Metabolic enhancers (e.g., carbamazepine) will decrease the plasma level of methylphenidate • High intake of acidifying agents (e.g., fruit juices, vitamin C) may decrease the efficacy of amphetamine preparations • Substance abuse, including alcohol and marijuana, may make management difficult; need to discontinue substances of abuse to optimize treatment outcomes • Side effects to medication • Psychosocial factors may affect response; nonpharmacological treatment approaches (e.g., behavior modification, psychotherapy, and education) can increase the probability of response

Drug Combinations in ADHD

Methylphenidate/Dexmethyl-phenidate/Dextroamphet-amine + Clonidine	• Additive effect on hyperactivity, aggression, mood lability, and sleep problems; studies indicate efficacy in 50–80% patients. Has been found helpful in patients with concomitant tic disorders, conduct disorder or oppositional defiant disorder. • **CAUTION:** 5 case reports of sudden death in combination with methylphenidate [monitor ECG, heart rate, and blood pressure with combination]
Psychostimulants + Antidepressants	• Tricyclics (imipramine, nortriptyline, and desipramine) useful in refractory patients or those with concomitant enuresis or bulimia; they may reduce abnormal movements in patients with tic disorders. There is an increase in the incidence of adverse effects, including cardiovascular, GI, anticholinergic effects, and weight gain; use caution in patients at risk of overdose • SSRIs or venlafaxine may be effective in adult patients with concomitant mood or anxiety disorders (e.g., PTSD) • Bupropion used to augment effects of psychostimulants and in patients with concomitant mood disorder, substance abuse, or conduct disorder. May cause dermatological reactions, exacerbate tics, and increase seizure risk
Atomoxetine + Stimulants	• Use in patients who can't tolerate stimulants alone, as the combination may permit lower doses of stimulant and allows robust coverage as well as coverage early and late in the day and in the summer • Monitor for increased blood pressure, tachycardia, and weight loss
Psychostimulants + Antipsychotics	• Second-generation antipsychotics (low doses of risperidone, olanzapine) have been found useful in patients with comorbid symptoms of dyscontrol, aggression, hyperactivity, and tics • Low doses of haloperidol, risperidone, and pimozide have been used in patients with concurrent Tourette's syndrome
Psychostimulants + Mood Stabilizers	• Combination used in patients with comorbid bipolar disorder, conduct disorder, impulsivity, and aggression; case reports in children include the use of lithium, carbamazepine, valproate, and gabapentin – the possibility of drug interactions should be considered (see Drug Interactions)
Psychostimulants + Buspirone	• Open studies suggest benefit in improving rage attacks, impulsivity, inattention, and disruptive behavior using doses of 15–30 mg daily

Clonidine (cont.)

Further Reading

- Bangs ME, Jin L, Zhang S, et al. Hepatic events associated with atomoxetine treatment for attention-deficit hyperactivity disorder. Drug Saf. 2008;31(4):345–354.
- Bangs ME, Tauscher-Wisniewski S, Polzer J, et al. Meta-analysis of suicide-related behavior events in patients treated with atomoxetine. J Am Acad Child Adolesc Psychiatry. 2008;47(2):209–218.
- Biederman J, Spencer TJ. Psychopharmacological interventions. Child Adolesc Psychiatr Clin N Am. 2008;17(2):439–458, xi.
- Buck, ML, Hofer KN, McCarthy, MW. New treatment options for attention-deficit/hyperactivity disorder (ADHD): Part I. Transdermal methylphenidate and lisdexamfetamine. Pediatric Pharmacotherapy. 2008;14(3)
- Canadian ADHD Practice Guidelines. CADDRA 2007/08. Available from: www.caddra.ca/english/phys_guide.html.
- Carlson GA, Dunn D, Kelsey D, et al. A pilot study for augmenting atomoxetine with methylphenidate: Safety of concomitant therapy in children with attention-deficit/hyperactivity disorder. Child Adolesc Psychiatry Ment Health. 2007;1(1):10.
- Findling RL. Evolution of the treatment of attention-deficit/hyperactivity disorder in children: A review. Clin Ther. 2008;30(5):942–957.
- Newcorn JH. Nonstimulants and emerging treatments in adults with ADHD. CNS Spectr. 2008;13(9 Suppl 13):12–16.
- Newcorn JH, Kratochvil CJ, Allen AJ, et al. Atomoxetine and osmotically released methylphenidate for the treatment of attention deficit hyperactivity disorder: Acute comparison and differential response. AM J Psychiatry. 2008;165(6):721-30.
- Palumbo DR, Sallee FR, Pelham WE Jr, et al. Clonidine for attention-deficit/hyperactivity disorder: I. Efficacy and tolerability outcomes. J Am Acad Child Adolesc Psychiatry. 2008;47(2):180–188.
- Polzer J. Meta-analysis of suicide-related behavior events in patients treated with atomoxetine. J Am Acad Child Adolesc Psychiatry. 2008;47(2):209–218.
- Rostain AL. Attention-deficit/hyperactivity disorder in adults: Evidence-based recommendations for management. Postgrad Med. 2008;120(3), 27–38.
- Scahill L, Carroll D, Burke K. Methylphenidate: Mechanism of action and clinical update. J Child Adolesc Psychiatr Nurs. 2004;17(2):85–86.
- Stein MA. Treating adult ADHD with stimulants. CNS Spectr. 2008;13(9 Suppl 13), 8–11.
- Volkow ND, Fowler JS, Wang G, et al. Mechanism of action of methylphenidate: Insights from PET imaging studies. J Atten Disord. 2002;6(Suppl 1):S31–S43.
- Wilens TE. Mechanism of action of agents used in attention-deficit/hyperactivity disorder. J Clin Psychiatry. 2006;67 Suppl 8:S32–S37.
- Wolraich ML, McGuinn L, Doffing M. Treatment of attention deficit hyperactivity disorder in children and adolescents: Safety considerations. Drug Saf. 2007;30(1):17–26.

☰ **Classification**	• Drugs for treatment of dementia can be classified as follows:

Chemical Class	Agent	Page
Cholinesterase inhibitor	Donepezil Tacrine Rivastigmine Galantamine	See p. 235
Aminoadamantane	Memantine	See p. 240

Cholinesterase Inhibitors

 Product Availability

Chemical Class	Generic Name	Trade Name⁽ᴬ⁾	Dosage Forms and Strengths
Piperidine	Donepezil	Aricept	Tablets: 5 mg, 10 mg
Acridine	Tacrine⁽ᴮ⁾	Cognex	Tablets: 10 mg, 20 mg, 30 mg, 40 mg
Carbamate	Rivastigmine	Exelon	Capsules: 1.5 mg, 3 mg, 4.5 mg, 6 mg Oral solution: 2 mg/ml
		Exelon Patch	Patch: 5 (9 mg/5 cm²), 10 (18 mg/10 cm²)
Phenanthrene alkaloid	Galantamine (Galanthamine)	Reminyl⁽ᶜ⁾, Razadyne⁽ᴮ⁾	Tablets: 4 mg, 8 mg, 12 mg Liquid: 4 mg/ml
		Reminyl ER⁽ᶜ⁾, Razadyne ER⁽ᴮ⁾	Extended release capsules: 8 mg, 16 mg, 24 mg

⁽ᴬ⁾ Generic preparations may be available, ⁽ᴮ⁾ Not marketed in Canada, ⁽ᶜ⁾ Not marketed in USA

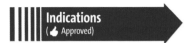 **Indications**
(👍 Approved)

- 👍 Symptomatic treatment of mild to moderate Alzheimer's dementia (AD); minor effect on the underlying neurodegenerative process
- 👍 Dementia of Parkinson's disease (rivastigmine – USA)
- 👍 Treatment of severe AD (donepezil – USA, Canada)
- • Data suggest efficacy in treatment of memory dysfunction following brain injury and in dementia of Parkinson's disease
- • No benefit of donepezil and galantamine on cognitive function in patients with vascular dementia
- • Galantamine and donepezil suggested to improve cognition and behaviors and stabilize or improve activities of daily living
- • Anecdotal reports suggest improvement, with donepezil, on neuropsychological tests of verbal fluency and attention in patients with schizophrenia; negative results reported in double-blind studies
- • Galantamine used to reverse neuromuscular blocking effects of curare-type muscle relaxants

Cholinesterase Inhibitors (cont.)

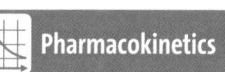 **General Comments**

- These drugs are suggested to ameliorate behavioral disturbances (such as apathy, depression, anxiety, disinhibition, aberrant motor behavior, delusions and hallucinations) as well as enhance cognition. Benefits are lost after drug withdrawal. Therapeutic response following re-initiation of therapy shown to be less than that obtained with initial therapy
- Double-blind placebo-controlled studies involving patients with mild to moderate Alzheimer's disease showed improvement (i.e., less decline in cognitive ability). Approximately 25% of patients had significantly improved attention, interest, orientation, communication and memory (controversy exists over whether cognition enhancers should be used routinely for dementia given their modest efficacy[2])
- Significant treatment benefits of donepezil demonstrated in early stage Alzheimer's disease and support initiating treatment early to improve daily cognitive functioning; shown to have additive effects with memantine in patients with moderate to severe Alzheimer's disease
- The improvement, on average, is modest and benefits may not be evident until 6–12 weeks of continuous treatment. In long-term studies patients receiving treatment with cholinesterase inhibitors still cross their baseline cognitive ability after 6 months of therapy and continue to decline thereafter
- Economic analyses suggest that treatment initiated in early stages of Alzheimer's disease may be cost neutral as a result of patients remaining in a less severe state of disease for a longer time and delayed institutionalization
- Failure to respond to one agent does not preclude response to another; open-label studies suggest that approximately 50% of patients experiencing loss of efficacy with one drug respond to subsequent treatment with another agent

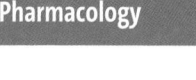 **Pharmacology**

- See chart on p. 244
- It is postulated that these compounds increase acetylcholine levels in the brain through inhibition of the enzyme acetylcholinesterase; clinical improvement occurs with between 40% and 70% cholinesterase inhibition (in preclinical studies they increased extracellular acetylcholine levels in the hippocampus and cerebral cortex)
- Nicotinic cholinergic receptors may regulate cognitive functions, such as attention, and may increase the release of neurotransmitters throughout the brain
- Cholinesterase inhibitors with dual inhibitory action (BuChE – butyrylcholinesterase; AChE – acetylcholinesterase) may be of greater value in more advanced stages of dementia

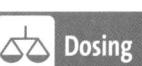 **Dosing**

- See chart on p. 242
- With galantamine and rivastigmine, treatment is started at lower doses with gradual dose escalation to minimize side effects
- Effects on cognition and functional activities are dose-dependent, while effects on behavioral disturbances are not
- Tacrine dose escalation is guided by transaminase (ALT) levels expressed as × ULN (upper level of normal) and measured bi-weekly for 16 weeks (see product monograph for details)
- Rivastigmine Patch 5 releases drug at a rate of 4.6 mg/24 h; Patch 10 releases drug at a rate of 9.5 mg/24 h. When switching from oral drug, Patch 5 is recommended for patients on less than 6 mg/day and Patch 10 can be used for patients on higher doses; apply patch on the next day following the last oral dose
- Patients who discontinued tacrine because of ALT elevation may be rechallenged upon return to normal limits; if rechallenged, AST should be monitored weekly for 16 weeks; the initial dose is 40 mg/day
- Patients who discontinue galantamine or rivastigmine for longer than several days should be re-started at the lowest daily dose (i.e., 4 mg bid for galantamine and 1.5 mg od or bid for rivastigmine) to reduce the possibility of severe vomiting; dosage should be titrated over a period of 2 months to the maintenance dose

Pharmacokinetics

- See chart, p. 242
- Duration of cholinesterase inhibition does not reflect plasma half-life of drug (e.g., rivastigmine half-life is 1–2 h, but cholinesterase inhibition lasts up to 10 h)
- Plasma rivastigmine levels are approximately 30% higher in elderly male patients than in young adults
- Rivastigmine Patch produces lower peak plasma levels than oral drug and steadier plasma levels

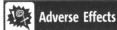 **Adverse Effects**

- See chart on pp. 243–244
- Most common adverse effects are due to cholinomimetic activity: nausea, vomiting, diarrhea, constipation, and anorexia – occur early in treatment and are associated with rapid dose titration
- Occur more often in patients over 85 years of age and in females
- Gastrointestinal symptoms (e.g., cramping, nausea, vomiting) are dose-dependent, occur more often during dose escalation and tend to resolve with time; they are associated more frequently with the nonselective inhibitor rivastigmine than with donepezil or galantamine [reported to respond to short-term use of propantheline (7.5–15 mg) or domperidone (10 mg tid) – caution due to anticholinergic effects]
- Other side effects (e.g., CNS, cardiovascular, respiratory) occur more often during the maintenance phase and are more commonly associated with rivastigmine and galantamine; these have no clear dose-dependence
- Skin reactions (redness, itching, irritation, swelling) can occur at application site of rivastigmine patch

| Tacrine |
- Elevation of liver transaminases is seen in approximately 50% of patients using dose of 160 mg/day; seen within the first 12 weeks of treatment. It returns to normal within 4–6 weeks after the discontinuation of tacrine; may not recur on drug rechallenge. Liver biopsy is not indicated in cases of uncomplicated ALT elevation. Tacrine must be discontinued if transaminase levels rise to over 5 times the upper limit of normal

 Discontinuation Syndrome

- Sudden worsening of cognitive function and behavior reported following drug withdrawal – suggest that dose be reduced by 25–50% every 1–2 weeks, with close monitoring

 Precautions

- Caution should be exercised if any of the following exists:
  - Known hypersensitivity to above compounds
  - History of syncope, bradycardia, bradyarrhythmia, sick sinus syndrome, hepatic or renal disease, obstructive urinary disease, conduction disturbances, congestive heart failure, coronary artery disease, asthma, COPD, ulcers or increased risk for ulcers or GI bleeding (concomitant use of NSAIDS or higher doses of ASA)
  - With galantamine: patients with supraventricular conduction disorders, or those taking drugs that significantly slow heart rate
  - Patient with low body weight, over 85 years of age and/or female, or with a comorbid disease
- Tacrine may have vagotonic effects on the SA and AV nodes leading to bradycardia and/or heart block. DO NOT USE in patients with conduction abnormalities, bradyarrhythmias, or sick sinus syndrome
- Anesthesia: possible exaggeration of muscle relaxation induced by succinylcholine-type drugs
- Epilepsy: reduction of seizure threshold

 Contraindications

- Tacrine is contraindicated in patients who were previously treated with the drug and developed treatment-associated jaundice confirmed by elevated total bilirubin > 3.0 mg/dl; or if there is known hypersensitivity to tacrine or acridine derivatives
- Galantamine is contraindicated in patients with severe hepatic and/or renal impairment (creatinine clearance < 9 ml/min)

 Toxicity

- Overdose can result in cholinergic crisis characterized by severe nausea, vomiting, salivation, sweating, bradycardia, hypotension followed by increasing muscle weakness, respiratory depression and convulsions

| Management |
- Institute general supportive measures
- Treatment: atropine sulfate 1 mg to 2 mg IV with subsequent doses depending on clinical response. The value of dialysis in overdosage is not known
- In asymptomatic rivastigmine overdose – hold drug for 24 h, then resume treatment. Because of the short half-life of rivastigmine, the value of dialysis in treatment of cholinergic crisis is unknown

 Pediatric Considerations

- No approved indications for use in children
- Open trials suggest that augmentation with donepezil may improve organization, mental efficiency and attention in treatment-refractory children and adolescents with ADHD or those with concomitant pervasive developmental disorders

 Geriatric Considerations

- Caution should be exercised and adverse events closely monitored when using donepezil in doses over 5 mg a day
- Galantamine plasma concentrations are 30–40% higher in the elderly than in healthy young subjects
- Galantamine reported to increase mortality in patients with mild cognitive impairment and should not be used

Cholinesterase Inhibitors (cont.)

- Women, over age 85, with low body weight are at high risk for adverse effects
- Use caution in patients with comorbid disease

 Use in Pregnancy
- Not recommended for women of childbearing potential, pregnant or nursing women

Breast Milk
- Effect unknown

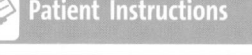 **Nursing Implications**
- Advise patients to take the drug as directed; increasing the dose will increase adverse effects while skipping doses will decrease the benefit of the drug
- Liver function should be monitored regularly in patients taking tacrine (i.e., every 2 weeks for the first 16 weeks, then monthly for two months, thereafter every 3 months)
- Advise patients not to stop the medication abruptly, as changes in behavior and/or concentration can occur
- Anticholinergic agents (including over-the-counter drugs, e.g., antinauseants) will reduce the effects of these drugs and should be avoided
- Rivastigmine patches should be kept sealed until use. Apply the first rivastigmine patch the day following the last oral dose. The location of the patch should be rotated and applied to the upper or lower back, upper arm, or chest; if there is potential for the patient to remove the patch, apply it onto an inaccessible area. Remove patch after 24 h, prior to applying the next dose – fold it in half with the adhesive sides on the inside and dispose of in waste container; wash hands after handling

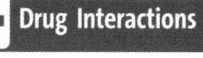 **Patient Instructions**
- For detailed patient instructions on cognition enhancers, see the Patient Information Sheet on p. 355

Drug Interactions
- Clinically significant interactions are listed below

DRUGS INTERACTING WITH DONEPEZIL

Class of Drug	Example	Interaction Effects
Antiarrhythmic	Quinidine	Inhibited metabolism of donepezil via CYP2D6
Anticholinergic	Benztropine, diphenhydramine	Antagonism of effects
Anticonvulsant	Carbamazepine, phenytoin, phenobarbital	Increased metabolism of donepezil resulting in decreased efficacy
Antidepressant	SSRI – paroxetine	May increase plasma level of donepezil by inhibiting metabolism via CYP2D6
Antifungal	Ketoconazole	Inhibited metabolism of donepezil via CYP3A4
Antipsychotic	Risperidone	Exacerbation of EPS; worsening of Parkinson's disease
Antitubercular drug	Rifampin	Increased metabolism of donepezil resulting in decreased efficacy
β-Blocker	Propranolol	May potentiate bradycardia
Bethanechol		Synergistic effects: increased nausea, vomiting and diarrhea
Dexamethasone		Increased metabolism of donepezil resulting in decreased efficacy
Neuromuscular blocker	Succinylcholine, suxamethonium	Prolonged neuromuscular blockade

DRUGS INTERACTING WITH TACRINE

Class of Drug	Example	Interaction Effects
Anticholinergic	Benztropine, chlorpheniramine	Antagonism of effects
Antidepressant	SSRI – fluvoxamine	Increased plasma level of tacrine; peak plasma level increased 5-fold and clearance decreased by 88% due to inhibited metabolism via CYP1A2
Antipsychotic	Haloperidol	Exacerbation of EPS
β-Blocker	Propranolol	May potentiate bradycardia
Bethanechol		Synergistic effects: increased nausea, vomiting and diarrhea
Cimetidine		Increased effects of tacrine (peak level by 54%)
Neuromuscular blocker	Succinylcholine, suxamethonium	Prolonged neuromuscular blockade
NSAID	Ibuprofen	Reports of delirium (with delusions, hallucinations and insomnia)
Riluzole		Elevated plasma level of both agents
Smoking		Decreased plasma level of tacrine due to induction of metabolism via CYP1A2
Theophylline		Increased plasma level of theophylline (2-fold)

DRUGS INTERACTING WITH RIVASTIGMINE

Class of Drug	Example	Interaction Effects
Anticholinergic	Benztropine, diphenhydramine	Antagonism of effects
β-Blocker	Propranolol	May potentiate bradycardia
Neuromuscular blocker	Succinylcholine, suxamethonium	Prolonged neuromuscular blockade
Nicotine		Increased clearance of rivastigmine by 23%

DRUGS INTERACTING WITH GALANTAMINE

Class of Drug	Example	Interaction Effects
Antiarrhythmic	Quinidine	Decreased clearance of galantamine by 25–30% due to inhibited metabolism via CYP2D6
Antibiotic	Erythromycin	Increased AUC of galantamine by 10% due to inhibited metabolism via CYP3A4
Anticholinergic	Benztropine, chlorpheniramine	Antagonism of effects
Antidepressant	Amitriptyline, fluoxetine, fluvoxamine Paroxetine	Decreased clearance of galantamine by 25–30% due to inhibited metabolism via CYP2D6 Increased AUC of galantamine by 40% due to inhibited metabolism via CYP2D6
Antifungal	Ketoconazole	Increased AUC of galantamine by 30% due to inhibited metabolism via CYP3A4
β-Blocker	Propranolol	May potentiate bradycardia
Cimetidine		Increased AUC of galantamine by 16%
Neuromuscular blocker	Succinylcholine, suxamethonium	Prolonged neuromuscular blockade

Memantine

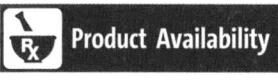
Product Availability

Chemical Class	Generic Name	Trade Name	Dosage Forms and Strengths
Aminoadamantane	Memantine	Namenda[A], Ebixa[B]	Tablet: 5 mg[A] 10 mg Solution[A]: 2 mg/ml

[A] not available in Canada, [B] not available in USA

Indications (♦ Approved)

♦ Symptomatic treatment of moderate to severe dementia of Alzheimer's type (memantine is not effective in mild AD)
- Double-blind studies report benefit on cognitive function in patients with vascular dementia[1]
- Reported to decrease delusions in moderate to severe Alzheimer's disease
- Memantine has demonstrated benefits for treatment of neuropathic pain in double-blind studies
- Post-analysis of 3 large randomized studies suggests that memantine decreases agitation/aggression and psychosis in patients with moderate to severe Alzheimer's disease[3]

General Comments

- Memantine has shown to have additive effects in patients with moderate to severe Alzheimer's disease
- Contradictory results reported when combined with cholinesterase inhibitors in patients with moderate to severe dementia
- Shown to modify the progressive symptomatic decline in global status, cognition, function and behavior in patients with moderate to severe Alzheimer's disease over 28-week trial
- Fewer viral infections reported with memantine in clinical trials (as compared to comparator drugs) due to its antiviral properties (it belongs to the same chemical class as amantadine)

Pharmacology

- Memantine has NMDA inhibitory properties thought to contribute to its clinical effectiveness, and preserves neuronal function by selectively blocking the excitotoxic effects associated with abnormal glutamate transmission
- Increases dopamine levels and reported to have antidyskinetic (antiparkinsonian) and antiviral properties

Dosing

- See chart, p. 242
- Starter packs available for easier dosage titration
- Bid administration recommended for doses above 10 mg; usual daily dose is 20 mg (see table p. 242)
- Reduce dose in patients with moderate renal impairment (CrCl 40–60 ml/min); AVOID in patients with severe impairment (< 9 ml/min)

Pharmacokinetics

- See chart, p. 242
- Food has no effect on absorption
- Crosses blood-brain barrier readily and is detectable in cerebrospinal fluid within 30 min of administration
- Alkalinization of urine (e.g., high antacid use or drastic diet change) can reduce renal elimination of memantine – monitor urine pH
- Minimal hepatic metabolism and minimal effect on CYP450 isoenzymes

Adverse Effects

- See chart, pp. 243–244
- Most common: confusion, agitation, insomnia, mild to moderate dizziness, and headaches
- Urinary incontinence and urinary tract infections reported

STOP Contraindications	• Not recommended in patients with severe renal impairment

Toxicity	• Overdose (up to 400 mg) resulted in CNS effects including restlessness, somnolence, stupor, visual hallucinations, seizures, and unconsciousness
Management	• Treatment: symptomatic • Elimination of memantine can be enhanced by acidification of urine

Pediatric Considerations	• Early data suggests benefit in children and adolescents with pervasive developmental disorders; case reports of decreasing disruptive behavior • Single-blind placebo-controlled trial suggests memantine improves social withdrawal in children with autism

Geriatric Considerations	• Caution in patients with decreased renal function • Monitor adverse effects closely

Use in Pregnancy	• Not teratogenic in animals; effects in humans unknown
Breast Milk	• Effect unknown

Nursing Implications	• Minimize the use of antacids (e.g., Milk of Magnesia, Al/Mg products) as alkalinization of urine (pH > 8) will reduce elimination and increase the effects of the drug – monitoring urine pH is recommended by some

Patient Instructions	• For detailed patient instructions on memantine, see Patient Information Sheet on p. 355

→← Drug Interactions	• Clinically significant interactions are listed below

Class of Drug	Example	Interaction Effects
Alkaline agent	Antacids, sodium bicarbonate, carbonic anhydrase inhibitors	Increased levels of memantine possible as elimination rate decreased significantly (by 80%) if pH > 8
Aminoadamantanes	Amantadine, rimantadine	Do not combine as adverse effects may be enhanced (additive effects on NMDA receptors)
Anesthetic	Ketamine	Do not combine as adverse effects may be enhanced (additive effects on NMDA receptors)
Anticonvulsant	Valproate	Synergistic effect in seizure suppression reported in animal studies
Antiinfective	Trimethoprim	Increased level of memantine due to competition for excretion via organic cation transporter-2 in the renal tubule
Hydrochlorothiazide		Reduced excretion of hydrochlorothiazide possible; bioavailability of hydrochlorothiazide reduced by 20%
Hypoglycemic agent	Metformin	Increased level of memantine due to competition for excretion via organic cation transporter-2 in the renal tubule
L-Dopa		Synergistic effect reported in animal studies

Comparison of Drugs for Treatment of Dementia

	Donepezil hydrochloride	Tacrine	Rivastigmine	Galantamine	Memantine
Pharmacology	Piperidine-based Reversible inhibitor of AChE AchE > BuChE Binds to acetylcholinesterase in the brain and has little effect on cholinesterase in serum, heart or small intestine	Acridine derivative Reversible non-selective inhibitor of AChE and BuChE	Carbamate derivative Reversible inhibitor of AChE and BuChE	Phenanthrene alkaloid Reversible inhibitor of AChE AChE > BuChE Allosteric modulator of central nicotinic receptors (may increase release of acetylcholine presynaptically)	Aminoadamantane class compound Moderate NMDA (*N*-methyl-D-aspartate) receptor channel blocker Releases dopamine
Dosing	Initial dose is 5 mg/day taken once daily; could be increased to 10 mg a day if no side effects are seen after 4–6 weeks of therapy. The maximum dose is 10 mg/day	Initial dose is 40 mg/day (10 mg qid) taken at regular intervals at least 1 h before meals for 6 weeks; ALT/SGPT must be monitored biweekly If there is no significant transaminase elevation, the dose can be increased to 80 mg/day (20 mg qid) The dose can be further increased to 120–160 mg/day at 6 week intervals if patient is tolerating treatment Dose titration and monitoring sequence should be repeated if patient suspends treatment for more than 4 weeks	Oral: Initial dose is 1.5 mg bid, given with meals for 4 weeks; increase by 1.5 mg bid every 4 weeks Usual maintenance dose: 3–6 mg bid (with meals) Patch: When switching from oral drug, Patch 5 is recommended for patients on less than 6 mg/day (do not increase dose for at least 4 weeks). Patch 10 can be used for patients on oral doses above 6 mg/day; apply patch on the next day following the last oral dose	Initial dose tabs: 4 mg bid with meals for 4 weeks; increase to 8 mg bid after 4 weeks; if no side effects occur, increase dose to 12 mg bid In moderate hepatic impairment: 4 mg od ER: initial dose is 8 mg a.m. for 4 weeks, increase to 16 mg a.m.; if no side effects occur, can increase to 24 mg a.m. after 4 weeks, if necessary (IR 4 mg bid = ER 8 mg/day)	Dose escalation (over 1 month): 5 mg od for 7 days, 5 mg bid for 7 days, 10 mg am and 5 mg in afternoon for 7 days, then 10 mg bid; can be taken with or without food In patients with CrCl < 60 ml/min, reduce dose to 5 mg bid (do not use if CrCl < 9 ml/min) Watch for confusion and hallucinations
Pharmacokinetics Bioavailability	100% and is independent of food or time of day	17–33%; food reduces bioavailability by 30–40%	36%; food delays absorption, lowers C_{max}, and increases AUC by 25%	90% (immediate release); food lowers C_{max} by 25% and delays T_{max} by 1.5 h ER: not affected by food	100% (food has no effect on absorption)
Peak plasma level	3–4 h	1–2 h	Oral = 1.4–2.6 h Patch = 10–16 h after first dose	Immediate release: 1 h ER = 4.5–5 h	3–8 h
Plasma protein binding	96%, predominantly to albumin	55–75%	40%	18%	approx. 45%
Plasma half-life	70–80 h in healthy adults; increases after multiple dose administration	2 to 4 h (independent of dose or plasma concentration)	Oral = 1–2 h (in both young and elderly) Patch = 3 h after patch removal	6–7 h	Elimination half-life 60–100 h
Liver disease	Clearance decreased by 20% in patients with liver cirrhosis	Clearance decreased with liver disease	Clearance decreased by 60% in patients with liver disease	Clearance decreased by 25–30% with liver disease	–
Renal disease	Renal impairment has no effect on clearance	Renal impairment has no effect on clearance	Clearance decreased by 65% in moderate renal impairment	In moderate and severe renal impairment AUC increased by 37% and 67%, respectively Clearance about 20% lower in females	Clearance dependent on renal function (see Dosing, above)

	Donepezil hydrochloride	Tacrine	Rivastigmine	Galantamine	Memantine
Metabolism	via CYP2D6 and 3A4 Four major metabolites, of which 2 are active	via CYP1A2 and 2D6 Has active metabolites	Metabolized by esterase enzymes – low risk of drug interactions Phenolic metabolite has approximately 10% of the activity of parent drug	via CYP2D6 and 3A4 (high risk for drug interactions)	Excreted renally (60–80%) Metabolized only to a minor extent – metabolites inactive Renal elimination rate decreased significantly in alkaline pH (> 8)
Adverse effects GI	5–10%: nausea, vomiting, diarrhea, gastric upset, constipation; > 2%: anorexia	10–30%: nausea, vomiting, diarrhea, gastric upset; 5–10%: anorexia, flatulence, constipation	10–30% nausea, vomiting, diarrhea, abdominal pain > 30% anorexia (with weight loss, especially in females)	10–30% nausea, vomiting 5–10% diarrhea 5–10% anorexia > 1% flatulence	> 5% diarrhea 2–10% constipation
CNS	5–10%: fatigue, headache; up to 18%: insomnia; 2–5%: abnormal dreams, nightmares, somnolence, agitation, activation, depression; < 2%: restlessness, aggression, irritability; < 1%: transient ischemic attack, hypokinesia, seizures Nightmares reported; manageable by switching from nighttime to morning dosing Rapid onset of manic symptoms in patients with a history of bipolar disorder reported Case report of delirium Worsening of parkinsonism and abnormal movements (restless legs, stuttering) reported Case reports of Pisa syndrome	2–10%: headache; 2–5%: nervousness, agitation, irritability, aggression, transient dysphoria, confusion, insomnia, somnolence, fatigue, depression, hallucinations, ataxia, tremor; < 2%: vertigo, paresthesias, seizures; < 1%: cerebrovascular accident, transient ischemic attack	2–10% headache > 5% sedation, asthenia > 2% anxiety, insomnia, aggression, hallucinations > 1% tremor, ataxia, abnormal gait cases of seizures Case report of Pisa syndrome	5–10% insomnia, headache, depression, fatigue, agitation 2–5% sedation, tremor < 1% paranoia, delirium, ataxia, vertigo, hypertonia, seizures	5–20% insomnia, agitation > 2% headache, confusion < 2% lethargy Reports of vivid dreams, nightmares and hallucinations
Cardiovascular	2–10%: dizziness < 2%: syncope, atrial fibrillation, hypotension; < 1%: arrhythmia, first degree AV block, congestive heart failure, symptomatic sinus bradycardia, supraventricular tachycardia, deep vein thromboses	> 10–20%: dizziness; < 2%: hypertension, hypotension; < 1%: heart failure, myocardial infarction, angina, atrial fibrillation, palpitations, tachycardia, bradycardia Heart block reported	10–20% dizziness 2–5% syncope	5–10% dizziness > 2% bradycardia, syncope (dose-related) > 1% chest pain < 1% edema, atrial fibrillation Case report of QTc prolongation	2–10% dizziness 2–5% syncope
Respiratory	> 5%: nasal congestion; < 2%: dyspnea; < 1%: pulmonary congestion, pneumonia, sleep apnea	> 5%: nasal congestion; < 2%: pharyngitis, sinusitis, bronchitis, pneumonia, dyspnea	> 2% nasal congestion < 2% dyspnea < 1% upper respiratory tract infections	> 2% nasal congestion	> 2% cough

Dementia Treatm.

Comparison of Drugs for Treatment of Dementia (cont.)

	Donepezil hydrochloride	Tacrine	Rivastigmine	Galantamine	Memantine
Special senses	< 2%: blurred vision; < 1%: dry eyes, glaucoma	< 2%: conjunctivitis < 1%: dry eyes, glaucoma	> 2% tinnitus	–	–
Skin	2–10% flushing	2–10%: hot flushes, rash	> 5% increased sweating Flushing, skin reactions (e.g., rash, redness, inflammation at site of patch application)	–	Cases of epidermal necrolysis
Urogenital	< 2%: pruritus and urticaria < 2%: frequent urination, nocturia; < 1%: prostatic hypertrophy; > 5%: incontinence	< 2%: increased sweating > 2%: frequent urination, incontinence, urinary tract infection; < 1%: haematuria, urinary retention	> 5% urinary tract infection > 2% frequent urination, incontinence	> 5% urinary tract infection > 2% hematuria > 1% incontinence < 1% urinary retention	> 5% incontinence > 2% urinary tract infections < 1% increased libido
Musculoskeletal	5–10%: muscle cramps, pain < 2% arthritis	> 5%: myalgia < 2% arthralgia, arthritis	< 1% arthralgia, myalgia, pain	5–10% muscle cramps	< 1% hypertonia
Liver	–	up to 50%: elevated ALT/SGPT	–	–	Elevated ALT/SGPT Case of liver failure
Other	< 2%: dehydration; < 1%: blood dyscrasias, jaundice, renal failure	< 2%: chills, fever, malaise, peripheral edema; < 1%: blood dyscrasias	< 1% dehydration, hypokalemia < 1% nose bleeds	2–5% anemia < 1% blood dyscrasias	Case of aplastic anemia Cases of pancreatitis and renal failure

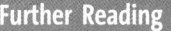 **Further Reading**

References

1 Baskys A, Hou AC. Vascular dementia: Pharmacological treatment approaches and perspectives. Clin Interv Aging. 2007;2(3):327–335.

2 Qaseem A, Snow V, Cross JT Jr, et al. Current Pharmacologic Treatment of Dementia: A Clinical Practice Guideline from the American College of Physicians and the American Academy of Family Physicians. Ann Intern Med. 2008;148(5):370–378.

3 Wilcock GK, Ballard CG, Cooper JA, et al. Memantine for agitation/aggression and psychosis in moderately severe to severe Alzheimer's disease: A pooled analysis of 3 studies. J Clin Psychiatry. 2008;69:341–348.

Additional Suggested Reading

• Academic Highlights. New paradigms in the treatment of Alzheimer's disease. J Clin Psychiatry. 2006;67(12):2002–2013.

• Alexopoulos GS, Jeste DV, Chung H, et al. The Expert Consensus Guideline Series: Treatment of dementia and its behavioral disturbances. Postgrad Med. Special Report. 2005;1–111.

• Birks J. Cholinesterase inhibitors for Alzheimer's disease. Cochrane Database Syst. Rev. 2006 Jan 25;CD 005593.

• Feldman HH, Pirttila T, Dartigues JF, et al. Analyses of mortality risk in patients with dementia treated with galantamine. Acta Neurol Scand. 2009;119(1):22–31.

• Geerts H, Grossberg GT. Pharmacology of acetylcholinesterase inhibitors and N-methyl-D-aspartate receptors for combination therapy in the treatment of Alzheimer's disease. J Clin Pharmacol. 2006;46 Suppl 1:S8–S16.

• Jann MW, Shirley KL, Small GW. Clinical pharmacokinetics and pharmacodynamics of cholinesterase inhibitors. Clin Pharmacokinetics. 2002;41(10):719–739.

• Mintzer JE. The search for better noncholinergic treatment options for Alzheimer's Disease. J Clin Psychiatry. 2003;64 Suppl 9:S18–S22.

• Moellentin D, Picone C, Leadbetter E. Memantine-induced myoclonus and delirium exacerbated by trimethoprim. Ann Pharmacother. 2008;42(3):443-447.

• Nelson, MW, Buchanan RW. Galantamine-induced QTc prolongation. J Clin Psychiatry. 2006;67(1):166–167.

• Robinson DM, Keating GM. Memantine: A review of its use in Alzheimer's Disease. Drugs. 2006;66(11):1515–1534.

• Rubey RN. The cholinesterase inhibitors. Int Drug Ther Newsl. 2003;38(11):81–87.

• Sano M. Noncholinergic treatment options for Alzheimer's Disease. J Clin Psychiatry. 2003;64 Suppl 9:S23–S28.

Product Availability

Chemical Class	Generic Name	Trade Name(A)	Dosage Forms and Strengths
Antiandrogen/Progestogen	Cyproterone	Androcur Androcur Depot	Tablets: 50 mg Injection (depot): 100 mg/ml
Progestogen	Medroxyprogesterone	Provera DepoProvera	Tablets: 100 mg Injection (depot): 50 mg/ml, 150 mg/ml
Luteinizing hormone-releasing hormone (LHRH)/gonadotropin-releasing hormone (GnRH) agonist	Leuprolide	Lupron Lupron Depot	Injection: 5 mg/ml Injection (depot): 1 mg/0.2 ml(B), 3.75 mg/vial, 7.5 mg/vial, 11.25 mg/vial, 15 mg/vial(B), 22.5 mg/vial, 30 mg/vial
	Goserelin	Zoladex LA Zoladex	Implant (depot): 10.8 mg/vial Implant (depot): 3.6 mg/vial

(A) Generic preparations may be available, (B) Not marketed in Canada

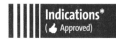 **Indications***
(👍 Approved)

* not approved

- Reduction of sexual arousal and libido (usually for sexual offenders)
- Inappropriate or disruptive sexual behavior in patients with dementia

💬 **General Comments**

- Pharmacotherapy should be combined with concurrent supportive or intensive psychotherapy, as well as treatment of any comorbid psychiatric conditions
- Medroxyprogesterone and cyproterone are used for partial sex drive reduction. LHRH (GnRH) agonists are used for more serious sexual difficulties in which ablation of testosterone of testicular origin is indicated
- Efficacy: 35–95%, depending on type of sexual problem and motivation of patient
- Medroxyprogesterone and cyproterone are not effective in some patients despite high doses and over 90% reduction of testosterone levels
- Leuprolide and goserelin may cause a transient increase (over 2 weeks or more) in luteinizing hormone and testosterone, followed by a dramatic decrease and suppression of the hormones (while not clinically significant, the transient hormone increase does not occur with LHRH antagonists)
- Seek consultation with an internist/endocrinologist prior to initiation of therapy; thereafter yearly consultation and bone density monitoring is recommended (see Monitoring Recommendations, p. 247)
- Longer-acting depot injections (e.g., leuprolide 30 mg q 4 months) have been found of benefit in high risk sex offenders
- Ablation of testosterone of nontesticular origin has been utilized in very high-risk offenders with adjunctive treatment with peripheral androgen blockers (e.g., finasteride)
- Inhibitors of adrenal androgen synthesis (e.g., abiraterone – small molecule inhibitor of cytochrome P17, a key enzyme in androgen synthesis) show promise as potent sex-drive reducing agents

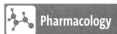 **Pharmacology**

- GnRH agonists interfere with synthesis of testosterone
- Lower plasma testosterone levels; androgen levels decline over 2 to 4 weeks; with medroxyprogesterone and cyproterone androgen levels may rise somewhat over time, without necessarily a parallel increase in sexual drive

Sex-Drive Depressants (cont.)

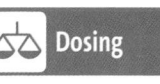 **Dosing**	• See p. 248 • GnRH agonist medication is relatively non-titratable in terms of testosterone suppression effects • Depot injections of medroxyprogesterone and cyproterone may initially be prescribed every 2 weeks with monitoring of serum testosterone and sexual self-report. Often, weekly injection schedule is necessary to achieve good behavioral control and testosterone suppression. Depot injection of LHRH agonists are available in 1–month, 3–month and 4–month preparations • Anaphylaxis, while reported in the literature with leuprolide, has rarely been observed in clinical practice; however, some clinicians feel that a test dose of short-acting leuprolide acetate is indicated
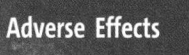 **Adverse Effects**	• See p. 247 • The main serious long-term side effects of LHRH is decreased bone density; other risk factors include smoking, alcohol use, low body mass index, and endocrine problems [Treatment with bisphosphonates, calcium, vitamin D, or even estrogens has been found to arrest or even reverse this side effect]
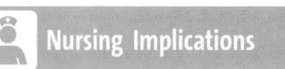 **Nursing Implications**	• Leuprolide: reconstitute drug only with 1 ml of diluent provided. Shake well. Suspension is stable for 24 h and can be stored at room temperature. Inject using 22 gauge needle (or larger). Injection may rarely cause irritation (burning, itching, and swelling) • Goserelin pellet is injected subcutaneously into the anterior abdominal wall • Drug must be taken consistently to maintain effect; report any changes in mood or behavior of patient to the physician
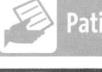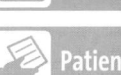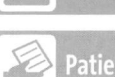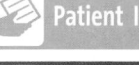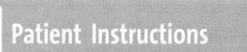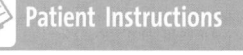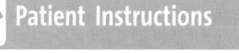 **Medicolegal Issues**	• As sex drive reduction is not an approved indication, formal patient consent (with an appropriate consent form) should be sought • Use of these drugs involves complex issues in regard to consent, as the patients are often involved with the legal system
Patient Instructions	• For detailed patient instructions on sex-drive-depressants, see the Patient Information Sheet on p. 357
Drug Interactions	• Clinically significant interactions are listed below

Class of Drug	Example	Interaction Effects
Rifampin		**INTERACTIONS WITH MEDROXYPROGESTERONE** Decreased plasma level of medroxyprogesterone due to increased metabolism
Alcohol		**INTERACTIONS WITH CYPROTERONE** Alcohol may reduce the antiandrogenic effect of cyproterone when used for hypersexuality
Finasteride		Additive effects on testosterone reduction

Comparison of Sex-Drive Depressants

	Cyproterone	Medroxyprogesterone	Leuprolide	Goserelin
Dosing	Oral: 100–500 mg/day Depot: 100–600 mg/week	Oral: 100–600 mg/day Depot: 100–700 mg/week	Depot: 3.75 – 7.5 mg/month; 11.25 or 22.5 mg q 3 months; 30 mg q 4 months	3.6 mg/month; or 10.8 mg q 3 months
Pharmacokinetics Peak plasma level Half-life	Oral: 3–4 h Depot: 3.4 h Oral: 33–42 h Depot: 4 days	Oral: not established Depot: few days Oral: 30 h Depot: not established Metabolized via CYP3A4	Not established	Not established 4.2 h (males); 2–3 h (females) half-life increased to 12 h in renal impairmen
Adverse effects CNS	Atrophy of seminiferous tubules with chronic use (possibly reversible if drug stopped) Gynecomastia (15–20%) [report that pretreatment with irradiation therapy will prevent this side effect] Decrease in body hair and sebum production, weight gain Decreased bone density Fatigue, depression (5–10%)	Decreased sperm count, hot flashes, sweating, impotence Increased appetite and weight gain Dyspnea, hypertension, edema, muscle cramps, GI upset Mild depression, lethargy, nervousness, insomnia, nightmares, headaches	Decreased sperm count, atrophy of seminiferous tubules, impotence Hot flashes (60%) Sweating, rash, edema (3%), nausea, other GI effects, loss of body hair, myalgia, spasms, lethargy, dyspnea Decreased bone density Anxiety, insomnia	Decreased sperm count, atrophy of seminiferous tubules, impotence Hot flashes Sweating, rash, edema (3%), nausea, other GI effects, loss of body hair, myalgia, spasms, dyspnea Decreased bone density Lethargy
Precautions	May impair carbohydrate metabolism, fasting blood glucose, and glucose tolerance test Hypercalcemia and changes in plasma lipids can occur Alcohol use may reduce the antiandrogenic effect Deep vein thrombosis and thromboembolism (smoking may increase risk)	May decrease glucose tolerance Monitor patients with conditions aggravated by fluid retention, e.g., asthma, migraine Deep vein thrombosis and thromboembolism (smoking may increase risk)		Transient elevation of BUN, creatinine, testosterone, and acid phosphatase reported
Contraindications	Liver disease, thromboembolic disorders Active pituitary pathology	Liver disease; thromboembolic disorders Active pituitary pathology	Hypersensitivity to drug Active pituitary pathology Disorders of bone demineralization (relative contraindication)	Hypersensitivity to drug Active pituitary pathology Disorders of bone demineralization (relative contraindication)
Toxicity	No reports	No reports	No reports	No reports

Comparison of Sex-Drive Depressants (cont.)

	Cyproterone	Medroxyprogesterone	Leuprolide	Goserelin
Lab Tests/Monitoring				
Pretreatment	Serum testosterone, prolactin, LH, FSH, liver function, Hb, WBC, glucose blood pressure, weight	Serum testosterone, prolactin, LH, FSH, liver function, Hb, WBC, glucose blood pressure, weight	Serum testosterone, prolactin, LH, FSH, ECG, BUN, creatinine, CBC, liver function, bone density scan	Serum testosterone, prolactin, LH, FSH, ECG, BUN, creatinine, CBC, liver function, bone density scan
Chronic	Testosterone: q 6 months LH, FSH, and prolactin: q 6 months Blood pressure, weight: q 3 months	Testosterone: q 6 months LH, FSH, and prolactin: q 6 months Blood pressure, weight	Testosterone: q 1 month, for 4 months, then q 6 months BUN, creatinine: q 6 months; LH, FSH, and prolactin: q 6 months Bone density: q 1 year	Testosterone: q 1 month for 4 months, then q 6 months BUN, creatinine: q 6 months LH, FSH, and prolactin: q 6 months Bone density: q 1 year

 Further Reading

- Bradford JMW. The neurobiology, neuropharmacology and pharmacological treatment of the paraphilias and compulsive sexual behaviour. Can J Psychiatry. 2001;46(1):26–34.
- Briken P, Hill A, Berner W. Pharmacotherapy of paraphilias with long-acting agonists of luteinizing hormone-releasing hormone. A systematic review. J Clin Psychiatry. 2003;64(8):890–897.
- Briken P, Kafka MP. Pharmacological treatments for paraphilic patients and sexual offenders. Curr Opin Psychiatry. 2007;20(6):609–613.
- Hsieh AC, Ryan CJ. Novel concepts in androgen receptor blockade. Cancer J. 2008;14(1):11–14.
- Saleh FM, Berlin FS. Sex hormones, neurotransmitters, and psychopharmacological treatments in men with paraphilic disorders. J Child Sex Abuse. 2003;12(3–4):233–253.

DRUGS OF ABUSE

General Comments

- This chapter gives a general overview of common drugs of abuse and is not intended to deal in detail with all agents, or be a complete guide to treatment
- Slang names of street drugs change rapidly and vary with country, region, and drug subculture
- Drugs of abuse can be classified as follows:

Chemical Class	Agent[A]	Page
Alcohol	Alcohol	See p. 252
Stimulants	Examples: Amphetamine, crystal meth Cocaine Sympathomimetics (incl. caffeine)	See p. 257
Hallucinogens	Examples: Lysergic acid diethylamide Cannabis Phencyclidine	See p. 262
Opiates/Narcotics	Examples: Morphine Heroin Pentazocine	See p. 269
Inhalants/Aerosols	Examples: Glue Paint thinner	See p. 273
Gamma hydroxy butyrate		See p. 275
Sedative/Hypnotics	Examples: Flunitrazepam Barbiturates* Benzodiazepines* Hypnotics*	See p. 277 See p. 174 See p. 158 See p. 174
Nicotine*	Examples: Cigarettes, cigars	

[A] Only includes examples of most commonly used substances; * Not dealt with specifically in this chapter

Definitions

Drug Abuse	• Acute or chronic intake of any substance that: (a) has no recognized medical use, (b) is used inappropriately in terms of its medical indications or its dose
Drug Dependence	
a) Behavioral aspects	• Craving or desire for repeated administration of a drug to provide a desired effect or to avoid discomfort
b) Physical aspects	• A physiological state of adaptation to a drug which usually results in development of tolerance to drug effects and withdrawal symptoms when the drug is stopped
Addiction	• intense persistent drug use associated with a strong desire to continue use, with disregard to consequences or personal harm
Tolerance	• Phenomenon in which increasing doses of a drug are needed to produce a desired effect, or effect intensity decreases with repeated use

Drugs of Abuse (cont.)

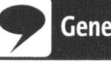 **General Comments**

- The effect which any drug of abuse has on an individual depends on a number of variables:
  1. dose (amount ingested, injected, sniffed, etc.)
  2. potency and purity of drug
  3. route of administration
  4. past experience of the user (this will predispose to selective behavioral response either on a pharmacologic or conditioning basis)
  5. present circumstances, i.e., environment, other people present, whether other drugs are taken concurrently
  6. personality and genetic predisposition of user
  7. age of user
  8. clinical status of user, i.e., type of psychiatric illness, degree of recent stress or loss, occurrence of a vulnerable phase of a circadian or ultradian rhythm, user's expectations, and present feelings
- Some users may have different experiences with the same drug on different occasions. They may encounter both pleasant and unpleasant effects during the same drug experience
- Many street drugs are adulterated with other chemicals, and may not be what the individual thinks they are; potency and purity of street drugs vary greatly
- It remains unclear whether drugs of abuse cause persistent psychiatric disorders in otherwise healthy individuals, or whether they precipitate latent psychiatric illness in predisposed individuals. Overall, in non-treatment community samples, it is estimated over 50% of drug users have at least one other psychiatric disorder and those with certain psychiatric disorders (e.g., bipolar disorder, schizophrenia) are more likely to abuse substances than the general population
- Dual diagnosis refers to the co-occurence of substance use disorder in a patient with a severe psychiatric illness. Substance abuse can occur during any phase of the psychiatric illness; it is associated with a variety of physical/psychosocial problems, and can destabilize treatment and lead to relapse
- Substance abuse has been associated with earlier onset of schizophrenia, decreased treatment responsiveness of positive symptoms and poor clinical functioning; similarly decreased treatment responsiveness in bipolar disorder can occur

 **Detection of Drugs of Abuse**

- Factors affecting detection of a drug in urine depend on dose and route of administration, drug metabolism, and characteristics of screening and confirmation assays; for instance:
  − Amphetamines in urine can be positive for up to 5 days
  − Marihuana (THC) in urine can be positive 2–4 days after acute use and for up to 1–3 months after chronic use
  − Cocaine can be positive, as its metabolite, in urine for up to 1.5 days after IV use, for up to 1 week with street doses used by different routes, and for up to 3 weeks after use of very high doses
  − Heroin can be positive, as its metabolite, in urine for up to 1.5 days when administered parenterally or intranasally

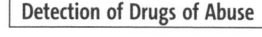 **Pharmacology**

- Research data have demonstrated that every drug of abuse increases dopamine activity in the nucleus accumbens of the brain; the increased dopamine is suggested to be associated with the pleasurable effects produced by the drug

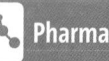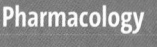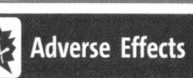 **Adverse Effects**

- See pharmacological/psychiatric effects under specific drugs
- Reactions are unpredictable and depend on the potency and purity of drug taken
- Psychiatric reactions secondary to drug abuse may occur more readily in individuals already at risk
- Renal, hepatic, cardiorespiratory, neurological, and gastrointestinal complications as well as encephalopathies can occur with chronic abuse of specific agents
- Intravenous drug users are at risk for infection, including cellulitis, hepatitis and AIDS
- Impurities in street drugs (especially if inhaled or injected) can cause tissue and organ damage (blood vessels, kidney, lungs, and liver)
- Psychological dependence can occur; the drug becomes central to a person's thoughts, emotions, and activities, resulting in craving
- Physical dependence can occur; the body adapts to the presence of the drug and withdrawal symptoms occur when the drug is stopped, resulting in addiction

- See specific agents
- Identification of drug(s) abused is important; toxicology may help in identification whenever multiple or combination drug use is suspected
- If 2 or more drugs have been chronically abused, withdraw one drug at a time, starting with the one that potentially represents the greatest problem: e.g., in alcohol/sedative abuse, withdraw the alcohol first

Treatment

Acute

- Treatment of substance use disorder presents special challenges in patients with a diagnosed psychiatric disorder and is best done with an integrated treatment program that combines pharmacotherapy with psychosocial interventions
- See specific agents
- The diagnosis of the type of substance abused can be difficult in an Emergency Room when a patient presents as floridly psychotic, intoxicated or delirious. Blood and urine screens take time, therefore diagnosis must include mental status, physical and neurological examination, as well as a drug history, whenever possible; collateral history should be sought
- In severe cases, monitor vitals and fluid intake
- Agitation can be treated conservatively by talking with the patient and providing reassurance until the drug wears off (i.e., "talking down"). When conservative approaches are inadequate or if symptoms persist, pharmacological intervention should be considered
- Avoid low-potency antipsychotics due to anticholinergic effects, hypotension, and tachycardia

Long-Term

- The presence of comorbid psychiatric disorders in substance abusers can adversely influence outcome in treatment of the substance abuse as well as the psychiatric disorder

Further Reading

- Antoniou T, Tseng AL. Interactions between recreational drugs and antiretroviral agents. Ann Pharmacother. 2002;36(10):1598–1613.
- Fiore MC, Jaén CR, Baker TB, et al. Treating tobacco use and dependence: 2008 update. US Department of Health and Human Services, 2008. Available from http://www.ncbi.nlm.nih.gov/books/bv.fcgi?rid=hstat2.chapter.28163 (Accessed March 16, 2009).

Alcohol

💬 **General Comments**	• Slang: Booze, hooch, juice, brew • Up to 50% of alcoholics meet the criteria for lifetime diagnosis of major depression • Related problems include withdrawal symptoms, physical violence, loss of control when drinking, surreptitious drinking, change in tolerance to alcohol, deteriorating job performance, change in social interactions, increased risk for stroke, and death from motor vehicle accidents
Pharmacological/ Psychiatric Effects	• Signs and symptoms are associated with blood alcohol level of approximately 34 mmol/L (higher in chronic users; 60–70 mmol/L) • Effects of a single drink occur within 15 min and last approximately 60 min, depending on amount taken; renal elimination is about 10 g alcohol per hour (about 30 ml (1 oz) whiskey or 1 bottle of regular beer). Blood alcohol level declines by 4–7 mmol per hour. • Tolerance decreases with age and with compromised brain function
Acute	• Disinhibition, relaxation, euphoria, agitation, drowsiness, impaired cognition, judgment, and memory, perceptual and motor dysfunction ☞ **Acute alcohol intake decreases hepatic metabolism of co-administered drugs by competition for microsomal enzymes**
Chronic	• Chronic use results in an increased capacity to metabolize alcohol and a concurrent CNS tolerance; psychological as well as physical dependence may occur; hepatic metabolism decreases with liver cirrhosis ☞ **Chronic alcohol use increases hepatic metabolism of co-administered drugs**
Physical	• Hand tremor, dyspepsia, diarrhea, morning nausea and vomiting, polyuria, impotence, pancreatitis, headache, hepatomegaly, peripheral neuropathy
Mental	• Memory blackouts, nightmares, insomnia, hallucinations, paranoia, intellectual impairment, dementia, Wernicke-Korsakoff syndrome, and other organic mental disorders • Chronic alcohol use by patients with schizophrenia suggested to be associated with more florid symptoms, more re-hospitalizations, poorer long-term outcome and increased risk of tardive dyskinesia
Pharmakokinetics	• Absorption occurs slowly from the stomach, and rapidly from the upper small intestine • Approximately 10% of ingested alcohol is eliminated by first-pass metabolism (less in females); percentage decreases as amount consumed increases • Alcohol is distributed in body fluids (is not fat soluble) and the blood alcohol level depends on gender, age, and body fluid volume/fat ratio • Metabolized in the liver primarily by alcohol dehydrogenase, CYP2E1 and CYP450 reductase (also by CYP3A4 and CYP1A2); activity of CYP2E1 is increased 10-fold in chronic heavy drinkers
☠ **Toxicity**	• Hazardous alcohol consumption: 3 standard drinks for females and 4 for males (standard drink = approximately 4 oz or 120 ml wine, 1 bottle of beer, 1.5 oz or 45 ml spirits); the legal blood alcohol concentration threshold for impaired driving in the Criminal Code of Canada is 80 mg in 100 ml blood (0.08 or 80 mg%) • Risk increases when combined with drugs with CNS depressant activity • Symptoms include: CNS depression, decreased or absent deep tendon reflexes, cardiac dysfunction, flushed skin progressing to cyanosis, hypoglycemia, hypothermia, peripheral vasodilation, shock, respiratory depression, and coma
D/C Discontinuation Syndrome	• Occurs after chronic use (i.e., drinking for more than 3 days, more than 500 ml of spirits or equivalent per day) • Most effects seen within 5 days after stopping
Mild Withdrawal	• Insomnia, irritability, headache • Usually transient and self-limiting
Severe Reactions	• Phase I: begins within hours of cessation and lasts 3–5 days. Symptoms: tremor, tachycardia, diaphoresis, labile BP, nausea, vomiting, anxiety • Phase II: perceptual disturbances (usually visual or auditory)

- Phase III: 10–15% untreated alcohol withdrawal patients reach this phase; seizures (usually tonic-clonic) last 0.5–4 min and can progress to status epilepticus
- Phase IV: Delirium tremens (DTs) usually occurs after 72 h; includes autonomic hyperactivity and severe hyperthermia; mortality rate of patients who reach phase IV is <1% because treatment is usually given early
- Wernicke's encephalopathy can occur in patients with thiamine deficiency

Protracted Abstinence Syndrome	- Patients may experience subtle withdrawal symptoms that can last from weeks to months – include sleep dysregulation, anxiety, irritability and mood instability - Cognitive impairment from chronic alcohol use will persist for several weeks after abstinence achieved - Individuals are at high risk for relapse during this period - Hepatic metabolism of co-administered drugs may decrease following abstinence from chronic alcohol use

 Precautions
- Increased risk of drug toxicity possible in patients with alcohol-induced liver impairment or cirrhosis
- Risk and type of drug-drug interaction varies with acute and chronic alcohol consumption

 Use in Pregnancy
- Drinking alcohol while pregnant increases the risk of problems in fetal development; fetal alcohol spectrum disorder (FASD) indicates full range of possible effects on the fetus; fetal alcohol syndrome (FAS) is characterized by severe effects of alcohol, including brain damage, facial deformities, and growth deficits. Infants should be reassessed and followed up regularly as early intervention improves long-term educational outcomes
- Withdrawal reactions reported; seen 24–48 hours after birth if mother is intoxicated at birth

Breast Milk
- Milk levels attain 90–95% of blood levels; prolonged intake can be detrimental

 Treatment
- In acute intoxication minimize stimulation; effects will diminish as blood alcohol level declines (rate of 4–7 mmol/L per hour)
- Withdrawal reactions following chronic alcohol use may require
  a) vitamin supplementation (thiamine 50 mg orally or IM for at least 3 days) to prevent or treat Wernicke-Korsakoff syndrome (level of evidence 3[1])
  b) benzodiazepine for symptomatic relief (to control agitation) and to prevent seizures (chlordiazepoxide, lorazepam, diazepam, or oxazepam); these drugs reduce mortality, reduce the duration of symptoms and are associated with fewer complications compared to antipsychotic drugs (level of evidence 1[1]); risk of transferring dependence from alcohol to benzodiazepine is small; loading dose strategy used with diazepam (i.e., patient dosed until light somnolence is achieved (level of evidence 3[1]); its long duration of action prevents breakthrough symptoms and possible withdrawal seizures)
  c) hydration and electrolyte correction
  d) high potency antipsychotic (e.g., haloperidol, zuclopenthixol) to treat behavior disturbances and hallucinations (level of evidence 3[1])
  e) beta-blockers may be considered for use in conjunction with benzodiazepines in select patients for control of persistent hypertension or tachycardia (level of evidence 3[1])
- SSRIs may be useful as treatment for late-onset alcoholics, or alcoholism complicated by comorbid major depression. Buspirone may have some utility for treating alcoholics with comorbid anxiety disorder
- Naltrexone and acamprosate reported to be effective adjuncts to treatment for relapse prevention following alcohol detoxification, see pp. 282 and 284; the efficacy of each is increased significantly when combined with psychosocial treatments
- See p. 279 for use of disulfiram in treatment

Alcohol (cont.)

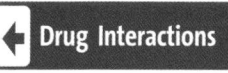 **Drug Interactions**

• Clinically significant interactions are listed below

Class of Drug	Example	Interaction Effects
Analgesic	Acetaminophen	Chronic excessive alcohol use increases susceptibility to acetaminophen-induced hepatotoxicity due to enhanced formation of toxic metabolites through CYP2E1 induction
	Salicylates	Increased gastric bleeding with ASA; reduced peak plasma concentration of ASA reported ASA may increase blood alcohol concentration by reducing ethanol oxidation by gastric alcohol dehydrogenase
	NSAIDs	Increased risk of gastric hemorrhage
Anesthetic	Propofol	Chronic consumption increases the dose of propofol required to induce anesthesia
	Enflurane, halothane	Chronic consumption increases risk of liver damage
Antibiotic	Cephalosporins, chloramphenicol, nitrofurantoin, griseofulvin	Disulfiram-like reaction with nausea, hypotension, flushing, headache, tachycardia
	Doxycycline	Chronic alcohol use induces metabolism and decreases plasma level of doxycycline
	Erythromycin	May increase gastric emptying leading to faster alcohol absorption in the small intestine
Anticoagulant	Warfarin	Chronic alcohol use induces warfarin metabolism and decreases hypoprothrombinemic effect Acute alcohol use can impair warfarin metabolism and may increase risk of hemorrhage
Anticonvulsant	Barbiturates, phenytoin	Additive CNS effects Decreased plasma level of ethanol Acute intoxication inhibits phenobarbital and phenytoin metabolism; chronic intoxication enhances metabolism
	Valproic acid, divalproex	Displaces alcohol from protein binding and potentiates intoxicating effect
Antidepressant	Tricyclic	Additive CNS and hypotensive effects Short-term or acute use reduces first-pass metabolism of the antidepressant and increases its plasma level Imipramine and desipramine clearance is increased in patients with chronic alcoholic dependence and during the first month after detoxification; delay in ethanol absorption with antidepressant use
	SSRI	Rate of fluvoxamine absorption increased by ethanol
	NaSSA	Additive CNS effects
	Irreversible MAOIs	Possible risk of hypertensive crisis with consumption of beer or wine, due to tyramine content (see p. 51)
Antifungal	Metronidazole, ketoconazole, furazolidone	Disulfiram-like reaction
Antipsychotic		Additive CNS effects Extrapyramidal side effects may be worsened by alcohol
Antitubercular drug	Isoniazid	Increased risk of hepatotoxicity Tyramine-containing alcoholic beverages may cause a hypertensive reaction (MAOI) Disulfiram-like reaction
Antiviral	Abacavir	Increased AUC of abacavir by 41%
Ascorbic acid		Increased ethanol clearance

Class of Drug	Example	Interaction Effects
Benzodiazepine	Lorazepam, alprazolam, diazepam	Potentiation of CNS effects Alprazolam reported to increase aggression in moderate alcohol drinkers Brain concentrations of various benzodiazepines altered by ethanol: triazolam and estazolam concentrations decreased, diazepam concentration increased, no change with chlordiazepoxide
Ca-channel blocker	Verapamil	Increased concentration of ethanol due to inhibited metabolism
Cardiovascular drug	Hydralazine, guanethidine, methyldopa, nitroglycerin	Increased dizziness or fainting upon standing up
Chloral hydrate		Additive CNS effects Increased plasma level of metabolite of chloral hydrate (trichloroethanol), which inhibits the metabolism of alcohol and increases blood alcohol levels
CNS depressants	Hypnotics, benzodiazepines, sedating antihistamines, muscle relaxants, valerian	Potentiation of CNS effects. Caution with high doses due to risk of respiratory depression Use of lorazepam in intoxicated individuals has been reported to decrease respiration
Disulfiram		Flushing, sweating, palpitations, headache due to formation of acetaldehyde (see p. 279)
H₂ blocker	Cimetidine, ranitidine	Inhibit alcohol dehydrogenase in the stomach, reduce first-pass metabolism of alcohol and increase gastric emptying Peak blood alcohol level increased by 92% with cimetidine and 34% with ranitidine – data contradictory (no effect with famotidine)
Hypoglycemic	Chlorpropamide, tolbutamide, glyburide	Flushing, sweating, palpitations, headache due to formation of acetaldehyde; disulfiram-like reaction Acute alcohol use decreases metabolism of tolbutamide; chronic use increases it Increased risk of hypoglycemia
Immunosuppressive	Methotrexate Pimecrolimus, tacrolimus	Increased risk of liver damage Facial flushing
Milk	Metformin	Possible increased levels of lactic acid in the blood after alcohol consumption Decreased ethanol absorption by delaying gastric emptying
Muscle relaxant	Carisoprodol, cyclobenzaprine, baclofen Metoclopramide	May produce opiate-like reaction with dizziness, weakness, confusion, agitation, and euphoria Increases absorption rate of alcohol by speeding gastric emptying
Narcotic	All opioids All slow-release opioids (Morphine sustained-release: Kadian) Methadone Propoxyphene	Additive CNS effects; caution with excessive doses due to risk of respiratory depression Alcohol can speed the release of opioids into the bloodstream by dissolving the slow-release system (not all products affected; no problems noted with Codeine Contin, Hydromorph Contin, MS Contin, and OxyContin). Use caution with other slow-release products Acute alcohol ingestion can slow methadone metabolism, increasing risk for toxicity Alcohol appears to increase bioavailability of propoxyphene by reducing first-pass metabolism
Nicotine	Smoking	Positive correlation reported between cigarette smoking and alcohol use; alcohol potentiates rewarding effects of nicotine
Nitrates	Isosorbide, nitroglycerin	Disulfiram-like reaction possible
NSAIDs	Naproxen, diclofenac, ibuprofen	Increased risk of gastric hemorrhage
Stimulant	Cocaine	Additive effects; increased heart rate; variable effect on blood pressure Reports of enhanced hepatotoxicity; increased risk of sudden death with combined use (18-fold) Combined use reported to increase risk-taking behavior and result in more impulsive decision making and poorer performance on tests of learning and memory
Tianeptine		Rate of tianeptine absorption decreased; plasma level decreased by 30%

Alcohol (cont.)

Further Reading

Reference

[1] Mayo-Smith MF, Beecher LH, Fischer TL, et al. Management of alcohol withdrawal delirium. An evidence-based practice guideline. Arch Intern Med. 2004;164(13):1405–1412.

Additional Suggested Reading

- Alcohol-related drug interactions. Pharmacist's Letter/Prescriber's Letter 2008;24(1):240106
- Anton RF. Pharmacologic approaches to the management of alcoholism. J Clin Psychiatry. 2001;62 Suppl 20:S11–S17.
- Centre for Addiction and Mental Health. Exposure to psychotropic medications and other substances during pregnancy and lactation: A handbook for health care providers. Toronto (Canada): Centre for Addiction and Mental Health; 2007.
- Kenna GA, McGeary JE, Swift RM. Pharmacotherapy, pharmacogenomics, and the future of alcohol dependence treatment, Part 1 and 2. Am J Health Syst Pharm. 2004;61(21):2272–2299, and 2004;61(22):2380–2388.
- National Institute on Alcohol Abuse and Alcoholism. Clinical Guidelines-Related Resources. Bethesda, MD: National Insitute on Alcohol Abuse and Alcoholism. Available from: www.niaaa.nih.gov/guide
- New South Wales Department of Health. National clinical guidelines for the management of drug use during pregnancy, birth and the early development years of the newborn. 2006. Available from http://www.health.nsw.gov.au/pubs/2006/pdf/ncg_druguse.pdf
- Sherwood Brown E. The challenges of dual diagnosis: Managing substance abuse in severe mental illness. J Clin Psychiatry. 2006;67(Suppl.7):S1–S35.
- Srisurapanant M, Jarusuraisin N. Opioid antagonists for alcohol dependence. Cochrane Database Syst. Rev. 2002;2:CD001867.
- Trachtenberg AI, Fleming MF. Diagnosis & treatment of drug abuse in family practice. National Institute On Drug Abuse. Available from www.drugabuse.gov/Diagnosis-Treatment/diagnosis.html.
- Weathermon R, Crabb DW. Alcohol and medication interactions. *Alcohol Res Health*. 1999;23(1):40–53.
- Wilkins JN. Traditional pharmacotherapy of alcohol dependence. J Clin Psychiatry. 2006;67(Suppl. 14):14–22.

Stimulants

 Pharmacological/ Psychiatric Effects

- Differ somewhat depending on type of drug taken, dose, and route of administration
- Effects occur rapidly, especially when drug used parenterally
- Acute toxicity reported with doses ranging from 5 to 630 mg of amphetamine; chronic users can ingest up to 1000 mg/day
- Following acute toxicity, psychiatric state usually clears within one week of amphetamine discontinuation

Physical
- Elevated BP, tachycardia, increased respiration and temperature, sweating, pallor, tremors, decreased appetite, dilated pupils, reduced fatigue, insomnia, increased sensory awareness, increased sexual arousal/libido combined with a delay in ejaculation

Mental
- Euphoria, exhilaration, alertness, improved task performance, exacerbation of obsessive-compulsive symptoms
- Methamphetamine reported to induce paranoia and hallucinations in non-schizophrenic subjects; flashbacks reported

High Doses
- Anxiety, excitation, panic attacks, grandiosity, delusions, visual, auditory and tactile hallucinations, paranoia, mania, delirium, increased sense of power, violence
- Fever, sweating, headache, flushing, pallor, hyperactivity, stereotypic behavior, cardiac arrhythmias, respiratory failure, loss of coordination, collapse, cerebral hemorrhage, convulsions, and death

Chronic Use
- Decreased appetite and weight, abdominal pain, vomiting, difficulty urinating, skin rash, increased risk for stroke, high blood pressure, irregular heart rate, impotence, headache, anxiety, delusions of persecution, violence
- Tolerance to physical effects occurs but vulnerability to psychosis remains
- Chronic high-dose use causes physical dependence; psychological dependence can occur even with regular low-dose use
- Recovery occurs rapidly after amphetamine withdrawal, but psychosis can sometimes become chronic

 Complications

- Exacerbation of hypertension or arrhythmias
- Strokes and retinal damage due to intense vasospasm, especially with "crack" and "ice"
- With methamphetamine cerebral side-effects reported include: vasculopathy with or without parenchymal infarction, hypertensive encephalopathy and hemorrhage

D/C Discontinuation Syndrome

- Anxiety, distorted sleep, chronic fatigue, irritability, difficulty concentrating, craving, depression, suicidal or homicidal ideation, and paranoid psychosis
- Nausea, diarrhea, anorexia, hunger, myalgia, diaphoresis, convulsions

Treatment

- Use calming techniques, reassurance, and supportive measures
- Supportive care of excess sympathomimetic stimulation may be required (e.g., BP, temperature); monitor hydration, electrolytes, and for possible serotonin syndrome
- For severe agitation and to prevent seizures, sedate with benzodiazepine (e.g., diazepam, lorazepam)
- For psychosis, use a high-potency antipsychotic (haloperidol); avoid low-potency antipsychotics
- Antidepressants (e.g., desipramine) can be used to treat depression following withdrawal, and to decrease craving. Positive results reported with propranolol and amantadine in patients with severe withdrawal symptoms from cocaine
- Several medications seem to be promising in the treatment of cocaine dependence including: GABA agents (topiramate, tiagabine, vigabatrin, baclofen), dopaminergic agents (disulfiram, cabergoline, amantadine); stimulant substitution trials suggest benefit with modafinil, and sustained-release formulations of methylphenidate and amphetamine (Caution re additive effects)

Stimulants (cont.)

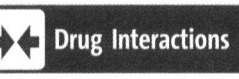 **Drug Interactions**   • Clinically significant interactions are listed below

GENERAL

Class of Drug	Example	Interaction Effects
Antipsychotics		Diminished pharmacological effects of stimulants
Irreversible MAOIs	Phenelzine	Severe palpitations, tachycardia, hypertension, headache, cerebral hemorrhage, agitation, seizures; **AVOID**. Serotonin syndrome reported with MDA, MDMA

AMPHETAMINES

Class of Drug	Example	Interaction Effects
Antidepressants	General	Enhanced antidepressant effect
	Tricyclics	Increased plasma level of amphetamine due to inhibited metabolism
Antihypertensive	Guanethidine	Reversal of hypotensive effects
Antipsychotic	Chlorpromazine	Increased plasma level of amphetamine due to inhibited metabolism
Urinary acidifiers	Ammonium chloride	Increased elimination of amphetamine due to decreased renal tubular reabsorption and increased elimination
Urinary alkalizers	Sodium bicarbonate	Prolonged pharmacological effects of amphetamine due to decreased urinary elimination of unchanged drug

COCAINE

Class of Drug	Example	Interaction Effects
Alcohol		Ethanol promotes the formation of a highly addicting metabolite, cocoethylene Reports of enhanced hepatotoxicity Increased heart rate; variable effect on blood pressure Increased risk of sudden death with combined use (18-fold) Combined use reported to result in more impulsive decision making and poorer performance on tests of learning and memory
Anticonvulsant	Carbamazepine	Augmentation of cocaine-induced increase in heart rate and diastolic BP
Antidepressant	Cyclic, SSRI Tricyclic: desipramine	Decreased craving Decreased seizure threshold Elevated heart rate and diastolic pressure by 20–30%; increased risk of arrhythmia
Antipsychotic	Flupenthixol	Decreased craving
Barbiturate		Reports of enhanced hepatotoxicity
β-Blocker		May increase the magnitude of cocaine-induced myocardial ischemia
Cannabis	Marihuana	Increased heart rate; blood pressure increased only with high doses of both drugs Increased plasma level of cocaine and increased subjective reports of euphoria

Catecholamine	Norepinephrine	Potentiation of vasoconstriction and cardiac stimulation
Disulfiram		Increased plasma level (3-fold) and half-life (60%) of cocaine with possible increased risk of cardiovascular effects
Mazindol		May decrease craving for cocaine Increased lethality and convulsant activity reported
Narcotics	Heroin, morphine	May potentiate cocaine euphoria
Yohimbine		Enhanced effect of cocaine on blood pressure

MDA/MDMA

Class of Drug	Example	Interaction Effects
Antidepressant	SSRI: fluoxetine	Diminished pharmacological effects of MDA
Protease inhibitor	Ritonavir	Case reports of increased plasma levels of MDMA due to inhibited metabolism via CYP2D6; death reported

Stimulant Agents

Drug	Comments
AMPHETAMINE, DEXTROAMPHETAMINE (Dexedrine, Dexampex, Biphetamine) Taken orally as tablet, capsule, sniffed, smoked, injected Slang: bennies, hearts, pep-pills, dex, beans, benn, truck-drivers, ice, jolly beans, black beauties, crank, pink football, dexies, crosses, hearts, LA turnaround	• Cause the release of amines (NE, 5-HT, DA) from central and peripheral neurons and inhibit their breakdown • Onset of action: 30 min after oral ingestion • Physical effects: increased heart rate, BP, metabolism, decreased appetite, weight loss, rapid breathing, tremor, loss of coordination • CNS effects: euphoria, increased energy and mental alertness, nervousness, anxiety, insomnia, irritability, restlessness, panic, impulsive or aggressive behavior • Active drug use usually terminated by a psychotic reaction, or by exhaustion with excessive sleeping • Tolerance and psychic dependence occurs with chronic use • Excessive doses can lead to heart failure, delirium, psychosis (can last up to 10 days), coma, convulsions, and death • Pregnancy: increase in premature births; withdrawal symptoms and behavioral effects (hyperexcitability) noted in offspring • Breast-feeding: irritability and poor sleeping pattern reported in infants

Stimulants (cont.)

Drug	Comments
METHAMPHETAMINE (Desoxyephedrine) – Crystal Meth (Desoxyn, Methampex) Powder: taken as tablets, capsules, liquid, injected, snorted, inhaled, smoked Slang: speed, meth, uppers, shit, moth, crank, crosses, methlies quick, jib, fire, chalk, glass, go fast, tweak Crystal ("ice") is methamphetamine washed in a solvent to remove inpurities – smoked in a glass pipe, "chased" on aluminium foil, or injected	• Synthetic drug related chemically to amphetamine and ephedrine; easily manufactured in 'home laboratories' from common household products • Enhances release of dopamine, norepinephrine, and serotonin and blocks uptake of these catecholamines[1] • Very rapid onset of action; can last 10–12 h • Powerful effects produced are referred to as a "rush." Used as a club drug at "raves" to increase alertness, energy, sociability, euphoria; has aphrodisiac effects and causes loss of inhibitions • A "run" refers to the use of the drug several times a day over a period of several days • "Ice" can be mixed with marihuana and smoked through a bong, or injected • Physical effects: tachycardia, tachypnea, diaphoresis, hyperthermia, mydriasis, hypertension; stroke reported • CNS effects: anxiety, agitation, confusion, insomnia, delirium, hallucinations, paranoia, violence; powerful psychological dependence and addiction occurs, particularly with "ice" • Chronic use can result in weight loss, bruxism, cardiovascular problems, decreases in lung function, pulmonary hypertension, rapid tooth decay ("meth mouth"), mood disturbances, decreased cognitive functioning, anxiety, psychosis with suicidal or homicidal thoughts; may persist for months after drug use is stopped; has been associated with neuronal damage • Users are at high risk of sexually transmitted and blood-borne diseases due to disinhibitory high-risk behaviors that can occur (e.g., shared needles, multiple partners, unprotected sex). "Ice" is especially sexually arousing and disinhibitory and described as "compulsive" or "obsessive" • Abuse of methamphetamine can produce impaired memory and learning, hyperawareness, hypervigilance, psychomotor agitation, irritability, aggression. Chronic intoxication (use) may result in a psychotic state with delusions, hallucinations, and delirium • Toxic effects: arrhythmias, hypertension, heart failure, hyperthermia, seizures, encephalopathy, rhabdomyolysis (see Complications p. 257) • After abrupt discontinuation withdrawal effects peak in 2–3 days and include GI distress, headache, depression, irritability and poor concentration • Methamphetamine exposure during pregnancy is associated with decreased growth in infants; withdrawal effects reported in newborns. Developmental delays can occur due to the drug's neurotoxic effects
COCAINE Extract from leaves of coca plant Leaves chewed, applied to mucous membranes, powder Taken orally, snorted, smoked, injected Slang: coke, coca, snow, flake, lady, toot, blow, big C, candy, crack, joy dust, stardust, rock, nose, boulders, bump, bianca, perico, nieve, soda "Crack": Free base cocaine	• Inhibits dopamine and serotonin reuptake – stimulates brain's reward pathway • Onset of action and plasma half-life varies depending on route of use (e.g., IV: peaks in 30 sec, half-life 54 min; snorting: peaks in 15–30 min, half-life 75 min). Metabolized via CYP3A4 • Crack is a free-based and more potent form of cocaine (volatilized and inhaled) • Often adulterated with amphetamine, ephedrine, procaine, xylocaine, or lidocaine • Used with heroin ("dynamite," "speedballs"), morphine ("whizbang") or marihuana ("cocoa puffs") for increased intensity • Used with flunitrazepam to moderate stimulatory effect • CNS effects: rapid euphoria, increased energy and mental alertness, insomnia, anxiety, agitation, delusion, hallucinations • Physical effects: nausea, vomiting, headaches, tachycardia, hypertension, chest pain, pyrexia, diaphoresis, mydriasis, ataxia, anorexia; tactile hallucinations ("coke bugs") occur • Perforation of the palate when swallowed repeatedly • Tolerance develops to some effects (appetite), but increased sensitivity (reverse tolerance) develops to others (convulsions, psychosis) • Powerful psychological dependence occurs; physical dependence seen in crack users; withdrawal symptoms can last for weeks or months • Depression commonly occurs after drug use; dysphoria promotes repetitive use • Chronic users can develop panic disorder, paranoia, dysphoria, irritability, assaultive behavior, paranoia and delirium • Snorting can cause stuffy, runny nose, eczema around nostrils, atrophy of nasal mucosa, bleeding, and perforated septum • Smokers are susceptible to respiratory symptoms and pulmonary complications • Sexual dysfunction is common

Drug	Comments
	• Chronic users of "crack" can develop microvascular changes in the eyes, lungs and brain; respiratory symptoms include asthma and pulmonary hemorrhage and edema • Dehydration can occur due to effect on temperature regulation, with possible hyperpyrexia • Toxic effects: hypertension, paroxysmal atrial tachycardia, hyperreflexia, irregular respiration, hyperthermia, seizures, unconsciousness, death; fatalities more common with IV use, or when cocaine-filled condoms are swallowed (by smugglers) then burst • Pregnancy: associated with spontaneous labor and abortion; increase in premature births; infants have lower weight, length, and head circumference, jitteriness, irritability, poor feeding, EEG abnormalities • Breast-feeding during cocaine intoxication reported to cause irritability, vomiting, diarrhea, tremulousness, and seizures in infants
KHAT (Catha edulis) Leaves chewed	• Grows as a bush in Africa and the Middle East; used by certain communities to attain religious euphoria • Cathinone is principal psychoactive agent • Symptoms occur within 3 h and last about 90 min • Acute symptoms include: euphoria, excitation, grandiosity, increased blood pressure, flushing • Chronic use can cause: anxiety, agitation, confusion, dysphoria, aggression, visual hallucinations, paranoia
METHYLPHENIDATE Tablets crushed and snorted, swallowed, injected; Slang: Vitamin R, R-ball, skippy, the smart drug, JIF, MPH	See pp. 216 • Large doses can cause psychosis, seizures, stroke, and heart failure
SYMPATHOMIMETICS Ephedrine, phenylpropanolamine, caffeine; taken as capsules, tablets; Slang: look alikes, Herbal Bliss, Cloud 9, Herbal X	• Known as Herbal Ecstasy and sold as "natural" alternative to Ecstasy • Misrepresented as amphetamines and sold in capsules or tablets that resemble amphetamines • Doses of ingredients vary widely • Reports of hypertension and seizures; death due to stroke can occur after massive doses

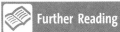 **Further Reading**

Reference

[1] Kish SJ. Pharmacologic mechanism of crystal meth. CMAJ. 2008;178(13):1679–1682.

Additional Suggested Reading

- Karila L, Gorelick D, Weinstein A, et al. New treatments for cocaine dependence: A focused review. Int J Neuropsychopharmacol. 2008;11(3):425–438.
- Maxwell JC. Emerging research on methamphetamine. Int. Drug Therapy Newsletter. 2006;41(3):17–24.
- Sofuoglu M, Kosten TR. Novel approaches to the treatment of cocaine addiction. CNS Drugs. 2005;19(1):13–25.

Hallucinogens

👨‍⚕️ **Pharmacological/ Psychiatric Effects**	• Differ somewhat depending on type of drug taken and route of administration (see specific agents below) • Effects occur rapidly and last from 30 min (e.g., DMT) to several days (e.g., PCP)
Physical	• Increased BP, tachycardia, dilated pupils, nausea, sweating, flushing, chills, hyperventilation, incoordination, muscle weakness, trembling, numbness • Cannabinoids may be effective for treating neuropathic pain (marketed in Canada under the name of Sativax or Cesamet [indicated for chemotherapy-induced nausea and vomiting]); mixed effects found on multiple sclerosis symptoms • Cannabinoids are being tested for treatment of obesity (rimonabant available in Europe)
Mental	• Alteration of perception and body awareness, impaired attention and short-term memory, disturbed sense of time, depersonalization, euphoria, mystical or religious experiences, grandiosity, anxiety, panic, visual distortions, hallucinations (primarily visual), erratic behavior, aggression
High Doses	• Confusion, restlessness, excitement, anxiety, emotional lability, panic, mania, paranoia, "bad trip" • Cardiac depression and respiratory depression (mescaline), hypotension, convulsions and coma (PCP)
Chronic Use	• Anxiety, depression, personality changes • Tolerance (tachyphylaxis) can occur with regular use (except with DMT); reverse tolerance (supersensitivity) has been described • "Woolly" thinking, delusions and hallucinations reported; may persist for months after drug discontinuation • Flashbacks – recurrent psychotic symptoms, may occur years after discontinuation • Cohort studies suggest that chronic use of cannabis by teenagers is associated with > 5-fold increase in risk of later-life depression and anxiety, as well as an increased risk of early-onset psychosis. Prolonged exposure to cannabis may cause an initial increase in synaptic dopamine and then lead to prolonged changes in the endogenous cannabinoid systems – may be more profound in adolescents • Regular (weekly) marihuana use has been associated with increased risk of tardive dyskinesia in schizophrenic patients on antipsychotics
D/C Discontinuation Syndrome	• Withdrawal symptoms identified in frequent cannabis users consist of one of two forms: weakness, hypersomnia, and psychomotor retardation, OR anxiety, restlessness, depression, and insomnia
👩‍⚕️ **Treatment**	• Provide reassurance and reduction of threatening external stimuli • Supportive care for excess CNS stimulation may be required; monitor hydration, electrolytes, and for possible serotonin syndrome • In severe cases, the "trip" should be aborted chemically as rapidly as possible. This reduces the likelihood of flashbacks or recurrences in the future; in mild cases "talking down" may be more appropriate • Use high-potency antipsychotic (e.g., haloperidol) for psychotic symptoms • Avoid low-potency antipsychotics with anticholinergic and α-adrenergic properties (e.g., chlorpromazine) to minimize hypotension, tachycardia, disorientation, and seizures • Use benzodiazepines (diazepam, lorazepam) to control agitation and to sedate, if needed • Propranolol and ascorbic acid may minimize effects of PCP and aid in its excretion

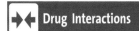
- Clinically significant interactions are listed below

CANNABIS/MARIHUANA

Class of Drug	Example	Interaction Effects
Antidepressant	Tricyclic: desipramine	Case reports of tachycardia, lightheadedness, mood lability, and delirium with combination Cardiac complications reported in children and adolescents
	MAOI: tranylcypromine	Caution: Cannabis increases serotonin levels and may result in a serotonin syndrome
Antipsychotic	Chlorpromazine, thioridazine	Drugs with anticholinergic and α-adrenergic properties can cause marked hypotension and increased disorientation
Barbiturate		Additive effect causing anxiety and hallucinations
Stimulant	Cocaine	Increased heart rate; blood pressure increased with high doses of both drugs; increased plasma level of cocaine and euphoria
Disulfiram		Synergistic CNS stimulation reported, hypomania
Lithium		Clearance of lithium may be decreased
Narcotic	Morphine	THC blocks excitation produced by morphine
Protease inhibitor	Indinavir, nelfinavir	Inhaled marihuana reported to reduce indinavir AUC by 17% and C_{max} of nelfinavir by 21%; no effect on viral load

KETAMINE

Class of Drug	Example	Interaction Effects
Protease inhibitor	Ritonavir, nelfinavir	Elevated levels of ketamine possible due to inhibited metabolism

LSD

Class of Drug	Example	Interaction Effects
Antidepressant	SSRI: fluoxetine	Grand mal seizures reported Recurrence or worsening of flashbacks reported with fluoxetine, sertraline, and paroxetine
Protease inhibitor	Ritonavir	Elevated levels of LSD possible due to inhibited metabolism

PCP

Class of Drug	Example	Interaction Effects
Acidifying agents	Cranberry juice, ammonium chloride	Increased excretion of PCP
Protease inhibitor	Ritonavir	Elevated levels of PCP possible due to inhibited metabolism

Hallucinogens (cont.)

Hallucinogenic Agents

Drug	Comments
CANNABIS **Marihuana** – crushed leaves, stems, and flowers of female hemp plant, *Cannabis sativa* Smoked (cigarettes or water pipe), swallowed Slang: grass, pot, joint, hemp, weed, reefer, smoke, Mary Jane, Indian hay, ace, ganja, gold, J, locoweed, shit, herb, Mexican, ragweed, bhang, sticks, blunt, dope, sinsemilla, skunk, Hydro (hydroponic marihuana) **Hashish** – resin from flowers and leaves; more potent than marihuana Smoked, cooked, swallowed Slang: hash, hash oil, weed oil, weed juice, honey oil, hash brownies, tea, black, solids, grease, smoke, boom, chronic, gangster, hemp	• Tetrahydrocannabinol (THC) is the active ingredient; 5–11% in marihuana and up to 28% in hashish • THC undergoes first pass metabolism to form psychoactive metabolite 11-OH-THC. Initial $T_{1/2}$ is 1–2h and elimination $T_{1/2}$ is 24–36 h. Metabolized by CYP2D6, 3A4, 2C9 and 2C19. Weak inhibitor of CYP1A2, 3A4, 2C9 and 2C19 • Effects occur rapidly and last up to several hours; accumulates in fat tissue for up to 4 weeks before being released back into bloodstream; effects may persist • THC may have beneficial effects in chemotherapy-induced nausea/vomiting (Cesamet) and for chronic neuropathic pain • Early data suggest THC may have some benefit in the treatment of tics in Tourette's syndrome and for chronic neuropathic pain • Tolerance and psychic dependence may occur; reverse tolerance (supersensitivity) described • Combined with other drugs including PCP ("killer weed"), opium ("o.j."), heroin ("A-bomb"), crack cocaine ("cocoa puffs"), or flunitrazepam to enhance effect • CNS effects: most users experience euphoria with feelings of self-confidence and relaxation; some become dysphoric, anxious, agitated and suspicious. Can cause psychotic symptoms with confusion, hallucinations, emotional lability (very prolonged or heavy use can cause serious and potentially irreversible psychosis) • Increased craving for sweets • Chronic use: bronchitis, weight gain, bloodshot eyes, loss of energy, apathy, "fuzzy" thinking, slow reaction time, impaired judgment, decreased testosterone in males; increased risk of depression, anxiety and schizophrenia • Link between cannabis use and early age at onset of psychosis suggested; results point to cannabis as a dangerous drug in young people at risk of developing psychosis[1] • Cannabis cigarettes have a higher tar content than ordinary cigarettes and are potentially carcinogenic • Pregnancy: can retard fetal growth, and cause mild withdrawal reactions in the infant; developmental problems in children born to cannabis-dependent parents have been reported in some studies • Breast-feeding: can reach high levels in breast milk
KETAMINE (Ketalar) General anesthetic in day surgery Taken orally as capsules, tablets, powder, crystals, and solution; injected, snorted, smoked Slang: K, special K, vitamin K, ket, green, jet, kit-kat, cat valiums, Ketalar SV	• NMDA receptor antagonist, prevents glutamate activation, inhibits reuptake of catecholamines (5-HT, NE, DA) • Related to PCP; used as a club drug at "raves" and involved in "date rapes"; most ketamine users are sporadic and poly-drug users • Doses of 60–100 mg injected; consciousness maintained at this dose, but get disorientation • Effects start within 60 sec (IV) and 10–20 min (PO) • Physical effects: increased heart rate and blood pressure, nausea, vomiting, increased muscle tone, nystagmus, stereotypic movements, impaired motor function, numbness; synthetic ketamine linked to serious urinary tract infections • CNS effects: dream-like state, depersonalization confusion, hostility, mild delirium, hallucinations, amnesia • Toxic effects: severe delirium, respiratory depression, loss of consciousness, catatonia

Drug	Comments
LYSERGIC ACID DIETHYLAMIDE (LSD) Semi-synthetic drug derived from ergot (grain fungus) White powder: used as tablet, capsule, liquid, snorted, smoked, inhaled, injected Slang: acid, cubes, purple haze, Raggedy Ann, sunshine, LBJ, peace pill, big D, blotters, domes, hits, tabs, doses, window-pane, microdot, boomers	• $5\text{-}HT_2$ receptor agonist • Used as a club drug at "raves" • Effects occur in less than 1 h and last 2–18 h • Physical effects: mydriasis, nausea, loss of appetite, muscle tension, hyperthermia, hypertension, weakness, numbness, tremors • CNS effects: can cause agitation, visual hallucinations, suicidal, homicidal, and irrational behavior and dysphoria; panic, psychotic reactions can last several days • Flashbacks occur without drug being taken • Tolerance develops rapidly; psychological dependence occurs • Combined with cocaine, mescaline, or amphetamine to prolong effects • Pregnancy: increased risk of spontaneous abortions; congenital abnormalities have been reported
MESCALINE From peyote cactus buttons; pure product rarely available Cactus buttons are dried, then sliced, chopped, or ground; used as powder, capsule, tablet, inhaled or injected Slang: mesc, peyote, buttons, cactus	• Effects occur slowly and last 10–18 h • Less potent than LSD, but cross-tolerance reported • Physical effects: high doses can cause: headache, dry skin, increased temperature and heart rate, hypotension or hypertension, numbness, tremors, cardiac and respiratory depression • CNS effects: anxiety, disorientation, impaired reality testing, chronic mental disorders and flashbacks reported • Dependence not reported but tolerance to effects occurs quickly
MORNING GLORY SEEDS Active ingredient is lysergic acid amide; 1/10th as potent as LSD Seeds eaten whole, or ground, mushed, soaked, and solution injected Slang: flying saucers, licorice drops, heavenly blue, pearly gates	• Effects occur after 30–90 min when seeds ingested and immediately when solution injected • Commercial seeds are treated with insecticides, fungicides, and other chemicals and can be poisonous
PEYOTE From cactus *Lophaphora williamsii* Dried, chewed, and swallowed, used as capsules, solution	• Used for centuries by native people of North and South America • Effects occur 1–2 h after ingestion • Geometric brilliant colors, weightlessness, time distortion, anxiety, panic, dizziness, severe nausea
PHENCYCLIDINE General anesthetic used in veterinary medicine; often misrepresented as other drugs Powder, chunks, crystals; used as tablets, capsules, liquid, inhaled, snorted, injected (IM or IV) Slang: PCP, angel dust, hog, horse tranquilizer, animal tranquilizer, peace pill, killer, weed, supergrass, crystal, "CJ," dust, rocket fuel, boat, love boat	• Glutamate agonist at NMDA receptor • Effects occur in a few minutes and can last several days to weeks (half-life 18 h) • Frequently sold on street as other drugs (easily synthesized); mis-synthesis yields a product that can cause abdominal cramps, vomiting, coma, and death • Physical effects: intermittent vomiting, drooling, loss of appetite, diaphoresis, miosis, nystagmus, hypertension and ataxia can occur • CNS effects: can cause apathy, estrangement, feelings of isolation, indifference to pain, delirium, disorientation with amnesia, schizophrenia-like psychosis, and violence (often self-directed); can feel intermittently anxious, fearful, to euphoric • Toxic effects: hypoglycemia, rhabdomyolysis, depression, delirium, CNS depression, coma; deaths have occurred secondary to uncontrollable seizures, or to hypertension resulting in intracranial hemorrhage • Flashbacks occur • Psychological dependence occurs • Pregnancy: signs of toxicity have been reported in newborns • Breast-feeding: drug concentrates in milk and detectable for weeks after heavy use

Hallucinogens (cont.)

Drug	Comments
PSILOCYBIN From *Psilocybe mexicana* mushroom Used as dried mushroom, white crystal, powder, capsule, injection; eaten raw, cooked or steeped as tea Slang: magic mushrooms, sacred mushrooms, mushroom, shroom, purple passion	• Chemically related to LSD and DMT • Effects occur within 30 min and last several hours • Pure drug rarely available; injection dangerous as foreign particles present • Physical effects: nausea • Mental effects: altered perceptions, nervousness, paranoia, flashbacks; chronic mental disorders reported • Tolerance develops rapidly; cross-tolerance occurs with LSD • Physical or psychological dependence not reported • Mistaken identity with "death-cap" (Amanita) mushroom can result in accidental poisoning
SALVIA DIVINORUM Member of the mint family Leaves chewed, or crushed and the juice ingested as tea, smoked Slang: diviner's sage, magic mint, Maria Pastora	• Main active ingredient is Salvinorin A; a potent kappa opioid agonist • Used in traditional spiritual practices by native people of Mexico • Effects, when taken orally, depend on the absorption of Salvinorin A through the oral mucosa as it is inactivated by the GI tract; when absorbed through oral mucosa, effects detected in 5–10 min, peak at 1 h and subside after 2 h. If inhaled, effects seen after 30 s, peak in 5–10 min and subside in 20–30 min • Taken in combination with cannabis to prolong effect • Physical effects: ataxia, incoherent speech, hysterical laughter, unconsciousness • CNS effects: altered perception; can cause dramatic, and sometimes frightening, hallucinogenic experiences with doses > 1 mg
TRYPTAMINES Soaked in parsley, dried and snorted or smoked, used as liquid (tea), injected Slang: lunch-hour drug, businessman's lunch, FOXY (= MeO-DIPT)	**DIMETHYLTRYPTAMINE (DMT), ALPHA-METHYLTRYPTAMINE (AMT), 5-METHYL-DI-ISOPROPYL-TRYPTAMINE (5-MeO-DIPT)** • Appear in nature in several plants in South America; easily synthesized • Monoamine oxidase inhibitors; interact with a variety of drugs and foods • Effects vary widely depending on amount ingested; occur almost immediately with DMT and last 30–60 min • Readily destroyed by stomach acids • Often mixed with marihuana • CNS effects: anxiety and panic frequent due to quick onset of effects; produce intense visual hallucinations, loss of awareness of surroundings

DRUGS WITH HALLUCINOGENIC AND STIMULANT PROPERTIES

Drug	Comments
2,5-dimethoxy-4-methylamphetamine (STP/DOM) Chemically related to both mescaline and amphetamine Used orally Slang: serenity, tranquility, peace	• Effects last 16–24 h • More potent than mescaline, but less potent than LSD • "Bad trips" occur frequently; prolonged psychotic reactions reported in people with psychiatric history • Tolerance reported; no evidence of dependence • Anticholinergic effects, exhaustion, convulsions, excitement, and delirium reported

Drug	Comments
3,4-methylene-dioxyamphetamine (MDA) Chemically related to both mescaline and amphetamine (synthetic drug) Used orally as liquid, powder, tablet; injection Slang: love drug	• Typical doses: 60–120 mg • Effects occur after 30–60 min (orally), or sooner if injected, and last about 8 h • CNS effects: hallucinations and perceptual distortions rare; feeling of peace and tranquility occurs • High doses: hyperreactivity to stimuli, agitation, hallucinations, violent and irrational behavior, delirium, convulsions, and coma
3,4-methylene-dioxymethamphetamine (MDMA) Powder, usually in tablets or capsules; may also be snorted or smoked, "bimped" or cooked on lollypops or pacifiers Slang: ecstasy; MDMA, "Adam," XTC, X, E, EVE, love drug, business man's special, clarity, lover's speed, hugs, beans Herbal Ecstasy: MDMA mixed with ephedrine	• Causes a calcium-dependent increase in serotonin release into the synaptic cleft and inhibits serotonin reuptake; increases levels of serotonin, norepinephrine and, to a smaller extent, dopamine; may decrease intracellular synthesis of serotonin if used long-term • Many MDMA products are contaminated with other compounds including dextromethorphan, caffeine, phenylpropanolamine, ephedra, MDA, PMA, ketamine, methylsalicylate • Typical dose varies from 50–150 mg, but amount of drug per tablet can be from 0 to 100 mg • Onset of effects 30–60 min; duration of action 3–6 h; half-life is about 8 h; metabolized primarily by CYP2D6 and may inhibit its own metabolism via CYP2D6; slow metabolizers of CYP2D6 may develop toxicity at moderate doses due to drug accumulation • Commonly used at "raves" • CNS effects: wakefulness, increases energy and decreases fatigue and sleepiness; creates feelings of euphoria and well-being together with de-realization, depersonalization, impaired memory and learning, and heightened tactile sensations (action believed to be mediated through release of serotonin) • Common physical effects include: increased blood pressure and heart rate, increased endurance and sexual arousal, salivation, mydriasis, bruxism, trismus, increased tension, headache, restless legs, blurred vision, dry mouth, urinary retention, nausea, and suppresses appetite, thirst and sleep • Severe physical reactions include: hypertension, tachycardia, dysrhythmia, hyperthermia, seizures; followed by hypotension, ischemic stroke, fatal brain hemorrhage, and coma; death can occur from excessive physical activity ("raves") that may result in disseminated intravascular coagulation, rhabdomyolysis, hyponatremia, acute renal and hepatic failure, and multiple organ failure • High doses can precipitate panic disorder, hallucinations, paranoid psychosis, aggression, and flashbacks • After-effects include: anorexia, drowsiness, muscle aches, generalized fatigue, irritability, anxiety, and depression (last 1–2 days due to half-life of drug of about 8 h) • Tolerance to euphoric effects with chronic use • Chronic regular use may result in mood swings, depression, impulsivity and lack of self-control, memory loss, and parkinsonism; can lead to psychological dependence • Suggested that chronic use can produce changes in serotonin function in the CNS and the development of progressive neurodegeneration. May also stress the immune system and increase susceptibility to infectious diseases
Benzylpiperazine (BZP) and 3-trifluoromethyphenylpiperazine (3-TFMPP) Slang: Peaq, Freq, PureRush, PureSpun	• Promoted as a special tonic and a "natural" alternative to more dangerous street drugs • Mechanism of action is believed to be similar to MDMA and the effects produced by BZP are comparable to those of amphetamine • Doses of 50–200 mg BZP ingested • Effects last 4–8 h • Metabolized via CYP2D6 and COMT • Physical effects: nausea, hyperthermia, increased blood pressure, dilated pupils, tingling skin, decreased appetite • CNS effects: alertness, increased euphoria, paranoia • With high doses: hallucinations, respiratory depression, renal toxicity, convulsions • Withdrawal effects include: nausea, headache, fatigue, hangover, confusion, insomnia
N-ethyl-3,4-methylene-dioxyamphetamine (MDE) Chemically related to MDMA (synthetic drug) Slang: Eve	• Effects as for MDMA (above) • Onset of effects within 30 min; duration of action 3–4 h

Hallucinogens (cont.)

Drug	Comments
NUTMEG Active ingredient related to trimethoxyamphetamine and to mescaline Seeds eaten whole, ground, powdered; sniffed	• Effects occur slowly and last several hours (duration of hallucinogenic effects is dose related) • Hallucinations are usually preceded by nausea, vomiting, diarrhea, and headache • Physical effects: lightheadedness, drowsiness, thirst, and hangover can occur
Paramethoxyamphetamine (PMA) Synthetic drug Used as powder, capsules	• Often sold as MDMA but has more pronounced hallucinogenic and stimulant effects • Metabolized by CYP2D6 • Physical effects: causes major increase in BP and pulse, hyperthermia, increased and labored breathing • Highly toxic; convulsions, coma, and death reported
Trimethoxyamphetamine (TMA) Synthetic drug related to mescaline Used orally, as powder, injection	• Effects occur after 2 h • Often misrepresented as MDA • More potent than mescaline • More toxic if injected or higher doses used • Can cause unprovoked anger and aggression

 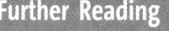 **Further Reading**

Reference

[1] González-Pinto A, Vega P, Ibáñez B, et al. Impact of Cannabis and other drugs on age at onset of psychosis. J Clin Psychiatry. 2008;69:1210–1216.

Additional Suggested Reading

• Centre for Addiction and Mental Health (Toronto, Canada). Information about drugs and addiction: Hallucinogens. Available from: http://www.camh.net/About_Addiction_Mental_Health/Drug_and_Addiction_Information/hallucinogens_dyk.html (Accessed March 13, 2008).

• Coulston CM, Perdices M, Tennant CC. The neuropsychology of cannabis and other substance use in schizophrenia: Review of the literature and critical evaluation of methodological issues. Aust NZ J Psychiatry. 2007;41(11):869–884.

• Fantegrossi WE, Murnane KS, Reissiq CJ. The behavioral pharmacology of hallucinogens. Biochem Pharmacol. 2008;75(1):17–33.

• Gahlinger PM. Club Drugs: MDMA, Gamma-Hydroxybutyrate (GHB), Rohypnol, and Ketamine. Am Fam Physician. 2004; 69(11):2619–2627.

• Lopez-Moreno JA, González-Cuevas G, Moreno JA, et al. The pharmacology of the endocannabinoid system: Functional and structural interactions with other neurotransmitter systems and their repercussions in behavioral addiction. Addict Biol. 2008;13(2):160–187.

• Teter CJ, Guthrie SK. A Comprehensive Review of MDMA and GHB: Two Common Club Drugs. Pharmacotherapy. 2001;21(12):1486–1513.

General Comments

- High rate of comorbidity, specifically depression, alcoholism, and antisocial personality disorder (often not clear if these are cause or effect)
- Prescription opiate abuse (e.g. codeine, oxycontin), in the general population, is relatively high in North America
- Polydrug use and co-dependence on benzodiazepines appears particularly common among individuals injecting opioids

Pharmacological/ Psychiatric Effects

- Differ somewhat depending on type of drug taken, the dose, the route of administration, and whether combined with other drugs
- Elderly more sensitive to effects and side effects of opiates

Physical

- Analgesia, "rush" sensation followed by relaxation, decreased tension, slow pulse and respiration, increased body temperature, dry mouth, constricted pupils, decreased GI motility

Mental

- Euphoria, state of gratification, sedation

High Doses

- Respiratory depression, cardiovascular complications, coma, and death

Chronic Use

- General loss of energy, ambition, and drive, motor retardation, attention impairment, sedation, slurred speech
- Tolerance and physical dependence; withdrawal
- Cross-tolerance occurs with other narcotics

D/C Discontinuation Syndrome

- Symptoms include: yawning, runny nose, sneezing, lacrimation, dilated pupils, vasodilation, tachycardia, elevated BP, vomiting and diarrhea, restlessness, tremor, chills, piloerection, bone pain, abdominal pain and cramps, anorexia, anxiety, irritability, insomnia
- Acute symptoms can last 10–14 days (longer with methadone)

Treatment

- Opioid withdrawal states are generally not life-threatening; "cold turkey" is acceptable to some addicts
- Non-narcotic alternatives (e.g., benzodiazepines, antipsychotics) usually do not work
- Drugs are prescribed for the following reasons:
  a) to reverse effects of toxicity using narcotic antagonists (e.g., naloxone, naltrexone – can precipitate withdrawal)
  b) to treat the immediate withdrawal reaction (e.g., clonidine, methadone)
  c) to aid in detoxification, or for maintenance therapy in a supervised treatment program (e.g., methadone, buprenorphine)

Drug Interactions

- Clinically significant interactions are listed below

OPIATES (GENERAL)

Class of Drug	Example	Interaction Effects
Antibiotic	Erythromycin, clarithromycin	Increased plasma concentration of fentanyl, alfentanyl due to inhibited metabolism via CYP3A4, resulting in prolonged analgesia and adverse effects
Antidepressant	MAOI, RIMA	Increased excitation, sweating and hypotension reported (especially with meperidine, pentazocine); may lead to development of encephalopathy, convulsions, coma, respiratory depression, and serotonin syndrome
Antihistamine	Tripelennamine, cyclizine	"Opiate high" reported in combination with opium; euphoria
CNS drugs	Alcohol, benzodiazepines	Additive CNS effects; can lead to respiratory depression
H_2 antagonist	Cimetidine	Enhanced effect of narcotic and increased adverse effects due to decreased metabolism; 22% decrease in clearance of meperidine
Narcotic antagonist	Naloxone, naltrexone	Will precipitate withdrawal reaction

Opiates/Narcotics (cont.)

Class of Drug	Example	Interaction Effects
Protease inhibitor	Ritonavir	Decreased clearance of narcotic due to inhibited metabolism resulting in increased plasma level (caution with fentanyl, alfentanyl, meperidine, propoxyphene)
Stimulant	Cocaine	May potentiate cocaine euphoria

Narcotic Agents

Drug	Comments
HEROIN Diacetylmorphine - synthetic derivative of morphine Injected (IV – "mainlining", or SC – "skin popping"), smoked, inhaled, taken orally Slang: "H", horse, junk, snow, stuff, lady, dope, shill, poppy, smack, scag, black tar, Lady Jane, white stuff, brown sugar, skunk, white horse	• Effects almost immediate following IV injection and last several hours; effects occur in 15–60 min after oral dosing • Risk of accidental overdose as street preparations contain various concentrations of heroin • Physical dependence and tolerance occur within 2 weeks; withdrawal occurs within 8–12 h after last dose peaks in 36–72 h and can last up to 10 days • Combined with flunitrazepam to enhance effects and to ameliorate heroin withdrawal • Physical effects: pain relief, nausea, constipation, staggering gait, respiratory depression • CNS effects: euphoria, drowsiness, confusion • Toxicity: sinus bradycardia or tachycardia, hypertension or hypotension, palpitations, syncope, respiratory depression, coma, and death • Pregnancy: high rate of spontaneous abortions, premature labor and stillbirths – babies are often small and have an increased mortality risk; withdrawal symptoms in newborn reported • Breast-feeding: tremors, restlessness, vomiting and poor feeding reported in infants
MORPHINE Principal active component of opium poppy Taken as powder, capsule, tablet, liquid, injected Slang: "M", dreamer, sweet Jesus, junk, morph, Miss Emma, monkey, white stuff	• Effects as for heroin, but slower onset and longer-acting • Effects occur in 15–60 min after oral dosing and last 1–8 h • Physical effects: pain relief, nausea, constipation; with high doses can get respiratory depression, unconsciousness, and coma • CNS effects: drowsiness, confusion, euphoria • Dependence liability high (second to heroin) due to powerful euphoric and analgesic effects
METHADONE (see p. 287) (Dolophine, Roxane, Methadol) Used as tablets, liquid, injected Slang: the kick pill, dolly, meth	• Drug used in withdrawal and detoxification from opiates, but subject to abuse • Effects occur 30–60 min after oral dosing, and last 7–48 h • Chronic use causes constipation, blurred vision, sweating, decreased libido, menstrual irregularities, joint and bone pain, sleep disturbances • Physical dependence and tolerance occur; withdrawal effects peak in 72–96 h and can last up to 14 days • Pregnancy: dosing needs should be reassessed (decreased between weeks 14 and 32 and increased prior to term); withdrawal effects reported in neonates • Breastfeeding: small amounts of methadone enter milk; nurse prior to taking dose or 2–6 h after
OPIUM Resinous preparation from unripe seed pods of opium poppy; available as dark brown chunks or as powder Soaked, taken as solution, smoked Slang: big O, black stuff, block, gum, hop	• Contains a number of alkaloids including morphine (6–12%) and codeine (0.5–1.5%) • Physical effects: nausea common, constipation; with high doses can get respiratory depression, unconsciousness, and coma • CNS effects: drowsiness, confusion, euphoria

Drug	Comments
CODEINE Methylmorphine Used orally, liquid, injected Slang: schoolboy, 3s, 4s, Captain Cody, Cody	• Naturally occurring alkaloid from opium poppy • Common ingredient of both prescription and over-the-counter analgesics and antitussives (e.g., Fiorinal-C, Tylenol #1, etc.) • Mixed with glutethimide (called loads, pacs, doors and fours, pancakes, and syrup) • Physical effects: pain relief, constipation • CNS effects: euphoria, drowsiness, confusion • Toxic effects: respiratory depression and arrest, decreased consciousness, coma, death • Tolerance develops gradually; physical dependence is infrequent; withdrawal will occur with chronic highdose use
DEXTROMETHORPHAN (Robitussin DM) Used orally Slang: robo, robo-trip, poor man's PCP	• Higher doses can cause agitation, euphoria, altered perceptions, ataxia, nystagmus, hypertension, tachycardia, visual disturbances, and disorientation; may progress to panic attacks, delusions, psychotic/manic behavior, hallucinations, paranoia, and seizures • If combination product abused (e.g. cough/cold preparation) must consider toxic effects of other ingredients
FENTANYL (Duragesic, Sublimaze) Slang: tango, cash, Apache, China girl, China white, dance fever, friend, goodfella, jackpot, murders, TNT	• Effects almost immediate following IV injection and last 30–60 min; with IM use, onset slower and duration of action is up to 120 min; exposing application site of fentanyl patch to an external heat source (e.g., heating pad, hot tub) can increase drug absorption and result in increased drug effect • Physical effects: dizziness, dry mouth, constipation, and GI distress • CNS effects: primarily sedation, confusion, euphoria occurs quickly • High doses can produce muscle rigidity (including respiratory muscles) respiratory depression, unconsciousness, and coma
HYDROCODONE (e.g., Novahistex DH)	• Related to codeine, but more potent • An ingredient in prescription antitussive preparations; sought by abuser due to easy availability and purity of product • Physical, CNS, and toxic effects as for codeine • Tolerance develops rapidly • Lethal dose: 0.5–1.0 g
HYDROMORPHONE (Dilaudid) Used orally Slang: juice, dillies	• Semisynthetic narcotic • At low doses side effects less common than with other narcotics; high doses more toxic due to strong respiratory depressant effect
LEVORPHANOL (Levo Dromoran)	• Synthetic narcotic analgesic with effects similar to morphine • High doses can produce cardiac arrhythmias, hypotension, respiratory depression, and coma
MEPERIDINE/PETHIDINE (Demerol) Synthetic opioid derivative Used orally, injected Slang: demmies, pain killer	• Metabolite (normeperidine) is highly toxic; may accumulate with chronic use and cause convulsions • High doses produce disorientation, hallucinations, respiratory depression, stupor, and coma • Risk of serotonin syndrome when used with various serotonergic agents (SSRIs, SNRIs, linazolid, etc.) and MAOIs

Opiates/Narcotics (cont.)

Drug	Comments
OXYCODONE (Percodan, Percocet, OxyContin) Semisynthetic derivative Used orally; tablets chewed, crushed and snorted, powder boiled for injection Slang: percs, OC, OXY, oxycotton, killers	• An ingredient in combination analgesic products and on its own (OxyContin) • Very high abuse potential • Physical effects: nausea, constipation; with high doses can get respiratory depression and coma • Mental effects: drowsiness, disorientation, euphoria
PENTAZOCINE (Talwin) Used orally, injected Slang: T's, big T, Tee, Tea	• Has both agonist and antagonist properties at opioid receptors • Repeated injections can result in tissue damage at injection site • Mixed with tripelennamine (called T's and blues)
PROPOXYPHENE (Darvon) Used orally, injected Slang: yellow football	• Synthetic narcotic analgesic • Abuse results in a state of euphoria • Repeated injections can cause damage to veins and local tissue • Tolerance to analgesic and euphoric effects develops gradually; chronic use results in physical dependence

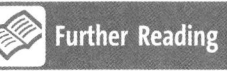 **Further Reading**

• Meehan WJ, Adelman SA, Rehman Z, et al. Opioid abuse. eMedicine; 2006 [Article updated: Apr 18, 2006]. Available from: http://www.emedicine.com/med/TOPIC1673.HTM
• Smelson DA, Dixon L, Craig T, et al. Pharmacological treatment of schizophrenia and co-occuring substance use disorders. CNS Drugs. 2008;22(11):903–916.

Inhalants/Aerosols

💬 General Comments
- High rate of psychopathology, specifically alcoholism, depression, and antisocial personality disorder, have been demonstrated in individuals with a history of solvent use
- Considered "poor man's" drug of abuse, is inexpensive and readily available; primarily used by children, and in third world countries to lessen hunger pain
- Fourth most commonly abused substance among teens in Canada; high use in Aboriginal populations
- Use is often episodic, and "fads" determine current inhalant of choice; users often abuse/misuse other drugs
- Nitrite abuse often associated with "club" scene; Amyl nitrite used to promote sexual excitement and orgasm; may cause a temporary loss of social inhibitions thereby leading to higher-risk sexual practices

Slang
- Glue, gassing, sniffing, chemo, snappers
- Amyl and butyl nitrates: pearls, poppers, rush, locker room, Bolt, Kix
- Nitrous oxides: laughing gas, balloons, whippets

Substances Abused
- Volatile gases: butane, propane, aerosol propellants
- Solvents: airplane glue, gasoline, toluene, printing fluid, cleaning solvents, benzene, acetone, spray paint ("chroming"), amyl nitrite ("poppers"), etc.
- Aerosols: deodorants, hair spray, freon
- Anesthetic gases: nitrous oxide (laughing gas), chloroform, ether

Methods of Use
- "Bagging" – pouring liquid or discharging gas into plastic bag or balloon
- "Sniffing" – holding mouth over container as gas is discharged
- "Huffing" – holding a soaked rag over mouth or nose
- "Torching" – inhaling fumes discharged from a cigarette lighter, then igniting the exhaled air

🧠 Pharmacological/ Psychiatric Effects
- Differ somewhat depending on type of drug taken
- Fumes sniffed, inhaled; use of plastic bag can lead to suffocation
- Inhaled product enters the bloodstream quickly via the lungs and CNS penetration is rapid – intoxication occurs within minutes and can last from a few minutes to an hour

Physical
- Drowsiness, dizziness, slurred speech, impaired motor function, muscle weakness, cramps, light sensitivity, headache, nausea or vomiting, salivation, sneezing, coughing, wheezing, decreased breathing and heart rate, hypotension, cramps
- Fatalities can arise from cardiac arrest or inhalation of vomit while unconscious

Mental
- Changing levels of awareness, impaired judgment and memory, loss of inhibitions, hallucinations, euphoria, excitation, vivid fantasies, feeling of invincibility, delirium

High Doses
- Loss of consciousness, convulsions, cardiac arrhythmia, seizures, death

Chronic Use
- Fatigue, chronic headaches, encephalopathy, hearing loss, visual impairment, sinusitis, rhinitis, laryngitis, weight loss, kidney and liver damage, bone marrow damage, cardiac arrhythmias, chronic lung disease
- Inability to think clearly, memory disturbances, depression, irritability, hostility, paranoia
- Tolerance develops to desired effect; psychological dependence is frequent

☠ Toxicity
- CNS: acute and chronic effects reported, e.g., ataxia, peripheral neuropathy
- Cardiac: an MI can occur, primarily with use of halogenated solvents
- Renal: acidosis, hypokalemia

Inhalants/Aerosols (cont.)

- Hepatic: hepatitis, hepatic necrosis
- Hematologic: bone marrow suppression primarily with benzene and nitrous oxide use
- Accidental suffocation from plastic bag used over the head

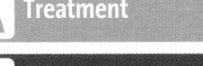 **Use in Pregnancy**	• Associated with increased risk of miscarriage, birth defects, low birth weight, and sudden infant death syndrome (SIDS); in a meta-analysis of 10 studies of maternal solvent exposure, 5 showed major malformations • There is some evidence that prenatal exposure may cause long-term neurodevelopmental impairments, such as deficits in cognitive, speech, and motor skills • Residual withdrawal symptoms reported in babies of mothers who used volatile substances during pregnancy. Symptoms in babies include excessive and high-pitched crying, sleeplessness, hyperreflexia, tremor, hypotonia, and poor feeding
Breast milk	• Risk of inhalants entering breast milk and exposing infant to adverse effects
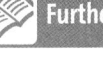 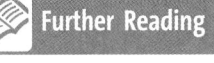 **Treatment**	• Effects are usually short-lasting; use calming techniques, reassurance
Drug Interactions	• Clinically significant interactions are listed below

Class of Drug	Example	Interaction Effects
CNS depressants	Alcohol, benzodiazepines, hypnotics, narcotics	Increased impairment of judgment, distortion of reality

Further Reading	• Centre for Addiction and Mental Health (Toronto, Canada). Resources for Professionals: Inhalants. Available from: http://www.camh.net/Publications/Resources_for_Professionals/Pregnancy_Lactation/per_inhalants.html (Accessed July 11, 2008).

Gamma-hydroxy Butyrate (GHB)/Sodium Oxybate

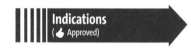

Indications
(👍 Approved)

👍 Approved (as Xyrem) for oral treatment of cataplexy and excessive daytime sleepiness for patients with narcolepsy

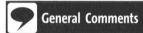

General Comments

- Xyrem is available in the US via the Xyrem Success Program®, using a centralized pharmacy 1-866-XYREM88 (1-866-997-3688)
- Prescribing and dispensing restrictions apply for use of Xyrem in patients with narcolepsy
- Xyrem is available as an oral solution containing 500 mg/ml
- Abused as a powder mixed in a liquid; usually sold in vials and taken orally; has a salty or soapy taste
- Used for its hallucinogenic and euphoric effects at raves (or dance parties)
- Has been used in Europe to treat alcohol dependency at a dose of 50 mg/kg/day – reported to reduce alcohol cravings and increase abstinence; also used for sedation and to treat opiate withdrawal
- Marketed as Xyrem in the USA for treatment of cataplexy in patients with narcolepsy – distributed as a "controlled drug" with generic name of sodium oxybate; improves nighttime sleep and reduces daytime sleep attacks and cataplexy at doses of 6–9 g/night; initial starting doses are recommended to be 4.5 g/night (divided into two doses of 2.25 g each). The second dose is taken 2.5–4 h after the first
- Xyrem, being a CNS depressant, should not be used with alcohol or other CNS depressants. Food significantly decreases the bioavailability of Xyrem. Therefore, the first dose should be taken at least 2 h after eating. Minimize variability in dose timing in relation to meals, and patients should not drive or operate machinery for at least 6 h after taking Xyrem
- Originally researched as an anesthetic; shown to have limited analgesic effects and increased seizure risk
- Promoted illegally as a health food product, an aphrodisiac and for muscle building
- Has been used in "date rapes" because it acts rapidly, produces disinhibition and relaxation of voluntary muscles and causes anterograde amnesia for events that occur under the influence of the drug
- Chronic use may result in tolerance and/or psychological dependence
- Products converted to GHB in the body include: gammabutyrolactone (GBL – also called Blue Nitro Vitality, GH Revitalizer, GHR, Remforce, Renew-trient and Gamma G – is sold in health food stores) and the industrial solvent butanediol (BD – also called tetramethylene glycol or Sucol B, and sold as Zen, NRG-3, Soma Solutions, Enliven, and Serenity)

Slang

- Liquid ecstasy, liquid X, liquid F, goop, GBH = Grievous Bodily Harm, Easy lay, Ghost Breath, G, Somatomax, Gamma-G, Growth Hormone Booster, Georgia home boy, nature's Quaalude, G-riffick, Soapy, Salty Water

Pharmacology

- Produced naturally in the body and is a metabolite of gamma aminobutyric acid (GABA); acts on $GABA_B$ receptor to potentiate gabaergic effects
- Reduces cataplexy
- Some effects of GHB are blocked by opioid receptor antagonists
- Shown to increase dopamine levels in the basal ganglia
- Stimulates slow-wave sleep (stages 3 and 4) and decreases stage 1 sleep; with continued use decreases REM sleep

Pharmacological/ Psychiatric Effects

- Deep sleep reported with doses of 2.0 g
- At 10 mg/kg produces anxiolytic effect, muscle relaxation, and amnesia
- At 20–30 mg/kg increases REM and slow-wave sleep
- Caution: doses > 60 mg/kg can result in anesthesia, respiratory depression, and coma

Pharmacokinetics

- Quickly absorbed orally; onset of action occurs within 30 min; peak plasma concentration reached in 20–60 min
- Elimination half-life approx. 20–30 min; no longer detected in blood after 2–8 h and in urine after 8–12 h

Gamma-hydroxy Butyrate (GBH)/Sodium Oxybate (cont.)

Adverse Reactions

Physical
- With high doses: high frequency of drop attacks – "victim" suddenly loses all muscular control and drops to the floor, unable to resist the "attacker"
- Drowsiness, dizziness, nausea, vomiting, headache, hypotension, bradycardia, hypothermia, ataxia, nystagmus, hypotonia, tremors, muscle spasms, seizures, decreased respiration; symptoms usually resolve within 7 h, but dizziness can persist up to 2 weeks
- Use of sodium oxybate in narcolepsy has been associated with headache, nausea, dizziness, sleepwalking, confusion and urinary incontinence; worsening of sleep apnea
- Use of high doses may lead to unconsciousness and coma (called "G-hold," – particularly dangerous in combination with alcohol)

Mental
- Feeling of well-being, lowered inhibitions, sedation, poor concentration, confusion, amnesia, euphoria, and hallucinations; can cause agitation and aggression

D/C Discontinuation Syndrome
- Symptoms occur 1–6 h after abrupt cessation and can last for 5–15 days after chronic use
- Initial symptoms include nausea, vomiting, insomnia, anxiety, confusion, and/or tremor; after chronic use, symptoms can include mild tachycardia and hypertension, and can progress to delirium with auditory and visual hallucinations

Toxicity
- Low therapeutic index; dangerous in combination with alcohol
- Overdoses can occur due to unknown purity and concentration of ingested product
- Symptoms: bradycardia, seizures, apnea, sudden (reversible) coma with abrupt awakening and violence
- Coma reported in doses > 60 mg/kg (4 g)
- Several deaths reported secondary to respiratory failure

Management
- No known antidote

Use in Pregnancy
- Schedule B drug

Breast milk
- Unknown

Drug Interactions
- Clinically significant interactions are listed below

Class of Drug	Example	Interaction Effects
Benzodiazepine	Diazepam	Has been used to treat GHB withdrawal; theoretically may worsen respiratory depression
CNS Depressant	Alcohol	Synergistic CNS depressant effects can occur, especially with high doses of GHB, leading to respiratory depression
Cannabis		Increased pharmacological effects
Protease inhibitor	Ritonavir–saquinavir combination	GHB toxicity – may cause bradycardia, respiratory depression and seizures
Stimulant	Amphetamines	Increased pharmacological effects

Further Reading
- Gahlinger PM. Club Drugs: MDMA, Gamma-Hydroxybutyrate (GHB), Rohypnol, and Ketamine. Am Fam Physician. 2004;69(11):2619–2627.
- Teter CJ, Guthrie SK. A Comprehensive Review of MDMA and GHB: Two Common Club Drugs. Pharmacotherapy. 2001;21(12):1486–1513.

Flunitrazepam (Rohypnol)

General Comments
- Used as a sedative/tranquilizer in some European countries
- Commonly used as a date-rape drug because it acts rapidly, produces disinhibition and relaxation of voluntary muscles, and causes anterograde amnesia for events that occur under the influence of the drug
- Alcohol potentiates the drug's effects

Slang
- Roofies, R-2s, Roches Dos, forget-me pill, Mexican Valium, roofinol, rope, rophies

Method of Use
- Purchased in doses of 1 and 2 mg (legal manufacturers have added blue or green dye to formulation to color beverages and make them murky); illegal manufacturing is common
- Ingested, snorted or injected
- Added to alcoholic beverages of unsuspecting victim

Pharmacology
- Fast-acting benzodiazepine, structurally related to clonazepam (not marketed in Canada or US)
- See p. 160
- Effects begin in 30 min; peak level within 2 h and lasts up to 8 h

Pharmacokinetics
- Effects begin in 30 min, peak within 2 h, and last up to 8 h

Adverse Reactions
- These reactions are reported following restoration of consciousness

Physical
- Dizziness, impaired motor skills, "rubbery legs," weakness, unsteadiness, visual disturbances, blood-shot eyes, slurred speech, and urinary retention
- Decreased blood pressure and pulse, slowed breathing; may lead to respiratory depression and arrest

Mental
- Rapid loss of consciousness and amnesia; residual symptoms include drowsiness, fatigue, confusion, impaired memory and judgment, reduced inhibition
- If some memory of the event remains, the "victim" may describe a disassociation of body and mind – a sensation of being paralyzed, powerless, unable to resist

Toxicity
- See Benzodiazepines p. 163

Drug Interactions
- See Benzodiazepines pp. 164–165

Further Reading
- Gahlinger PM. Club Drugs: MDMA, Gamma-Hydroxybutyrate (GHB), Rohypnol, and Ketamine. Am Fam Physician. 2004; 69(11):2619–2627.
- Teter CJ. Club drugs. Part I and II. Int Drug Ther Newsl. 2003;38(7+8):49–64.

TREATMENT OF SUBSTANCE USE DISORDERS

☰ Classification

- Drugs available for treatment of substance use disorders may be classified as follows:

Substance Use Disorder	Agent	Page
Alcohol dependence	♦ Disulfiram[B] ♦ Acamprosate[B]	See p. 279 See p. 282
Alcohol/opioid dependence	♦ Naltrexone	See p. 284
Opioid dependence	♦ Methadone ♦ Buprenorphine (Subutex) ♦ Buprenorphine/Naloxone (Suboxone)[B]	See p. 287 See p. 292 See p. 292
Nicotine dependence	Bupropion (Zyban) Varenicline tartrate (Champix/Chantix in the US)* Nicotine replacement therapies (nicotine patches, gum, lozenges, inhalers)*	See p. 16
Heroin and nicotine withdrawal	Clonidine	See p. 230

♦ Approved indication, [B] Not marketed in Canada, * Treatment indicated only for nicotine dependence (e.g., nicotine replacement therapies and varenicline) have not been included in this edition of the handbook

💬 General Comments

- In patients with co-morbid disorders (diagnosed psychiatric disorder and a substance-use disorder) simultaneous treatment is suggested for each disorder, regardless of the status of the comorbid condition; experts disagree as to whether it is necessary to wait for abstinence from the substance abused before treating the psychiatric condition[1]
- Treatment of comorbid conditions is often guided by clinical consensus rather than randomized clinical trials

📖 Further Reading

Reference

1 Watkins KE, Hunter SB, Burnam MA, et al. Review of treatment recommendations for persons with a co-occurring affective or anxiety and substance use disorder. Psychiatr Serv. 2005;56(8):913–926.

Additional Suggested Reading

- American Psychiatric Association. Practice guideline and resources for treatment of patients with substance use disorders, 2nd ed. Am J Psychiatry 2006;163(8 Suppl); 1–276. Available from: http://www.psychiatryonline.com/pracGuide/pracGuideTopic_5.aspx (Accessed November 20, 2008)
- Faragon JJ, Piliero PJ. Drug interactions associated with HAART: Focus on treatments for addiction and recreational drugs. The Aids Reader. 2003;13(9):433–434, 437–441, 446–450.
- McRae A. Pharmacotherapy of substance use disorders. Int Drug Ther Newsl. 2004;39(4):25–30.
- Swift RM. Can medication successfully treat substance addiction? Psychopharmacology Update. 2001;12(1):4–5.

Disulfiram

Product Availability

Chemical Class	Generic Name	Trade Name(A)	Dosage Forms and Strengths
	Disulfiram(B)	Antabuse	Tablets: 250 mg, 500 mg

(A) Generic preparations may be available, (B) Not marketed in Canada

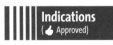

Indications (👍 Approved)

- 👍 Deterrent to alcohol use/abuse (level of evidence 2[1])
- Double-blind and open studies suggest benefit in decreasing cocaine use (by decreasing the "rush" and "high" from cocaine) and increasing abstinence in patients with comorbid alcohol abuse (caution – see Drug Interactions p. 280)[1]

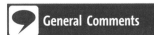
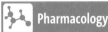

General Comments

- Acts as an aversive agent or psychological deterrent; clinical efficacy is limited due to poor compliance (efficacy is dependent on adherence to treatment)
- Disulfiram treatment should be part of a comprehensive alcohol management program that includes psychosocial support (level of evidence 1[1])

Pharmacology

- Inhibits alcohol metabolism by irreversibly inhibiting the oxidation of acetaldehyde, by competing with the cofactor nicotinamide adenine dinucleotide for binding sites on aldehyde dehydrogenase; the accumulating acetaldehyde produces an unpleasant reaction consisting of headache, sweating, flushing, choking, nausea, vomiting, tachycardia, and hypotension; response is proportional to the dose and amount of alcohol ingested; can occur 10–20 min after alcohol ingestion and may last for several hours
- Increases brain dopamine concentrations by inhibiting dopamine catabolizing enzymes, dopamine-beta-hydroxylase

Dosing

- 125–500 mg daily (h.s.)

Pharmacokinetics

- Highly lipid soluble; bioavailability 80%
- Onset of action: 3–12 h
- Duration of action: up to 14 days
- Metabolized in the liver to active metabolites via CYP3A4/5, 1A2, 2B6, 2E1 and FMO3 (flavin monooxygenase); elimination is slow and about 20% of the drug remains in the body up to 2 weeks after ingestion
- Selectively inhibits CYP2E1 with both acute and chronic administration; with chronic use, other enzymes (e.g., CYP1A2, 3A4 and P-gp) may also be inhibited

Adverse Effects

- Drowsiness and lethargy frequent, depression, disorientation, restlessness, excitation, psychosis
- Physical effects: Neurological toxicity can occur proportional to dose and duration of therapy (e.g., central and peripheral neuropathy, movement disorders); optic neuritis, headaches, dizziness, skin eruptions (up to 5% risk), impotence, garlic-like taste, blood dyscrasias
- Transient elevated liver function tests reported in up to 30% of individuals; hepatitis is rare. Baseline liver function test recommended and repeat periodically, and at first symptoms or sign of liver dysfunction

Precautions

- Do not give to intoxicated individuals or within 36 h of alcohol consumption
- Do not administer without patient's knowledge
- If alcohol reaction occurs, general supportive measures should be used; in severe hypotension, vasopressor agents may be required

Contraindications

- Cardiac and pulmonary disorders, liver disease, renal disorders, epilepsy, diabetes mellitus; psychotic conditions including depression
- Use of alcohol-containing products

Disulfiram (cont.)

 Toxicity
- Alcohol reaction is proportional to dose of drug and alcohol ingested; severe reactions may result in respiratory depression, cardiovascular collapse, arrhythmias, convulsions, and death; supportive measures may involve oxygen, vitamin C, antihistamines or ephedrine

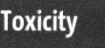 **Pediatric Considerations**
- For detailed information on the use of disulfiram in this population, please see the *Clinical Handbook of Psychotropic Drugs for Children and Adolescents* (2007)
- Double-blind and open studies suggest benefit in decreasing cocaine use and increasing abstinence in patients with comorbid drug abuse

 Geriatric Considerations
- Cardiovascular tolerance decreases with age, thus increasing the severity of the alcohol reactions

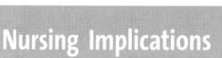 **Use in Pregnancy**
- Possible teratogenicity: report of limb reduction anomalies

Breast Milk
- Unknown

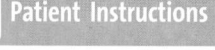 **Nursing Implications**
- The patient should be made aware of purpose of medication and educated about the consequences of drinking; informed consent to treatment is recommended
- The patient should avoid all products (food and drugs) containing alcohol, including tonics, cough syrups, mouth washes, and alcohol-based sauces; exposure to alcohol-containing rubs or organic solvents may also trigger a reaction
- Reactions can occur up to 6 days after a dose
- Daily uninterrupted therapy must be continued until the patient has established a basis for self-control
- Drug should not be used alone, without proper motivation and supportive therapy; disulfiram will not cure alcoholism, but acts as a motivational aid
- Encourage patient to carry an identification card stating the name of the drug they are taking

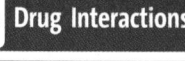 **Patient Instructions**
- For detailed patient instructions on disulfiram, see the Patient Information Sheet on p. 358

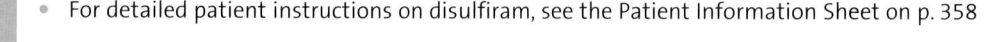 **Drug Interactions**
- Clinically significant interactions are listed below

Class of Drug	Example	Interaction Effects
Antiarrhythmic	Amiodarone	Increased amiodarone levels due to inhibited metabolism via CYP3A4
Antibiotic	Clarithromycin	Case of toxic epidermal necrolysis likely secondary to competitive inhibition via CYP3A4
Anticoagulant	Warfarin, coumarins	Increased PT ratio or INR response due to reduced metabolism
Anticonvulsant	Phenytoin	Increased anticonvulsant blood levels and toxicity due to reduced metabolism
Antidepressant Cyclic Irreversible MAOIs	Amitriptyline, desipramine Tranylcypromine	Increased plasma level of antidepressant due to reduced metabolism; neurotoxicity reported with combination Report of delirium, psychosis with combination
Antipsychotic	Clozapine	Inhibited metabolism and increased plasma level of clozapine
Antitubercular Drug	Isoniazid	Unsteady gait, incoordination, behavioral changes reported due to reduced metabolism of isoniazid
Benzodiazepine	Diazepam, alprazolam chlordiazepoxide, triazolam	Increased activity of benzodiazepine due to decreased clearance (oxazepam, temazepam, and lorazepam not affected)

Class of Drug	Example	Interaction Effects
Caffeine		Reduced clearance of caffeine by 24–30%
Cocaine		Increased plasma level (3- to 6-fold) and half-life (by 60%) of cocaine; increased risk of cardiovascular effects
Metronidazole		Acute psychosis, ataxia, and confusional states reported
Narcotic	Methadone	Decreased clearance of methadone
Paraldehyde		Alcohol-like reaction can occur as paraldehyde is metabolized to acetaldehyde
Protease inhibitor	Ritonavir solution Amprenavir solution	Alcohol-like reaction reported (as formulation contains alcohol) Toxicity reported – formulation contains propylene glycol; metabolism inhibited
St. John's Wort		Alcohol-like reactions reported
Theophylline	Oxtriphylline, theophylline	Increased plasma level of theophyllines due to reduced metabolism via aldehyde hydrogenase

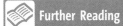 **Further Reading**

Reference

[1] American Psychiatric Association. Practice guideline and resources for treatment of patients with substance use disorders, 2nd ed. Am J Psychiatry 2006;163(8 Suppl); 1–276. Available from: http://www.psychiatryonline.com/pracGuide/pracGuideTopic_5.aspx (Accessed November 20, 2008)

Additional Suggested Reading

- Malcolm R, Olive MF, Lechner W. The safety of disulfiram for the treatment of alcohol and cocaine dependence in randomized clinical trials; guidance for clinical practice. Expert Opin Drug Saf. 2008;7(4):459–472.
- Soghoian S, Weiner SW, Diaz-Alcala JE. Toxicity, Disulfiram. eMedicine; 2007 [Article updated: Aug 20, 2008]. Available from: http://www.emedicine.com/emerg/TOPIC151.HTM (Accessed November 20, 2008)
- Wilkens, JN. Neurobiology and pharmacotherapy for alcohol dependence: Treatment options. New York, NY: Medscape, 2007. Available from: http://www.medscape.com/viewarticle/552196

Acamprosate

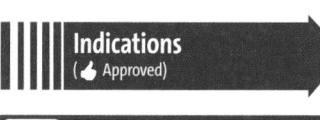 **Product Availability**

Chemical Class	Generic Name	Trade Name	Dosage Forms and Strengths
Calcium acetyl-homotaurine	Acamprosate calcium	Campral	Delayed-release enteric-coated tablets: 333 mg (equiv. to 300 mg acamprosate)

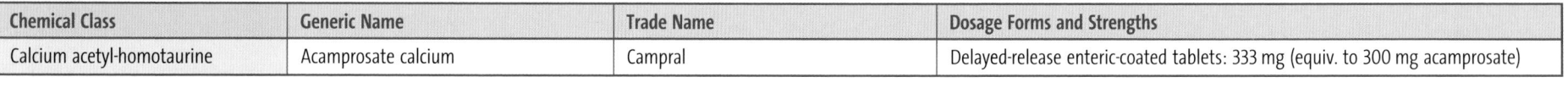 **Indications** (👍 Approved)

- 👍 Maintenance of abstinence from alcohol; reduces alcohol cravings and prevents relapse (level of evidence 1[1])

General Comments

- Meta-analyses have shown that patients treated with acamprosate had significantly higher continuous abstinence rates than those on placebo
- May not be effective in patients who are actively drinking at the start of treatment or in patients who abuse other substances; it is not effective for acute withdrawal and does not treat delirium tremens. Initiate treatment as soon as possible after alcohol withdrawal; treatment should be maintained for 1 year and continued during relapses
- Acamprosate treatment should be part of a comprehensive alcohol management program that includes psychosocial support (level of evidence 1[1])
- Mixed results seen with combination with naltrexone as to increased efficacy and success of abstinence (see Interactions p. 283); acamprosate appears more useful in achieving abstinence as it reduces dysphoric effects that trigger some patients to resume drinking, while naltrexone controls alcohol consumption by reducing the pleasurable effects of alcohol
- Has been used in combination with disulfiram to increase abstinence

Pharmacology

- Restores glutamate tone and modulates neuronal hyperexcitability during withdrawal from alcohol
- Weak inhibitor of presynaptic GABA B receptors in the nucleus accumbens

Dosing

- Adults > 60 kg: 666 mg tid; < 60 kg: 666 mg bid; to minimize GI effects can initiate more gradually, i.e., 333 mg tid and increase dose by 1 tablet per week until target dose is reached
- Hepatic disorders: no dosage adjustment needed
- Renal dysfunction: give 333 mg tid if creatinine clearance (CrCl) is 30–50 ml/min; avoid in patients with CrCl < 30 ml/min

Pharmacokinetics

- Food decreases absorption of acamprosate; C_{max} decreased by 42% and AUC by 23%
- Bioavailability = 11%; peak plasma level = 3–8 h
- Has low protein binding
- Half-life = 20–33 h
- Is not degraded by the liver and is primarily excreted as unchanged drug by the kidneys – not involved in CYP-450 interactions

Adverse Effects

- Common: nausea, flatulence and diarrhea (dose-related and decreases over time), headache, asthenia, pruritus
- Depression, anxiety, insomnia and suicidal ideation reported
- Less common: vomiting, dizziness, fluctuations in libido, maculopapular rash
- Acute renal failure reported

Precautions

- Use of acamprosate does not diminish withdrawal symptoms

Contraindications

- Avoid in severe renal insufficiency (CrCl < 30 ml/min)

| **Toxicity** | • Diarrhea reported after overdose of 56 g |
| | • Provide supportive treatment |

| **Pediatric Considerations** | • Not recommended |

| **Geriatric Considerations** | • Use caution and avoid in patients with renal impairment |

| **Use in Pregnancy** | • Category C drug; teratogenic effects seen in animal studies – not recommended in humans |
| Breast Milk | • Not known if excreted in human milk |

Nursing Implications	• Acamprosate treatment should be part of a comprehensive alcohol management program that includes psychosocial support
	• As tablets are enteric-coated, they should not be broken or chewed, but swallowed whole
	• Monitor patients for symptoms of depression or suicidal thinking
	• Diarrhea occurs commonly during therapy, is dose-related, and generally transient

| **Patient Instructions** | • For detailed patient instruction on acamprosate, see the Patient Information Sheet on p. 359 |

| **Drug Interactions** | • Clinically significant interactions are listed below |

Class of Drug	Example	Interaction Effects
Naltrexone		Rate and extent of absorption of acamprosate increased; C_{max} increased by 33% and AUC by 25%

Further Reading

Reference

[1] American Psychiatric Association. Practice guideline and resources for treatment of patients with substance use disorders, 2nd ed. Am J Psychiatry 2006;163(8 Suppl); 1–276. Available from: http://www.psychiatryonline.com/pracGuide/pracGuideTopic_5.aspx (Accessed November 20, 2008)

Additional Suggested Reading

• Gage A. Acamprosate efficacy in alcohol-dependent patients: Summary of results from three pivotal trials. Am J Addict. 2008;17(1):70–76.
• Mason BJ. Acamprosate in the treatment of alcohol dependence. Expert Opin Pharmacother. 2005; 6(12):2103–2115.
• Rosenthal RN, Brady KT, Petros L, et al. Advances in the treatment of alcohol dependence. J Clin Psychiatry. 2007;68(7):1117–1127.

Naltrexone

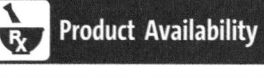

Product Availability

Chemical Class	Generic Name	Trade Name[A]	Dosage Forms and Strengths
	Naltrexone	ReVia Vivitrol[B]	Tablets: 25 mg[B], 50 mg, 100 mg[B] Extended-release injection: 380 mg

[A] Generic preparations may be available, [B] Not available in Canada

Indications
(👍 Approved)

- 👍 Adjunct in the treatment of alcohol dependence (level of evidence 1[1])
- 👍 Adjunct in the treatment of opiate addiction (level of evidence 1[1])
- Used in rapid opiate detoxification from methadone in combination with clonidine or trazodone
- Reported benefit in impulse-control disorders, e.g., binge-eating behavior in females with bulimia, trichotillomania, kleptomania; double-blind and open trials suggest benefit in treating pathological gambling, with good long-term outcomes reported
- Treatment of repetitive self-injurious behavior, hyperactivity, temper tantrums and stereotypic behavior of autism
- Decreased drinking and alcohol craving reported in patients with schizophrenia and comorbid alcohol dependence
- Used in combination with antidepressants in patients with comorbid alcohol dependence and depression
- Open trial suggests benefit in treating adolescent sexual offenders with doses of 100–200 mg/day

General Comments

- Recommended to be used together with psychosocial interventions (level of evidence 1[1])
- Metaanalyses have shown variable effects on abstinence: have shown a moderate decrease in the number of heavy drinking days; may be more effective in males with a family history of alcoholism; double-blind study suggests that it may not have long-term benefits in men with chronic severe alcohol dependence
- Patient compliance plays a significant role in the efficacy of naltrexone
- Mixed results seen with combination with acamprosate as to increased efficacy and success of abstinence (see interaction p. 286); naltrexone controls alcohol consumption while acamprosate more useful in achieving abstinence
- Does not attenuate craving for opioids or suppress withdrawal symptoms; patients must undergo detoxification before starting the drug
- Does not produce euphoria
- Pretreatment with oral naltrexone is not required prior to use of the extended-release injection

Pharmacology

- Synthetic long-acting antagonist at various opiate receptor sites in the CNS; highest affinity for the μ opioid receptor – inhibits the positive reinforcement of increased B-endorphins during alcohol use
- Blocks the craving mechanism in the brain producing less of a high from alcohol; stops the reinforcing effect of alcohol by blocking the opioid system – promotes abstinence and reduces risk for relapse

Dosing

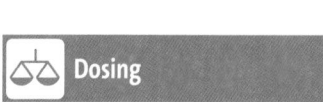

Oral

- Alcohol dependence: begin at 25 mg/day and increase to 50 mg/day over several days to minimize side effects
- Opioid dependence: initiate dose at 12.5 to 25 mg/day and monitor for withdrawal signs; increase dose gradually based on response. Maintenance dose can be given every 2 to 3 days to a total of 350 mg weekly
- Dosage requirements in impulse-control disorders may be higher (up to 200 mg/day)

Injection

- The extended-release injection is formulated as microspheres and 380 mg is administered by IM injection into the gluteal muscle every 4 weeks

Pharmacokinetics

Oral

- Rapidly and completely absorbed from the GI tract
- Undergoes extensive first-pass metabolism; only about 20% of drug reaches the systemic circulation
- Widely distributed; 21–28% is protein bound
- Onset of effect occurs in 15–30 minutes in chronic morphine users
- Duration of effect is dose-dependent; blockade of opioid receptors lasts 24–72 h
- Metabolized in liver (not via CYP-450); major metabolite, 6-b-naltrexone is active as an opiate antagonist
- Elimination half-life is 96 h; excreted primarily by the kidneys
- Dose adjustment not required in mild to moderate liver or renal impairment

Injection

- First peak occurs 2 h post injection; second peak occurs 2–3 days later; onset of effect seen within 48 h
- Elimination half-life is 5–10 days and is dependent on the erosion of the polymer; plasma concentrations are sustained for at least 30 days

Adverse Effects

- Common with oral naltrexone: nausea and vomiting (approx 10%), dysphoria
- Common with extended-release injection: nausea, headache, fatigue, pain; and tenderness at injection site, pruritus or indurations
- GI effects – abdominal pain, cramps, anorexia and weight loss; women are more sensitive to GI side effects
- CNS effects: insomnia, anxiety, depression, confusion, nervousness, fatigue; case reports of naltrexone-induced panic attacks
- Physical effects: headache (6.6%), joint and muscle pain or stiffness
- Dose-related elevated enzymes and hepatocellular injury reported; increased ALT and AST associated with concurrent use of NSAIDs, ASA or acetaminophen, liver function tests recommended at start of treatment and monthly for the first 6 months
- Eosinophilia
- Cases of allergic pneumonia reported with injection

D/C Discontinuation Syndrome

- No data available

Precautions

- Since naltrexone is an opiate antagonist, do not give to patients who have used narcotics in the previous 10 days – may result in symptoms of opiate withdrawal
- Do not use in patients with liver disorders; baseline liver function tests recommended; repeat monthly for 6 months. Liver toxicity has been reported in very obese individuals on high doses and in combination with NSAIDs, ASA, and acetaminophen
- Attempts to overcome blockade of naltrexone with high doses of opioid agonists (e.g., morphine) may lead to respiratory depression and death

Contraindications

- Patients receiving opioids, or those in acute opioid withdrawal
- Acute hepatitis or liver failure

Toxicity

- No experience in humans; 800 mg dose for 1 week showed no evidence of toxicity

Pediatric Considerations

- Has been studied in children for aggression, self-injurious behavior, autism and mental retardation (dose: 0.5–2 mg/kg/day)
- Effects noted within first hour of administration

Geriatric Considerations

- No data

Naltrexone (cont.)

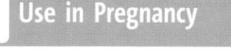
Use in Pregnancy

- No adequate well-controlled studies done

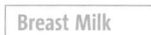
Breast Milk

- Naltrexone and its primary metabolite 6-b-naltrexone are excreted into breast milk in very low concentrations

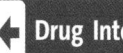
Nursing Implications

- Naltrexone should be used in conjunction with established psychotherapy or self-help programs
- As naltrexone does not attenuate craving for opioids or suppress withdrawal symptoms, compliance problems may occur; individuals must undergo detoxification prior to starting drug
- Patients should be advised to carry documentation stating that they are taking naltrexone
- Advise patients not to self-medicate with NSAIDs, acetaminophen, or aspirin
- Advise patients receiving extended-release injections of naltrexone that administration of large doses of opioids may lead to serious adverse effects, coma or death
- Advise patients to report shortness of breath, coughing or wheezing to their physician
- Vivitrol injection must be diluted only with the supplied diluent and administered with needle provided in kit. Store kit in the refrigerator; can be kept at room temperature for no more than 7 days. Once diluted, the injection should be administered IM right away (alternating buttocks); pain on injection possible; monitor patients for rash or indurations at injection site
- Should a patient miss a scheduled appointment for receiving injectable naltrexone, the next dose of injection can be given as soon as possible

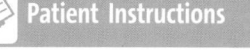
Patient Instructions

- For detailed patient instructions on naltrexone, see the Patient Information Sheet on p. 360

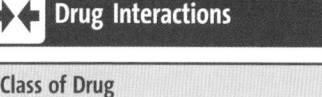
Drug Interactions

- Clinically significant interactions are listed below

Class of Drug	Example	Interaction Effects
Acamprosate		Rate and extent of absorption of acamprosate increased; C_{max} increased by 33% and AUC by 25%
Antipsychotic	Chlorpromazine	Lethargy, somnolence with combination
Narcotic	Codeine, morphine	Decreased efficacy of narcotic

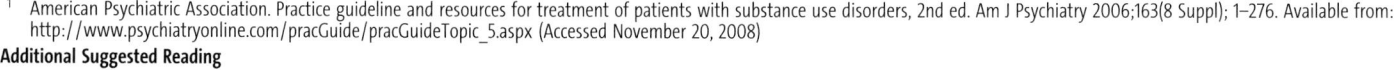
Further Reading

Reference
[1] American Psychiatric Association. Practice guideline and resources for treatment of patients with substance use disorders, 2nd ed. Am J Psychiatry 2006;163(8 Suppl); 1–276. Available from: http://www.psychiatryonline.com/pracGuide/pracGuideTopic_5.aspx (Accessed November 20, 2008)

Additional Suggested Reading
- Grant JE, Kim SW, Hartman BK. A double-blind, placebo-controlled study of the opiate antagonist naltrexone in the treatment of pathological gambling urges. J Clin Psychiatry 2008;69:783–789.
- Minozzi S, Amato L, Vecchi S, et al. Oral naltrexone maintenance treatment for opioid dependence. Cochrane Database of Systematic Reviews 2006, Issue 1. Art. No.: CD001333. DOI: 10.1002/14651858.CD001333.pub2.
- National Institute for Health and Clinical Excellence (NICE). Technology appraisal TA 115: Drug misuse – Naltrexone: Naltrexone for the management of opioid dependence. London, UK: NICE; 2007. Available from: www.nice.org.uk/TA115 (Accessed November 21, 2008).
- Rosenthal RN, Brady KT, Petros L, et al. Advances in the treatment of alcohol dependence. J Clin Psychiatry. 2007; 68(7):1117–1127.
- Symons FJ, Thompson A, Rodriguez MC. Self-injurious behavior and the efficacy of naltrexone treatment: A quantitative synthesis. Ment Retard Dev Disabil Res Rev. 2004;10:193–200.

Methadone

Product Availability

Chemical Class	Generic Name	Trade Name(A)	Dosage Forms and Strengths
	Methadone	Roxane(B), Metadol(C) Dolophine(B), Metadol(C)	Bulk powder Oral liquid: 1 mg/ml(C), 5 mg/5 ml(B), 10 mg/5 ml(B), 10 mg/ml Tablets: 1 mg(C), 5 mg, 10 mg, 25 mg(C), 40 mg(B) (dispersible) Injection(B): 10 mg/ml

(A) Generic preparations may be available, (B) Not marketed in Canada, (C) Not marketed in USA

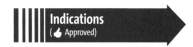

Indications
(👍 Approved)

- 👍 A substitute drug in narcotic analgesic dependence therapy (level of evidence 1[1])
- 👍 Treatment of severe pain

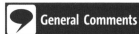

General Comments

- Useful drug in opiate-dependent patients who desire maintenance opiate therapy and who relapse with alternative interventions, because:
  - effective orally and can be administered once daily, due to its long half-life
  - suppresses withdrawal symptoms of other narcotic analgesics
  - suppresses chronic craving for narcotics without developing tolerance
  - does not produce euphoria in users already tolerant to euphoric effects of narcotic analgesics
- Patients receiving methadone remain in treatment longer, demonstrate a decreased use of illicit opiates, show decreased antisocial behavior and maintain social stability
- Methadone is a narcotic and its prescribing, dispensing and usage is governed by Federal regulations (regulations vary in different countries). It is prepared as a liquid, mixed with orange juice. Most patients receive their methadone, on a daily basis, from the pharmacy and are required to drink the contents of the bottle in the presence of the pharmacist. Some patients (who are stable on their medication) are permitted to carry several days' supply of methadone

Pharmacology

- A synthetic opiate acting on the mu-opiate receptor; blocks reinforcing euphorigenic effects of other administered opiates
- Analgesic and sedative properties – similar in degree to morphine, but with a longer duration of action

Dosing

- Initially 30–40 mg/day, given once daily; increase by 10 mg every 2–3 days to a stable maintenance dose; doses > 100 mg are rarely needed for control of symptoms
- Oral methadone doses are approximately twice the intravenous dose (due to decreased bioavailability)
- Patients vary in dosage requirements; dosage is adjusted to control abstinence symptoms without causing marked sedation or respiratory depression
- In rare cases patients who are rapid metabolizers of methadone may require a divided (split) dose rather than one single daily dose; this situation should be carefully evaluated and monitored for toxicity and respiratory depression

Pharmacokinetics

- Bioavailability: 70–80%
- Peak plasma level: 2–3 h
- 70–85% protein bound
- Half-life: 13–55 h (average: 25 h); half-life increases with repeated dosing. Note: $T_{1/2}$ is longer than methadone's duration of action (4–8 h); drug accumulates if taken too frequently
- Metabolized by the liver primarily via CYP3A4 and 2D6, with minor elimination via CYP2C19 – see Interactions pp. 289–290
- Inhibits P-gp

Methadone (cont.)

- Plasma level measurements are not considered useful, except in specific circumstances where stabilization has posed difficulties (threshold range suggested to be 150–220 ng/ml)
- Urine testing may be done to detect illicit drug use and/or compliance with methadone

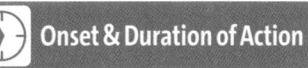

Onset & Duration of Action

- Onset of effect: 30–60 minutes
- Duration of action increases with chronic use

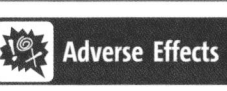

Adverse Effects

CNS Effects

- Drowsiness, insomnia, euphoria, dysphoria, confusion, cognitive impairment, depression and weakness; tolerance develops to sedating and analgesic effects
- With chronic use: sleep disturbances
- Headache

Anticholinergic Effects

- Sweating, flushing
- Chronic constipation

Cardiovascular Effects

- Dizziness, lightheadedness
- Cases of QT prolongation and torsades de pointes – increased risk with higher doses (> 150 mg/day), drug accumulation, in patients with pre-existing heart disease, in combination with drugs that increase the QT interval, or with drugs that decrease the metabolism of methadone via CYP3A4 (see Interactions p. 289) [baseline ECG recommended; repeat periodically and if dose increased > 150 mg/day]

GI Effects

- Nausea, vomiting, decreased appetite
- Weight changes

Urogential and Sexual Effects

- Impotence, ejaculatory problems

Other Adverse Effects

- Rarely, pulmonary edema and respiratory depression
- With chronic use: menstrual irregularities, pain in joints and bones

D/C Discontinuation Syndrome

- Rapid withdrawal can result in opiate withdrawal syndrome, which includes CNS effects: restlessness, agitation, insomnia, headache; Autonomic effects: increased blood pressure, heart rate, body temperature and respiration, lacrimation, perspiration, congestion, itching, "gooseflesh"; Neurological effects: muscle twitching, cramps, tremors, seizures; GI effects: nausea, vomiting, diarrhea, anorexia
- Symptoms may begin 24–48 h after the last dose, peak in 72 h, and may last for 6–7 weeks
- If no dosing changes occurred, consider drug interaction as a potential cause of withdrawal symptoms

Management

- Reinstitute dose to previous level; restabilize patient and monitor while tapering dose at a slower rate
- Clonidine may ameliorate withdrawal symptoms

⚠ Precautions

- Methadone has a high physical and psychological dependence liability, therefore withdrawal symptoms will occur on abrupt discontinuation – decrease the dose slowly
- Prior to prescribing methadone, a baseline ECG should be done; repeat within 30 days of treatment and annually, or if patient has unexplained syncope or seizures. Consider discontinuing drug if QTc interval is > 500 ms. Avoid methadone in patients with a history of structural heart disease, arrhythmia or syncope
- Methadone can build up in the body if dosed too frequently, with high doses or in combination with drugs that decrease its metabolism – caution re possible QT prolongation. Peak respiratory depressant effects occur later, and persist longer than peak analgesic effects

Toxicity	• With excessive doses can get shallow breathing, pinpoint pupils, flaccidity of skeletal muscles, low blood pressure, slowed heart rate, cold and clammy skin; can progress to cyanosis, coma, severe respiratory depression, circulatory collapse and cardiac arrest
Pediatric Considerations	• For detailed information on the use of methadone in this population, please see the *Clinical Handbook of Psychotropic Drugs for Children and Adolescents* (2007) • Has been used for postoperative pain in children at doses of 0.2 mg/kg; longer duration of action than with morphine. Drug must be tapered (by 5–10% every 1–2 days) if used for longer than 5–7 days; the patient must be continually assessed for withdrawal symptoms
Geriatric Considerations	• No data
Use in Pregnancy	• Methadone treatment throughout pregnancy reduces risk of perinatal and infant mortality in heroin-dependent women, and is not associated with adverse postnatal development • Dosing needs should be assessed during pregnancy: decreased between weeks 14 and 32, increased prior to term, reduced following birth, and reassessed regularly • Short-term withdrawal effects reported in approximately 60% of infants (not dose-related); no long-term effects demonstrated
Breast Milk	• A small amount of methadone enters breast milk; nurse prior to a dose of methadone, or 2–6 h after dose
Nursing Implications	• Methadone must be prescribed in sufficient doses, on a maintenance basis, to prevent relapse; long-term treatment may be required. Premature withdrawal may lead to relapse • Methadone is a narcotic and must be prescribed according to Federal regulations. It is prepared as a liquid mixed in orange juice. Many patients pick up their methadone, from the pharmacy, on a daily basis, and drink the medication in the presence of the pharmacist. Some patients (who are stable on their medication) are permitted to carry several days' supply of methadone • Each time the patient is to be medicated, he/she should be assessed for impairment (i.e., drowsiness, slurred speech, forgetfulness, lack of concentration, disorientation and ataxia); patients should not be medicated if they appear impaired or smell of alcohol – the physician should be contacted as to management of the patient • Encourage patients to carry a card in their wallet stating that they are taking methadone
Patient Instructions	• For detailed patient instructions on methadone, see the Patient Information Sheet on p. 361
Drug Interactions	• Clinically significant interactions are listed below

Class of Drug	Example	Interaction Effects
Alcohol		Acute alcohol use can decrease methadone metabolism and increase the plasma level – may result in intoxication and respiratory depression Chronic alcohol use can induce methadone metabolism and decrease the plasma level
Antacid	Al/Mg antacids	Decreased absorption of methadone
Antiarrhythmic	Quinidine	Possible risk of QT prolongation
Anticonvulsant	Phenytoin, carbamazepine, barbiturates	Decreased plasma level of methadone due to enhanced metabolism (by 50% with phenytoin) – may cause opioid withdrawal
Antidepressant Cyclic SSRI	 Desipramine, amitriptyline Fluvoxamine	 Increased plasma level of desipramine (by about 108%) due to increased metabolism via CYP2D6 Increased giddiness, euphoria; suspected potentiation of methadone's "euphoric" effects – abuse with amitriptyline reported Increased plasma level of methadone by 20–100% with fluvoxamine, due to decreased clearance
Antifungal	Fluconazole	Increase in methadone peak and trough plasma levels by 27% and 48% respectively; clearance decreased by 24%

Methadone (cont.)

Class of Drug	Example	Interaction Effects
Antipsychotic	Risperidone	Case reports of precipitation of narcotic withdrawal symptoms (mechanism unclear)
Antitubercular	Isoniazid	Decreased clearance and increased plasma level of methadone
	Rifampin	Decreased plasma level of methadone (by up to 50%) due to enhanced metabolism – may cause withdrawal symptoms
Antiviral	Efavirenz, nevirapine	Increased clearance of methadone and decreased total concentration (AUC) (by up to 60% with efavirenz and nevirapine) via enzyme induction – withdrawal symptoms reported within 7–10 days
	Didanosine, stavudine	Decreased bioavailability of antiretrovirals due to increased degradation in GI tract by methadone (C_{max} and AUC decreased by 66% and 63%, respectively, for didanosine, and by 44% and 25% for stavudine)
	Zidovudine (AZT)	Inhibited metabolism of AZT by methadone (AUC increased by 43%)
	Abacavir	Abacavir levels decreased by 34%, however clearance remained the same Methadone plasma level increased by 23% – may result in withdrawal
	Delavirdine	Likely to increase methadone levels via inhibition of metabolizing enzymes
Benzodiazepine	Diazepam, clonazepam	Enhanced risk of respiratory depression
	Diazepam	"Opiate high" reported with combined use
Buprenorphine		Decreased metabolism of methadone through inhibition of CYP3A4
Disulfiram		Decreased clearance of methadone
Grapefruit juice		Decreased metabolism of methadone through inhibition of CYP3A4 and P-gp
H₂ antagonist	Cimetidine	Decreased clearance of methadone
Hypnotic	Zolpidem	Decreased metabolism of methadone through inhibition of CYP3A4
Narcotic	Pentazocine, nalbuphine, butorphanol	Occurrence of withdrawal symptoms due to partial antagonist effects of these narcotics
	Morphine	Efficacy of narcotic analgesic reduced; dosage may need to be increased
Protease inhibitor	Ritonavir	Variable effects on clearance of methadone reported
	Amprenavir	AUC, C_{max}, and C_{min} of amprenavir decreased by 30%, 27%, and 25%, respectively Methadone levels decreased an average of 35% with amprenavir/abacavir combination
	Indinavir	Variable effects reported on C_{max} of indinavir Reduced AUC of methadone by 40%
	Nelfinavir	AUC of nelfanavir metabolite decreased by 53% – significance unknown
	Lopinavir/ritonavir	Methadone AUC decreased by 36% due to increased clearance (attributed to lopinavir) – may result in withdrawal
	Ritonavir/saquinavir	Displacement from protein binding of methadone and decrease in AUC of both R-methadone and S-methadone
St. John's Wort		Decreased plasma level of methadone; symptoms of withdrawal reported
Stimulant	MDMA	Decreased metabolism of methadone through inhibition of CYP2D6
Urine acidifier	Ascorbic acid	Increased elimination of methadone
Urine alkalizer	Sodium bicarbonate	Decreased elimination of methadone

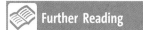 **Further Reading**

Reference

[1] American Psychiatric Association. Practice guideline and resources for treatment of patients with substance use disorders, 2nd ed. Am J Psychiatry 2006;163(8 Suppl); 1–276. Available from: http://www.psychiatryonline.com/pracGuide/pracGuideTopic_5.aspx (Accessed November 20, 2008)

Additional Suggested Reading

- Bomsien S, Skopp G. An in vitro approach to potential methadone metabolic-inhibition interactions. Eur J Clin Pharmacol. 2007;63(9):821–827.
- Ehret GB, Desmeules JA, Broers B. Methadone-associated long QT syndrome: Improving pharmacotherapy for dependence on illegal opioids and lessons learned for pharmacology. Expert Opin Drug Saf. 2007;6(3):289–303.
- Krantz MJ, Martin J, Stimmel B, et al. QTc interval screening in methadone treatment: The CSAT Consensus Guideline. Ann Intern Med. 2009;150(6):387–395.
- Leavitt SB. Methadone-Drug Interactions, 3rd ed. (November 2005).Available from: http://www.atforum.com/SiteRoot/pages/addiction_resources/Drug_Interactions.pdf
- National Institute for Health and Clinical Excellence (NICE). Technology appraisal TA 114: Drug misuse – methadone and buprenorphine: Methadone and buprenorphine for managing opioid dependence. London, UK: NICE, 2007 . Available from: www.nice.org.uk/TA114
- Office of Canada's Drug Strategy, Health Canada. Literature review – methadone maintenance treatment. Ottawa, Canada: Health Canada, 2002. Available from: http://www.hc-sc.gc.ca/hl-vs/pubs/adp-apd/methadone/index_e.html (Accessed November 21, 2008).
- Toombs JD, Kral LA. Methadone treatment for pain states. Am Fam Physician. 2005;71(7):1353–1358.

Buprenorphine

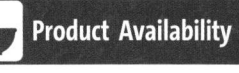 **Product Availability**

Chemical Class	Generic Name	Trade Name	Dosage Forms and Strengths
	Buprenorphine	Subutex	Sublingual tablets: 0.4 mg[c] 2 mg, 8mg
	Buprenorphine HCl/Naloxone HCl	Suboxone	Sublingual tablets: 2 mg/0.5 mg, 8 mg/2 mg

[c] Not marketed in USA

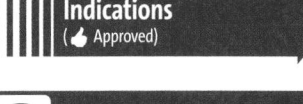 **Indications**
(Approved)

- Treatment of opioid addiction (level of evidence 1[1]); used alone or together with naloxone
- Significant decrease in cocaine use noted in patients with comorbid cocaine/opioid dependence
- Analgesic for moderate to severe pain

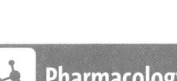 **General Comments**

- Subutex may be better tolerated by patients during the first few days of treatment; Suboxone is preferred for maintenance treatment due to presence of naloxone in a 4:1 formulation – intended to deter intravenous abuse as it causes withdrawal symptoms if crushed or taken IV
- Reduces use and craving for opioids; should be combined with concurrent behavior therapies and psychosocial programs
- Considered as effective as moderate doses of methadone; methadone is considered the treatment of choice in patients with higher levels of physical dependence
- Improvement noted in psychosocial adjustment and social functioning
- Causes minimal withdrawal symptoms due to partial agonist activity
- Other formulations of buprenorphine (i.e., injection) are not approved for the treatment of opioid addiction

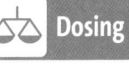 **Pharmacology**

- If switching to Suboxone from methadone maintenance, it is recommended that the methadone dose be tapered down to 30 mg or less prior to starting buprenorphine, to minimize withdrawal symptoms[1]
- Buprenorphine is a partial µ-opiate receptor agonist and κ-opiate receptor antagonist (naloxone is an opiate antagonist)
- Agonist effects increase linearly with increasing doses of buprenorphine, to a plateau or "ceiling effect"; at high doses will act as an antagonist and can precipitate withdrawal symptoms – less risk of fatal overdose

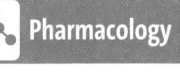 **Dosing**

- 4–24 mg (buprenorphine) sublingually (or 4–24 mg buprenorphine/1–6 mg naloxone) given once daily; due to long half-life, some patients can be dosed every 2 days
- Phases of treatment:
  - Induction Phase: individual has abstained from opioids for 12–24 h and is in early stages of withdrawal: 8 mg buprenorphine can be administered sublingually on day 1, and 16 mg on day 2; from day 3 onward continue with the dose given on day 2
  - Stabilization Phase: patient has discontinued or greatly reduced drug of abuse, and has no more cravings and few side effects; dose of buprenorphine can be adjusted in increments/decrements of 2–4 mg to a level that suppresses both cravings and withdrawal effects (4–24 mg/day)
  - Maintenance Phase: patient is on a stable dose of buprenorphine (or combination) and is doing well; the patient may require indefinite maintenance therapy, or the drug may be gradually withdrawn

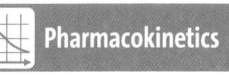 **Pharmacokinetics**

- Sublingual buprenorphine provides moderate bioavailability while sublingual naloxone bioavailability is poor; therefore buprenorphine's opioid agonist effects predominate
- Peak effects seen in 3–4 h after dosing; C_{max} and AUC increase in a linear fashion with dose increases
- Buprenorphine is highly bound to plasma proteins (96%) – primarily to α and β globulin; naloxone is 45% protein bound to albumin
- Metabolized by CYP3A4 to active metabolite, norbuprenorphine, and other metabolites; phase 2 metabolism via UGT1A1, 1A3
- Strong inhibitor of CYP3A4

- Buprenorphine half-life = 24–60 h (37 h mean); naloxone half-life = 1.1 h (mean)
- Use with caution in patients with hepatic dysfunction; no dosage adjustment required in renal disease

 Adverse Effects

- Most common in first 2–3 days of therapy and are dose-related; after the first dose, patient may experience some withdrawal symptoms
- Common: headache, insomnia, anxiety, nausea, abdominal pain, constipation, sweating and various pain
- No evidence of significant effects on cognitive or psychomotor performance
- Increase in liver enzymes; cases of hepatitis, hepatic necrosis, hepatic failure; monitor liver function tests periodically

 D/C Discontinuation Syndrome

- Very high doses can cause respiratory depression, which may be delayed in onset and more prolonged than with other opioids; reversal with naloxone is more difficult due to buprenorphine's very tight binding to opioid receptors[1]
- Withdrawal syndrome reported in patients on chronic therapy and with naloxone combination
- Causes milder withdrawal than full opioid antagonists (e.g., methadone), onset may be delayed
- Symptoms include: nausea/vomiting, diarrhea, muscle aches/cramps, sweating, lacrimation, rhinorrhea, dilated pupils, yawning, craving, mild fever, dysphoric mood, insomnia, and irritability

 Precautions

- Higher doses of buprenorphine can precipitate withdrawal in opioid-dependent individuals
- Chronic administration produces opiate-type dependence, characterized by withdrawal upon abrupt discontinuation or rapid taper
- Buprenorphine can be abused; if sublingual combination tablets are crushed and injected by opioid-dependent individual, naloxone effect predominates and can precipitate a withdrawal syndrome
- Use with caution in patients with compromised respiratory function or liver disorder

 Toxicity

- Safer in overdose than pure agonists due to poor bioavailability and ceiling effect of agonist action
- Symptoms include: pinpoint pupils, sedation, and hypotension; respiratory depression and deaths have been reported, particularly when buprenorphine was misused intravenously, or in combination with alcohol or other opioids
- Treatment: symptomatic
  - monitor for respiratory depression
  - naloxone may not be effective in reversing respiratory depression

 Pediatric Considerations

- Not recommended in children under age 16

 Geriatric Considerations

- No data

 Use in Pregnancy

- Teratogenic effects reported in animal studies; effects in humans unknown
- Neonatal withdrawal has been reported on days 1–8 after birth; symptoms include hypertonia, tremor, agitation, myoclonus, and rarely apnea, bradycardia, and convulsions; extended follow-up of infants, including full developmental pediatric assessment at 2 years, is suggested

Breast Milk

- Buprenorphine passes into mother's milk; breastfeeding is not recommended

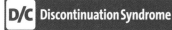 **Nursing Implications**

- Buprenorphine is a narcotic and considered to be a controlled substance
- Buprenorphine should be used in conjunction with behavior/psychosocial therapies
- The tablets should not be handled, but tipped directly in the mouth from a medicine cup; they should be placed (all together) under the tongue until dissolved (takes 2–10 min); drinking fluids prior to taking the tablets may speed up the dissolution process[1]; chewing or swallowing them reduces the bioavailability of the drug; the patient should not drink for at least 5 min so as to allow the drug to be absorbed
- Educate patient about not increasing his/her dose without physician approval, as high doses can precipitate a withdrawal syndrome; misuse/abuse may result in toxicity
- Serious CNS consequences may occur if buprenorphine is combined with benzodiazepines, hypnotics, or alcohol

Buprenorphine (cont.)

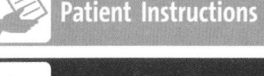

Patient Instructions

- For detailed patient instructions on buprenorphine, see the Patient Information Sheet on p. 362

Drug Interactions

- Clinically significant interactions are listed below

Class of Drug	Example	Interaction Effects
Antibacterial	Rifampin	Decreased level of buprenorphine possible due to increased metabolism via CYP3A4
Antibiotic	Erythromycin	Increased levels of buprenorphine possible due to inhibited metabolism via CYP3A4
Anticonvulsant	Carbamazepine, phenytoin, phenobarbital	Decreased levels of buprenorphine possible due to increased metabolism via CYP3A4
Antifungal	Ketoconazole	Increased Cmax and AUC of buprenorphine reported due to inhibited metabolism via CYP3A4
Anxiolytic	Benzodiazepine	Respiratory depression, coma and death reported when intravenous or high doses of buprenorphine used in combination
CNS Depressant	Alcohol, antipsychotics	CNS depression; deaths have been reported in combination
Narcotic	Morphine, meperidine, fentanyl	Low doses of buprenorphine antagonize analgesic effects High doses are synergistic; increase risk of CNS and respiratory depression
	Methadone	Can precipitate withdrawal
Protease Inhibitor	Ritonavir, indinavir, saquinavir	Increased level of buprenorphine possible due to inhibited metabolism via CYP3A4

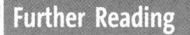

Further Reading

Reference

[1] American Psychiatric Association. Practice guideline and resources for treatment of patients with substance use disorders, 2nd ed. Am J Psychiatry 2006;163(8 Suppl); 1–276. Available from: http://www.psychiatryonline.com/pracGuide/pracGuideTopic_5.aspx (Accessed November 20, 2008)

Additional Suggested Reading

- Isaac P, Janecek E, Kalvik A, et al. A new treatment for opioid dependence. Pharmacy Connection. 2008;15(1):3237.
- Mattick RP, Kimber J, Breen C, et al. Buprenorphine maintenance versus placebo or methadone maintenance for opioid dependence. Cochrane Database of Systematic Reviews 2008, Issue 2. Art. No.: CD002207. DOI: 10.1002/14651858.CD002207.pub3.
- National Institute for Health and Clinical Excellence (NICE). Technology appraisal TA 114: Drug misuse – methadone and buprenorphine: Methadone and buprenorphine for managing opioid dependence. London, UK: NICE, 2007 . Available from: www.nice.org.uk/TA114
- Substance Abuse and Mental Health Services Administration (SAMHSA). About buprenorphine therapy. Available from: http://buprenorphine.samhsa.gov. Accessed Dec 1, 2008.
- Sung S, Conry, JM. Role of buprenorphine in the management of heroin addiction. Ann Pharmacother. 2006;40(3):501–505.
- U.S. Food and Drug Adminstration - Center for Drug Evaluation and Research. Subutex (buprenorphine hydrochloride) and Suboxone tablets (buprenorphine hydrochloride and naloxone hydrochloride). Available from: www.fda.gov/cder/drug/infopage/subutex_suboxone. Accessed Dec 1, 2008.

NEW UNAPPROVED TREATMENTS OF PSYCHIATRIC DISORDERS

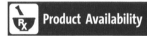 **Product Availability**

Biochemical theories on the etiology of specific psychiatric disorders have initiated investigations of various drugs/chemicals that may influence brain neurotransmitters and thereby play a role in the treatment of psychiatric disorders. Several drugs traditionally used to treat medical conditions have been found to be of benefit in ameliorating or preventing symptoms of certain psychiatric disorders. This section presents a summary of some of these drugs and their uses. **As a rule, unapproved treatments should be reserved for patients highly resistant to conventional therapies. Clinicians should always be cognizant of medicolegal issues when prescribing drugs for non-approved indications.**

	Anxiety Disorders	Depression	Bipolar Disorder (cycling)	Mania	Schizophrenia	Dementia	Antisocial Behavior/ Aggression	ADHD	Drug Dependence Treatment
Allopurinol (p. 303)				PR/S	PR/S	PR			
Anticonvulsants (p. 300)									
Phenytoin	PR	PR					C/P		
Pregabalin	+								
Tiagabine	+								
Vigabatrin	PR								
β-Blockers, e.g., propranolol, atenolol, pindolol (p. 296)	+	+/S/C			C/S		+		
Bromocriptine (p. 298)		+							
Cyproheptadine (p. 302)					C				
Estrogen/progesterone (p. 302)		+/S				PR	+		
Guanfacine (p. 297)								+	
Modafinil (p. 299)		PR/S						+	PR (cocaine)
Pramipexole (p. 300)		+/S							
Prazosin (p. 298)	PR								
Selegiline (p. 304)		see p. 56			PR	C/S		+	
Testosterone (p. 303)		PR/S/C							
Thyroid hormones (p. 297)	PR/S	S	C/S						
Tramadol (p. 302)	PR								

C = contradictory results, P = partial improvement, + = positive, S = synergistic effect, PR = preliminary data

Clinical Handbook of Psychotropic Drugs, 18th Edition, © 2009 Hogrefe & Huber Publishers

New Treatments

Adrenergic Agents

| β-Blockers e.g., propranolol | Have membrane-stabilizing effect and GABA-mimetic activity; presynaptic 5-HT_{1A} antagonist |

Antisocial Behavior/Aggression

- Propranolol dose: 80–960 mg/day, pindolol 10–60 mg/day
- Response may take up to 8 weeks
- Useful in controlling rage, violence, irritability, and aggression due to a number of causes (e.g., autism, ADHD, PTSD); usefulness of propranolol in SDAT is limited by short-term efficacy and contraindication for use in frail elderly
- May be effective in controlling aggressive behavior in children and adolescents with organic brain dysfunction; meta-analysis suggests β-blockers show good evidence for efficacy for management of agitation and aggression in patients with acquired brain injury
- Rebound rage reactions on drug withdrawal reported; taper dose gradually

Fleminger S, Greenwood RJ, Oliver DL. Pharmacological management for agitation and aggression in people with acquired brain injury. Cochrane Database Syst Rev. 2006 Oct 18;(4):CD003299.
Peskind ER, Tsuang DW, Bonner LT, et al. Propranolol for disruptive behaviors in nursing home residents with probable or possible Alzheimer disease: A placebo-controlled study. Alzheimer Dis Assoc Disord. 2005;19(1):23–28.

Anxiety Disorders

- Propranolol dose: up to 320 mg/day
- Beneficial for somatic or autonomically mediated symptoms of anxiety (e.g., tremor, palpitations) as seen in performance anxiety and acute panic
- Propranolol and pindolol may augment effects of SSRIs in panic disorder
- Efficacy reported in adults and children with posttraumatic stress disorder – early administration reported to treat intrusive memories and reduce severity of later symptoms
- Positive response also reported with atenolol (50 mg/day) for performance anxiety
- Pindolol 2.5–7.5 mg/day reported to augment response to SSRIs in OCD and panic disorder

Davidson JR. Pharmacotherapy of social anxiety disorder: What does the evidence tell us? J Clin Psychiatry. 2006;67(Suppl.12):S20–S26.
Debiec J, LeDoux JE. Disruption of reconsolidation but not consolidation of auditory fear conditioning by noradrenergic blockade in the amygdala. Neuroscience. 2004;129:267–272.
Glannon W. Psychopharmacology and Memory. J Med Ethics. 2006;32(2):74–78.
Pitman RK, Sanders KM, Zusman RM, et al. Pilot study of secondary prevention of posttraumatic stress disorder with propranolol. Biol Psychiatry. 2002;51(2):189–192.
Vaiva G, Ducrocq F, Jezequel K, et al. Immediate treatment with propranolol decreases posttraumatic stress disorder two months after trauma. Biol Psychiatry. 2003;54(9):947–949.

Depression

- Pindolol dose: 2.5 mg bid to 5 mg tid (5-HT_{1A} and $5\text{-HT}_{1B/1D}$ receptor blocker)
- Meta-analysis concluded that pindolol accelerates antidepressant response but doesn't increase the effectiveness of SSRIs in nonresponsive patients; data contradictory as lack of efficacy in some studies may be related to dose used and insufficient CNS 5-HT_{1A} receptor occupancy
- β-blockers are used to treat akathisia caused by SSRI antidepressants

Artigas F, Adell A, Celada P. Pindolol augmentation of antidepressant response. Curr Drug Targets. 2006;7(2):139–147.
Ballesteros J, Callado LF. Effectiveness of pindolol plus serotonin uptake inhibitors in depression: A meta-analysis of early and late outcomes from randomised controlled trials. J Affect Disord. 2004;79:137–147.
Brousse G, Schmitt A, Chereau I, et al. [Interest of the use of pindolol in the treatment of depression: review] [Article in French]. Encephale. 2003;29(4.1):338–350.

Schizophrenia

- Propranolol: 120–640 mg/day; pindolol 5 mg tid
- May be useful in controlling aggressive behavior in schizophrenic patients; nadolol reported to decrease overall psychotic symptoms and extrapyramidal side effects in aggressive schizophrenic patients; pindolol decreased the number and severity of aggressive acts
- May be beneficial in acute schizophrenia; may increase plasma level of antipsychotic; contradictory results seen
- Some response seen on negative symptoms
- Efficacy may be related to treatment of antipsychotic-induced akathisia; improvement reported in tardive akathisia
- When combined with clozapine β-blockers may have additive effects on weight gain and serum lipids

- Case reports of encephalopathy with doses over 1000 mg of propranolol

Baymiller SP, Ball P, McMahon RP, et al. Serum glucose and lipid changes during the course of clozapine treatment: the effect of concurrent beta-adrenergic antagonist treatment. Schizophr Res. 2003;59(1):49–57.

Caspi N, Modai I, Barak P, et al. Pindolol augmentation in aggressive schizophrenic patients: a double-blind crossover randomized study. Int Clin Psychopharmacol. 2001;16(2):111–115.

Guanfacine

Antihypertensive; α_{2A} agonist

ADHD

- Dose: 0.5–9 mg/day given bid
- Children metabolize guanfacine faster than adults and may require more frequent dosing (2–3 times a day)
- Studies suggest efficacy in patients nonresponsive to other medication or in patients with prominent impulsivity, aggression, hyperactivity, or co-morbid tic disorders
- Retrospective review of 80 cases showed benefit on hyperactivity, inattention, insomnia, and tics in 24% of children aged 3–18 with pervasive developmental disorders
- Efficacy reported in double-blind studies for adult ADHD
- Case reports of induced mania
- Common side effects: fatigue, sedation, and modest reductions in blood pressure and heart rate
- May cause withdrawal effects if stopped abruptly

Posey DJ, McDougle CJ. Guanfacine and guanfacine extended release: Treatment for ADHD and related disorders. CNS Drug Rev. 2007;13(4):465–474.

Posey DJ, Puntney JI, Sasher TM, et al. Guanfacine treatment of hyperactivity and inattention in pervasive developmental disorders: A retrospective analysis of 80 cases. J Child Adolesc Psychopharmacol. 2004;14(2):233–241.

Scahill L, Chappell PB, Kim YS, et al. A placebo-controlled study of guanfacine in the treatment of children with tic disorders and attention deficit hyperactivity disorder. Am J Psychiatry. 2001;158(7):1067–1074.

Taylor FB, Russo J. Comparing guanfacine and dextroamphetamine for the treatment of adult attention-deficit/hyperactivity disorder. J Clin Psychopharmacol. 2001;21(2):223–228.

Thyroid Hormones

Modulate adrenergic receptor function and permit a given concentration of catecholamines to be more effective; metabolic enhancers

Anxiety Disorders

- Dose: liothyronine 0.025 mg/day
- Open trial showed that addition of liothyronine to an SSRI reduced hyperarousal and depressive symptoms in 4 out of 5 patients with PTSD

Agid O, Shalev AY, Lerer B. Triiodothyronine augmentation of selective serotonin reuptake inhibitors in posttraumatic stress disorder. J Clin Psychiatry. 2001;62(3):169–173.

Friedman MJ, Wang S, Jalowiec JE, et al. Thyroid hormone alterations among women with posttraumatic stress disorder due to childhood sexual abuse. Biol Psychiatry. 2005;57(10):1186–1192.

Depression

- Dose: liothyronine (T_3): 0.005–0.05 mg/day, L-thyroxine (T_4) 0.15–0.5 mg/day
- In refractory depression, may potentiate effects of antidepressants; positive effects seen in up to 60% of refractory patients within 2 weeks – may be more beneficial in women than in men; suggested that treatment be discontinued if no response seen after 3 weeks
- Meta-analysis of 8 studies (4 double-blind) of T_3 augmentation showed an absolute response rate of 23% in patients refractory to tricyclics; evidence for augmentation of SSRIs is more limited and contradictory
- Suggested T_3 may actually be treating subclinical hypothyroidism
- Transitory side effects can include: sweating, shaking, nervousness, anxiety, and tachycardia
- May exacerbate mania
- Negative results reported when T_3 added to T_4 therapy in hypothyroid patients with depressive symptoms

Abraham G, Milev R, Lawson JS. T3 augmentation of SSRI resistant depression. J Affect Disord. 2006;91(2–3):211–215.

Cooper-Kazaz R, Apter JT, Cohen R, et al. Combined treatment with sertraline and liothyronine in major depression: A randomized, double-blind, placebo-controlled trial. Arch Gen Psychiatry. 2007;64(6):679–688.

Cooper-Kazaz R, Lerer B. Efficacy and safety of triiodothyronine supplementation in patients with major depressive disorder treated with specific serotonin reuptake inhibitors. Int J Neuropsychopharmacol. 2008;11(5):685–699.

Iosifescu DV, Nierenberg AA, Mischoulon D, et al. An open study of triiodothyronine augmentation of selective serotonin reuptake inhibitors in treatment-resistant major depressive disorder. J Clin Psychiatry. 2005;66(8):1038–1042.

New Treatments

Adrenergic Agents (cont.)

Lojko D, Rybakowski JK. L-thyroxine augmentation of serotonergic antidepressants in female patients with refractory depression. J Affect Disord. 2007;103(1–3):253–256.

Nierenberg AA, Fava M, Trivedi MH, et al. A comparison of lithium and T3 augmentation following two failed medication treatments for depression: a STAR*D report. Am J Psychiatry. 2006;163(9):1519–1530.

Sawka AM, Gerstein HC, Marriott MJ, et al. Does a combination regimen of thyroxine (T4) and 3,5,3'-triiodothyronine improve depressive symptoms better than T4 alone in patients with hypothyroidism? Results of a double-blind, randomized, controlled trial. J Clin Endocrinol Metab. 2003;88(10):4551–4555.

Sintzel F, Mallaret M, Bouquerol T. [Potentializing of tricyclics and serotoninergics by thyroid hormones in resistant depressive disorders] [Article in French]. Encephale. 2004;30(3):267–275.

Bipolar Disorder	• Dose: L-thyroxine: 0.3–0.5 mg/day

- Dose: L-thyroxine: 0.3–0.5 mg/day
- Controversial results seen
- May be treating unidentified hypothyroidism
- High dose of L-thyroxine reported to be an effective adjunctive maintenance treatment of prophylaxis-resistant mood disorder
- Reported to alleviate symptoms and increase cycle length in rapid-cycling female patients; adjunctive to other therapies of bipolar disorder
- Recommended to regularly assess bone mineral density in postmenopausal women on chronic T_4 therapy

Bauer M, Berghöfer A, Bschor T, et al. Supraphysiological doses of L-thyroxine in the maintenance treatment of prophylaxis-resistant affective disorders. Neuropsychopharmacology. 2002;27(4):620–628.

Bauer M, London ED, Silverman DH, et al. Thyroid, brain and mood modulation in affective disorder: insights from molecular research and functional brain imaging. Pharmacopsychiatry. 2003;36(Suppl. 3):S215–S221.

Gyulai L, Bauer M, Garcia-Espana F, et al. Bone mineral density in pre-and post-menopausal women with affective disorder treated with long-term L-thyroxine augmentation. J Affect Disord. 2001;66(2–3):185–191.

Prazosin

α_1-adrenergic antagonist

Anxiety Disorders	• Dose: up to 10.5 mg/day

- Dose: up to 10.5 mg/day
- A review of double-blind cross-over studies, open trials, and chart reviews suggests benefit in ameliorating sleep disturbances and nightmares in individuals with PTSD
- Daytime prazosin reported to decrease distress related to trauma cues
- Hypotension was the main side effect reported

Boehnlein JK, Kinzie JD. Pharmacologic reduction of CNS noradrenergic activity in PTSD: The case for clonidine and prazosin. J Psychiatr Pract. 2007;13(2):72–78.

Dierks MR, Jordan JK, Sheehan AH. Prazosin treatment of nightmares related to posttraumatic stress disorder. Ann Pharmacother. 2007;41(6):1013–1017.

Taylor HR, Freeman MK, Cates ME. Prazosin for treatment of nightmares related to posttraumatic stress disorder. Am J Health Syst Pharm. 2008;65(8):716–722.

Taylor FB, Lowe K, Thompson C, et al. Daytime prazosin reduces psychological distress to trauma specific cues in civilian trauma posttraumatic stress disorder. Biol Psychiatry. 2006;59(7):577–581.

Dopaminergic Agents

Bromocriptine

Biphasic effect hypothesized: Acts on presynaptic autoreceptors to inhibit dopaminergic transmission at lower doses, while acting as a dopamine postsynaptic receptor agonist at high doses

Depression	• Dose: 2.5–60 mg/day (doses up to 220 mg/day have been used)

- Dose: 2.5–60 mg/day (doses up to 220 mg/day have been used)
- Response seen after 4–14 days therapy
- Several double-blind studies show beneficial effect; may alleviate depressive recurrence in patients who initially responded to SSRIs; up to 57% of treatment-refractory patients responded in open trials; may alleviate SSRI-induced apathy syndrome
- Case reports of efficacy as augmentation therapy with cyclic antidepressants
- Hypomania has been reported

Nierenberg AA, Dougherty D, Rosenbaum JF. Dopaminergic agents and stimulants as antidepressant augmentation strategies. J Clin Psychiatry. 1998;59(Suppl 5):60–63.

Wada T, Kanno M, Aoshima T, et al. Dose-dependent augmentation effect of bromocriptine in a case with refractory depression. Prog Neuropsychopharmacol Biol Psychiatry. 2001;25(2):457–462.

Modafanil

Psychostimulant which blocks the dopamine transporter and increases dopamine; activates neurons and increases the release of histamine, dopamine NE and 5-HT; may work by reducing GABA release and increasing the release of glutamate

Depression

- Dose: 100–400 mg/day
- Review of double-blind, open label, and retrospective studies suggests modafinil may improve residual fatigue and sedation in patients receiving antidepressants; may enhance executive function, decrease sleepiness, and improve concentration, mood, and motivation
- Double-blind and open-label studies showed benefit in patients with atypical depression
- Placebo-controlled trial suggests modafinil plus a mood stabilizer may be more effective for treating bipolar depression without increasing the risk of mania
- Main side effects include headache and nausea; weight loss reported
- Has a low abuse potential
- Induces CYP1A2, 2B6 and 3A4; may decrease levels of drugs metabolized by these enzymes

DeBattista C, Doghramji K, Menza MA, et al. Adjunct modafinil for the short-term treatment of fatigue and sleepiness in patients with major depressive disorder: a preliminary double-blind, placebo-controlled study. J Clin Psychiatry. 2003;64(9):1057–1064.

Dunlop BW, Crits-Christoph P, Evans DL, et al. Coadministration of modafinil and a selective serotonin reuptake inhibitor from the initiation of treatment of major depressive disorder with fatigue and sleepiness: A double-blind, placebo-controlled study. J Clin Psychopharmacol. 2007;27(6):614–619.

Fava M, Thase EM, DeBattista C, et al. Modafinil augmentation of selective serotonin reuptake inhibitor therapy in MDD partial responders with persistent fatigue and sleepiness. Ann Clin Psychiatry. 2007;19(3):153–159.

Frye MA, Grunze H, Suppes T, et al. A placebo-controlled evaluation of adjunctive modafinil in the treatment of bipolar depression. Am J Psychiatry. 2007;164(8):1242–1249.

Fava M, Thase ME, DeBattista C. A multicenter, placebo-controlled study of modafinil augmentation in partial responders to selective serotonin reuptake inhibitors with persistent fatigue and sleepiness. J Clin Psychiatry. 2005;66(1):85–93.

Lam JY, Freeman MK, Cates ME. Modafinil augmentation for residual symptoms of fatigue in patients with a partial response to antidepressants. Ann Pharmacother. 2007;41(6):1005–1012.

Lundt L. Modafinil treatment in patients with seasonal affective disorder/winter depression: An open-label pilot study. J Affect Disord. 2004;81(2):173–178.

Ninan PT, Hassman HA, Glass SJ, et al. Adjunctive modafinil at initiation of treatment with a selective serotonin reuptake inhibitor enhances the degree and onset of therapeutic effects in patients with major depressive disorder and fatigue. J Clin Psychiatry. 2004;65(3):414–420.

Price CS, Taylor FB. A retrospective chart review of the effects of modafinil on depression as monotherapy and as adjunctive therapy. Depress Anxiety. 2005;21(4):149–153.

Schwartz TL, Azhar N, Cole K, et al. An open-label study of adjunctive modafinil in patients with sedation related to serotonergic antidepressant therapy. J Clin Psychiatry. 2004;65(9):1223–1227.

Stahl SM, Zhang L, Damatarca C, et al. Brain circuits determine destiny in depression: a novel approach to the psychopharmacology of wakefulness, fatigue, and executive dysfunction in major depressive disorder. J Clin Psychiatry. 2003;64(Suppl 14):6–17.

Vaishnavi S, Gadde K, Alamy S, et al. Modafinil for atypical depression: Effects of open-label and double-blind discontinuation treatment. J Clin Psychopharmacol. 2006;26(4):373–378.

ADHD

- Dose: 100–425 mg/day in divided doses
- Beneficial results reported in open and double-blind trials of children, aged 5–15 – may be useful for inattention, hyperactivity/impulsivity and oppositional behavior, or when anorexia limits the use of stimulants
- Good response reported in double-blind placebo-controlled study of modafinil (mean dose 206.8 mg/day) compared with dextroamphetamine, in adults

Amiri S, Mohammadi MR, Nouroozinejad GH, et al. Modafinil as a treatment for attention-deficit/hyperactivity disorder in children and adolescents: A double blind, randomized clinical trial. Prog Neuro-psychopharmacol Biol Psychiatry. 2008;32(1):145–149.

Ballon JS, Feifel D. A systematic review of modafinil: Potential, clinical uses and mechanisms of action. J Clin Psychiatry. 2006;67(4):554–566.

Biederman J, Pliszka SR. Modafinil improves symptoms of attention-deficit/hyperactivity disorder across subtypes in children and adolescents. J Pediatr. 2008;152(3):394–399.

Biederman J, Swanson JM, Wigal SB, et al. Efficacy and safety of modafinil film-coated tablets in children and adolescents with attention-deficit/hyperactivity disorder: results of a randomized, double-blind, placebo-controlled, flexible-dose study. Pediatrics. 2005;116(6):e777–e784.

Swanson JM, Greenhill LL, Lopez FA, et al. Modafinil film-coated tablets in children and adolescents with attention-deficit/hyperactivity disorder: Results of a randomized, double-blind, placebo-controlled, fixed-dose study followed by abrupt discontinuation. J Clin Psychiatry. 2006;67(1):137–147.

Cocaine Dependence

- Dose: 200–400 mg
- A review and meta-analysis of stimulant treatment for cocaine dependance reports contradictory results as to benefit of modafinil in decreasing euphoria associated with cocaine use
- Long-term cravings or withdrawal symptoms not helped

Castells X, Casas M, Vidal X, et al. Efficacy of central nervous system stimulant treatment for cocaine dependence: A systematic review and meta-analysis of randomized controlled clinical trials. Addiction. 2007;102(12):1871–1887.

Dopaminergic Agents (cont.)

Dackis CA, Kampman KM, Lynch KG, et al. A double-blind, placebo-controlled trial of modafinil for cocaine dependence. Neuropsychopharmacology. 2005;30(1):205–211.
Dackis CA, O'Brien C. Glutamatergic agents for cocaine dependence. Ann N Y Acad Sci. 2003;1003:328–345.

Pramipexole

Depression

D_2/D_3 dopamine receptor agonist; neuroprotective and exerts beneficial effects on sleep architecture

- Dose: 0.375–3 mg/day
- A review of open and one double-blind studies suggests efficacy in bipolar and unipolar depression, used alone or in combination with TCAs or SSRIs – has a large effect size (0.6–1.1) with a low short-term rate of manic switching in bipolar patients (1% mania and 5% hypomania)
- Double-blind study showed improvement in 60% bipolar II depressed patients when added to lithium therapy
- Preliminary data suggest pramipexole may augment antidepressants in treatment-refractory patients
- High incidence of nausea; sedation and dizziness reported

Aiken CB. Pramipexole in psychiatry: A systematic review of the literature. J Clin Psychiatry. 2007;68(8):1230–1236.
Goldberg JF, Burdick KE, Endick CJ. Preliminary randomized, double-blind, placebo-controlled trial of pramipexole added to mood stabilizers for treatment-resistant bipolar depression. Am J Psychiatry. 2004;161(3):564–566.
Zarate CA, Payne JL, Singh J, et al. Pramipexole for bipolar II depression: a placebo-controlled proof of concept study. Biol Psychiatry. 2004;56(1):54–60.

GABA-Agents/Anticonvulsants

Phenytoin

Anticonvulsant; stabilizes membranes, has 5-HT potentiating and GABA-agonist properties

Antisocial Behavior/Aggression
- Dose: 100–600 mg/day
- Contradictory results seen in ability to alter emotional lability, impulsivity, irritability, and aggression when used alone or with neuroleptics (high doses may produce deterioration in behavior); greater benefit in reducing impulsive aggressive acts
- Reports of behavior improvement in adults and children with EEG abnormalities

Stanford MS, Helfritz LE, Conklin SM, et al. A comparison of anticonvulsants in the treatment of impulsive aggression. Exp Clin Psychopharmacol. 2005;13(1):72–77.
Stanford MS, Houston RJ, Mathias CW, et al. A double-blind placebo-controlled crossover study of phenytoin in individuals with impulsive aggression. Psychiatry Res. 2001;103(2–3):193–203.

Anxiety Disorders
- Open label study of 9 adults reported significant reduction in PTSD symptoms; no change seen in severity of depression or anxiety

Bremner JD, Mletzko T, Welter S, et al. Treatment of posttraumatic stress disorder with phenytoin: An open-label pilot study. J Clin Psychiatry. 2004;65(11):1559–1564.

Depression
- Double-blind study comparing phenytoin (200–400 mg/day) to fluoxetine (up to 20 mg/day) demonstrated similar efficacy in patients with MDD

Nemets B, Bersudsky Y, Belmaker RH. Controlled double-blind trial of phenytoin vs. fluoxetine in major depressive disorder. J Clin Psychiatry. 2005;66(5):586–590.

Pregabalin

Anxiety Disorders
- Dose 150–600 mg/day
- Double-blind studies report efficacy in treating moderate to severe GAD and social anxiety disorder
- Onset of action occurs in about 1 week and is maintained long-term
- Efficacy comparable to benzodiazepines and venlafaxine, with less cognitive and psychomotor impairment than benzodiazepines

- Transient sedation and dizziness reported; mild withdrawal symptoms observed

Bandelow B, Wedekind D, Leon T. Pregabalin for the treatment of generalized anxiety disorder: A novel pharmacologic intervention. Expert Rev Neurother. 2007;7(7):769–781.

Feltner D, Wittchen H-U, Kavoussi R, et al. Long-term efficacy of pregabalin in generalized anxiety disorder. Int Clin Psychopharmacol. 2008;23(1):18–28.

Montgomery SA, Tobias K, Zornberg GL, et al. Efficacy and safety of pregabalin in the treatment of generalized anxiety disorder: A 6-week, multicenter, randomized, double-blind, placebo-controlled comparison of pregabalin and venlafaxine. J Clin Psychiatry. 2006;67(5):771–782.

Owen RT. Pregabalin: Its efficacy, safety and tolerability profile in generalized anxiety. Drugs Today. 2007; 43(9):601–610.

Pohl RB, Feltner DE, Fieve RR, et al. Efficacy of pregabalin in the treatment of generalized anxiety disorder: double-blind, placebo-controlled comparison of BID versus TID dosing. J Clin Psychopharmacol. 2005;25(2):151–158.

Tiagabine

Anticonvulsant; selective GABA reuptake inhibitor

Anxiety Disorders

- Dose: up to 16 mg/day
- Contradictory results seen in controlled and open trials in GAD, PTSD, and panic disorder
- Common side effects include dizziness, headache, nausea, fatigue, and sedation
- Does not interact with alcohol

Connor KM, Davidson JR, Weisler RH, et al. Tiagabine for posttraumatic stress disorder: Effects of open-label and double-blind discontinuation treatment. Psychopharmacology (Berl). 2006;184(1):21–25.

Mula M, Pini S, Cassano GB. The role of anticonvulsant drugs in anxiety disorders: A critical review of the evidence. J Clin Psychopharmacol. 2007;27(3):263–272.

Pollack MH, Roy-Byrne PP, Van Ameringen M, et al. J Clin Psychiatry. 2005;66(11):1401–1408.

Pollack MH, Tiller J, Xie F, et al. Tiagabine in adult patients with generalized anxiety disorder: Results from 3 randomized, double-blind, placebo-controlled, parallel-group studies. J Clin Psychopharmacol. 2008;28(3):308–316.

Schwartz TL, Azhar N, Husain J, et al. An open-label study of tiagabine as augmentation therapy for anxiety. Ann Clin Psychiatry. 2005;17(3):167–172.

Depression

- Dose: 4–20 mg/day
- Open-label study suggests tiagabine useful in treating depressive disorder with anxiety

Carpenter LL, Schecter JM, Tyrka AR, et al. Open-label tiagabine monotherapy for major depressive disorder with anxiety. J Clin Psychiatry. 2006;67(1):66–71.

Bipolar Disorder

- Dose: up to 12 mg/day
- 8 of 12 with rapid-cycling, mixed, or hypomanic presentation responded to open trial of adjunctive tiagabine at 1–8 mg/day; side effects limited response (i.e., episodes of syncope and seizures)
- Open label studies and case reports of improvement in bipolar disorder and schizoaffective disorder bipolar type, when used as adjunctive drug
- Negative data as to response in refractory BD or in mania

Grunze H, Erfurth A, Marcuse A, et al. Tiagabine appears not to be efficacious in the treatment of acute mania. J Clin Psychiatry. 1999;60(11):759–762.

Kaufman KR. Adjunctive tiagabine treatment of psychiatric disorders: Three cases. Ann Clin Psychiatry. 1998;10(4):181–184.

Schaffer LC, Schaffer CB, Howe J. An open case series on the utility of tiagabine as an augmentation in refractory bipolar outpatients. J Affect Dis. 2002;71(1–3):259–263.

Suppes T, Chisholm KA, Dhavale D, et al. Tiagabine in treatment refractory bipolar disorder: a clinical case series. Bipolar Disord. 2002;4(5):283–289.

Vasudev A, MacRitchie K, Rao SNK, et al. Tiagabine in the treatment of acute affective episodes in bipolar disorder: Efficacy and acceptability. Cochrane Database of Systematic Reviews 2006, Issue 3. Art. No.: CD004694. DOI: 10.1002/14651858.CD004694.pub2.

Young AH, Geddes JR, Macritchie K, et al. Tiagabine in the treatment of acute affective episodes in bipolar disorder: Efficacy and acceptability. Cochrane Database Syst Rev. 2006 Jul 19;3:CD004694.

Vigabatrin

Irreversible GABA transaminase inhibitor

Anxiety Disorders

- Dose: 250–500 mg/day
- Preliminary data suggest efficacy for symptoms of panic disorder and in decreasing startle response and improving sleep in patients with PTSD

MacLeod AD. Vigabatrin and posttraumatic stress disorder. J Clin Psychopharmacol. 1996;16(2):190–191.

Zwanzger P, Baghai T, Boerner RJ, et al. Anxiolytic effects of vigabatrin in panic disorder. J Clin Psychopharmacol. 2001;21(5):539–540.

Serotonin Antagonists

Cyproheptadine	5-HT$_{2A}$ and 5-HT$_{2C}$ antagonist

Schizophrenia

- Dose: 12–24 mg/day
- Contradictory data suggest beneficial effects on negative symptoms of schizophrenia when added to a typical antipsychotic
- Improvement of clozapine-withdrawal syndrome noted; may be related somewhat to stabilizing sleep architecture
- Studies report efficacy in antipsychotic-induced akathisia (see pp. 126–131)

Akhondzadeh S, Mohammadi MR, Amini-Nooshabadi H, et al. Cyproheptadine in treatment of chronic schizophrenia: A double-blind, placebo-controlled study. J Clin Pharm Ther. 1999;24(1):49–52.

Chaudhry IB, Soni SD, Hellewell JS, et al. Effects of the 5-HT antagonist cyproheptadine on neuropsychological function in chronic schizophrenia. Schizophr Res. 2002;53(1–2):17–24.

Fischel T, Hermesh H, Aizenberg D, et al. Cyproheptadine versus propranolol for the treatment of acute neuroleptic-induced akathisia: A comparative double-blind study. J Clin Psychopharmacol. 2001;21(6):612–615.

Opioid Antagonists/Agonists

Tramadol	Atypical central-acting opioid analgesic with µ-receptor activity; weakly inhibits reuptake of NE and 5-HT

Anxiety disorders

- Dose: mean of 254 mg/day
- Open-label study and case series suggest some benefit in treatment-refractory OCD

Koran LM, Aboudjaoude E, Bullock KD, et al. Double-blind treatment with oral morphine in treatment-resistant obsessive-compulsive disorder. J Clin Psychiatry. 2005;66(3):353–359.

Hormones

Estrogens & Progesterone	*Estrogens* increase central bioavailability of norepinephrine, serotonin and acetylcholine; may increase binding sites on platelets for antidepressants; alters dopamine synthesis, increases its turnover, and modulates dopamine receptor sensitivity. *Progesterone* enhances serotonergic activity (chronic estrogen use augments activity of progesterone in CNS)

Antisocial Behavior/Aggression

- Dose: conjugated estrogens 0.625–3.75 mg/day; diethylstilboestrol 1–2 mg/day; transdermal estrogen 100 micrograms/day
- Used in elderly males with dementia exhibiting aggressive behavior (results contradictory)
- Feminizing effects and risk of thrombosis minimal with low doses; peripheral edema has been reported

Eriksson CJP, von der Pahlen B, Sarkola T, et al. Oestradiol and human male alcohol-related aggression. Alcohol Alcohol. 2003;38(6):589–596.

Hall KA, Keks NA, O'Connor DW. Transdermal estrogen patches for aggressive behavior in male patients with dementia: A randomized, controlled trial. Int Psychogeriatr 2005;17(2):165–178.

Shelton PS, Brooks VG. Estrogen for dementia-related aggression in elderly men. Ann Pharmacother. 1999;33(7–8):808–812.

Depression

- Dose: transdermal estrogen 100 micrograms/day; conjugated estrogens 0.625 mg/day for 21 days followed by progesterone 5 mg/day
- Found useful when used alone in perimenopausal women with mild to moderate depression
- Data contradictory when used in combination with antidepressant in some refractory female patients (post-menopausal women more likely to respond); may accelerate antidepressant response
- Maximum clinical effect may take up to 4 weeks to occur
- Estradiol patches (100 micrograms/day) and sublingual 17β-estradiol reported effective in treating severe postpartum depression (data contradictory)

Ahoka A, Kaukoranta J, Wahlbeck K, et al. Estrogen deficiency in severe postpartum depression: successful treatment with sublingual physiologic 17beta-estradiol: a preliminary study. J Clin Psychiatry. 2001;62(5):332–336.

Cohen LS, Soares CN, Poitras JR, et al. Short-term use of estradiol for depression in perimenopausal and postmenopausal women: a preliminary report. Am J Psychiatry. 2003;160(8):1519–1522.

Kumar R, McIvor RJ, Davies RA, et al. Estrogen administration does not reduce the rate of recurrence of affective psychosis after childbirth. J Clin Psychiatry. 2003;64(2):112–118.

Morgan ML, Cook IA, Rapkin AJ, et al. Estrogen augmentation of antidepressants in perimenopausal depression: a pilot study. J Clin Psychiatry. 2005;66(6):774–780.

Rasgon NL, Altshuler LL, Fairbanks LA, et al. Estrogen replacement therapy in the treatment of major depressive disorder in perimenopausal women. J Clin Psychiatry. 2002;63(Suppl 7):45–48.

Rasgon NL, Dunkin J, Fairbanks L, et al. Estrogen and response to sertraline in postmenopausal women with major depressive disorder: A pilot study. J Psychiatr Res. 2007;41(3–4):338–343.

Dementia	

- Estrogen promotes cholinergic activity, reduces neuronal loss, improves blood flow, and reduces cholesterol
- Studies suggest a protective effect of estrogen therapy on age of onset of Alzheimer's disease – improvement noted in memory and attention; women with a history of long-term use had the lowest risk – data contradictory as recent studies in women over age 65 suggest estrogen and progesterone can increase the risk for probable dementia and may not prevent cognitive decline
- Estrogen may help cognitive functioning of women not carrying the APOE epsilon 4 allele

Asthana S, Baker LD, Craft S, et al. High-dose estradiol improves cognition for women with AD: results of a randomized study. Neurology. 2001;57(4):605–612.

Burkhardt MS, Foster JK, Laws SM, et al. Oestrogen replacement therapy may improve memory functioning in the absence of APOE epsilon4. J Alzheimers Dis. 2004;6(3):221–228.

Farquhar C, Marjoribanks J, Lethaby A, et al. Long term hormone therapy for perimenopausal and postmenopausal women. Cochrane Database Syst Rev. 2005 Jul 20;3:CD004143.

MacLennan AH, Henderson VW, Paine B, et al. Hormone therapy, timing of initiation, and cognition in women aged older than 60 years: The REMEMBER pilot study. Menopause. 2006;13(1):28–36.

Rapp SR, Espeland MA, Shumaker SA, et al. Effect of estrogen plus progestin on global cognitive function in postmenopausal women: the Women's Health Initiative Memory Study: a randomized controlled trial. JAMA. 2003;289(20):2663–2672.

Resnick SM, Maki PM, Rapp SR, et al. Effects of combination estrogen plus progestin hormone treatment on cognition and affect. J Clin Endocrinol Metab. 2006;91(5):1802–1810.

Testosterone

Depression	

- Testosterone concentrations (total, free, and bioavailable) reported to be lower in males over the age of 45 with MDD
- Dose: 400 mg im every 2 weeks; testosterone transdermal gel 1% (10 mg/day)
- Early data suggests benefit as augmentation strategy in men, with low-normal serum testosterone, refractory to SSRIs
- Gel improved psychological and somatic symptoms of depression, in double-blind study, in men with low testosterone levels
- Negative results reported in double-blind study of hypogonodal men with MDD

Dikobe AM, van Staden CW, Reif S, et al. Deficient testosterone levels in men above 45 years with major depressive disorder – an age-matched case control study. SAJP. 2007;13(3):96-100.

McIntyre RS, Mancini D, Eisfeld BS, et al. Calculated bioavailable testosterone levels and depression in middle-aged men. Psychoneuroendocrinology. 2006;31(9):1029-1035.

Pope HG, Cohane GH, Kanayama G, et al. Testosterone gel supplementation for men with refractory depression: a randomized, placebo-controlled trial. Am J Psychiatry. 2003;160(1):105–111.

Seidman SN. The aging male: androgens, erectile dysfunction, and depression. J Clin Psychiatry. 2003;64(Suppl 10):31–37.

Seidman SN, Roose SP. The sexual effects of testosterone replacement in depressed men: Randomized, placebo-controlled clinical trial. J Sex Marital Ther. 2006;32(3):267–273.

Shores MM, Sloan KL, Matsumoto AM, et al. Increased incidence of diagnosed depressive illness in hypogonadal older men. Arch Gen Psychiatry. 2004;61(2):162–167.

Miscellaneous

Allopurinol

Xanthine oxidase inhibitor – suggested to increase adenosine, a neuromodulator of dopaminergic and glutamatergic systems. May have neuroprotective effect due to antioxidant properties

Schizophrenia/Mania	

- Dose 300 mg od-bid
- Double-blind studies and case series suggest the addition of allopurinol to an antipsychotic in treatment-refractory patients results in improvement in positive symptoms
- Randomized DB data suggests allopurinol and lithium is more effective than lithium plus placebo for treating mania (e.g., lower YMRS scores) at day 21 and 28
- Early data suggest allopurinol may be helpful in aggressive patients with neurological disorders or dementia
- Skin rash seen in 3% of patients; early leukocytosis, eosinophilia, and increased aminotransferase activity reported

Miscellaneous (cont.)

Brunstein MG, Ghisolfi ES, Ramos FLP, et al. A clinical trial of adjuvant allopurinol therapy for moderately refractory schizophrenia. J Clin Psychiatry. 2005;66:213–219.

Lara DR, Cruz MRS, Xavier F, et al. Allopurinol for the treatment of aggressive behaviour in patients with dementia. Int Clin Psychopharmacol. 2003;18(1):53–55.

Machado-Vieira R, Soares JC, Lara DR et al. A double-blind, randomized, placebo-controlled 4-week study on the efficacy and safety of the purinergic agents allopurinol and dipyridamole adjunctive to lithium in acute bipolar mania. J Clin Psychiatry. 2008 69(8)1237–1245.

Selegiline	**Inhibitor of MAO-B, possibly nonselective at higher doses; stimulates nitric oxide production, increases catecholamines and adrenergic stimulation Transdermal preparation inhibits CNS MAO-A and -B enzymes but avoids inhibition of intestinal and hepatic MAO-A enzymes – avoids sensitivity to dietary tyramine** (see p. 56 for use in MDD)

ADHD

- Positive effects on ADHD and tic symptoms reported in double-blind placebo controlled cross-over studies and in open trials
- May have a preferential effect on symptoms of inattention

Akhondzadeh S, Tavakolian R, Davari-Ashtiani R, et al. Selegiline in the treatment of attention deficit hyperactivity disorder in children: A double blind and randomized trial. Prog Neuropsychopharmacol Biol Psychiatry. 2003;27(5):841–845.

Mohammadi MR, Ghanizadeh A, Alaghband-rad J, et al. Selegiline in comparison with methylphenidate in attention deficit hyperactivity disorder children and adolescents in a double-blind, randomized clinical trial. J Child Adolesc Psychopharmacol. 2004;14(3):418–425.

Rubinstein S, Malone MA, Roberts W, et al. Placebo-controlled study examining effects of selegiline in children with attention-deficit/hyperactivity disorder. J Child Adolesc Psychopharmacol. 2006;16(4):404–415.

Dementia

- Dose: 5 mg bid
- Contradictory data as to improvement in cognitive function, behavior and activities of daily living in patients with Alzheimer's disease; combination with Vitamin E 2000 IU/day may improve response
- Synergistic benefit on cognitive impairment reported in combination with donepezil
- Meta-analysis of studies suggests some improvement in memory and cognition but no benefit on activities of daily living or emotions of Alzheimer's disease
- May slow down the progression of Alzheimer's disease of moderate severity; suggested to reduce the concentration of free radicals and other neurotoxins
- Well tolerated with few side effects: primarily dizziness and orthostatic hypotension

Birks J, Flicker L. Selegiline for Alzheimer's disease. Cochrane Database Syst Rev. 2003;1:CD000442.

Thomas T. Monoamine oxidase-B inhibitors in the treatment of Alzheimer's disease. Neurobiol Aging. 2000;21(2):343–348.

Tsunekawa H, Noda Y, Mouri A, et al. Synergistic effects of selegiline and donepezil on cognitive impairment induced by amyloid beta (25–35). Behav Brain Res. 2008;190(2):224–232.

Wilcock GK, Birks J, Whitehead JGE, et al. The effect of selegiline in the treatment of people with Alzheimer's disease: a meta-analysis of published trials. Int J Geriatr Psychiatry. 2002;17(2):175–183.

Schizophrenia

- Case report and both open-label trials report improvement of negative symptoms associated with augmentation of antipsychotic with low-dose oral selegiline; double-blind studies show variable results in patients with schizoprenia

Amiri A, Noorbala AA, Nejatisafa AA, et al. Efficacy of selegiline add on therapy to risperidone in the treatment of the negative symptoms of schizophrenia: A double-blind randomized placebo-controlled study. Human Psychopharmacol. 2008;23(2):79–86.

Fohey KD, Hieber R, Nelson LA. The role of selegiline in the treatment of negative symptoms associated with schizophrenia. Ann Pharmacother. 2007;41(5):851–856.

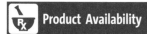 **Product Availability**

Herbal (natural) health products have been traditionally used by many cultures to treat a variety of psychiatric conditions. Very few of these products, however, have been subjected to scientific scrutiny through standardized research methods. Clinicians should always be cognizant of medicolegal issues when recommending herbal products for non-approved indications.

CAUTION: Quality control of herbal/natural products is variable, depending on the preparation used. As these products are not standardized in North America, the amount of active constituents can vary between preparations, and some products may be adulterated with other herbs, chemicals and drugs.

Drug	Anxiety	Depression	Bipolar Disorder	Sleep Disorders	Schizophrenia	Alzheimer's Dementia	ADHD
Ginkgo Biloba (p. 306)					PR/S	+(C)	
Inositol (p. 306)	PR						
Kava Kava (p. 307)	+						
Melatonin (p. 307)				+(C)			
Omega 3 Fatty Acids (p. 308)			PR		PR/C	PR	PR/C
S-Adenosyl-methionine (p. 309)		P					
St. John's Wort (p. 309)	PR	+*					
Valerian (p. 310)				+(C)			
Vitamins (p. 311) Vitamin B6 Vitamin C Vitamin E					PR/S PR/S PR/S	+	

C = contradictory results, P = partial improvement, + = positive, PR = preliminary data, S = synergistic effect; * Mild to moderate depression only

Herbal and "Natural" Products (cont.)

Ginkgo Biloba	Active ginkgolides obtained from the nuts and leaves of the oldest deciduous tree in the world (ginkgo – also called Maidenhair tree or kew tree) Standardized products contain flavone glycosides (24%) and terpenoids (6%) Increases vasodilation and peripheral blood flow in capillary vessels and end arteries; may have antioxidant action (free radical scavenger); may increase cholinergic transmission by inhibiting acetylcholinesterase; may have anticonvulsant activity through elevation of GABA levels
Alzheimer's Dementia	• Dose: 120–240 mg/day in divided doses; 1–3 months treatment, at full dose, required for full therapeutic effect • A number of controlled studies suggest that ginkgo extracts can improve vascular perfusion and decrease thrombosis; used in dementia, chronic cerebrovascular insufficiency and cerebral trauma. Improvement noted in memory, concentration, fatigue, anxiety and depressed mood; data contradictory • Meta-analysis suggests evidence of improvement in cognition and functioning in patients with cognitive impairment and dementia – results inconsistent • Randomized controlled trials suggest improvement in memory impairment caused by Alzheimer's and vascular dementia – trials show inconsistent results • Side effects are rare and include: agitation/nervousness, emotional lability, depression, headache, dizziness, palpitations, GI upset and contact dermatitis; spontaneous bruising and bleeding have been reported. Very large doses may cause restlessness, diarrhea, nausea and vomiting. Cases of seizure reported (ginkgo may reduce GABA levels) • Inhibits platelet adhesions; caution in patients on anticoagulants, NSAIDs, or ASA, due to possible enhanced effect and risk of bleeding • Interactions: inhibitor of CYP2C9 and inducer of CYP2C19; may interact with drugs metabolized by these isoenzymes: decreases omeprazole levels up to 42%; may inhibit metabolism of warfarin; may potentiate drugs that lower the seizure threshold Birks J, Grimley EJ. Cochrane Database Syst Rev. 2002;4:CD 003120. Mazza M, Capuano A, Bria P, et al. Eur J Neurol. 2006;13(9):981–985. Mintzer JE. J Clin Psychiatry. 2003;64 Suppl 9:S18–S22. Scott GN, Elmer GW. Am J Health Syst Pharm. 2002;59(4):339–347. Scott GN. Pharmacist's Letter 2005;21:210910. Solomon PR, Adams F, Silver A, et al. JAMA. 2002;288(7):835–840.
Schizophrenia	• Dose: 360 mg/day (given tid) • Double-blind trial suggests that ginkgo biloba may enhance the effects of haloperidol, on both positive and negative symptoms, in treatment-refractory patients, and may reduce EPS Atmaca M, Tezcan E, Kuloglu M, et al. Psychiatry Clin Neurosci. 2005;59(6):652–656. Zhang XY, Zhou DF, Zhang PY, et al. J Clin Psychiatry. 2001;62(11):878–883.
Inositol	Simple isomer of glucose and a precursor of a "second messenger" system (the phosphotidyl-inositol cycle) used by various receptors including α, and 5-HT$_2$
Anxiety Disorders	• 6–18 g/day • Double-blind study suggests benefit in treatment of panic disorder • Preliminary data suggest efficacy in treating phobic disorders, obsessive-compulsive disorder, and trichotillomania • May aggravate symptoms of ADHD in children Carley PD, et al. Metab Brain Dis. 2004;19(1–2):125–134. Palatnik A, Frolov K, Fux M, et al. J Clin Psychopharmacol. 2001;21(3):335–339. Seedat S, Stein D, Harvey B. J Clin Psychiatry. 2001;62(1):60–61.

Kava Kava

Made from the roots of *Piper methysticum*; active ingredients felt to be kavalactones.
May have activity at GABA receptor, antagonize dopamine, and block voltage dependent sodium ion channels
Slang name: AWA.

Anxiety Disorders

- Dose: 60–240 mg kavalactones daily
- Used throughout the Pacific Islands as a ceremonial drink to induce relaxation and sleep and to decrease anxiety; may have anticonvulsant and muscle relaxant activity
- Meta-analysis of placebo-controlled studies suggests benefit in the treatment of anxiety, tension and agitation
- Studies suggest benefit for sleep disturbances associated with anxiety
- Does not adversely affect cognition, mental acuity or coordination
- Adverse effects are rare at lower doses, and include: gastric discomfort, dizziness, and, with chronic use, yellow skin discoloration; at doses above 400 mg/day: dry flaking skin, red eyes, facial puffiness, muscle weakness, dystonic reactions, dyskinesias, and choreoathetosis
- Liver dysfunction has been reported; use with caution in patients with a history of liver disease – periodic liver function tests recommended
- May potentiate other CNS depressants (including alcohol and benzodiazepines), causing increased side effects and toxicity

Lehrl S. J Affect Disord. 2004;78(2):101–110.
Pittler MH, Ernst E. Cochrane Database Syst Rev. 2003;1:CD003383.
Witte S, Loew D, Gaus W. Phytother Res. 2005;19(3):183–188.

Melatonin

Hormone produced by the pineal gland involved in regulation of circadian rhythms
- Dietary supplement in the USA, not regulated by FDA with regard to purity, efficacy or safety; ramelteon approved in USA (see p. 174)

Sleep Disorders

- Dose: 0.3–10 mg/day (0.3 mg = physiological dose) taken 30–120 min before bedtime; exogenous melatonin does not appear to affect endogenous production or secretion of melatonin
- Peak plasma concentrations achieved within 60 min; metabolized by the liver; elimination half-life = 20–50 min
- Promotes sleep onset and minimizes nighttime awakenings without producing drowsiness; not associated with rebound insomnia or withdrawal effects
- Hypnotic effect not fully established, as studies show inconsistent results (due to different populations and variable doses used in trials); shown to decrease sleep latency and increase total sleep time in some studies; may be more effective given 2 h before bedtime, or may exert hypnotic effect only when endogenous concentrations of melatonin are low
- Useful in circadian-based sleep disorders (e.g., jet lag) – can shift circadian rhythms at a rate of 1–2 h/day with taken when physiological plasma levels of melatonin are low (i.e., noon to bedtime)
- May be useful in elderly, who have decreased nocturnal secretion of melatonin; found not to be effective in patients with sleep disturbances and dementia
- Doses up to 50 mg hs used to alter sleep architecture in narcolepsy–increases REM sleep and dreaming
- May be helpful for medically ill patients with insomnia for whom conventional hypnotics may be problematic
- May facilitate withdrawal from benzodiazepines (which can decrease nocturnal melatonin production)
- Early data suggest it may be beneficial in multidisabled children (with neurological or behavioral disorders) with severe insomnia in doses of 2–10 mg, and in Asperger's disorder
- Double-blind study showed benefit in children with idiopathic chronic sleep-onset insomnia – reduces time to sleep onset and minimizes night-time awakenings
- Shown to improve sleep efficiency in patients with schizophrenia, in double-blind study
- Adverse effects are rare: abdominal cramps with high doses, fatigue, headache, dizziness and increased irritability; very high doses (> 75 mg) can exacerbate depression, cause coagulation abnormalities, and inhibit ovulation
- Not recommended in individuals with autoimmune disorders since melatonin may play a role in immune function, and in patients with vascular disorders as it may cause vasoconstriction

Herbal Products

Herbal and "Natural" Products (cont.)

- Interactions: increased melatonin levels with fluvoxamine due to inhibited metabolism via CYP1A2 or 2C9 – endogenous melatonin secretion increased; melatonin reduces the antihypertensive effect of slow-release nifedipine. Caution in patients taking warfarin or other agents that affect coagulation

Buck ML. Pediatr Pharm. 2003;9(11):1–5.
Buscemi N, Vandermeer B, Hooton N, et al. J Gen Intern Med. 2005;20(12):1151–1158.
Malhotra S, Sawhney G, Pandhi P. MedGenMed. 2004 April 13;6(2):46.
Paavonen EJ, Nieminen-von Wendt T, Vanhala R, et al. J Child Adolesc Psychopharmacol. 2003;13(1):83–95.
Smits MG, van Stel HF, van der Heijden K, et al. J Am Acad Child Adolesc Psychiatry. 2003;42(11):1286–1293.
Weiss MD, Wasdell MB, Bomben MM, et al. J Am Acad Child Adolesc Psychiatry. 2006;45(5):512–519.

Omega 3 Polyunsaturated Fatty Acids

Contained in fish oil (e.g., mackerel, halibut, salmon), green leafy vegetables, nuts, flaxseed oil and canola oil; may affect cell membrane composition at neuron synapses and interfere with signal transduction; may also affect monoamine oxidase
Include: arachidonic acid (AA), eicosapentaenoic acid (EPA), docosapentaenoic acid (DPA), and docosahexaenoic acids (DHAs)

Bipolar Disorder

- Preliminary double-blind study suggests that patients with BD who took supplements of fish oil, in addition to their usual medication, had longer remission than those on placebo
- Epidemiological data suggest a relationship between consumption of seafood and decreased lifetime prevalence of depression, bipolar I and II disorder, and bipolar spectrum disorder; contradictory data reported as to efficacy and dosage in depressed and rapid-cycling BD
- Meta-analysis of randomized studies demonstrates benefit of omega-3-fatty acids (particularly EPA and DHA) in unipolar and bipolar depression; potential benefit suggested in MDD and BD
- Case reports of induced hypomania, mania or mixed states with supplements of omega 3 fatty acids

Freeman MP, Hibbeln JR, Wisner KL, et al. J Clin Psychiatry. 2006;67(12):1954–1967.
Hibbeln JR. Lancet 1998;351:1213.
Int Drug Ther Newsl. 2000;35(10):73.
Noaghiul S, Hibbeln JR. Am J Psychiatry. 2003;160(12):2222–2227.
Osher Y, Bersudsky Y, Belmaker RH. J Clin Psychiatry. 2005;66(6):726–729.
Pomerantz JM. Drug Benefit Trends. 2001;13(6):2–3.

Schizophrenia

- Preliminary data suggest a relationship between high consumption of omega 3 fatty acids and less severe symptoms of schizophrenia; E-EPA (ethyleicosapentanoate) suggested to inhibit phospholipase A_2, an enzyme found to be overactive in patients with schizophrenia and may be responsible for depletion of arachidonic acid from brain and red cell phospholipids in these patients – meta-analysis suggests that benefit in schizophrenia is inconclusive
- Reported to decrease PANSS scores and symptoms of tardive dyskinesia; triglyceride levels elevated with clozapine were decreased with daily doses of 2–4 g of EPA
- Supplementation of a mixture of EPA/DHA (180:120 mg) in combination with vitamins E and C (400 IU:500 mg) bid for 4 months reported to significantly reduce psychopathology in schizophrenic patients
- Review of double-blind studies suggest E-EPA, (at a dose of 2g/day) can augment effects of clozapine in treatment-refractory patients

Arvindakshan M, Ghate M, Ranjekar PK, et al. Schizophr Res. 2003;62(3):195–204.
Emsley R, Myburgh C, Oosthuizen P, et al. Am J Psychiatry. 2002;159(9):1596–1598.
Fenton WS, Dickerson F, Boronow J, et al. Am J Psychiatry. 2001;158(12):2071–2074.
Freeman MP, Hibbeln JR, Wisner KL, et al. J Clin Psychiatry. 2006;67(12):1954–1967.
Kontaxakis VP, Ferentinos PP, Havaki-Kontaxakis BJ, et al. Eur Psychiatry. 2005;20:409–415.
Peet M, Horrobin DF, Study Group E-EM. J Psychiatr Res. 2002;36(1):7–18.
Pomerantz JM. Drug Benefit Trends. 2001;13(6):2–3.

Alzheimer's Dementia	• Data suggest a relationship between high consumption of unsaturated fatty acids and a decreased risk of cognitive impairment

Kalmijn S, Launer LJ, Ott A, et al. Ann Neurol. 1997;42:776–782.
Morris MC, Evans DA, Bienias JL, et al. Arch Neurol. 2003;60(7):940–946.
Pomerantz JM. Drug Benefit Trends. 2001;13(6):2–3.
Solfrizzi V, Colacicco AM, Introno AD, et al. Neurobiol Aging. 2006;27(11):1694–1704.

ADHD	• Administered as efamol (evening primrose oil) or docosahexaenoic acid (DHA)
	• Suggested that relative deficiencies in highly unsaturated fatty acids may be implicated in some of the behavioral and learning problems associated with ADHD; has been suggested that efamol may improve or compensate for zinc deficiency
	• Contradictory results reported in double-blind studies with psychostimulants (d-amphetamine) in children with ADHD; augmentation studies also inconclusive

Arnold LE, Pinkham SM, Votolato N. J Child Adolesc Psychopharmacol. 2000;10(2):111–117.
Hirayama S, Hamazaki T, Terasawa K. Eur J Clin Nutr. 2004;58(3):467–473.
Richardson AJ, Puri BK. Prog Neuropsychopharmacol Biol Psychiatry. 2002;26(2):233–239.
Voigt R, Llorente A, Jensen C, et al. J Pediatr. 2001;139(2):189–196.

S-Adenosylmethionine (SAMe)

Naturally occurring brain methyl group donor in the methylation process, increasing membrane fluidity and influencing both monoamine and phospholipid metabolism; may increase the turnover of serotonin, norepinephrine, and dopamine

Depression	• Dose: 150–2400 mg/day
	• Meta-analysis of all studies suggests comparable efficacy to tricyclic antidepressants
	• Rapid onset reported; response may depend on folate and vitamin B_{12} levels
	• May augment effects of other antidepressants – caution as to increased serotonergic effects; DO NOT COMBINE with MAOIs
	• Few adverse effects: nausea with higher doses; may induce mania in bipolar patients

Alpert JE, Papakostas G, Mischoulon D, et al. J Clin Psychopharm. 2004;24(6):661–664.
Papakostas GI, Alpert JE, Fava M. Curr Psychiatry Rep. 2003;5(6):460–466.
Pies R. J Clin Psychiatry. 2000;61(11):815–820.

St. John's Wort

Active ingredients thought to be the naphthodianthrone, hypericum, hyperforin, and other flavonoids; standardized products contain 0.3% hypericin (approximately equivalent to 2–4 g of dried herb); affects number of systems; hyperforin and adhyperforin reported to inhibit reuptake of serotonin, norepinephrine, dopamine, GABA, and L-glutamate

Depression	• Dose: 300–1800 mg/day in divided doses (amount and potency of active ingredients in commercial products in North America vary widely)
	• Meta-analysis of clinical trials suggests efficacy in patients with mild to moderate depression; lack of data regarding long-term use
	• Double-blind studies suggests comparable efficacy in major depression to SSRIs (data contradictory)
	• Double-blind study of 250 mg hypericum extract showed equal efficacy to 150 mg imipramine, with fewer adverse effects, in mild to moderate depression
	• Postmarketing surveillance reports efficacy and good tolerability in 101 children, under age 12, with mild to moderate depression
	• Adverse effects are rare: GI problems, dry mouth, sedation, fatigue, headache, anxiety, restlessness, constipation, hair loss, paresthesias, erythema, photosensitivity and hypersensitivity reactions; cases of mania and hypomania in bipolar patients, including irritability, disinhibition, agitation, anger, decreased concentration, and disrupted sleep
	• Contraindicated in pregnancy, lactation, cardiovascular disease and pheochromocytoma
	• Due to possible MAOI activity, use caution with foods containing tyramine and with sympathomimetic or serotonergic drugs
	• Interactions
	– Potent inducer of CYP3A4; IA2 and/or the p-glycoprotein transporter; reported to decrease plasma level of cyclosporin, resulting in rejection of transplanted organ; also reported to decrease plasma level of indinavir (57% decrease in AUC), digoxin (up to 25% decrease in AUC), theophylline, irinotican, amiodarone, amitriptyline, alprazolam, methadone, and warfarin; breakthrough bleeding and cases of pregnancy reported in patients on oral contraceptives; may interact with other drugs metabolized by these enzymes

Herbal and "Natural" Products (cont.)

— May increase levels of serotonin in the CNS; several cases of serotonin syndrome reported in combination with serotonergic drugs

Findling RL, McNamara NK, O'Riordan MA, et al. J Am Acad Child Adolesc Psychiatry. 2003;42(8):908–914.
Gelenberg AJ (Ed.). Biol Ther in Psychiatry. 2000;23(6):22–24.
Hammerness P, Basch E, Ulbricht C, et al. Psychosomatics. 2003;44(4):271–282.
Hypericum Depression Trial Study Group. JAMA. 2002;287(4):1807–1814.
Knuppel L, Linde K. J Clin Psychiatry. 2004;65(11):1470–1479.
Muller WE. Pharmacol Res. 2003;47(2):101–109.
Scott GN, Elmer GW. Am J Health Syst Pharm. 2002;59(4):339–347.
Shelton RC, Keller MB, Gelenberg AJ, et al. JAMA. 2001;285:1978–1986.
Stevinson C, Ernst E. BJOG. 2000;107(7):870–876.
Szegedi A, Kohnen R, Dienel A, et al. BMJ. 2005;330(7490):503.
Woelk H. Br Med J. 2000;321:536–539.

Anxiety Disorders

- Efficacy reported in seasonal affective disorder
- Open trial suggests efficacy in obsessive compulsive disorder (not supported by double-blind study)
- Double-blind study demonstrated efficacy in somatoform disorders
- Case reports suggest benefit for GAD

Kobak KA, Taylor L, Bystritsky A, et al. Int Clin Psychopharmacol. 2005;20(6):299–304.
Kobak KA, Taylor L, Futterer R, et al. J Clin Psychopharmacol. 2003;23(5):531–532.
Volz HP. Psychopharmacology (Berl). 2002;164(3):294–300.

Valerian

VALERIAN consists of the roots, rhizomes (underground stems), and stolons from the plant *Valeriana officinalis*. Active ingredients associated with sedative properties thought to be valepotriates, mono and sesquiterpenes (e.g., valerenic acid) and pyridine alkaloids; the composition and relative proportions of these compounds vary between species. Interacts with central GABA receptors; causes CNS depression and muscle relaxation

Sleep Disorders

- Dose: 200–1200 mg/day; usual dose 400–900mg
- Several placebo-controlled cross-over studies show improvement in sleep quality, decrease in sleep latency, and a decrease in the number of awakenings; response better in females and individuals less than 40 years of age; some studies did not show benefit. A systematic review[1] of clinical trials suggests valerian has a mild hypnotic effect with improved sleep, but there are insufficient well-designed trials to be certain
- Double-blind cross-over polysomnographic evaluation of two preparations of valerian (*V. edulis* and *V. officinalis*) over four nights showed that both increased REM sleep and decreased stages 1–2; *V. edulis* also decreased the number of waking episodes
- Preliminary data report benefit for stress-induced insomnia
- Preliminary data report benefit on sleep latency and quality in children with hyperactivity
- Adverse effects include nausea, excitability, blurred vision, headache, morning lethargy, pruritus, and vivid dreams
- Will potentiate the effects of other CNS drugs
- Liver dysfunction reported; use with caution in patients with a history of liver disease – periodic liver function tests recommended
- Four cases of hepatotoxicity reported when valerian combined with herbal product, skullcap
- Withdrawal symptoms, including delirium, reported after abrupt discontinuation of chronic use
- A couple of systematic reviews of Valerian use for sleep find that it is safe and, relative to available pharmacological therapies, of limited benefit for sleep

[1] Stevinson C, Ernst E. Valerian for insomnia: A systematic review of randomized clinical trials. Sleep Med. 2000;1:91–99.
Bent S, Padula A, Moore D, et al. Am J Med. 2006;119(12):1005–1012.
Francis AJ, Dempster RJ. Phytomedicine. 2002;9(4):273–279.
Herrera-Arellano A, Luna-Villegas G, Cuevas-Uriostegui L, et al. Planta Med. 2001;67(8):695–699.
Poyares DR, Guilleminault C, Ohayon MM, et al. Prog Neuropsychopharmacology Biol Psychiatry. 2002;26(3):539–545.

Taibi DM, Landis CA, Petry H, et al. Sleep Med Rev. 2007;11(3):209–230.
Wheatly D. Hum Psychopharmacology. 2001;16(4):353–356.
Ziegler G, Ploch M, Miettinen-Baumann A, et al. Eur J Med Res. 2002;7(11):480–486.

Vitamins

Schizophrenia

- Reports that ascorbic acid (Vitamin C) in doses up to 8 g/day may antagonize dopamine neurotransmission and potentiate the activity of the antipsychotic (may antagonize the metabolism of the antipsychotic)
- Doses of vitamin E of 600 IU/day reported to reduce severity of acute EPS in patients treated with antipsychotics; doses of up to 1600 IU daily reported useful in decreasing symptoms of tardive dyskinesia (anti-oxidant) data contradictory; suggest Vitamin E may protect against worsening of tardive dyskinesia only. Combination of Vitamins E and C (400 IU:500 mg) plus omega 3 fatty acids reported to decrease psychopathology in schizophrenic patients
- Vitamin B_6 may act as an antioxidant and free radical scavenger; double-blind study reported benefit of Vitamin B_6 in doses of up to 400 mg/day for treatment of tardive dyskinesia and parkinsonism secondary to antipsychotic drugs; no therapeutic effect seen on psychotic symptoms; double-blind study using 600 mg bid reported to improve acute antipsychotic-induced akathisia

Adler LA, Edson R, Lavori P, et al. Biol Psychiatry. 1998;43:868–872.
Arvindakshan M, Ghate M, Ranjekar PK, et al. Schizophr Res. 2003;62(3):195–204.
Dorfman-Etrog P, Hermesh H, Prilipko L, et al. Eur Neuropsychopharmacology. 1999;9(6):475–477.
Int Drug Ther Newsletter. 1999;34(1):3.
Lerner V, Bergman J, Statsenko N, et al. J Clin Psychiatry. 2004;65(11):1550–1554.
McGrath J, Soares-Weiser K. Cochrane Database Syst Rev. 2001;4:CD000209.
Michael N, Sourgens H, Arolt V, et al. Neuropsychobiology. 2002;46 Suppl 1:28–30.
Miodownik C, Cohen H, Kotler M, et al. Harefuah. 2003;142(8–9):592–596, 647.

Alzheimer's Dementia

- Vitamin E shown to reduce cell death associated with beta-amyloid protein
- Conflicting information on whether increased antioxidant intake decreases the risk of developing Alzheimer's disease – reduced prevalence reported in individuals who used Vitamin C and E supplements with or without additional multivitamins
- Vitamin E at 2000 IU/day reported to slow down the progression of Alzheimer's disease of moderate severity due to antioxidant effect on neuronal cells; no improvement in cognitive function occurred
- Combination of at least 1000 IU daily with donepezil or with selegiline up to 5 mg daily showed a significantly lower rate of cognitive decline

Campbell J, et al. On Pharmacists Association. 2003;2(3):23–28.
Klatte ET, Scharre DW, Nagaraja HN, et al. Alzheimer Dis Assoc Disord. 2003;17(2):113–116.
Sano M. J Clin Psychiatry. 2003;64 Suppl 9:23–28; Zandi PP. Arch Neurol. 2004;61:82–88.

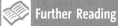

Further Reading

- Facts and Comparisons. The Review of Natural Products (updated loose-leaf binder). Facts and Comparisons Publ., St. Louis, MO.
- Manber R, Allen JJB, Morris MM. Alternative treatments for depression: Empirical support and relevance to women. J Clin Psychiatry. 2002;63(7):628–640.
- Pies R. Adverse neuropsychiatric reactions to herbal and over-the-counter "antidepressants." J Clin Psychiatry. 2002;61(11):815–820.
- Scott GN, Elmer GW. Update on natural product-drug interactions. Am J Health Syst Pharm. 2002;59(4):339–347.

GLOSSARY

ADHD	Attention deficit hyperactivity disorder
Agranulocytosis	Reduction of neutrophil white blood cells to very low levels
Akathisia	Inability to relax, compulsion to change position, motor restlessness
Akinesia	Absence of voluntary muscle movement
Alopecia	Hair loss
Amenorrhea	Absence of menstruation
Anorexia	Lack of appetite for food
Anterocollis	Forward spasm of the neck
Anticholinergic	Block effects of acetylcholine
Antiemetic	Helps prevent nausea and vomiting
Arrhythmia	Any variation of the normal rhythm (usually of the heart beat)
Arteriosclerosis	Hardening and degeneration of the arteries due to fibrous tissue formation
Arthralgia	Pain in the joints
Asterixis	Spots before the eyes
Asthenia	Weakness, fatigue
Ataxia	Incoordination, especially the inability to coordinate voluntary muscular action
Atherosclerosis	Degeneration of the walls of the arteries due to fatty deposits
Atypical Depression	As per DSM IV-TR, patient has mood reactivity and at least 2 of the following symptoms: increased appetite or weight, hypersomnia, leaden paralysis and a long-standing pattern of extreme sensitivity to perceived interpersonal rejection
AUC	Area under the concentration vs time curve (on graph depicting drug in the plasma after a single dose) – represents the extent of systemic exposure of the body to the drug
Autonomic	The part of the nervous system that is functionally independent of thought control (involuntary)
BD	Bipolar disorder
Ballismus	Jerking, twisting
Bioavailability	Amount of drug available to acton receptors (depends on amount absorbed, first-pass metabolism, distribution, protein-binding, and clearance)
Bipolar I Disorder	Cyclical mood disorder with depression alternating with mania or mixed mania
Bipolar II Disorder	Cyclical mood disorder with depression alternating with hypomania
Blepharospasm	Forceful sustained eye closure
BMI (body mass index)	Weight (in kg) divided by height (in m^2)
Bradycardia	Abnormally slow heart beat
Bruxism	Teeth clenching, grinding
Cataplexy	Loss of muscletone and collapse
Category C drug	There may be fetal risk based on animal studies; no data of harm to humans
Category D drug	Evidence suggests there may be a risk to human fetus

Choreiform	Purposeless, uncontrolled sinuous movements,
Choreoathetosis	Slow, repeated, involuntary sinuous movements or twitching of muscles
Chronic brain syndrome	Irreversible damage to brain cells = dementia
Clearance	Rate at which drug is removed from a unit of blood plasma (depends on rate of metabolism by liver and eliminiation from body)
CNS	Central nervous system
CNS depression	Drowsiness, ataxia, incoordination, slowing of respiration which in severe cases may lead to coma and death
Cortex	The external layer (superficial gray matter) of the brain
Coryza	"Head cold," acute catarrhal inflammation of nasal mucosa
Cycloplegia	Paralysis of accommodation of the eye
CYP	Cytochrome P450 enzymes, involved in drug metabolism
DA	Dopamine
DDAVP	Desmopressin acetate
Dermatitis	Inflammation of the skin
Diaphoresis	Perspiration
Diplopia	Double vision
DLPFC	dorsolateral prefrontal cortex
Dysarthria	Impaired, difficult speech
Dysgeusia	Unpleasant taste
Dyspepsia	Pain or discomfort in upper abdomen or chest (gas, feeling of fullness, or burning pain)
Dysphagia	Difficulty in swallowing
Dyskinesia	Abnormal movements, i.e., twitching, grimacing, spasm
Dystonia	Disordered muscle tone leading to spasms or postural change
ECG	Electrocardiogram (tracing of electrical activity of the heart muscle)
ECT	Electroconvulsive therapy, "shock therapy"
EEG	Electroencephalogram (tracing of electrical activity of the brain)
Edema	Swelling of body tissues due to accumulation of fluid
Elimination	Excretion or removal of drug (and/or metabolites) from the body, usually by the kidneys
Emesis	Vomiting
Endocrine	A gland that secretes internally, a ductless gland
Endogenous depression	Depression from within; in DSM-IV, called major depression
Enzyme	Organic compound that acts upon specific fluids, tissues, or chemicals in the body to facilitate chemical action
Enuresis	Involuntary discharge of urine
Eosinophilia myalgia syndrome (EMS)	Connective tissue disease with eosinophilia and myalgia (Eosinophils are blood cells that are usually in low quantities)
Epigastric	Referring to the upper middle region of the abdomen

Epistaxis	Nose bleed
Exacerbation	Increase in severity of symptoms or disease
Extrapyramidal	Refers to certain nuclei of the brain close to the pyramidal tract
Extrapyramidal syndrome	Parkinsonian-like effects of drugs
Fasciculation	Twitching of muscles
Fibrosis	Formation of fibrous or scar tissue
First-pass effect	Drugs absorbed from the intestine first pass through the liver; a portion of the drug is metabolized before it can act on receptors
FSH	Follicle stimulating hormone
GABA	Gamma-amino butyric acid; an inhibitory neurotransmitter
Galactorrhea	Excretion of milk from breasts
GI	Gastrointestinal
Glaucoma	Increased pressure within the eye
Glomerular	Pertaining to small blood vessels of the kidney that serve as filtering structures in the excretion of urine
Gynecomastia	Increase in breast size in males
Half-life	Time required to decrease the plasma concentration of a drug by 50% (depends on drug clearance and volume of distribution)
Histological	Pertaining to microscopic tissue anatomy
Hypercalcemia	An excessive amount of calcium in the blood
Hyperkinetic	Abnormal increase in activity
Hyperparathyroidism	Increased secretion of the parathyroid
Hyperreflexia	Increased action of the reflexes
Hypertension	High blood pressure
Hyperthyroid	Excessive activity of the thyroid gland
Hypertrophy	Enlargement
Hypnotic	Inducing sleep
Hypospadias	Developmental abnormality in males in which the urethra opens on the under surface of the penis or in the perineum
Hypotension	Low blood pressure
Hypothyroid	Insufficiency of thyroid secretion
Induration	Area of hardened tissue
INR	International Normalization Ratio; measures coagulation of blood
Jaundice	Yellow skin caused by excess of bile pigment
Kindling	Epileptogenesis caused by adaptive changes in neurons producing repeated electrical discharges
LDH	Lactic dehydrogenase (an enzyme)
LH	Luteinizing hormone
Libido	Drive or energy usually associated with sexual interest
Limbic system	A system of brain structures common to the brains of all mammals (deals with emotions)
Leukocytosis	Increase in the white blood cells in the blood
Leukopenia	Decrease in the white blood cells in the blood
Macrosomia	Birth weight of infant > 4 kg
MAOI	Monoamine oxidase (an enzyme) inhibitor
Manic depressive psychosis	Conspicuous mood swings ranging from normal to elation or depression, or alternating of the two; in DSM-IV, called bipolar affective disorder
MDD	Major depressive disorder
Metabolism	Process by which liver converts a fat-soluble drug into one that is water-soluble and can be excreted by the kidneys. Most psychotropic drugs are metabolized by cytochrome P450 enzymes
Metabolites	By-products of metabolism by liver cytochrome enzymes to create more water-soluble agents. Some metabolites are pharmacologically active
Micrographia	Decrease in size of hand writing; may be a form of akinesia
Miosis	Constricted pupils
Myalgia	Tenderness or pain in muscles
Mydriasis	Dilated pupils
Narcolepsy	Condition marked by an uncontrollable desire to sleep
Nephritis	Inflammation of the kidneys
Nystagmus	Involuntary movement of the eyeball or abnormal movement on testing
OCD	Obsessive compulsive disorder
Oculogyric crisis	Rolling up of the eyes and the inability to focus
Occipital	In the back part of the head
Ophthalmoplegia	Paralysis of the extraocular eye muscles
Opisthotonus	Arching (spasm) of the body due to contraction of back muscles
Orthostatic hypotension	Faintness caused by suddenly standing erect (leading to a drop in blood pressure)
Osteomalacia	Rickets
PANSS	Positive and negative syndrome scale used in the diagnosis and monitoring of symptoms of schizophrenia
Palinopsia	Visual perseveration, "tracking" or shimmering
Papilledema	Edema of the optic disc
Paresthesia	Feeling of "pins and needles," tingling or stiffness in distal extremities
Parkinsonism	A condition marked by mask-like facial appearance, tremor, change in gait and posture (resembles Parkin-son's disease)
Perioral	Around the mouth
Peripheral neuropathy	Pathological changes in the peripheral nervous system
Petechiae	Small purplish hemorrhagic spots on skin
P-gp	P-glycoprotein; a protein that transports molecules through cell membranes (e.g., in and out of specific body organs)
Photophobia	Sensitivity of the eyes to light
Photosensitivity	Light sensitive
Piloerection	"Goose-bumps" or hair standing up
Pisa syndrome	A condition where an individual leans to one side
PMS	Premenstrual syndrome
Polydipsia	Excessive drinking
Polyuria	Excessive urination
Postural hypotension	Lowered blood pressure caused by a change in position
Priapism	Abnormal, continued erection of the penis
Prostatic hypertrophy	Enlargement of the prostate gland

Glossary (cont.)

Pruritus	Itching
Psychosis	A major mental disorder of organic or emotional origin in which there is a departure from normal patterns of thinking, feeling and acting; commonly characterized by loss of contact with reality
Psychomotor excitement	Physical and emotional overactivity
Psychomotor retardation	Slowing of physical and psychological reactions
Pyloric	Referring to the lower opening of the stomach
Rabbit syndrome	Tremor of the lower lip
RDBCT	Randomized double-blind controlled trial
Retardation	Slowing
Retrocollis	Spasm of neck muscles causing the head to twist up and back
Schizophrenia	A severe disorder of psychotic depth characterized by a retreat from reality with delusions and hallucinations
Sedative	Producing calming of activity or excitement
Serotonin syndrome	Hypermetabolic syndrome resulting from serotonergic excess. Symptoms include: disorientation, confusion, agitation, tremor, myoclonus, hyperreflexia, twitching, shivering, ataxia, hyperactivity
SIADH	Syndrome of in appropriate secretion of antidiuretic hormone
Sialorrhea	Excessive flow of saliva
Somnambulism	Sleep-walking
Stereotypic	Rhythmic and repetitive
Syncope	A sudden loss of strength or fainting
Tachycardia	Abnormally rapid heart rate
Tachyphylaxis	Tolerance to effects
Tardive dyskinesia	Persistent dyskinetic movements that appear late in neuroleptic therapy
Tardive dystonia	Persistent abnormal muscle tone that appears late in neuroleptic therapy
Therapeutic index	Ratio of median lethal dose of a drug to its median effective dose: i.e.,

$$\text{therapeutic index} = \frac{\text{median lethal dose}}{\text{median effective dose}}$$

Tinnitus	A noise in the ears (ringing, buzzing, or roaring)
Torticollis	Spasm on one side of the neck causing the head to twist
Tortipelvis	Twisting of pelvis due to muscles pasm
Tracking	A reaction in which the medication leaves the original injection site and moves to another

TRH	Thyrotropin-releasing hormone, releases TSH and prolactin
Trismus	Severe spasm of the muscles of the jaw resembling tetanus (lock jaw); jaw clenching
TSH	Thyroid-stimulating hormone
UGT	Uridine diphosphate glucuronosyltransferase, enzyme involved in drug metabolism
Ulceration	An open lesion on the skin or mucous membrane
Vasoconstrictor	Causes narrowing of the blood vessels
Volume of distribution (Vd)	The extent to which a drug is distributed throughout the body (influenced by drug properties and the patient)
Wernicke-Korsakoff syndrome	Syndrome characterized by confusion, ataxia, ophthalmoplegia, recent memory impairment and confabulation

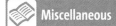 **Miscellaneous**

- Bezchlibnyk-Butler KZ, Virani AS. Clinical Handbook of Psychotropic Drugs for Children and Adolescents (2nd ed.). Cambridge, MA: Hogrefe & Huber, 2007.
- Flockhart DA. Drug interactions: Cytochrome P-450 drug-interaction table. Indiana University School of Medicine. Available from: http://medicine.iupui.edu/flockhart/table.htm. (Accessed December 1, 2008).
- Human P450 Metabolism Database: www.gentest.com/human_p450_database/srchh450.asp (Dec. 2003).
- Lesher BA. Pharmacogenomics: An update. Pharmacist's Letter/Practitioner's Letter. 2005;21(7):210701.
- Misra M, Papakostas GI, Klibanski A. Effects of psychiatric disorders and psychotropic medications on prolactin and bone metabolism. J Clin Psychiatry. 2004;65(12):1607–1618.
- Oesterheld JR, Osser DN, Sandson NB. P450, UGT and P-gp drug interactions. Available from: www.mhc.com/Cytochromes/. (January 2004) (Accessed December 1, 2008).
- Pies RW. Pharmacological approaches to psychotropic-induced weight loss. Int Drug Ther Newsletter. 2002;37(7):49–53.
- Posey DJ. Practical pharmacotherapeutic management of autism: A review and update of commonly prescribed drugs. Int Drug Ther Newsletter. 2002;37(1):1–6.
- Ramshaw L, Roberge J (eds.). Psychiatric medications: A practical guide to psychotropics. Toronto: Linacre, 2001
- Robinson GE. Women and psychopharmacology. Medscape Women's Health Journal. 2002;7(1):1–8.

PATIENT INFORMATION SHEETS

This section in the *Clinical Handbook of Psychotropic Drugs* contains information that may be passed on to patients about some of the most frequently used psychotropic medications. The sheets reproduced on the following pages, designed to be easily understood by patients, give details on such matters as the uses of the drug, how quickly it starts working, how long it should be taken, side effects and what to do if they occur, what to do if a dose is forgotten, drug interactions, and precautions. Information sheets such as these of course cannot replace a proper consultation with and advice from the physician or other medical professional, but can serve as a useful tool to enhance compliance, improve efficacy, and enhance safety. The authors and the publisher would welcome feedback and suggestions from readers (for contact addresses, see the front of the book). Information sheets are included here on the drugs and classes of drug shown at the right.

Contents

Patient Information on Selective Serotonin Reuptake Inhibitor (SSRI) Antidepressants

The name of your medication is _____.

What is this drug used for?

SSRI antidepressants are used in the treatment of a number of disorders including:

- Major depressive disorder, depression associated with Manic Depressive Illness (Bipolar Disorder)
- Obsessive compulsive disorder
- Panic disorder
- Bulimia
- Social phobia
- Premenstrual dysphoria or depression
- Post-traumatic stress disorder

These drugs have also been found effective in several other disorders, including dysthymia and impulsive or aggressive behavior, though they are currently not approved for these indications. Ask your doctor if you are not sure why you are taking this drug.

How quickly will the drug start working?

Antidepressants begin to improve sleep and appetite and to increase energy within about one week; however, feelings of depression may take from 4 to 6 weeks to improve. Because antidepressants take time to work, **do not decrease or increase the dose or stop the medication** without discussing this with your doctor.

Improvement in symptoms of obsessive compulsive disorder, panic disorder and bulimia also occur gradually.

How long should you take this medication?

This depends on what type of illness you have and how well you do.

Following the first episode of depression it is recommended that antidepressants be continued for a minimum of one year; this decreases the chance of being ill again. The doctor may then decrease the drug slowly and monitor for any symptoms of depression; if none occur, the drug can gradually be stopped.

For individuals who have had several episodes of depression, antidepressant medication should be continued indefinitely.

DO NOT STOP taking your medication if you are feeling better, without first discussing this with your doctor.

Long-term treatment is generally recommended for obsessive compulsive disorder, panic disorder and bulimia.

What side effects may happen?

Side effects may happen with any drug. They are not usually serious and do not happen to everyone. Side effects may sometimes occur before beneficial effects of the medication are noticed. If you think you may be having a side effect, speak to your doctor or pharmacist as they can help you decrease it or cope with it.

Common side effects that should be reported to your doctor at the **NEXT VISIT** include:

- Feeling sleepy or tired – This problem goes away with time. Use of other drugs that make you drowsy will worsen the problem. Avoid driving a car or operating machinery if drowsiness persists.
- Energizing/agitated feeling – Some individuals may feel nervous or have difficulty sleeping for a few days after starting this medication. Report this to your doctor; he/she may advise you to take the medication in the morning.
- Headache – This tends to be temporary and can be managed by taking pain medicine (such as aspirin, acetaminophen) when required. If the headache persists or is "troubling", contact your doctor.
- Nausea or heartburn – If this happens, take the medication with food.
- Muscle tremor, twitching – Speak to your doctor as this may require a change in your dosage.
- Changes in sex drive or sexual performance – Discuss this with your doctor.
- Blurred vision – This usually happens when you first start the drug and tends to be temporary. Reading under a bright light or at a distance may help; a magnifying glass can be of temporary use. If the problem lasts more than a few weeks, let your doctor know.
- Dry mouth – Sour candy and sugarless gum help increase saliva in your mouth. Do not drink sweet drinks like colas as they may give you cavities and increase your weight. Drink water and brush your teeth regularly.
- Constipation – Drink plenty of water and try to increase the amount of fiber in your diet (like fruit, vegetables or bran). Some individuals find a bulk laxative (e.g., Metamucil, Fibyrax) or a stool softener (Colace, Surfak) helps regulate their bowels. If these remedies are not effective, speak to your doctor or pharmacist.
- Nightmares – Can be managed by changing the time you take your drug – speak with your doctor.
- Loss of appetite.

Rare side effects you should report to your doctor **RIGHT AWAY** include:

- Sore mouth, gums, or throat
- Skin rash or itching, swelling of the face
- Any unusual bruising or bleeding, increased nosebleeds or blood in your stool
- Nausea, vomiting, loss of appetite, feeling tired, weak, feverish or like you have the flu
- Yellow tinge in the eyes or to the skin; dark-colored urine (pee)
- Going 24 h or more without peeing
- Tingling in the hands and feet, severe muscle twitching
- Severe agitation, restlessness, irritability, or thoughts of suicide
- Switch in mood to an unusual state of happiness, excitement, irritability, or problems sleeping

Let your doctor know **right away** if you miss your period or think you may be **pregnant**, plan to become pregnant, or are breastfeeding.

What should you do if you forget to take a dose of your medication?

If you take your total dose of antidepressant in the morning and you forget to take it for more than 6 h, skip the missed dose and continue with your schedule the next day. **DO NOT DOUBLE THE DOSE**. If you take the drug several times a day, take the missed dose when you remember, then continue with your regular schedule.

Is this drug safe to take with other medication?

Because SSRI antidepressant drugs can change the effect of other medication, or may be affected by other medication, always check with your doctor or pharmacist before taking other drugs, including those you can buy without a prescription, such as cold remedies and herbal preparations. Always inform any doctor or dentist that you see that you are taking an antidepressant drug.

Precautions/Considerations

1. Do not change your dose or stop the drug without talking to your doctor.
2. Take your drug with meals or with water, milk, orange or apple juice; avoid grapefruit juice as it may change the effect of the drug in your body.
3. If you are taking a controlled-release medication (e.g., Paxil CR), swallow it whole. Do not crush or chew the tablet, as this will affect the controlled release of the medication.
4. This drug may impair the mental and physical abilities required for driving a car or operating machinery. Avoid these activities if you feel drowsy or slowed down.
5. This drug may increase the effects of alcohol, making you more sleepy, dizzy and light-headed.
6. Do not stop your drug suddenly as this may result in withdrawal symptoms such as muscle aches, chills, tingling in your hands or feet, nausea, vomiting, and dizziness.
7. Report any changes in mood or behavior to your physician.
8. This drug may interact with medication prescribed by your dentist, so let him/her know the name of the drug you are taking.
9. Store your medication in a clean, dry area at room temperature. Keep all medication out of the reach of children.

If you have any questions regarding this medication, please ask your doctor, pharmacist, or nurse.

Bupropion belongs to a class of antidepressants called Selective Norepinephrine Dopamine Reuptake Inhibitors (NDRI).

What is this drug used for?

Bupropion is mainly used in the treatment of Major Depressive Disorders and depression associated with Manic Depressive Illness (Bipolar Disorder). It has also been approved in the management of smoking cessation.

Though not approved for these indications, bupropion has also been found useful in children and adults with Attention Deficit Hyperactivity Disorder, and has been used as an add-on treatment to increase the effects of other classes of antidepressants Ask your doctor if you are not sure why you are taking this drug.

How quickly will the drug start working?

Bupropion is usually prescribed twice a day, morning and evening, or once a day if you are using an extended-release tablet. It begins to improve sleep and appetite and to increase energy within about one week; however, feelings of depression may take from 4–6 weeks to improve. Because antidepressants take time to work, **do not decrease or increase the dose or stop the medication** without discussing this with your doctor. Improvement in smoking cessation/withdrawal also occurs over a period of 6 weeks.

How long should you take this medication?

This depends on what type of illness you have and how well you do.

Following the first episode of depression it is recommended that antidepressants be continued for a minimum of one year; this decreases the chance of being ill again. The doctor may then decrease the drug slowly and monitor for any symptoms of depression; if none occur, the drug can gradually be stopped.

For individuals who have had several episodes of depression, antidepressant medication should be continued indefinitely.

DO NOT STOP taking your medication if you are feeling better, without first discussing this with your doctor.

Use of bupropion for smoking cessation is recommended as a one-time treatment for a period of 6 weeks.

What side effects may happen?

Side effects may happen with any drug. They are not usually serious and do not happen to everyone. Side effects may sometimes occur before beneficial effects of the medication are noticed. If you think you may be having a side effect, speak to your doctor or pharmacist as they can help you decrease it or cope with it.

Common side effects that should be reported to your doctor at the **NEXT VISIT** include:
- Energizing/agitated feeling – Some individuals may feel nervous or have difficulty sleeping for a few days after starting this medication. Report this to your doctor; he/she may advise you to take the medication in the morning.
- Vivid dreams or nightmares – This can occur at the start of treatment.
- Headache – This can be managed by taking pain medicine (e.g., aspirin, acetaminophen) as required. If the headache persists or is "troubling" contact your doctor.
- Muscle tremor, twitching – Speak to your doctor as this may require a change in your dosage.
- Nausea or heartburn – If this happens, take the medication with food.
- Loss of appetite.
- Dry mouth – Sour candy and sugarless gum help increase saliva in your mouth. Do not drink sweet drinks like colas as they may give you cavities and increase your weight. Drink water and brush your teeth regularly.
- Sweating – You may sweat more than usual; frequent showering, use of deodorants and talcum powder may help.
- Blood pressure – A slight increase in blood pressure can occur with this drug. If you are taking medication for high blood pressure, tell your doctor, as this medication may have to be adjusted.

Rare side effects you should report to your doctor **RIGHT AWAY** include:
- Persistent, troubling headache
- Seizures; these usually occur with high doses – should you have a seizure, stop taking your drug and contact your physician
- Chest pain, shortness of breath
- Sore mouth, gums, or throat
- Skin rash or itching, swelling of the face
- Nausea, vomiting, loss of appetite, fatigue, weakness, fever, or flu-like symptoms
- Muscle pain and tenderness or joint pain accompanied by fever and rash
- Yellow tinge in the eyes or to the skin; dark-colored urine (pee)
- Tingling in the hands and feet, severe muscle twitching
- Severe agitation, restlessness, irritability, or thoughts of suicide
- **Switch in mood to an unusual state of happiness, excitement, irritability, or problems sleeping**

Let your doctor know **right away** if you miss your period or think you may be **pregnant**, plan to become pregnant, or are breastfeeding.

What should you do if you forget to take a dose of your medication?

If you forget to take the morning dose of antidepressant by more than 4 hours, skip the missed dose and continue with your schedule for the evening dose. **DO NOT DOUBLE THE DOSE** as seizures may occur.

Is this drug safe to take with other medication?

Because antidepressant drugs can change the effect of other medication, or may be affected by other medication, always check with your doctor or pharmacist before taking other drugs, including those you can buy without a prescription such as cold remedies and herbal preparations. Always inform any doctor or dentist that you see that you are taking an antidepressant drug.

Precautions/Considerations

1. Do not change your dose or stop the drug without talking to your doctor.
2. Do not chew or crush the tablet, but swallow it whole.
3. If you have been told by your doctor to break a bupropion sustained release tablet in half, do so just prior to taking this medication; throw out the second half unless you can use it within 24 hours (store the half tablet in a tightly-closed container away from light).
4. Do not stop your drug suddenly as this may result in withdrawal symptoms such as muscle aches, chills, tingling in your hands or feet, nausea, vomiting, and dizziness.
5. Report any changes in mood or behavior to your physician.
6. Inform your doctor of all medications you are taking including all drugs prescribed by any physician, as well as over-the-counter and herbal preparations.
7. This drug may interact with medication prescribed by your dentist, so let him/her know the name of the drug you are taking.
8. It is best not to drink alcohol at all, or to drink very moderately while taking bupropion. The risk of seizures is increased if you drink a lot of alcohol and suddenly stop.
9. Store your medication in a clean, dry area at room temperature and away from high humidity. Keep all medication out of the reach of children.

If you have any questions regarding this medication, please ask your doctor, pharmacist, or nurse.

The name of your medication is _____. It belongs to a class of antidepressants called Selective Serotonin and Norepinephrine Reuptake Inhibitors (SNRI).

What is this drug used for?

SNRIs are primarily used in the treatment of Major Depressive Disorders, depression associated with Manic Depressive Illness (Bipolar Disorder), for Generalized Anxiety Disorder or Social Anxiety Disorder, and Panic Disorder in adults.

Though not approved for these indications, some of these drugs have also been found effective in several other disorders including obsessive compulsive disorder, premenstrual dysphoric disorder, pain syndromes, and in children and adults with Attention Deficit Hyperactivity Disorder. Ask your doctor if you are not sure why you are taking this drug.

How quickly will the drug start working?

SNRIs begin to improve sleep and appetite and to increase energy within about one week; however, feelings of depression may take from 4 to 6 weeks to improve. Because antidepressants take time to work, **do not decrease or increase the dose or stop the medication** without discussing this with your doctor.

Improvement in symptoms of obsessive compulsive disorder, panic disorder and social phobia also occur gradually over several weeks.

How long should you take this medication?

This depends on what type of illness you have and how well you do.

Following the first episode of depression it is recommended that antidepressants be continued for a minimum of one year; this decreases the chance of being ill again. The doctor may then decrease the drug slowly and monitor for any symptoms of depression; if none occur, the drug can gradually be stopped. For individuals who have had several episodes of depression, antidepressant medication should be continued indefinitely.

DO NOT STOP taking your medication if you are feeling better, without first discussing this with your doctor.

Long-term treatment is generally recommended for obsessive compulsive disorder, panic disorder, and social phobia.

What side effects may happen?

Side effects may happen with any drug. They are not usually serious and do not happen to everyone. Side effects may sometimes occur before beneficial effects of the medication are noticed. If you think you may be having a side effect, speak to your doctor or pharmacist as they can help you decrease it or cope with it.

Common side effects that should be reported to your doctor at the **NEXT VISIT** include:

- Energizing/agitated feeling – Some individuals may feel nervous or have difficulty sleeping for a few days after starting this medication. Report this to your doctor; he/she may advise you to take the medication in the morning.
- Headache – This can be managed by taking pain medicine (e.g., aspirin, acetaminophen) as required. If the headache persists or is "troubling" contact your doctor.
- Nausea or heartburn – If this happens, take the medication with food.
- Dry mouth – Sour candy and sugarless gum help increase saliva in your mouth. Do not drink sweet drinks like colas as they may give you cavities and increase your weight. Drink water and brush your teeth regularly.
- Constipation – Drink plenty of water and try to increase the amount of fiber in your diet (like fruit, vegetables or bran). Some individuals find a bulk laxative (e.g., Metamucil, Fibyrax) or a stool softener (Colace, Surfak) helps regulate their bowels. If these remedies are not effective, speak to your doctor or pharmacist.
- Sweating – You may sweat more than usual; frequent showering, use of deodorants and talcum powder may help.
- Blood pressure – A slight increase in blood pressure can occur with this drug. If you are taking medication for high blood pressure, tell your doctor, as this medication may have to be adjusted.
- Changes in sex drive or sexual performance – Discuss this with your doctor.

Rare side effects you should report to your doctor **RIGHT AWAY** include:

- Persistent, troubling headache
- Sore mouth, gums, or throat
- Skin rash or itching, swelling of the face
- Nausea, vomiting, diarrhea, loss of appetite, feeling tired, weak, feverish, or like you have the flu
- Yellow tinge in the eyes or to the skin; dark-colored urine (pee)
- Tingling in the hands and feet, severe muscle twitching, tremor, shivering, loss of balance
- Racing heart/pulse
- Severe agitation, restlessness, anxiety, panic, irritability, or thoughts of suicide
- **Switch in mood to an unusual state of happiness, excitement, irritability, or problems sleeping**

Let your doctor know **right away** if you miss your period or think you may be **pregnant**, plan to become pregnant, or are breastfeeding.

What should you do if you forget to take a dose of your medication?

If you take your total dose of antidepressant in the morning and you forget to take it for more than 6 h, skip the missed dose and continue with your schedule the next day. **DO NOT DOUBLE THE DOSE.** If you take the drug several times a day, take the missed dose when you remember, then continue with your regular schedule.

Is this drug safe to take with other medication?

Because antidepressant drugs can change the effect of other medication, or may be affected by other medication, always check with your doctor or pharmacist before taking other drugs, including those you can buy without a prescription such as cold remedies and herbal preparations. Always inform any doctor or dentist that you see that you are taking an antidepressant drug.

Precautions/Considerations

1. Do not change your dose or stop the drug without talking to your doctor.
2. Do not chew or crush the sustained-release tablet (Effexor XR), but swallow it whole.
3. This drug may impair the mental and physical abilities required for driving a car or operating machinery. Avoid these activities if you feel drowsy or slowed down.
4. This drug may increase the effects of alcohol, making you more sleepy, dizzy and light-headed.
5. Do not stop your drug suddenly as this may result in withdrawal symptoms such as muscle aches, chills, tingling in your hands or feet, nausea, vomiting, and dizziness.
6. Report any changes in mood or behavior to your physician.
7. This drug may interact with medication prescribed by your dentist, so let him/her know the name of the drug you are taking.
8. Store your medication in a clean, dry area at room temperature. Keep all medication out of the reach of children.

If you have any questions regarding this medication, please ask your doctor, pharmacist, or nurse.

The name of your medication is _____.

What is this drug used for?

SARI antidepressants are used in the treatment of Major Depressive Disorder and depression associated with Manic Depressive Illness (Bipolar Disorder). Though currently not approved for these indications, these drugs have also been found effective in several other disorders including dysthymia, premenstrual dysphoria or depression, social phobia, posttraumatic stress disorder, acute and chronic insomnia as well as disruptive and impulsive behavior. Ask your doctor if you are not sure why you are taking this drug.

How quickly will the drug start working?

Antidepressants begin to improve sleep and appetite and to increase energy within about one week; however, feelings of depression may take from 4–6 weeks to improve. Because antidepressants take time to work, **do not decrease or increase the dose or stop the medication** without discussing this with your doctor. Improvement in symptoms of premenstrual dysphoria or impulsive behavior also occur gradually.

How long should you take this medication?

This depends on what type of illness you have and how well you do.

Following the first episode of depression it is recommended that antidepressants be continued for a minimum of one year; this decreases the chance of being ill again. The doctor may then decrease the drug slowly and monitor for any symptoms of depression; if none occur, the drug can gradually be stopped. For individuals who have had several episodes of depression, antidepressant medication should be continued indefinitely.

DO NOT STOP taking your medication if you are feeling better, without first discussing this with your doctor.

What side effects may happen?

Side effects may happen with any drug. They are not usually serious and do not happen to everyone. Side effects may sometimes occur before beneficial effects of the medication are noticed. If you think you may be having a side effect, speak to your doctor or pharmacist as they can help you decrease it or cope with it.

Common side effects that should be reported to your doctor at the **NEXT VISIT** include:

- Feeling drowsy or tired – This problem goes away with time. Use of other drugs that make you drowsy will worsen the problem. Avoid driving a car or operating machinery if drowsiness persists.
- Energizing/agitated feeling – Some individuals may feel nervous or have difficulty sleeping for a few days after starting this medication.
- Headache – This tends to be temporary and can be managed by taking pain medicine (such as aspirin, acetaminophen) when required. If the headache persists or is "troubling" contact your doctor.
- Nausea or heartburn – If this happens, take the medication with food.

- Muscle tremor, twitching – Speak to your doctor as this may require a change in your dosage.
- Changes in sex drive or sexual performance – Though rare, should this problem occur, discuss it with your doctor.
- Dry mouth – Sour candy and sugarless gum help increase saliva in your mouth. Do not drink sweet drinks like colas as they may give you cavities and increase your weight. Drink water and brush your teeth regularly.
- Loss of appetite.

Rare side effects you should report to your doctor **RIGHT AWAY** include:

- Sore mouth, gums, or throat
- Skin rash or itching, swelling of the face
- Any unusual bruising or bleeding
- Nausea, vomiting, loss of appetite, feeling tired, weak, feverish, or like you have the flu
- Persistent abdominal pain, pale stools
- Yellow tinge in the eyes or to the skin; dark-colored urine (pee)
- Tingling in the hands and feet, severe muscle twitching
- Severe agitation, restlessness, irritability, or thoughts of suicide
- **Switch in mood to an unusual state of happiness, excitement, irritability, or problems sleeping**

Let your doctor know **right away** if you miss your period or think you may be **pregnant**, plan to become pregnant, or are breastfeeding.

What should you do if you forget to take a dose of your medication?

If you take your total dose of antidepressant in the morning and you forget to take it for more than 6 h, skip the missed dose and continue with your schedule the next day. **DO NOT DOUBLE THE DOSE**. If you take the drug several times a day, take the missed dose when you remember, then continue with your regular schedule.

Is this drug safe to take with other medication?

Because SARI antidepressant drugs can change the effect of other medication, or may be affected by other medication, always check with your doctor or pharmacist before taking other drugs, including those you can buy without a prescription such as cold remedies and herbal preparations. Always inform any doctor or dentist that you see that you are taking an antidepressant drug.

Precautions/Considerations

1. Do not change your dose or stop the drug without talking to your doctor.
2. Take your drug with meals or with water, milk, orange or apple juice; avoid grapefruit juice as it may change the effect of the drug in your body.
3. This drug may impair the mental and physical abilities required for driving a car or operating machinery. Avoid these activities if you feel drowsy or slowed down.
4. This drug may increase the effects of alcohol, making you more sleepy, dizzy and lightheaded.

5. Do not stop your drug suddenly as this may result in withdrawal symptoms such as muscle aches, chills, tingling in your hands or feet, nausea, vomiting, and dizziness.
6. Report any changes in mood or behavior to your physician.
7. This drug may interact with medication prescribed by your dentist, so let him/her know the name of the drug you are taking.
8. Store your medication in a clean, dry area at room temperature. Keep all medication out of the reach of children.

If you have any questions regarding this medication, please ask your doctor, pharmacist, or nurse.

Patient Information on Mirtazapine

Mirtazapine belongs to a class of antidepressants called Noradrenergic/Specific Serotonergic Antidepressants (NaSSA)

What is this drug used for?

Mirtazapine is primarily used in the treatment of Major Depressive Disorders, depression associated with Manic Depressive Illness (Bipolar Disorder).

Though not approved for these indications, mirtazapine has also been found effective in several anxiety disorders including obsessive compulsive disorder, panic disorder, generalized anxiety disorder, posttraumatic stress disorder and premenstrual dysphoria. Ask your doctor if you are not sure why you are taking this drug.

How quickly will the drug start working?

Mirtazapine begins to improve sleep and appetite and to increase energy within about one week; however, feelings of depression may take from 4 to 6 weeks to improve. Because antidepressants take time to work, **do not decrease or increase the dose or stop the medication** without discussing this with your doctor.

Improvement in symptoms of anxiety disorder also occur gradually over several weeks.

How long should you take this medication?

This depends on what type of illness you have and how well you do.

Following the first episode of depression it is recommended that antidepressants be continued for a minimum of one year; this decreases the chance of being ill again. The doctor may then decrease the drug slowly and monitor for any symptoms of depression; if none occur, the drug can gradually be stopped. For individuals who have had several episodes of depression, antidepressant medication should be continued indefinitely.

DO NOT STOP taking your medication if you are feeling better, without first discussing this with your doctor.

Long-term treatment is generally recommended for anxiety disorders.

What side effects may happen?

Side effects may happen with any drug. They are not usually serious and do not happen to everyone. Side effects may sometimes occur before beneficial effects of the medication are noticed. If you think you may be having a side effect, speak to your doctor or pharmacist as they can help you decrease it or cope with it.

Common side effects that should be reported to your doctor at the **NEXT VISIT** include:

- Feeling sleepy or tired – This problem goes away with time. Use of other drugs that make you drowsy will worsen the problem. Avoid driving a car or operating machinery if drowsiness persists.
- Dry mouth – Sour candy and sugarless gum help increase saliva in your mouth. Do not drink sweet drinks like colas as they may give you cavities and increase your weight. Drink water and brush your teeth regularly.
- Constipation – Drink plenty of water and try to increase the amount of fiber in your diet (like fruit, vegetables or bran). Some individuals find a bulk laxative (e.g., Metamucil, Fi-

byrax) or a stool softener (Colace, Surfak) helps regulate their bowels. If these remedies are not effective, speak to your doctor or pharmacist.

- Increased appetite and weight gain – Monitor your food intake and try to avoid foods with a high fat content (e.g., cakes and pastry).
- Joint pain or worsening of arthritis – Discuss this with your doctor.

Rare side effects you should report to your doctor **RIGHT AWAY** include:

- Sore mouth, gums, or throat, mouth ulcers
- Skin rash or itching, swelling of the face
- Nausea, vomiting, loss of appetite, feeling tired, weak, feverish or like you have the flu
- Yellow tinge in the eyes or to the skin; dark-colored urine (pee)
- Severe agitation, restlessness, irritability, or thoughts of suicide
- **Switch in mood to an unusual state of happiness, excitement, irritability, or problems sleeping**

Let your doctor know **right away** if you miss your period or think you may be **pregnant**, plan to become pregnant, or are breastfeeding.

What should you do if you forget to take a dose of your medication?

If you take your total dose of antidepressant at bedtime and you forget to take your medication, skip the missed dose and continue with your schedule the next day. **DO NOT DOUBLE THE DOSE.** If you take the drug several times a day, take the missed dose when you remember, then continue with your regular schedule.

Is this drug safe to take with other medication?

Because antidepressant drugs can change the effect of other medication, or may be affected by other medication, always check with your doctor or pharmacist before taking other drugs, including those you can buy without a prescription such as cold remedies and herbal preparations. Always inform any doctor or dentist that you see that you are taking an antidepressant drug.

Precautions/Considerations

1. Do not change your dose or stop the drug without talking to your doctor.
2. This drug may impair the mental and physical abilities required for driving a car or operating machinery. Avoid these activities if you feel drowsy or slowed down.
3. This drug may increase the effects of alcohol, making you more sleepy, dizzy and light-headed.
4. Do not stop your drug suddenly as this may result in withdrawal symptoms such as muscle aches, chills, tingling in your hands or feet, nausea, vomiting, and dizziness.
5. Report any changes in mood or behavior to your physician.
6. This drug may interact with medication prescribed by your dentist, so let him/her know the name of the drug you are taking.
7. Store your medication in a clean, dry area at room temperature. Keep all medication out of the reach of children.

If you have any questions regarding this medication, please ask your doctor, pharmacist, or nurse.

✍ Patient Information on Cyclic Antidepressants

The name of your medication is _____.

What is this drug used for?

Cyclic antidepressants are primarily used in the treatment of major depressive disorders and depression associated with Manic Depressive Illness (Bipolar Disorder).

Certain drugs in this class have also been found effective in several other disorders including obsessive compulsive disorder, panic disorder, bulimia, social phobia, premenstrual dysphoria, as well as management of chronic pain conditions (e.g., migraines) and bed-wetting in children. Ask your doctor if you are not sure why you are taking this drug.

How quickly will the drug start working?

Antidepressants begin to improve sleep and appetite and to increase energy within about one week; however, feelings of depression may take from 4 to 6 weeks to improve. Because antidepressants take time to work, **do not decrease or increase the dose or stop the medication** without discussing this with your doctor.

Improvement in symptoms of obsessive compulsive disorder, panic disorder and bulimia, pain management and enuresis also occur gradually.

How long should you take this medication?

This depends on what type of illness you have and how well you do.

Following the first episode of depression it is recommended that antidepressants be continued for a minimum of one year; this decreases the chance of being ill again. The doctor may then decrease the drug slowly and monitor for any symptoms of depression; if none occur, the drug can gradually be stopped.

For individuals who have had several episodes of depression, antidepressant medication should be continued indefinitely.

DO NOT STOP taking your medication if you are feeling better, without first discussing this with your doctor.

Long-term treatment is generally recommended for obsessive compulsive disorder, panic disorder, bulimia, pain management and enuresis.

What side effects may happen?

Side effects may happen with any drug. They are not usually serious and do not happen to everyone. Side effects may sometimes occur before beneficial effects of the medication are noticed. If you think you may be having a side effect, speak to your doctor or pharmacist as they can help you decrease it or cope with it.

Common side effects that should be reported to your doctor at the **NEXT VISIT** include:

- Feeling drowsy or tired – This problem goes away with time. Use of other drugs that make you drowsy will worsen the problem. Avoid driving a car or operating machinery if drowsiness persists.

- Energizing/agitated feeling – Some individuals may feel nervous or have difficulty sleeping for a few days after starting this medication. Report this to your doctor; he/she may advise you to take the medication in the morning.
- Blurred vision – This usually happens when you first start the drug and tends to be temporary. Reading under a bright light or at a distance may help; a magnifying glass can be of temporary use. If the problem lasts more than a few weeks, let your doctor know.
- Dry mouth – Sour candy and sugarless gum help increase saliva in your mouth. Do not drink sweet drinks like colas as they may give you cavities and increase your weight. Drink water and brush your teeth regularly.
- Constipation – Drink plenty of water and try to increase the amount of fiber in your diet (like fruit, vegetables or bran). Some individuals find a bulk laxative (e.g., Metamucil, Fibyrax) or a stool softener (Colace, Surfak) helps regulate their bowels. If these remedies are not effective, speak to your doctor or pharmacist.
- Headache – This tends to be temporary and can be managed by taking pain medicine (aspirin, acetaminophen) when required.
- Nausea or heartburn – If this happens, take the medication with food.
- Dizziness – Get up from a lying or sitting position slowly; dangle your legs over the edge of the bed for a few minutes before getting up. Sit or lie down if dizziness persists or if you feel faint, then contact your doctor.
- Sweating – You may sweat more than usual; frequent showering, use of deodorants and talcum powder may help.
- Muscle tremor, twitching – Speak to your doctor as this may require a change in your dosage.
- Changes in sex drive or sexual performance – Discuss this with your doctor.
- Nightmares – Can be managed by changing the time you take your drug – speak with your doctor.

Rare side effects you should report to your doctor **RIGHT AWAY** include:

- Sore mouth, gums, or throat
- Skin rash or itching, swelling of the face
- Nausea, vomiting, loss of appetite, fatigue, weakness, fever, or flu-like symptoms
- Yellow tinge in the eyes or to the skin; dark-colored urine (pee)
- Going 24 hours or more without peeing
- Inability to have a bowel movement (more than 2–3 days)
- Tingling in the hands and feet, severe muscle twitching
- Severe agitation, restlessness, irritability or thoughts of suicide
- **Switch in mood to an unusual state of happiness, excitement, irritability, or problems sleeping**

Let your doctor know **as soon as possible** if you miss your period or suspect you may be **pregnant**.

What should you do if you forget to take a dose of your medication?

If you take your total dose of antidepressant in the morning and you forget to take it for more than 6 h, skip the missed dose and continue with your schedule the next day. **DO NOT DOUBLE THE DOSE**. If you take the drug several times a day, take the missed dose when you remember, then continue with your regular schedule.

Is this drug safe to take with other medication?

Because antidepressant drugs can change the effect of other medication, or may be affected by other medication, always check with your doctor or pharmacist before taking other drugs, including those you can buy without a prescription such as cold remedies and herbal preparations. Always inform any doctor or dentist that you see that you are taking an antidepressant drug.

Precautions/Considerations

1. Do not change your dose or stop the drug without talking to your doctor.
2. Take your drug with meals or with water, milk, orange or apple juice; avoid grapefruit juice as it may change the effect of the drug in your body.
3. Avoid taking high-fiber foods (e.g., bran) or laxatives (e.g., psyllium) together with your medication, as this may reduce the antidepressant effect.
4. This drug may impair the mental and physical abilities required for driving a car or operating machinery. Avoid these activities if you feel drowsy or slowed down.
5. This drug may increase the effects of alcohol, making you more sleepy, dizzy and light-headed.
6. Avoid exposure to extreme heat and humidity since this drug may affect your body's ability to regulate temperature.
7. Do not stop your drug suddenly as this may result in withdrawal symptoms such as muscle aches, chills, tingling in your hands or feet, nausea, vomiting, and dizziness.
8. Report any changes in mood or behavior to your physician.
9. This drug may interact with medication prescribed by your dentist, so let him/her know the name of the drug you are taking.
10. Store your medication in a clean, dry area at room temperature. Keep all medication out of the reach of children.

If you have any questions regarding this medication, please ask your doctor, pharmacist, or nurse.

Patient Information on Moclobemide

The name of your medication is moclobemide. It belongs to a class of antidepressants called RIMA (Reversible Inhibitor of Monoamine Oxidase-A).

What is this drug used for?

Moclobemide is primarily used in the treatment of major depressive disorders and depression associated with Manic Depressive Illness (Bipolar Disorder). It has also been approved in the management of chronic dysthymia.

Though not approved for these indications, moclobemide has also been found effective in seasonal affective disorder and social phobia. Ask your doctor if you are not sure why you are taking this drug.

How quickly will the drug start working?

Moclobemide begins to improve sleep and appetite and to increase energy within about one week; however, feelings of depression may take from 4–6 weeks to improve. Because antidepressants take time to work, **do not decrease or increase the dose or stop the medication** without discussing this with your doctor. Improvement in symptoms of seasonal affective disorder and social phobia also occur gradually.

When should I take this medication?

Moclobemide is usually prescribed to be taken twice daily, morning and evening. Take this drug after meals to minimize side effects. If a meal is missed, the drug should still be taken, but a large meal should not be eaten for at least 1 hour.

How long should you take this medication?

This depends on what type of illness you have and how well you do.

Following the first episode of depression it is recommended that antidepressants be continued for a minimum of 1 year; this decreases the chance of being ill again. The doctor may then decrease the drug slowly and monitor for any symptoms of depression; if none occur, the drug can gradually be stopped. For individuals who have had several episodes of depression, antidepressant medication should be continued indefinitely.

DO NOT STOP taking your medication if you are feeling better, without first discussing this with your doctor.

Long-term treatment is generally recommended for social phobia; while cyclical therapy may be effective for seasonal affective disorder.

What side effects may happen?

Side effects may happen with any drug. They are not usually serious and do not happen to everyone. Side effects may sometimes occur before beneficial effects of the medication are noticed. If you think you may be having a side effect, speak to your doctor or pharmacist as they can help you decrease it or cope with it.

Common side effects that should be reported to your doctor at the **NEXT VISIT** include:

- Energizing/agitated feeling – Some individuals may feel nervous or have difficulty sleeping for a few days after starting this medication. Report this to your doctor; he/she may advise you to take the medication in the morning and afternoon (rather than the evening).
- Headache – This can be managed by taking pain medicine (e.g., aspirin, acetaminophen) as required. If the headache persists or is "troubling" contact your doctor.
- Dizziness – Get up from a lying or sitting position slowly; dangle your legs over the edge of the bed for a few minutes before getting up. Sit or lie down if dizziness persists or if you feel faint, – then call the doctor.
- Nausea or heartburn – If this happens, take the medication with food.
- Sweating – You may sweat more than usual; frequent showering, use of deodorants and talcum powder may help.

Rare side effects you should report to your doctor **RIGHT AWAY** include:
- Persistent, throbbing headache
- Sore mouth, gums, or throat
- Skin rash or itching, swelling of the face
- nausea, vomiting, loss of appetite, feeling tired, weak, feverish, or like you have the flu
- Yellow tinge in the eyes or to the skin; dark-colored urine
- Severe agitation, restlessness, irritability, or thoughts of suicide
- **Switch in mood to an unusual state of happiness, excitement, irritability, or problems sleeping**

Let your doctor know **right away** if you miss your period or think you may be **pregnant**, plan to become pregnant, or are breastfeeding.

Treatment with moclobemide does NOT require special diet restrictions as with other MAOI's. However, you should avoid eating excessive amounts of aged, overripe cheeses or yeast extracts. If a **hypertensive reaction** (high blood pressure) should occur, the symptoms usually come on suddenly, so be alert for these signs:

- Severe, throbbing headache which starts at the back of the head and moves toward the front. Often nausea and vomiting occur at the same time
- Stiff neck
- Heart palpitations, fast heart beat, chest pain
- Sweating, cold and clammy skin
- Enlarged (dilated) pupils of the eyes
- Sudden unexplained nose bleeds

If a combination of these symptoms does occur, **contact your doctor IMMEDIATELY**; if you are unable to do so, go to the Emergency Department of your nearest hospital.

Moclobemide should always be taken after meals to avoid any food-related side effects (e.g., headaches).

What should you do if you forget to take a dose of your medication?

If you take your total dose of antidepressant in the morning and you forget to take it for more than 6 hours, skip the missed dose and continue with your schedule the next day.

DO NOT DOUBLE THE DOSE. If you take the drug several times a day, take the missed dose when you remember, then continue with your regular schedule.

Is this drug safe to take with other medication?

Because antidepressant drugs can change the effect of other medication, or may be affected by other medication, always check with your doctor or pharmacist before taking other drugs, including those you can buy without a prescription such as cold remedies and herbal preparations. Always inform any doctor or dentist that you see that you are taking the antidepressant drug moclobemide.

Precautions/Considerations

1. Do not increase or decrease your dose without consulting your doctor.
2. Do not stop your drug suddenly as this may result in withdrawal symptoms such as muscle aches, chills, tingling in your hands or feet, nausea, vomiting, and dizziness.
3. Report any changes in mood or behavior to your physician.
4. This drug may interact with medication prescribed by your dentist, so let him/her know the name of the drug you are taking.
5. Take no other medication (including drugs you buy without a prescription or herbal products) without consulting with your doctor or pharmacist. Avoid all products containing dextromethorphan (DM).
6. Store your medication in a clean, dry area at room temperature. Keep all medication out of the reach of children.

If you have any questions regarding this medication, please ask your doctor, pharmacist, or nurse.

Patient Information on Monoamine Oxidase Inhibitor (MAOI) Antidepressants

The name of your medication is _____.

What is this drug used for?

This medication is primarily used in the treatment of major depressive disorders and depression associated with Manic Depressive Illness (Bipolar Disorder). It has also been approved in the management of atypical depression, phobic anxiety states or social phobia.

Though not approved for these indications, MAOIs have also been found effective in dysthymia, panic disorder and obsessive-compulsive disorder. Ask your doctor if you are not sure why you are taking this drug.

How quickly will the drug start working?

MAOIs begin to improve sleep and appetite and to increase energy within about one week; however, feelings of depression may take from 4 to 6 weeks to improve. Because antidepressants take time to work, **do not decrease or increase the dose or stop the medication** without discussing this with your doctor.

Improvement in symptoms of atypical depression, phobic anxiety or social phobia, dysthymia, panic disorder and obsessive-compulsive disorder also occur gradually.

How long should you take this medication?

This depends on what type of illness you have and how well you do.

Following the first episode of depression it is recommended that antidepressants be continued for a minimum of one year; this decreases the chance of being ill again. The doctor may then decrease the drug slowly and monitor for any symptoms of depression; if none occur, the drug can gradually be stopped. For individuals who have had several episodes of depression, antidepressant medication should be continued indefinitely.

DO NOT STOP taking your medication if you are feeling better, without first discussing this with your doctor. Long-term treatment is generally recommended for atypical depression, phobic anxiety or social phobia, dysthymia, panic disorder or obsessive-compulsive disorder.

What side effects may happen?

Side effects may happen with any drug. They are not usually serious and do not happen to everyone. Side effects may sometimes occur before beneficial effects of the medication are noticed. If you think you may be having a side effect, speak to your doctor or pharmacist as they can help you decrease it or cope with it.

Common side effects that should be reported to your doctor at the **NEXT VISIT** include:

- Feeling sleepy or tired – This problem goes away with time. Use of other drugs that make you drowsy will worsen the problem. Avoid driving a car or operating machinery if drowsiness persists.
- Energizing/agitated feeling – Some individuals may feel nervous or have difficulty sleeping for a few days after starting this medication. Report this to your doctor; he/she may advise you to take the medication in the morning and afternoon (rather than the evening).

- Headache – This can be managed by taking pain medicine (e.g., aspirin, acetaminophen) as required. If the headache persists or is "troubling" contact your doctor.
- Dizziness – Get up from a lying or sitting position slowly; dangle your legs over the edge of the bed for a few minutes before getting up. Sit or lie down if dizziness persists or if you feel faint – then call the doctor.
- Nausea or heartburn – If this happens, take the medication with food.
- Dry mouth – Sour candy and sugarless gum help increase saliva in your mouth. Do not drink sweet drinks like colas as they may give you cavities and increase your weight. Drink water and brush your teeth regularly.
- Blurred vision – This usually happens when you first start the drug and tends to be temporary. Reading under a bright light or at a distance may help; a magnifying glass can be of temporary use. If the problem lasts more than a few weeks, let your doctor know.
- Constipation – Drink plenty of water and try to increase the amount of fiber in your diet (like fruit, vegetables or bran). Some individuals find a bulk laxative (e.g., Metamucil, Fibyrax) or a stool softener (Colace, Surfak) helps regulate their bowels. If these remedies are not effective, speak to your doctor or pharmacist.
- Muscle tremor, twitching, jerking – Speak to your doctor as this may require a change in your dosage.
- Sweating – You may sweat more than usual; frequent showering, use of deodorants and talcum powder may help.
- Loss of appetite.

Rare side effects you should report to your doctor **RIGHT AWAY** include:

- Persistent, throbbing headache
- Sore mouth, gums, or throat
- Skin rash or itching, swelling of the face
- Nausea, vomiting, loss of appetite, feeling tired, weak, feverish, or like you have the flu
- Yellow tinge in the eyes or to the skin; dark-colored urine (pee)
- Going 24 hours or more without peeing
- Severe agitation, restlessness, irritability or thoughts of suicide
- **Switch in mood to an unusual state of happiness, excitement, irritability, or problems sleeping**

Let your doctor know **right away** if you miss your period or think you may be **pregnant**, plan to become pregnant, or are breastfeeding.

Caution

Certain foods and drugs contain chemicals which are broken down by the enzyme monoamine oxidase. Since this drug inhibits this enzyme, these chemicals increase in the body and may raise the blood pressure and cause a severe reaction called a **hypertensive crisis**.

Listed below are the foods and drugs which should be **avoided** while taking this drug.

Do not eat the following foods:

- All matured or aged cheeses (Cheddar, Brick, Blue, Stilton, Camembert, Roquefort)
- Broad bean pods (e.g., Fava Beans)
- Concentrated yeast extracts ("Marmite")
- Sausage (if aged, especially salami, mortadella, pastrami, summer sausage), other unrefrigerated fermented meats, game meat that has been hung, aged liver
- Dried salted fish, pickled herring
- Sauerkraut
- Soy sauce or soybean condiments, tofu
- Packet soup (especially miso)
- Tap (draft) beer, alcohol-free beer
- Improperly stored or spoiled meat, poultry, or fish

Wait for 14 days after stopping a MAOI drug before restarting to eat the above foods.

Hypertensive reactions have been reported, by some individuals, with the following foods; try small portions to determine if these foods will cause a reaction:

- Smoked fish, caviar, snails, tinned fish, shrimp paste
- Yogurt
- Meat tenderizers
- Meat extract ("Bovril," "Oxo")
- Homemade red wine, Chianti, canned/bottled beer, sherry, champagne
- Cheeses (e.g., Parmesan, Muenster, Swiss, Gruyere, Mozzarella, Feta)
- Pepperoni
- Overripe fruit, avocados, raspberries, bananas, plums, canned figs and raisins, orange pulp, tomatoes
- Oriental foods
- Spinach, eggplant

It is SAFE to use the following foods, in moderate amounts (only if fresh):

- Cottage cheese, cream cheese, farmer's cheese, processed cheese, Cheez Whiz, ricotta, Havarti, Boursin, Brie without rind, Gorgonzola
- Liver (as long as it is fresh), fresh or processed meats, poultry or fish (e.g., hot dogs, bologna)
- Spirits, liquor (in moderation)
- Soy milk
- Sour cream
- Salad dressings
- Worcestershire sauce
- Yeast-leavened bread

Make sure all food is fresh, stored properly, and eaten soon after being purchased. Never touch food that is fermented or possibly "off." Avoid restaurant sauces, gravy and soup.

Do not use the following drugs, which you can buy without a prescription, unless you have spoken to your doctor or pharmacist:

- Cold remedies, decongestants (including nasal sprays and drops), some anti-histamines and cough medicine
- Narcotic painkillers (e.g., products containing codeine)
- All stimulants including pep-pills (Wake-ups, Nodoz), or appetite suppressants
- Anti-asthma drugs (Primatine P)
- Sleep aids and Sedatives (Sominex, Nytol)
- Yeast, dietary supplements (e.g., Ultrafast, Optifast)

It is SAFE to use:

- Plain ASA (aspirin), acetaminophen (e.g., Tylenol), or ibuprofen (e.g., Motrin, Advil)
- Antacids (e.g., Tums, Maalox)
- Throat lozenges

If a **hypertensive reaction** (high blood pressure) should occur, the symptoms usually come on suddenly, so be alert for these signs:

- Severe, throbbing headache which starts at the back of the head and radiates forward; often the headache is accompanied by nausea and vomiting
- Stiff neck
- Heart palpitations, fast heart beat, chest pain
- Sweating, cold and clammy skin
- Enlarged (dilated) pupils of the eyes
- Sudden unexplained nose bleeds

If a combination of these symptoms does occur, **contact your doctor IMMEDIATELY**; if you are unable to do so, go to the Emergency Department of your nearest hospital.

What should you do if you forget to take a dose of your medication?

If you take your total dose of antidepressant in the morning and you forget to take it for more than 6 h, skip the missed dose and continue with your schedule the next day. **DO NOT DOUBLE THE DOSE**. If you take the drug several times a day, take the missed dose when you remember, then continue with your regular schedule.

Is this drug safe to take with other medication?

Because antidepressant drugs can change the effect of other medication, or may be affected by other medication, always check with your doctor or pharmacist before taking other drugs, including those you can buy without a prescription such as cold remedies and herbal preparations. Always inform any doctor or dentist that you see that you are taking an antidepressant drug.

Precautions/Considerations

1. Do not increase or decrease your dose without consulting your doctor.
2. Be aware of foods which you cannot eat while taking this medication.
3. Take no other medication (including those you can buy without a prescription or herbal products) without speaking with your doctor or pharmacist. Avoid all products containing dextromethorphan (DM).
4. This drug may interact with medication prescribed by your dentist, so let him/her know the name of the drug you are taking.
5. This drug may impair the mental and physical abilities required for driving a car or operating other machinery. Avoid these activities if you feel drowsy or slowed down.
6. Do not stop your drug suddenly as this may result in withdrawal symptoms such as muscle aches, chills, tingling in your hands or feet, nausea, vomiting, and dizziness.
7. Report any changes in mood or behavior to your physician.
8. Store your medication in a clean, dry area at room temperature. Keep all medication out of the reach of children.

If you have any questions regarding this medication, please ask your doctor, pharmacist, or nurse.

Patient Information on the Antidepresssant Transdermal Selegiline

The name of your medication is selegiline. It belongs to a class of antidepressants called MAO-B (monoamine oxidase-B) inhibitors.

What is this drug used for?

Selegiline transdermal (EMSAM) comes as a skin patch and is used to treat major depression. The skin patch delivers the medicine through your skin and into your bloodstream.

Your doctor will prescribe a dose of EMSAM based on your condition; he/she may change your dose if needed. Ask your doctor if you are not sure why you are taking this drug.

How quickly will the drug start working?

Though selegiline may begin to improve sleep and appetite and to increase energy within about one week, feelings of depression may take from 4 to 6 weeks to improve.

How long should you take this medication?

This depends on what type of illness you have and how well you do.

Following the first episode of depression it is recommended that antidepressants be continued for a minimum of one year; this decreases the chance of being ill again. The doctor may then decrease the drug slowly and monitor for any symptoms of depression; if none occur, the drug can gradually be stopped. For individuals who have had several episodes of depression, antidepressant medication should be continued indefinitely.

DO NOT STOP taking your medication if you are feeling better, without first discussing this with your doctor. Long-term treatment is generally recommended for atypical depression, phobic anxiety or social phobia, dysthymia, panic disorder or obsessive-compulsive disorder.

How do you use the transdermal patch?

Carefully read and follow the instructions, which are given to you with the patch.

1. EMSAM should be applied to dry, intact skin on the upper torso (below the neck and above the waist), upper thigh or the outer surface of the upper arm. A new application site should be selected with each new patch to avoid re-application to the same area.
2. Apply the patch at approximately the same time each day to an area of skin that is not hairy, oily, irritated, broken, scarred or calloused. Do not place the patch where your clothing is tight which could cause the patch to rub off.
3. Only one EMSAM patch should be worn at a time. Carefully dispose of used patches, as instructed.
4. Avoid exposing the EMSAM application site to external sources of direct heat, such as heating pads or electric blankets, heat lamps, saunas, hot tubs, heated water beds, and prolonged direct sunlight.

What side effects may happen?

Side effects may happen with any drug. They are not usually serious and do not happen to everyone. Side effects may sometimes occur before beneficial effects of the medication are noticed. If you think you may be having a side effect, speak to your doctor or pharmacist as they can help you decrease it or cope with it.

Common side effect that should be reported to your doctor at the **NEXT VISIT** include:

- Itching, skin rash or other skin reactions at the site of application of patch; change the site where you apply the patch regularly
- Dizziness, lightheadedness – get up from lying or sitting positions slowly. Let the doctor know if the dizziness occurs frequently, or you feel faint
- Stomach upset, diarrhea – if these symptoms continue, the doctor may need to adjust the dose
- Headache – this tends to be temporary and can be managed by taking pain medicine (Aspirin, acetaminophen, ibuprofen) as required. If the headache persists or is "troubling", contact your doctor.
- Dry mouth, sore throat – Sour candy and sugarless gum help increase saliva in your mouth. Do not drink sweet drinks like colas as they may give you cavities and help put on weight. Drink water and brush your teeth regularly.
- Sleeping difficulties – some individuals may feel nervous or have difficulty sleeping for a few days after starting this medication. The doctor may advise you to remove the patch at bedtime if your sleeping difficulties continue

Rare side effects you should report to your doctor **RIGHT AWAY** include:

- Sudden onset of severe headache, nausea, stiff neck, a fast heartbeat or a change in the way your heart beats (palpitations), a lot of sweating, and confusion. **If you suddenly have these symptoms, get medical care right away**
- High fever or sweating
- Tremors, muscle stiffness, or movements you cannot control
- Convulsions (or seizures)
- Increased anxiety, agitation, increase in suicidal thoughts
- Switch in mood to an unusual state of happiness, excitement, irritability
- Symptoms which indicate that you may have too much selegiline in your body include: excitement, irritability, nervousness, insomnia, dizziness, severe headache, hallucinations, sweating, light-headedness, fainting, or seizures

Let your doctor know **right away** if you miss your period or think you may be **pregnant**, plan to become pregnant, or are breastfeeding.

Caution

Certain foods and drugs contain chemicals which are broken down by the enzyme monoamine oxidase. Since this drug inhibits this enzyme, these chemicals increase in the body and may raise the blood pressure and cause a severe reaction called a **hypertensive crisis**.

Listed below are the foods and drugs which should be **avoided** while taking this drug.

Do not eat the following foods:

- All matured or aged cheeses (Cheddar, Brick, Blue, Stilton, Camembert, Roquefort)
- Broad bean pods (e.g., Fava Beans)
- Concentrated yeast extracts ("Marmite")
- Sausage (if aged, especially salami, mortadella, pastrami, summer sausage), other unrefrigerated fermented meats, game meat that has been hung, aged liver
- Dried salted fish, pickled herring

- Sauerkraut
- Soy sauce or soybean condiments, tofu
- Packet soup (especially miso)
- Tap (draft) beer, alcohol-free beer
- Improperly stored or spoiled meat, poultry, or fish

Wait for 14 days after stopping a MAOI drug before restarting to eat the above foods.

Hypertensive reactions have been reported, by some individuals, with the following foods; try small portions to determine if these foods will cause a reaction:

- Smoked fish, caviar, snails, tinned fish, shrimp paste
- Yogurt
- Meat tenderizers
- Meat extract ("Bovril," "Oxo")
- Homemade red wine, Chianti, canned/bottled beer, sherry, champagne
- Cheeses (e.g., Parmesan, Muenster, Swiss, Gruyere, Mozzarella, Feta)
- Pepperoni
- Overripe fruit, avocados, raspberries, bananas, plums, canned figs and raisins, orange pulp, tomatoes
- Oriental foods
- Spinach, eggplant

It is SAFE to use the following foods, in moderate amounts (only if fresh):

- Cottage cheese, cream cheese, farmer's cheese, processed cheese, Cheez Whiz, ricotta, Havarti, Boursin, Brie without rind, Gorgonzola
- Liver (as long as it is fresh), fresh or processed meats, poultry or fish (e.g., hot dogs, bologna)
- Spirits, liquor (in moderation)
- Soy milk
- Sour cream
- Salad dressings
- Worcestershire sauce
- Yeast-leavened bread

Make sure all food is fresh, stored properly, and eaten soon after being purchased. Never touch food that is fermented or possibly "off." Avoid restaurant sauces, gravy and soup.

Do not use the following drugs, which you can buy without a prescription, unless you have spoken to your doctor or pharmacist:

- Cold remedies, decongestants (including nasal sprays and drops), some anti-histamines and cough medicine
- Narcotic painkillers (e.g., products containing codeine)
- All stimulants including pep-pills (Wake-ups, Nodoz), or appetite suppressants
- Anti-asthma drugs (Primatine P)
- Sleep aids and Sedatives (Sominex, Nytol)
- Yeast, dietary supplements (e.g., Ultrafast, Optifast)

It is SAFE to use:

- Plain ASA (aspirin), acetaminophen (e.g., Tylenol), or ibuprofen (e.g., Motrin, Advil)
- Antacids (e.g., Tums, Maalox)
- Throat lozenges

If a **hypertensive reaction** should occur, the symptoms usually come on suddenly, so be alert for these signs:

- Severe, throbbing headache which starts at the back of the head and radiates forward; often the headache is accompanied by nausea and vomiting
- Stiff neck
- Heart palpitations, fast heart beat, chest pain
- Sweating, cold and clammy skin
- Enlarged (dilated) pupils of the eyes
- Sudden unexplained nose bleeds

If a combination of these symptoms does occur, **contact your doctor IMMEDIATELY**; if you are unable to do so, go to the Emergency Department of your nearest hospital.

What should you do if you forget to take a dose of your medication?

Should you forget to apply the patch at your usual time in the morning, apply it as soon as you remember to do so, unless it is almost time for the next dose. Replace this patch with a new one on the following day, at your usual time. **Do not** use extra medicine (or use more than one patch) to make up the missed dose.

Is this drug safe to take with other medication?

Because selegiline can change the effect of other medication, or may be affected by other medication, always check with your doctor of pharmacist before taking other drugs, including those you can buy without a prescription such as cold remedies and herbal preparations. Always inform any doctor or dentist that you see that you are using selegiline patches.

Precautions/Considerations

1. It is important that you understand how to use and apply an EMSAM Patch. **Read the instruction provided with your medication carefully, and ask your physician, nurse or pharmacist if there is something that you do not understand.**
2. Use EMSAM exactly as prescribed by your doctor. **Use only one patch at a time.** Change the patch once a day (every 24 hours). Choose a time of day that works best for you. Do not stop the drug suddenly without discussing this with your doctor.
3. Do not take other medicines while using EMSAM or for 2 weeks after you stop using it unless your doctor has told you it is okay.
4. Do not drive or operate dangerous machinery until you know how the selegiline patch affects you. It may reduce your judgment, ability to think, or coordination. Drinking alcoholic beverages is not recommended while using this drug.
5. Tell your doctor if you plan to have surgery. Also, tell your surgeon that you take EMSAM. EMSAM should be stopped 10 days before you have elective surgery.
6. Avoid exposing the EMSAM application site to external sources of direct heat, such as heating pads or electric blankets, heat lamps, saunas, hot tubs, heated waterbeds, and prolonged direct sunlight.
7. Store your medication in a clean, dry area at room temperature, in its sealed pouch until use. **Keep the patch out of the reach of children and away from pets.**

If you have any questions regarding this medication, please ask your doctor, pharmacist, or nurse.

Patient Information on Electroconvulsive Therapy (ECT)

What is ECT used for?

ECT is a procedure used primarily to treat patients with severe Depression. It has also been found effective in the manic phase of Manic Depressive Illness (Bipolar Affective Disorder), and in some patients with Schizophrenia.

What is the ECT procedure?

ECT is given to the patient while he/she is under anesthetic which has put them to sleep; a muscle relaxant is also given to relax the muscles, bones and joints.

ECT involves passing a small, controlled electric current between two metal discs (electrodes) which are applied on the surface of the scalp. The two electrodes may be placed on one side of the head for unilateral ECT or on both sides of the forehead for bilateral ECT. The electric current passes between the two electrodes and through part of the brain in order to stimulate the brain; that electrical stimulation induces a convulsion or seizure which usually lasts from 20–90 s.

The procedure takes approximately 10 minutes from the time the anesthetic is given until its effect wears off. Oxygen is given throughout this time and the patient is monitored continuously by the physician. The treatment is not painful and the electric current and seizure are not felt by the patient.

How does ECT work?

As is the case with many medical treatments, the actual way that ECT relieves symptoms of illness is not totally understood. It is believed that ECT affects some of the chemicals which transfer impulses or messages between nerve cells in the brain, perhaps more strongly and quickly than some medications. The treatment may correct some of the biochemical changes which accompany the illness.

How effective is ECT?

Studies comparing the effectiveness of ECT and drug therapy in depression have consistently shown that ECT is the most effective treatment of depression, especially in patients whose illness does not respond adequately to drug treatment.

The total number of treatments required to get the full benefit from ECT may range from 6 to 20, depending on the patient's diagnosis and response to treatment. In some patients, a response may be seen after 3 treatments, however a full course is generally recommended to obtain a full response. Some patients require periodic treatments to maintain their improvement.

How safe is ECT and what are the potential side effects?

ECT is considered safe when given according to modern standards. It has been shown to be safe when given to elderly patients as well as during pregnancy, with proper monitoring. Side effects that can occur include the following:

- Memory – The most common side effect seen following ECT is some degree of memory loss. Recovery from that memory loss begins a few weeks after treatment and is usually complete in most patients after 6 to 9 months. There may be a permanent loss of memory for details of some events, particularly those which occurred some time before and during the

weeks the treatment was given. Also, there may be some difficulty learning and remembering new information for a short period after ECT. However, the ability to acquire new memories recovers completely, usually a few months after treatment. A very small number of patients report severe problems with memory that remain for months or years.

- Confusion – Some patients experience a brief period of confusion after waking from the anesthetic.
- Headache – Common, but not usually severe.
- Muscle aches – Usually temporary.
- Increased heart rate and blood pressure – This can occur during treatment and last for several minutes. Monitoring of patients during and following ECT includes temperature, pulse, blood pressure and electrocardiogram (ECG).
- Prolonged seizure – Occurs rarely; seizure activity is monitored during the procedure by an electroencephalogram (EEG). Rarely a patient may have a spontaneous seizure following the ECT.
- Dental injury (e.g., broken teeth) or bone fractures – Occur very rarely.

The risk of death is very rare (2 to 4 per 100,000 treatments) and is similar to that seen with any treatment given under a general anesthetic.

What else do I need to know about the ECT procedure?

1. Make sure that you understand the information that has been provided to you by your doctor or nurse regarding ECT; ask them to explain anything about the treatment which you do not understand.
2. Do not eat or drink anything for approximately 8 hours before each treatment (and nothing after midnight).
3. Any essential medication (e.g., for high blood pressure) which your physician has told you must be taken before ECT, should be swallowed only with a very small sip of water.
4. Any other medication which you usually take in the morning should not be taken until after the ECT procedure.

Patient Information on Bright Light Therapy (BLT)

What is Bright Light Therapy used for?

Bright Light Therapy is a procedure used primarily to treat patients with a form of Depression called a Seasonal Affective Disorder.

It has also been used to treat milder "winter blues," premenstrual syndrome, and some sleeping disorders.

How do you use Bright Light Therapy?

There are a number of different BLT products on the market, including *light visors*, *standard light boxes*, or *dawn simulators* (your physician will tell you what units may be best for you). These units deliver up to 10,000 lux units of illumination; it is of upmost importance that only UV-filtered light be used.

You will wear the visor, or sit near the light source for a period of 20 to 60 minutes each day during the time of year when you typically experience symptoms of seasonal depression. (Your physician will tell you when to begin using the light source and whether to use it in the early morning or evening.)

It is not necessary for you to glance directly at the light source; you may read, eat, or perform other activities during exposure.

How does Bright Light Therapy work?

As in the case of many medical treatments, the actual way that BLT relieves symptoms of depression is not totally understood. Several theories have been suggested related primarily to an effect on the "light-dark" hormone melatonin, and to the ability of bright light to re-set the body's internal clock.

How effective is Bright Light Therapy?

Studies comparing the effectiveness of BLT and drug therapy in seasonal affective disorder have consistently shown that BLT is the most effective treatment for this form of depression. Most patients begin to see improvement in their symptoms after 1–3 weeks of daily exposure to the light.

How safe is Bright Light Therapy and what are the potential side effects?

BLT is considered a very safe procedure and studies over several years have shown no damage to the eyes from the light source.

Side effects that can occur include:

- Nausea – if severe, use an antinauseant (e. g., dimenhydrinate) prior to light exposure
- Headache – acetaminophen can be used
- Itchy or stinging eyes – this tends to occur early in treatment and goes away with time. If it continues to be bothersome, sit further away from the light source or decrease the time you spend under the light until the problem no longer occurs.
- Skin irritation – tends to occur in people with sensitive skin, or blondes and redheads. You may need to decrease your exposure to the light until the skin problem resolves; then you can gradually increase the time spent under the light.

- Nervousness – let your doctor know if this problem continues. If you feel stimulated or anxious following BLT, contact your doctor before continuing with the treatment.

What else do I need to know about Bright Light Therapy?

- Light should be used under supervision from your doctor.
- Ensure you understand how, when, and for how long you are to use the light visor or standard light box. Ask your doctor to explain anything about the treatment that you do not understand.
- Do not overuse BLT.
- As medication can interact with BLT, ensure your doctor is aware of all medication you are taking, including drugs you can buy without a prescription and herbal preparations.

Patient Information on Repetitive Transcranial Magnetic Stimulation (rTMS)

What is rTMS used for?

rTMS is a procedure used primarily to treat patients with depression, though there is increasing evidence that it can reduce auditory hallucinations (voices) in patients with schizophrenia.

How do you use rTMS?

A wire coil (encased in insulated plastic) is held over the skull and an electrical current is pulsed through the coil to generate a magnetic field that stimulates the brain. Individuals are awake and alert throughout the procedure and there is no recovery period once the treatment is finished. No anesthetic is required during this procedure. Depending on the type of rTMS given, each treatment may take anywhere from 15 to 45 minutes and is repeated on a daily basis for 10 to 20 days.

How does rTMS work?

As in the case of many medical treatments, the actual way that rTMS relieves symptoms of depression is not understood.

It is thought that rTMS may stimulate certain brain chemicals (serotonin and dopamine) that are important in stabilizing mood, or may alter the excitability of part of the brain called the cortex.

How effective is rTMS?

Studies comparing the effectiveness of rTMS to other forms of treatment of depression, including electroconvulsive therapy, suggest that rTMS is an effective treatment for depression. Most patients begin to see improvement in their symptoms after a few sessions.

How safe is rTMS and what are the potential side effects?

rTMS is considered a very safe procedure; however, as with all forms of treatment, side effects can occur in certain individuals.

Side effects that can occur include:

- Headache – acetaminophen or aspirin can be used, but are usually not necessary
- Pain around the site of coil placement can occur with each magnetic pulse if very high intensity stimulation is used – let your doctor know
- Loss of hearing sensitivity is possible if hearing protection is not used – use of foam earplugs during the procedure should prevent this effect
- Worsening depression, or the appearance of hypomania are rare – if your mood becomes unusually sad or elevated following rTMS, contact your doctor

The long-term effects of exposure to high-power magnetic fields are not known; however, the magnetic field strength of rTMS is similar to that of an MR (magnetic resonance) imaging scanner. To date no health hazards have been identified for patients or staff who have been exposed to the magnetic fields of an MR scanner.

What else do I need to know about rTMS?

1. Make sure you understand the information that has been provided to you by your doctor or nurse regarding rTMS. Ask your doctor to explain anything about the treatment that you do not understand.
2. Ensure your doctor is aware of all medication you are taking, including drugs you can buy without a prescription and herbal preparations. Some medications may increase the risk of seizures during some types of rTMS.

Patient Information on Antipsychotic Drugs

The name of your medication is _____.

What is this drug used for?

The main use of this drug is to treat psychosis. Psychosis can be a part of many illnesses like schizophrenia, major depression, and bipolar disorder (Manic Depression). Ask your doctor if you are not sure why you are taking it.

What symptoms will this drug help control?

Symptoms of psychosis may not be the same for each person. Some symptoms of psychosis that this drug can help with are:
- Hearing voices, seeing things, or smelling, tasting or feeling things that are not real (hallucinations).
- Feeling that someone is trying to hurt you or is following you, or that people are talking about you, or that you have special powers or are famous (delusions).
- Finding it hard to think clearly, having thoughts that are speeded up, or feeling like you don't have control of your thoughts.
- Becoming easily upset or over excited.
- Showing no interest in yourself or others.

The doctor may choose to use this medications for reasons not listed here. If you are not sure why this drug is being prescribed for you, please ask the doctor.

How quickly will the drug start working?

Some symptoms of psychosis may get better before others. Over the first few weeks you may find that you sleep better and have less mood changes (feel too angry, sad or happy, or have too much energy). Slowly over the next 2–8 weeks, hallucinations or delusions fade away and your thoughts become more clear. Other symptoms like having no interest in yourself or others may get better slowly over 6 months or more.

Because antipsychotics take time to work, do NOT change your dose or stop your medication without talking to your doctor.

How long should you take this medication?

This depends on what type of illness you have and how well you do.

If you are taking this drug to treat psychosis for the first time and do well on it, your doctor will likely want you to stay on it for at least 1–2 years. This will help stop you from getting sick again. If you have had symptoms of psychosis for many years or symptoms that go away but then come back, you may need to stay on this drug for a long time. Talk with your doctor about how long you should stay on it.

How do you take this drug?

Antipsychotic drugs come in different forms:
- Fast-acting injection – used to control symptoms quickly
- Liquid form or quick–melting tablet – Used for people who can't swallow tablets easily
- Tablets – The most common way to take this drug

- Long-acting or depot injection – drug is given in an injection once every 2 to 4 weeks. This is helpful if you can't remember to take your drug every day.

What side effects may happen?

Side effects may happen with any drug. They are not usually serious and do not happen to everyone. Side effects may sometimes occur before beneficial effects of the medication are noticed. Many side effects get better or go away over time. If you think you may be having a side effect, speak to your doctor or pharmacist as they can help you decrease it or cope with it.

Common side effects of some antipsychotic drugs that you should tell your doctor about **RIGHT AWAY** are:

Extrapyramidal Side Effects (or EPS): There are different kinds of EPS. Try not to be scared if these happen to you because they can be treated.
- One kind, called dystonia, can make your muscles stiff. This can make your neck tip back or turn to the side, or cause your eyes to roll back up in your head, or make your tongue feel bigger than normal making it hard to swallow. This kind of EPS most often happens in the first week that you start to take antipsychotc drugs. Call your doctor right away if you think you have this and s/he will give you another medicine that should make you feel better within 10 to 15 minutes.
- Another kind of EPS, called akathisia, may make you feel restless, fidgety, or unable to sit still.
- Another kind of EPS, called parkinsonism, may make your hands shake, or your body feel stiff and slow.

Common side effects that you should tell your doctor about at the **NEXT VISIT** include:
- Feeling sleepy or tired – this usually goes away over time. Be careful driving or during times when you need to be wide awake.
- Feeling dizzy – you may find you get dizzy or feel faint when you get up too fast from sitting or lying down. Getting up more slowly or sitting on the side of your bed with your feet on the floor before getting up will help. This side effect usually goes away over time.
- Dry mouth – Sugarless hard candy or gum, ice cubes, or popsicles can help. Do NOT drink sweet drinks like colas to help your dry mouth as they may give you cavities or may cause you to put on weight. Brush your teeth daily and visit your dentist regularly.
- Blurred vision – May happen when you first start to take this drug and may last for 1–2 weeks. Reading under a bright light or moving the book further away to read may help. If the problem lasts more than a few weeks let your doctor know.
- Constipation – Drink water, try to increase the amount of fibre (like fruits, vegetables, or bran) in your diet, and exercise your tummy muscles. Some people find that taking a bulk laxative containing psyllium (like Metamucil®) works. If this does not work or if you go more than 3 days without having a bowel movement call your doctor or pharmacist.
- Weight gain – The best way to limit weight gain is to watch how much you eat and avoid eating fatty foods (like cakes, ice cream) or foods high in sugar (like colas). Exercise can also help. Your doctor may check your weight, cholesterol (a type of body fat) and sugar levels from time to time.
- Increased thirst or peeing more often – Let your doctor know. Your doctor may want to check your blood sugar.
- Nausea or heartburn – Try taking your drug with food if this happens.

- Effects in women – Some antipsychotic drugs may cause changes in how regular your monthly periods are or cause you to miss your period. It may also cause your breasts to leak milk. Let your doctor know if this happens to you as these effects can be treated.
- Tardive Dyskinesias – May occur in people who have taken some antipsychotic drugs, usually after taking them for many years. Tardive dyskinesias happen when some of your body muscles, usually in your face (lips and tongue), move on their own, without you making them do so. Your doctor will check you often for any signs of tardive dyskinesia as picking them up early and taking action (depending on how you are doing, your doctor may decide to stop your drug or change to another drug) can help increase the chance that this side effect will go away.

Rare side effects you should tell your doctor about **RIGHT AWAY** are:
- Skin rash or itching
- Really bad headache
- Constant dizziness or fainting, breathing too fast or feeling like your heart is skipping or missing beats.
- Fever, nausea, vomiting, appetite loss, or feeling tired, confused, really thirsty, weak, or like you have a flu.
- Sore mouth, gums, or throat.
- Yellow tinge in the eyes or to the skin or dark coloured pee.
- Going 24 hours or more without peeing.
- Going more than 2 or 3 days without having a bowel movement.
- Fever (high temperature) with muscle stiffness.
- Sudden weakness or numbing in the face, arms, or legs or difficulty seeing or talking.

Let your doctor know **right away** if you miss your period or think you may be **pregnant**, plan to become pregnant, or are breastfeeding.

What should you do if you forget to take a dose of your medication?

If it is almost time for your next dose, just skip the missed one. Do NOT take two doses at the same time.

Is this drug safe to take with other medication?

Antipsychotic drugs can change the effect of other drugs that you are taking, or they may be affected by other drugs. Always check with your doctor or pharmacist before taking any drugs, including those that you are taking or plan to take, those you can buy without a prescription (like cold remedies), and herbals (like St. John's Wort, ginseng, and many others).

What else should I know about antipsychotic drugs?

1. Do not change your dose or stop it without talking to your doctor.
2. Take your drug with meals or with water, milk, or orange juice. Do NOT take it with apple juice or grapefruit juice as these may change the amount of drug in your body.
3. If you take ziprasidone (Geodon®), make sure you take your tablets with meals. If you take risperidone liquid (Risperdal® Oral solution), do NOT take it with colas or with tea.
4. If you take paliperidone (Invega), you may see some of the tablet in your stool. This is normal because the tablet does not dissolve all the way.
5. Do not break or crush your drug unless you have been told to do it by your doctor.
6. This drug may increase the effects of alcohol, making you more sleepy and less alert.
7. This drug may affect your body's ability to control body temperature, so avoid places that are very hot and humid like saunas.

8. Antacids (like Diovol, Maalox, amphogel, etc.) may lower the amount of drug in your body. Take your antacid at least 2 hours before or 1 hour after taking your antipsychotic drug to avoid this.
9. Some people may get bad sunburn even without being in direct sun a long time. Avoid direct sun, wear protective clothes and use sunscreen.
10. Drinking a lot of caffeine (coffee, teas, colas, etc.) can cause you to become easily upset or jittery and make it harder for this drug to work.
11. Cigarette smoking can change the amount of drug in your body so let your doctor know if you smoke, or if you stop smoking or change how much you smoke.
12. Stopping your drug all of a sudden ("cold turkey") may make you ill. Talk to your doctor or pharmacist first about how to stop it safely.
13. Keep your antipsychotic drugs in a clean, dry area at room temperature. Keep all medication out of the reach of children.

If you have any questions about antipsychotic drugs, please ask your doctor, pharmacist, or nurse.

Patient Information on Clozapine

Clozapine belongs to the class of drugs called **antipsychotics**.

What is this drug used for?

The main use of this drug is to treat psychosis. Psychosis can be a part of many illnesses like schizophrenia, or bipolar disorder (Manic Depression). Clozapine is most often used in people when other antipsychotic drugs don't work well enough. Ask your doctor if you are not sure why you are taking it.

What symptoms will this drug help control?

Symptoms of psychosis may not be the same for each person. Some symptoms of psychosis that this drug can help with are:

- Hearing voices, seeing things, or smelling, tasting or feeling things that are not real (hallucinations).
- Feeling that someone is trying to hurt you or is following you, or that people are talking about you, or that you have special powers or are famous (delusions).
- Finding it hard to think clearly, having thoughts that are speeded up, or feeling like you don't have control of your thoughts.
- Becoming easily upset or over excited.
- Showing no interest in yourself or others.

How quickly will the drug start working?

Some symptoms of psychosis may get better before others. Over the first few weeks you may find that you sleep better and have less mood changes (feel too angry, sad or happy, or have too much energy). Slowly over the next 2–8 weeks, hallucinations or delusions fade away and your thoughts become clearer. Other symptoms like having no interest in yourself or others may get better slowly over 6 months or more.

Because antipsychotics take time to work, do NOT change your dose or stop your medication without talking to your doctor.

How long should you take this medication?

People who take clozapine have often had symptoms of psychosis for a long time and may need to stay on this drug long term. Your doctor may change your dose from time to time based on how well you are doing and on the results of blood tests that you have.

DO NOT CHANGE the dose or STOP taking clozapine without talking to your doctor first. Stopping clozapine all at once ("cold turkey") may cause you to feel ill.

Why do I need blood tests with clozapine?
Why can I only get 1 or 2 weeks' supply at a time?

Clozapine can cause a rare side effect called agranulocytosis. This can happen in 1 out of every 100 people that take clozapine. It causes the number of white blood cells (a type of cell in your blood) to drop too low. This makes it harder for your body to fight off an infection. Blood tests must be done every 1–2 weeks so your doctor can check your white blood cells. It is also very important to call your doctor if you get any signs of infection such as fever, sore throat or mouth sores. Always let your doctor and pharmacist know you are taking clozapine before taking other drugs.

What side effects may happen?

Side effects may happen with any drug. They are not usually serious and do not happen to everyone. Side effects may sometimes occur before beneficial effects of the medication are noticed. Many side effects get better or go away over time. If you think you may be having a side effect, speak to your doctor or pharmacist as they can help you decrease it or cope with it.

Common side effects that you should tell your doctor about at the **NEXT VISIT** include:

- Feeling sleepy or tired – this usually goes away over time. Be careful driving or during times when you need to be wide awake.
- Feeling dizzy – you may find you get dizzy or feel faint when you get up too fast from sitting or lying down. Getting up more slowly or sitting on the side of your bed with your feet on the floor before getting up will help. This side effect usually goes away over time.
- Dry mouth – Sugarless hard candy or gum, ice cubes, or popsicles can help. Do NOT drink sweet drinks like colas to help your dry mouth as this may give you cavities. Brush your teeth daily and visit your dentist regularly.
- Blurred vision – May happen when you first start to take this drug and may last for 1–2 weeks. Reading under a bright light or moving the book further away to read may help. If the problem lasts more than a few weeks let your doctor know.
- Constipation – Drink water, try to increase the amount of fibre (like fruits, vegetables, or bran) in your diet, and exercise your tummy muscles. Some people find a bulk laxative like Metamucil® helps. If this does not work or if you go more than 3 days without having a bowel movement call your doctor or pharmacist.
- Drooling – Often occurs at night. Use a towel on the pillow when sleeping. If you also drool when awake, talk to your doctor about other ways to deal with this.
- Weight gain – The best way to limit weight gain is to watch how much you eat and avoid eating fatty foods (like cakes, ice cream) or foods high in sugar (like colas). Exercise can also help. Your doctor may check your weight, cholesterol (a type of body fat) and sugar levels from time to time.
- Increased thirst or peeing more often – Let your doctor know. Your doctor may want to check your blood sugar.
- Nausea or heartburn – Try taking your drug with food if this happens.

Rare side effects you should tell your doctor about **RIGHT AWAY** are:
- Sore mouth, gums, or throat
- Feeling tired or weak, fever or flu-like, or other signs of having an infection
- Feeling like your heart is beating to fast, chest pain, or problems breathing.
- Having a blackout, fit or seizure
- Skin rash or itching
- Really bad headache
- Constant dizziness or fainting
- Yellow tinge in the eyes or to the skin or dark coloured pee.

- Going 24 hours or more without peeing.
- Going more than 2 or 3 days without having a bowel movement.

Tardive Dyskinesias: This is a group of side effects that may occur in people who have taken some antipsychotic drugs, usually after taking them for many years. Tardive dyskinesias happen when some of your body muscles, usually in your face (lips and tongue), move on their own, without you making them do so. The chance of this happening with clozapine is very low and sometimes clozapine may be used to help treat it.

Let your doctor know **right away** if you miss your period or think you may be **pregnant**, plan to become pregnant, or are breastfeeding.

What should you do if you forget to take a dose of your medication?

If it is almost time for your next dose, just skip the missed one. Do NOT take two doses at the same time.

Is this drug safe to take with other medication?

Clozapine can change the effect of other drugs that you are taking, or it may be affected by other drugs. Always check with your doctor or pharmacist before taking any drugs, including those that you are taking or plan to take, those you can buy without a prescription (like cold remedies), and herbals (like St. John's Wort, ginseng, and many others).

What else should I know about clozapine?

1. Do not change your dose or stop it without talking to your doctor.
2. Take clozapine with meals or with water, milk, or orange juice. Do NOT take it with grapefruit juice as it may change the amount of drug in your body.
3. Do not break or crush clozapine unless you have been told to do it by your doctor.
4. Clozapine may increase the effects of alcohol, making you more sleepy and less alert.
5. Clozapine may affect your body's ability to control body temperature, so avoid places that are very hot and humid like saunas.
6. Antacids (like Diovol, Maalox, amphogel, etc.) may lower the amount of clozapine in your body. Take your antacid at least 2 hours before or 1 hour after taking clozapine to avoid this.
7. Drinking a lot of caffeine (coffee, teas, colas, etc.) can cause you to become easily upset or jittery and make it harder for clozapine
8. Cigarette smoking can change the amount of clozapine in your body so let your doctor know if you smoke, or if you stop smoking or change how much you smoke.
9. Stopping your drug all of a sudden ("cold turkey") may make you ill. Talk to your doctor or pharmacist first about how to stop it safely.
10. Keep your antipsychotic drugs in a clean, dry area at room temperature. Keep all medication out of the reach of children.

If you have any questions about clozapine, please ask your doctor, pharmacist, or nurse.

Patient Information on Antiparkinsonian Agents for Treating Extrapyramidal Side Effects

The name of your medication is _____.

What is this drug used for?

This drug is called an antiparkinsonian drug. It is used to treat a group of side effects, known as Extrapyramidal Side Effects or EPS, that can happen when taking antipsychotic drugs. EPS affects your muscles and can cause:

- Muscle spasms or tightening (This usually happens in the neck – can make your neck tip back or turn to the side; eyes – can make your eyes to roll back up in your head; or tongue – can make your tongue feel bigger than normal making it hard to swallow).
- Muscle stiffness, tremors or shaking, and a shuffling walk
- Feeling restless or unable to sit still

How quickly will the drug start working?

When given by injection, this drug works very fast, usually in 10 or 15 minutes. When swallowed as a pill, the drug should make you feel better within 1 hour.

How long should you take this medication?

Many people only take this drug for 2–3 weeks to prevent or treat an EPS when an antipsychotic drug is first started. Your doctor may lower the dose of this drug to see if any signs of EPS return; if not, you may be able to stop this drug. Do not change the dose of this drug without talking to your doctor first.

Some people may need to take this drug for a longer time, because they are more "sensitive" or more likely to get EPS. Other people only have to take it for short periods from time to time. (e.g., for 1 week after getting an antipsychotic by injection).

What side effects may happen?

Side effects may happen with any drug. They are not usually serious and do not happen to everyone. Side effects may sometimes occur before beneficial effects of the medication are noticed. Many side effects get better or go away over time. If you think you may be having a side effect, speak to your doctor or pharmacist as they can help you decrease it or cope with it.

Common side effects than can occur with antiparkinsonian drugs are:

- Dry mouth – Sugarless hard candy or gum, ice cubes, or popsicles can help. Do NOT drink sweet drinks like colas to help your dry mouth as this may give you cavities and cause you to put on weight. Brush your teeth daily and visit your dentist regularly.
- Blurred vision – May happen when you first start to take this drug and may last for 1–2 weeks. Reading under a bright light or moving the book further away to read may help. If the problem lasts more than a few weeks let your doctor know.
- Constipation – Drink water, try to increase the amount of fibre (like fruits, vegetables, or bran) in your diet, and exercise your tummy muscles. Some people find taking a bulk laxative containing psyllium (like Metamucil®) works. If this does not work or if you go more than 3 days without having a bowel movement call your doctor or pharmacist.
- Feeling sleepy or tired – this usually goes away over time. Be careful driving or during times when you need to be wide awake.

- Nausea or heartburn – Try taking your drug with food if this happens.

Less common side effects that you should tell your doctor about **RIGHT AWAY** are:
- Feeling confused, having memory loss or noticing an increase in your psychosis symptoms.
- Going more than 3 days without having a bowel movement.
- Going a day without peeing.
- Getting a skin rash

Let your doctor know **right away** if you miss your period or think you may be **pregnant**, plan to become pregnant, or are breastfeeding.

Is this drug safe to take with other medication?

Antiparkinsonian drugs can change the effect of other drugs that you are taking, or they may be affected by other drugs. Always check with your doctor or pharmacist before taking any drugs, including those that you are taking or plan to take, those you can buy without a prescription (like cold remedies), and herbals (like St. John's Wort, ginseng, and many others).

What else should I know about antiparkinsonian drugs?

1. Do not change your dose or stop it without talking to your doctor.
2. This drug may increase the effects of alcohol, making you more sleepy and less alert.
3. This drug may affect your body's ability to control body temperature, so avoid places that are very hot and humid like saunas.
4. Keep your antiparkinsonian drugs in a clean, dry area at room temperature. Keep all medication out of the reach of children.

If you have any questions about this drug, please ask your doctor, pharmacist, or nurse.

Patient Information on Benzodiazepine Antianxiety Drugs (Anxiolytics)

The name of your medication is _____.

What is this drug used for?

This medication is used to **treat symptoms of anxiety.** Anxiety is a normal human response to stress and is considered necessary for effective functioning and coping with daily activities. It may, however, be a symptom of many other disorders, both medical and psychiatric. There are many different types of anxiety and there are many different approaches to treating it. Anxiolytics can help relieve the symptoms of anxiety but will not get rid of its cause. In usually prescribed doses, they help to calm and relax the individual; in high doses these drugs may be used to induce sleep.

Benzodiazepines may also be used as muscle relaxants, to stop seizures, and before some diagnostic procedures. Ask your doctor if you are not sure why you are taking this drug.

How quickly will the drug start working?

Anxiolytic drugs can reduce agitation and induce calm or sedation usually within an hour. Sometimes they have to be given by injection, or dissolved under the tongue, for a quicker effect.

How long should you take this medication?

Anxiety is usually self-limiting; often when the cause of anxiety is treated or eliminated, symptoms of anxiety will decrease. Therefore, anxiolytics are usually prescribed for a limited period of time. Many individuals take the medication only when needed (during periods of excessive stress) rather than on a daily basis. Tolerance or loss of effectiveness can occur in some individuals if they are used continuously beyond 4 months. If you have been taking the medication for a continuous period of time, the physician may try to reduce the dose of this drug slowly to see if the anxiety symptoms return; if not, the dosage may be further reduced and you may be advised to stop using this medication. **Do not increase the dose or stop the drug without consulting with your doctor.** Some patients need to use an anxiolytic drug for longer time periods, because of the type of anxiety they may be experiencing. Others require it only from time to time, i.e., as needed.

What side effects may happen?

Side effects may happen with any drug. They are not usually serious and do not happen to everyone. Side effects may sometimes occur before beneficial effects of the medication are noticed. Many side effects get better or go away over time. If you think you may be having a side effect, speak to your doctor or pharmacist as they can help you decrease it or cope with it.

Common side effects that should be reported to your doctor at the **NEXT VISIT** include:

- Feeling sleepy and tired – This problem goes away with time, or when the dose is reduced. Use of other drugs that make you drowsy will worsen the problem. Avoid driving a car or operating machinery if drowsiness persists.
- Muscle incoordination, weakness or dizziness – Inform your doctor; an adjustment in your dosage may be needed.
- Forgetfulness, memory lapses – Inform your doctor.
- Slurred speech – An adjustment in your dosage may be needed.
- Nausea or heartburn – If this happens, take the medication with food.

Less common side effects that you should report to your doctor **RIGHT AWAY** include:

- Disorientation, confusion, worsening of memory, blackouts, difficulty learning new things, or amnesia
- Nervousness, excitement, restlessness, or any behavior changes
- Incoordination leading to falls
- Skin rash

Let your doctor know **right away** if you miss your period or think you may be **pregnant**, plan to become pregnant, or are breastfeeding.

Is this drug safe to take with other medication?

Because these drugs can change the effect of other medication, or may be affected by other medication, always check with your doctor or pharmacist before taking other drugs, including those you can buy without a prescription such as cold remedies and herbal preparations. Always inform any doctor or dentist that you see that you are taking these drugs.

Precautions/Considerations

1. Do not change your dose or stop the drug without talking to your doctor.
2. Take your medication with meals or with water, milk, orange or apple juice. Avoid grapefruit juice as it may change the effects of the drug in your body.
3. Check with your doctor or pharmacist before taking other drugs, including drugs you can buy without a prescription such as cold remedies and herbal preparations.
4. If you are taking the extended-release alprazolam (Xanax XR®) or clorazepate (Tranxene SD), do not cut, crush, or chew the tablet, but swallow it whole. Take this drug at the same time in relation to your meals (preferably in the morning).
5. This drug may impair the mental and physical abilities required for driving a car or operating machinery. Avoid these activities if you feel drowsy or slowed down.
6. This drug may increase the effects of alcohol, making you more sleepy, dizzy and lightheaded.
7. Do not stop taking the drug suddenly, especially if you have been on the medication for a number of months or have been taking high doses. Anxiolytics need to be withdrawn gradually to prevent withdrawal reactions.
8. Drinking a lot of caffeine (coffee, tea, colas, etc.) can cause you to become easily upset or jittery and make it harder for this drug to work.
9. Store your medication in a clean, dry area at room temperature. Keep all medication out of the reach of children.

If you have any questions regarding this medication, please ask your doctor, pharmacist, or nurse.

Buspirone is an anti-anxiety drug (anxiolytic).

What is this drug used for?

Buspirone is used to **treat symptoms of chronic anxiety.** Anxiety is a normal human response to stress and is considered necessary for effective functioning and coping with daily activities. It may, however, be a symptom of many other disorders, both medical and psychiatric. There are many different types of anxiety and there are many different approaches to treating it.

Though not approved for these indications, buspirone has also been found effective in other conditions, including posttraumatic stress disorder, social phobia, body dysmorphic disorder, agitation, irritability, aggression, and antisocial behavior, and as an aid in smoking cessation and alcohol withdrawal. It has been used alone or in combination with antidepressants in the treatment of depression and obsessive compulsive disorder. Ask your doctor if you are not sure why you are taking this drug.

How quickly will the drug start working?

Buspirone causes a gradual improvement in symptoms of anxiety and can reduce agitation and induce calm usually within 1 to 2 weeks. The maximum effect is seen after 3–4 weeks.

Improvement in symptoms of other disorders, for which buspirone may be prescribed, occur gradually over several weeks.

How long should you take this medication?

This depends on what type of illness you have and how well you do.

Anxiety is usually self-limiting; often when the cause of anxiety is treated or eliminated, symptoms of anxiety will decrease. Therefore, anxiolytics are usually prescribed for a limited period of time. To maintain effectiveness, buspirone cannot be taken only when needed (during periods of excessive stress), but needs to be taken on a daily basis. The physician may try to reduce the dose of this drug to see if the anxiety symptoms return; if not, the dosage may be further reduced and you may be advised to stop using this medication. **Do not increase the dose or stop the drug without consulting with your doctor.** Some patients need to use an anxiolytic drug for longer time periods, because of the type of anxiety they may be experiencing.

Long-term treatment is generally recommended for certain other indications such as social phobia, body dysmorphic disorder or antisocial behavior.

What side effects may happen?

Side effects may happen with any drug. They are not usually serious and do not happen to everyone. Side effects may sometimes occur before beneficial effects of the medication are noticed. If you think you may be having a side effect, speak to your doctor or pharmacist as they can help you decrease it or cope with it.

Common side effects that should be reported to your doctor at the **NEXT VISIT** include:

- Feeling sleepy and tired – This problem goes away with time, or when the dose is reduced. Avoid driving a car or operating machinery if drowsiness persists.
- Headache – tends to be temporary and can be managed by taking pain medicine (e.g., aspirin, acetaminophen) when required.
- Nausea or heartburn – If this happens, take the medication with food.
- Dizziness, lightheadedness – sit or lie down; if symptoms persist, contact your doctor.
- Energized/agitated feeling – some individuals may feel nervous for a few days after starting this medication. Report this to your doctor.
- Tingling or numbing in fingers or toes – report this to your doctor.

Less common side effects that you should report to your physician **RIGHT AWAY** include:

- Severe agitation, excitement or any changes in behavior.

Let your doctor know **right away** if you miss your period or think you may be **pregnant**, plan to become pregnant, or are breastfeeding.

What should you do if you forget to take a dose of your medication?

If you take your total dose of buspirone at bedtime and you forget to take your medication, skip the missed dose and continue with your schedule the next day. **DO NOT DOUBLE THE DOSE.** If you take the drug several times a day, take the missed dose when you remember, then continue with your regular schedule.

Is this drug safe to take with other medication?

Because this drug can change the effect of other medication, or may be affected by other medication, always check with your doctor or pharmacist before taking other drugs, including those you can buy without a prescription such as cold remedies and herbal preparations. Always inform any doctor or dentist that you see that you are taking this drug.

Precautions/Considerations

1. Do not increase your dose without consulting your doctor.
2. Take your medication at the same time each day in relation to your meals (i.e., always with or without food).
3. Take your medication with water, milk, orange or apple juice. Avoid grapefruit juice as it may change the effects of the drug in your body.
4. Drinking a lot of caffeine (coffee, tea, colas, etc.) can cause you to become easily upset or jittery and make it harder for this drug to work.
5. Check with your doctor or pharmacist before taking other drugs, including drugs you can buy without a prescription or herbal remedies.
6. Store your medication in a clean, dry area at room temperature. Keep all medication out of the reach of children.

If you have any questions regarding this medication, please ask your doctor, pharmacist, or nurse.

Patient Information on Hypnotics/Sedatives

The name of your medication is _____.

What is this drug used for?

This medication is used to **treat sleep problems,** such as problems falling asleep or remaining asleep for a reasonable number of hours or waking up often during the night. Sleeping problems occur in most individuals from time to time. If, however, sleeping problems persist, this may be a symptom of some other disorder, either medical and psychiatric.

A person may have difficulty in falling asleep because of stress or anxiety felt during the day, pain, physical discomfort or changes in daily routine (e.g., jet-lag, changes in work shifts, etc.) Any disease that causes pain (e.g., ulcers) or breathing difficulties (e.g., asthma or a cold) can interfere with continuous sleep. Stimulant drugs, including caffeine, may also contribute to problems falling asleep; other medications may change sleep patterns when they are stopped (e.g., antidepressants, antipsychotics). Sleep will improve when these causes have been identified, corrected, or treated.

Problems remaining asleep may be due to age, as older people tend to sleep less at night. Certain disorders, including depression, may also affect sleep.

Hypnotic/sedatives are similar to antianxiety drugs, but tend to cause more drowsiness and incoordination; therefore, sometimes antianxiety drugs are given to treat sleep problems.

How quickly will the drug start working?

Hypnotics/sedatives can induce calm or sedation usually within an hour. As some drugs act quickly, take the medication just prior to going to bed and relax in bed until the drug takes effect.

How long should you take this medication?

Sleep problems are usually self-limiting; often when the cause of sleep difficulties is treated or eliminated, sleep will improve. Therefore, hypnotic/sedatives are usually prescribed for a limited period of time. Many individuals take the medication only when needed (during periods of insomnia) rather than on a daily basis. It is suggested that once you have slept well for 2 or 3 nights in a row, try to get to sleep without taking the sedative/hypnotic. Tolerance or loss of effectiveness can occur in some individuals if they are used every day beyond four months. Individuals taking hypnotics for long periods of time have a risk of developing dependence – they may have difficulty stopping the medication and may experience withdrawal symptoms.

If you have been taking the medication every day for a period of time, the physician may try to reduce the dose of this drug slowly to see if sleeping problems persist; if not, the dosage may be further reduced and you may be advised to stop using this medication. **Do not increase the dose or stop the drug without consulting with your doctor.**

Some patients need to use a sedative/hypnotic drug for longer time periods, because of the type of problems they may be experiencing. Others require it only from time to time, i.e., PRN.

What side effects may happen?

Side effects may happen with any drug. They are not usually serious and do not happen to everyone. Side effects may sometimes occur before beneficial effects of the medication are noticed. If you think you may be having a side effect, speak to your doctor or pharmacist as they can help you decrease it or cope with it.

Common side effects that you should report to your doctor at the **NEXT VISIT** include:
- Morning hangover, feeling sleepy and tired – This problem may lessen with time; inform your doctor. Use of other drugs that make you drowsy will worsen the problem. Avoid driving a car or operating machinery if drowsiness persists.
- Muscle incoordination, weakness, lightheadedness or dizziness – Inform your doctor; a change in your dosage may be needed.
- Forgetfulness, memory lapses – Inform your doctor.
- Slurred speech – A change in your dosage may be needed.
- Nausea or heartburn – If this happens, take the medication with food.
- Bitter taste – Can occur with certain drugs (e.g., zopiclone). Avoid milk in the morning to lessen this effect.

Less common side effects that you should report to your physician **RIGHT AWAY** include:
- Disorientation, confusion, worsening of your memory, periods of blackouts, or amnesia
- Nervousness, excitement, agitation, hallucinations or any behavior changes
- Worsening of depression, suicidal thoughts
- Incoordination leading to falls
- Skin rash

Let your doctor know **right away** if you miss your period or think you may be **pregnant**, plan to become pregnant, or are breastfeeding.

Is this drug safe to take with other medication?

Because these drugs can change the effect of other medication, or may be affected by other medication, always check with your doctor or pharmacist before taking other drugs, including those you can buy without a prescription such as cold remedies and herbal preparations. Always inform any doctor or dentist that you see that you are taking these drugs.

Precautions/Considerations

1. Do not increase your dose without consulting your doctor.
2. Check with your doctor or pharmacist before taking other drugs, including drugs you can buy without prescription, such as cold remedies and herbal preparations.
3. Speak to your doctor if you begin having sleeping problems after starting any new medication (e.g., for a medical condition).
4. This drug may impair the mental and physical abilities required for driving a car or operating machinery. Avoid these activities if you feel drowsy or slowed down.
5. This drug may increase the effects of alcohol, making you more sleepy, dizzy and lightheaded.

6. Take your medication about half an hour before bedtime; do not smoke in bed afterwards.
7. Do not stop taking the drug suddenly, especially if you have been on the medication for a number of months or have been taking high doses. Hypnotics/sedatives need to be withdrawn gradually to prevent withdrawal reactions.
8. Drinking a lot of caffeine (coffee, tea, colas, etc.) can cause you to become easily upset or jittery and make it harder for this drug to work.
9. Store your medication in a clean, dry area at room temperature. Keep all medication out of the reach of children.
10. If you are prescribed Ambien CR, do not split, crush or chew the tablet, but swallow it whole.

Some nondrug methods to help you sleep include:

1. Avoid taking caffeine-containing drinks or foods (e.g., chocolate) after 6 pm and avoid heavy meals several hours before bedtime. A warm glass of milk is effective for some people.
2. Napping and sleeping during the day will make restful sleep at night difficult. Keep active during the day and exercise regularly.
3. Engage in relaxing activities prior to bedtime such a reading, listening to music or taking a warm bath. Strenuous exercise (e.g., jogging) immediately before bedtime may make it difficult to get to sleep.
4. Establish a routine or normal pattern of sleeping and waking.
5. Use the bed and bedroom only for sleep and sexual activity.
6. Minimize external stimulation which might disturb sleep. If necessary, use dark shades over windows or wear ear plugs.
7. Once in bed, make sure you are comfortable (i.e., not too hot or cold); use a firm mattress.
8. Relaxation techniques (e.g., muscle relaxation exercises, yoga) may be helpful in decreasing anxiety and promoting sleep
9. If you have problems getting to sleep, rather than toss and turn in bed, have some warm milk, read a book, listen to music, or try relaxation techniques until you again begin to feel tired.
10. Don't worry about the amount of sleep you are getting as the amount will vary from day to day. The more you worry the more anxious you will get and this may make it harder for you to fall asleep.

If you have any questions regarding this medication, please ask your doctor, pharmacist, or nurse.

Patient Information on L-Tryptophan

L-tryptophan is an amino acid, a natural body chemical.

What is this drug used for?

L-tryptophan is used primarily as an add-on therapy to treat symptoms of acute mania or depression, and in the long-term control or prophylaxis of Manic Depressive Illness (Bipolar Disorder).

Though not approved for these indications, L-tryptophan has also been found to be useful as a sedative in insomnia and in behavior disturbances, such as chronic aggression or antisocial behavior. Ask your doctor if you are not sure why you are taking this drug.

How quickly will the drug start working?

Control of manic symptoms may require up to 14 days of treatment. Because L-tryptophan takes time to work, **do not decrease or increase the dose or stop the medication** without discussing this with your doctor.

Improvement in sleep disorders tends to occur relatively quickly (with the first dose). Benefits in behavior disturbances occur gradually.

How long should you take this medication?

This depends on what type of illness you have and how well you do.

L-tryptophan is often prescribed to increase the effectiveness of an antidepressant, an antipsychotic or another mood stabilizer. Long-term treatment is generally recommended for recurring depression or mood disorder.

As sleep problems are usually self-limiting, many individuals take L-tryptophan only when needed (during periods of insomnia). Long-term treatment is generally recommended for treatment of behavior disturbances.

What side effects may happen?

Side effects may happen with any drug. They are not usually serious and do not happen to everyone. Side effects may sometimes occur before beneficial effects of the medication are noticed. If you think you may be having a side effect, speak to your doctor or pharmacist as they can help you decrease it or cope with it.

Common side effects that should be reported to your doctor at the **NEXT VISIT** include:

- Feeling sleepy and tired, difficulty concentrating – This problem goes away with time. Use of other drugs that make you drowsy will worsen the problem. Avoid driving a car or operating machinery if drowsiness persists.
- Problems with balance or unsteadiness, incoordination – Discuss this with your doctor as this may require a change in your dosage.
- Nausea or heartburn – If this happens, take the medication with food.

- Dry mouth – Sour candy and sugarless gum help increase saliva in your mouth. Do not drink sweet drinks like colas as they may give you cavities and help put on weight. Drink water and brush your teeth regularly.

Rare side effects you should report to your doctor **RIGHT AWAY** include:
- Muscle twitches, tremor, incoordination, shivering, confusion
- Sore mouth, gums, or throat, mouth ulcers or sores
- Skin rash or itching, swelling of the face
- Vomiting, stomach pain
- Feeling tired, weak, feverish or like you have the flu
- Yellowing of the skin or eyes, darkening of urine (pee)
- Severe dizziness
- Switch in mood to an unusual state of happiness, excitement, irritability

Let your doctor know **right away** if you miss your period or think you may be **pregnant**, plan to become pregnant, or are breastfeeding.

What should you do if you forget to take a dose of your medication?

If you take your total dose of L-tryptophan in the evening and you forget to take it that evening, skip the missed dose and continue with your schedule the next day. **DO NOT DOUBLE THE DOSE**. If you take the drug several times a day, take the missed dose when you remember, then continue with your regular schedule.

Is this drug safe to use with other medication?

Because L-tryptophan can change the effect of other medication, or may be affected by other medication, always check with your doctor or pharmacist before taking other drugs, including those you can buy without a prescription. Always inform any doctor or dentist you see that you are taking this drug.

Precautions/Considerations

1. Do not change your dose or stop the drug without speaking to your doctor.
2. This drug may impair the mental and physical abilities and reaction time required for driving a car or operating other machinery. Avoid these activities if you feel drowsy or slowed down.
3. Let your doctor know before starting any protein-reduced diets as these can interfere with the action of this medication.
4. Report any changes in mood or behavior to your physician.
5. Store your medication in a clean, dry area at room temperature. Keep all medication out of the reach of children.

If you have any questions regarding this medication, please ask your doctor, pharmacist, or nurse.

Patient Information on Lithium

Lithium is classified as a mood stabilizer. It is a simple element, found in nature, and is also present in small amounts in the human body.

What is this drug used for?

Lithium is used primarily to treat symptoms of acute mania and in the long-term control or prevention of Manic Depressive Illness (Bipolar Disorder).

Though not approved for these indications, lithium has also been found to augment the effects of antidepressants in depression and obsessive compulsive disorder, and is useful in the treatment of cluster headaches, as well as chronic aggression or impulsivity. Ask your doctor if you are not sure why you are taking this drug.

How does the doctor decide what dose (how many milligrams) to prescribe?

The dose of lithium is different for every patient and is based on how much lithium is in the blood, as well as the response to treatment. The doctor will measure the lithium level in the blood on a regular basis during the first few months. The lithium level that is usually found to be effective for most patients is between 0.6 and 1.2 mmol/l (mEq/l).

You may initially take your medication several times a day (2 or 3); after several weeks, the doctor may decide to prescribe the drug once daily. It is important to drink 8–12 cups of fluid daily when on lithium (e.g., water, juice, milk, broth, etc.).

On the morning of your lithium blood test, take the morning dose of lithium **after** the test to avoid inaccurate results.

How quickly will the drug start working?

Control of manic symptoms may require up to 14 days of treatment. Because lithium takes time to work, **do not decrease or increase the dose or stop the medication** without discussing this with your doctor.

Improvement in symptoms of depression, obsessive compulsive disorder, cluster headaches, as well as aggression/impulsivity also occur gradually.

DO NOT STOP taking your medication if you are feeling better, without first discussing this with your doctor.

How long should you take this medication?

This depends on what type of illness you have and how well you do.

Following the first episode of mania it is recommended that lithium be continued for a minimum of one year; this decreases the chance of being ill again. The doctor may then decrease the drug slowly and monitor for any symptoms; if none occur, the drug can gradually be stopped.

For individuals who have had several episodes of mania or depression, lithium may need take be continued indefinitely.

Long-term treatment is generally recommended for recurring depression, obsessive-compulsive disorder, cluster headaches or aggression/impulsivity.

DO NOT STOP taking your medication if you are feeling better, without first discussing this with your doctor.

What side effects may happen?

Side effects may happen with any drug. They are not usually serious and do not happen to everyone. Side effects may sometimes occur before beneficial effects of the medication are noticed. If you think you may be having a side effect, speak to your doctor or pharmacist as they can help you decrease it or cope with it.

Common side effects that should be reported to your doctor at the **NEXT VISIT** include:

- Feeling tired, difficulty concentrating – This problem usually goes away with time. Use of other drugs that make you drowsy will worsen the problem. Avoid driving a car or operating machinery if drowsiness persists.
- Nausea or heartburn – If this happens, take the medication with food. If vomiting or diarrhea occur and persist for more than 24 hours, call your doctor.
- Muscle tremor, weakness, shakiness, stiffness – Speak to your doctor as this may require a change in your dosage.
- Changes in sex drive or sexual performance – Discuss this with your doctor.
- Weight changes – Watch the type of food you eat; avoid foods with high fat content (e.g., cakes and pastry).
- Increased thirst and increase in how often you pee – Discuss this with your doctor.
- Skin changes, e.g., dry skin, acne, rashes.

Side effects you should report RIGHT AWAY, as they may indicate the amount of lithium in the body is higher than it should be, include:

- Loss of balance
- Slurred speech
- Visual disturbances (e.g., double-vision)
- Nausea, vomiting, stomach ache
- Watery stools, diarrhea (more than twice a day)
- Abnormal general weakness or drowsiness
- Marked trembling (e.g., shaking that interferes with holding a cup), muscle twitches, jaw shaking

IF THESE OCCUR CALL YOUR DOCTOR RIGHT AWAY. If you cannot reach your doctor, stop taking the lithium until you get in touch with him. Drink plenty of fluids and snack on salty foods (e.g., chips, crackers). If symptoms continue to get worse, or if they do not clear within 12 hours, go to the Emergency Department of the nearest hospital. A clinical check-up and a blood test may show the cause of the problem.

Rare side effects you should report to your doctor **RIGHT AWAY** include:

- Sore mouth, gums, or throat
- Skin rash or itching, swelling of the face
- Nausea, vomiting, loss of appetite, feeling tired, weak, feverish, or like you have the flu
- Swelling of the neck (goitre)

- Abnormally frequent need to pee and increased thirst (e.g., having to get up in the night several times to pass urine)

Let your doctor know **right away** if you miss your period or think you may be **pregnant**, plan to become pregnant, or are breastfeeding.

What should you do if you forget to take a dose of your medication?

If you take your total dose of lithium in the morning or evening and you forget to take it for more than 6 hours, skip the missed dose and continue with your schedule the next day. **DO NOT DOUBLE THE DOSE**. If you take the drug several times a day, take the missed dose when you remember, then continue with your regular schedule.

Is this drug safe to take with other medication?

Because lithium can change the effect of other medication, or may be affected by other medication, always check with your doctor or pharmacist before taking other drugs, including over-the-counter medication such as cold remedies and herbal preparations. Always inform any doctor or dentist that you see that you are taking lithium.

Precautions/Considerations

1. Do not change your dose or stop the drug without talking to your doctor.
2. This drug may impair the mental and physical abilities and reaction time required for driving a car or operating other machinery. Avoid these activities if you feel drowsy or slowed down.
3. Do not stop your drug suddenly as this may result in withdrawal symptoms such as anxiety, irritability and changes in mood.
4. Report any changes in mood or behavior to your physician.
5. It is important to drink 8–12 cups of fluids daily (e.g., water, juice, milk, broth, etc.)
6. Limit the number of caffeinated liquids you drink (e.g., coffee, tea, colas), and avoid excessive alcohol use.
7. To treat occasional pain, avoid the use of nonsteroidal anti-inflammatory drugs (e.g., ibuprofen or Motrin, Advil) as they can affect the blood level of lithium and may result in toxicity. Acetaminophen is a safer alternative.
8. Do not change your salt intake during your treatment, without first speaking to your doctor (e.g., avoid no-salt or low-salt diets).
9. If you have the flu, especially if vomiting or diarrhea occur, check with your doctor regarding your lithium dose.
10. Use extra care in hot weather and during activities that cause you to sweat heavily (e.g., hot baths, saunas, exercising). The loss of too much water and salt from your body may lead to changes in the level of lithium in your body.
11. Tablets or capsules of lithium should be swallowed whole; do not chew or crush them.
12. Store your medication in a clean, dry area at room temperature. Keep all medication out of the reach of children.

If you have any questions regarding this medication, please ask your doctor, pharmacist, or nurse.

Patient Information on Anticonvulsant Mood Stabilizers

The name of your medication is _____.

What is this drug used for?

Anticonvulsants can be used to treat symptoms of acute mania and in the long-term control or prevention of Manic Depressive Illness (Bipolar Disorder).

They are also used to treat seizure disorders as well as certain pain syndromes (e.g., trigeminal neuralgia – carbamazepine; migraines – valproate).

Though not approved for these indications, these drugs have has also been found to be useful in the treatment of several other conditions, including: add-on therapy with antidepressants to treat depression, add-on therapy with antipsychotics to treat schizophrenia, withdrawal reactions from alcohol or sedative/hypnotics, and in behavior disturbances, such as chronic aggression or impulsivity. Ask your doctor if you are not sure why you are taking this drug.

How does the doctor decide what dose (how many milligrams) to prescribe?

The dose (amount in milligrams) of the medication is different for every patient and is based on the amount of drug in the blood (for some of these drugs) as well as your response to treatment. You may initially take your medication several times a day (2 or 3); after several weeks, the doctor may decide to prescribe the drug once daily.

How often will you need to have blood levels done with carbamazepine and valproate?

The doctor will measure the drug level in the blood on a regular basis during the first few months until the dose is stable. Thereafter, drug levels will be done at least once a year or whenever there is a change in drug therapy.

What do the blood levels mean?

The carbamazepine level that is usually found to be effective for most patients is between 17 and 50 umol/l (4–12 ug/ml). The valproate level that is usually found to be effective for most patients is between 350 and 700 umol/l (50–100 ug/ml).

On the morning of your blood test, take the morning dose of your medication **after** the test to avoid inaccurate results.

Blood levels do not need to be done with lamotrigine, topiramate, or gabapentin.

How quickly will the drug start working?

Control of manic symptoms or stabilization of mood may require up to 14 days of treatment. Because these medications need time to work, **do not decrease or increase the dose or stop the medication** without discussing this with your doctor.

Improvement in seizures, pain symptoms, as well as aggression/impulsivity also occur gradually.

How long should you take this medication?

This depends on what type of illness you have and how well you do. Following the first episode of mania it is recommended that these drugs be continued for a minimum of one year; this decreases the chance of being ill again. The doctor may then decrease the drug slowly and monitor for any symptoms; if none occur, the drug can gradually be stopped. For individuals who have had several or severe episodes of mania or depression, medication may need to be continued indefinitely.

Long-term treatment is generally recommended for recurring depression, seizure disorder and aggression/impulsivity.

What side effects may happen?

Side effects may happen with any drug. They are not usually serious and do not happen to everyone. Side effects may sometimes occur before beneficial effects of the medication are noticed. If you think you may be having a side effect, speak to your doctor or pharmacist as they can help you decrease it or cope with it.

Common side effects that should be reported to your doctor at the **NEXT VISIT** include:

- Feeling sleepy, tired, difficulty concentrating – This problem usually goes away with time. Use of other drugs that make you drowsy will worsen the problem. Avoid driving a car or operating machinery if drowsiness persists.
- Dizziness – Get up from a lying or sitting position slowly; dangle your legs over the edge of the bed for a few minutes before getting up. Sit or lie down if dizziness persists or if you feel faint – then call the doctor.
- Problems with balance or unsteadiness – Discuss this with your doctor as this may require a change in your dosage.
- Blurred vision – This usually happens when you first start the drug and tends to be temporary. Reading under a bright light or at a distance may help; a magnifying glass can be of temporary use. If the problem lasts more than a few weeks, let your doctor know.
- Dry mouth – Sour candy and sugarless gum help increase saliva in your mouth. Do not drink sweet drinks like colas as they may give you cavities and help put on weight. Drink water and brush your teeth regularly.
- Nausea or heartburn – If this happens, take the medication with food. If vomiting or diarrhea occur and last for more than 24 hours, call your doctor.
- Muscle tremor – Speak to your doctor as this may require a change in your dosage.
- Changes in hair texture, hair loss (valproate).
- Changes in your menstrual cycle (valproate).
- Changes in sex drive or sexual performance – Discuss this with your doctor.
- Weight changes – Watch the type of food you eat; avoid foods with high fat content (e.g., cakes and pastry).
- Periods of hyperventilation or rapid breathing.

Rare side effects you should report to your doctor **RIGHT AWAY** include:

- Sore mouth, gums, or throat, mouth ulcers, or sores
- Skin rash or itching, swelling of the face, skin blistering or crusting (especially with carbamazepine and lamotrigine)

- Severe stomach pain, nausea, vomiting, loss of appetite
- Feeling tired, weak, feverish, or like you have the flu
- Feeling confused or disoriented
- Easy bruising, bleeding, appearance of splotchy purplish darkening of the skin
- Yellowing of the skin or eyes, darkening of urine (pee)
- Unusual eye movements
- Sudden blurring of vision and/or painful or red eyes
- Feeling very dizzy or falling/fainting

Let your doctor know **right away** if you miss your period or think you may be **pregnant**, plan to become pregnant, or are breastfeeding.

What should you do if you forget to take a dose of your medication?

If you take your total dose of medication in the morning or bedtime and you forget to take it for more than 6 hours, skip the missed dose and continue with your schedule the next day. **DO NOT DOUBLE THE DOSE**. If you take the drug several times a day, take the missed dose when you remember, then continue with your regular schedule.

Is this drug safe to take with other medication?

Because these drugs can change the effect of other medication, or may be affected by other medication, always check with your doctor or pharmacist before taking other drugs, including those you can buy without a prescription such as cold remedies and herbal preparations. Always inform any doctor or dentist that you see that you are taking this drug.

Precautions/Considerations

1. Do not change your dose or stop the drug without speaking with your doctor.
2. Avoid drinking grapefruit juice while on *carbamazepine* as it can change the effect of carbamazepine in your body.
3. If your are on *liquid carbamazepine*, do not mix it with any other liquid medication. The liquid form of *valproic acid* should not be mixed with carbonated beverages, such as soda pop; this may cause an unpleasant taste or mouth irritation.
4. Unless you are prescribed a chewable tablet, capsules or tablets should be swallowed whole; do not break, chew or crush them.
5. These drugs may impair the mental and physical abilities and reaction time required for driving a car or operating other machinery. Avoid these activities if you feel drowsy or slowed down.
6. Do not stop your drug suddenly as this may result in withdrawal symptoms such as anxiety, irritability and changes in mood.
7. To treat occasional pain, avoid the use of ASA (aspirin and related products) if you are taking *divalproex* or *valproic acid,* as it can affect the amount of this drug in your body; acetaminophen (Tylenol) or ibuprofen (Motrin, Advil) are safer alternatives.
8. *Gabapentin* should not be taken within 2 hours of an antacid (e.g., Tums, Rolaids, Maalox).
9. If you are taking *topiramate,* drink plenty of fluids before and during activities such as exercise or exposure to warm temperatures. Avoid the regular use of antacids (e.g., Tums, Maalox).
10. Report any changes in mood or behavior to your physician.
11. Store your medication in a clean, dry area at room temperature. Keep all medication out of the reach of children.

If you have any questions regarding this medication, please ask your doctor, pharmacist, or nurse.

The name of your medication is _____.

What is this drug used for?

Psychostimulants are primarily used in the treatment of Attention Deficit Hyperactivity Disorder (ADHD) in children and adults. These drugs are also approved for use in Parkinson's Disease and Narcolepsy (a sleeping disorder).

Though they are currently not approved for this indication, psychostimulants have been found useful as add-on therapy in the treatment of depression. Ask your doctor if you are not sure why you are taking this drug.

How quickly will the drug start working?

Some response to psychostimulants is usually noted within the first week of treatment of ADHD and tends to increase over the next 3 weeks.

How does the doctor decide on the dosage?

Psychostimulants come in various preparations including short-acting and slow-release (i.e., spansules or extended-release) forms as well as a skin patch (Daytrana – available in the US). The dose is based on the body weight and is usually given several times a day. Take the drug exactly as prescribed; **do not increase or decrease the dose without speaking to your doctor.**

How long should you take this medication?

Psychostimulants are usually prescribed for a period of several years. Some clinicians may prescribe "drug holidays" to individuals on this medication (i.e., the drug is not taken at certain times such as weekends, vacations, etc.), in situations when side effects may be of concern.

What side effects may happen?

Side effects may happen with any drug. They are not usually serious and do not happen to everyone. Side effects may sometimes occur before beneficial effects of the medication are noticed. If you think you may be having a side effect, speak to your doctor or pharmacist as they can help you decrease it or cope with it.

Common side effects that should be reported to your doctor at the **NEXT VISIT** include:

- Energizing/agitated feeling, excitability – Some individuals may feel nervous or have difficulty sleeping for a few days after starting this medication. If you are taking the medication in the late afternoon or evening, the physician may decide to prescribe it earlier in the day.
- Increased heart rate and blood pressure – Speak to your doctor.
- Headache – This tends to be temporary and can be managed by taking pain medicine (aspirin, acetaminophen) when required. If the headache persists or is "troubling", contact your doctor. Blood pressure should be checked.
- Nausea or heartburn – If this happens, take the medication with food or milk.

- Dry mouth – Sour candy and sugarless gum help increase saliva in your mouth. Do not drink sweet drinks like colas as they may give you cavities and help put on weight. Drink water and brush your teeth regularly.
- Loss of appetite, weight loss – Taking the medication after meals, eating smaller meals more frequently or drinking high calorie drinks may help.
- Blurred vision – This usually happens when you first start the drug and tends to be temporary. Reading under a bright light or at a distance may help; a magnifying glass can be of temporary use. If the problem lasts more than a few weeks, let your doctor know.
- Respiratory symptoms including sore throat, coughing, or sinus pain.
- Decreased growth.

Rare side effects you should report to your doctor **RIGHT AWAY** include:

- Fast or irregular heart beat
- Muscle twitches, tics or movement problems
- Persistent throbbing headache
- Sore mouth, gums, or throat
- Skin rash or itching, swelling of the face
- Any unusual bruising or bleeding, appearance of splotchy purplish darkening of the skin
- Tiredness, weakness, fever, or feeling like you have the flu, associated with nausea, vomiting, loss of appetite
- Yellow tinge in the eyes or to the skin; dark-colored urine (pee)
- Severe agitation or restlessness
- **A switch in mood to an unusual state of happiness or irritability; fluctuations in mood**

Let your doctor know **right away** if you miss your period or think you may be **pregnant**, plan to become pregnant, or are breastfeeding.

What should you do if you forget to take a dose of your medication?

If you take the psychostimulant 2–3 times a day and forget to take a dose by more than 4 hours, skip the missed dose and continue with your regular schedule. **DO NOT DOUBLE THE DOSE.**

The skin patch (Daytrana) is placed on the body in the moring and removed after 9 hours.

Is this drug safe to take with other medication?

Because psychostimulants can change the effect of other medication, or may be affected by other medication, always check with your doctor or pharmacist before taking other drugs, including those you can buy without a prescription such as cold remedies and herbal preparations. Always inform any doctor or dentist that you see that you are taking a psychostimulant drug.

Precautions/Considerations

1. This medication should not be used in patients who have high blood pressure, heart disease or abnormalities, hardening of the arteries, or an overactive thyroid.
2. Do not change your dose or stop the drug without talking to your doctor.
3. Do not chew or crush the tablets or capsules unless told to do so by your doctor.

4. If you have difficulty swallowing medication, the doctor may prescribe a capsule which can be opened and the beads can be sprinkled in applesauce and swallowed without chewing.

5. If you are prescribed the skin patch (Daytrana), it should be applied to clean, dry skin on the hip immediately upon removal from the protective pouch. Skin should not be exposed to external heat (e.g., heating pads, hot tubs); used patches need to be discarded carefully, according to package instructions.

6. If you take Concerta, you may see some of the tablet in your stool. This is normal because the tablet does not dissolve all the way but the contents of the tablet are fully absorbed.

7. Use caution while driving or performing tasks requiring alertness as these drugs can mask symptoms of fatigue and impair concentration.

8. Report to your doctor any changes in sleeping or eating habits or changes in mood or behavior.

9. Unless instructed otherwise, do not stop your drug suddenly as this may result in withdrawal symptoms that include changes in mood and behavior.

10. This drug may interact with medication prescribed by your dentist, so let him/her know the name of the drug you are taking.

11. Store your medication in a clean, dry area at room temperature. Keep all medication out of the reach of children.

If you have any questions regarding this medication, please ask your doctor, pharmacist, or nurse.

Atomoxetine is used primarily in the treatment of Attention Deficit Hyperactivity Disorder (ADHD) in children and adults.

How quickly will the drug start working?

Some response to atomoxetine is usually noted within the first 3–4 weeks of treatment of ADHD.

How does the doctor decide on the dosage?

Atomoxetine comes in a capsule; the dose is based on your body weight and how well it works for you. The capsule is usually given once or twice a day, with or without food. Do not increase or decrease the dose without speaking to your doctor.

How long should you take this medication?

Atomoxetine is usually prescribed for a period of several months to years.

What side effects may happen?

Side effects may happen with any drug. They are not usually serious and do not happen to everyone. Side effects may sometimes occur before beneficial effects of the medication are noticed. If you think you may be having a side effect, speak to your doctor or pharmacist as they can help you decrease it or cope with it.

Common side effects that should be reported to your doctor at the **NEXT VISIT** include:

- Increased anxiety, agitation or excitability – Some individuals may feel nervous or have difficulty sleeping for a few days after starting this medication.
- Headache – This tends to be temporary and can be managed by taking pain medicine (e.g., acetaminophen) when required. If the headache persists or is "troubling", contact your doctor.
- Nausea, abdominal pain, vomiting – try taking your medication with food; if symptoms persist, speak to your doctor.
- Loss of appetite, weight loss – Try eating small meals several times a day.
- Feeling sleepy and tired – The problem goes away with time, however, your doctor may suggest you take your medication at bedtime. Use of other drugs that make you drowsy will worsen the problem. Avoid operating machinery if drowsiness persist.
- Dry mouth – Sour candy and sugarless gum help increase saliva in your mouth. Do not drink sweet drinks like colas as they may give you cavities and help put on weight. Drink water and brush your teeth regularly.
- Dizziness – Get up from a lying or sitting position slowly; dangle your legs over the edge of the bed for a few minutes before getting up. Sit or lie down if dizziness persists or if you feel faint, then contact your doctor.
- Difficulty remembering things – Speak to your doctor.

Rare side effects you should report to your doctor **RIGHT AWAY** include:

- Fast or irregular heart beat.
- Skin rash with swelling, itching.
- Soreness of the mouth, gums or throat.
- Any unusual bruising or bleeding, appearance of splotchy purplish darkening of the skin.
- Tenderness on the right side of your abdomen, fatigue, weakness, fever or flu-like symptoms accompanied by nausea, vomiting or loss of appetite.
- Yellow tinge in the eyes or to the skin; dark-colored urine.
- Severe agitation, restlessness or irritability.
- **Switch in mood to an unusual state of happiness, excitement, irritability, a marked disturbance in sleep or thoughts of suicide.**

Let your doctor know **as soon as possible** if you miss your period or suspect you may be pregnant.

What should you do if you forget to take a dose of your medication?

If you take atomoxetine more than once a day and you forget to take a dose by more than 6 hours, skip the missed dose and continue with your regular schedule. **DO NOT DOUBLE THE DOSE.**

Is this drug safe to take with other medication?

Because atomoxetine can change the effect of other medication, or may be affected by other medication, always check with your doctor or pharmacist before taking other drugs, including those you can buy without a prescription such as cold remedies and herbal preparations. Always inform any doctor or dentist that you see that you are taking atomoxetine.

Precautions/Considerations

1. This medication should not be used in patients who have high blood pressure, heart disease or abnormalities, harding of the arteries, or an overactive thyroid.
2. Report to your doctor any changes in sleeping or eating habits or changes in mood or behavior.
3. Do not change your dose or stop the drug without speaking with your doctor.
4. Use caution while performing tasks requiring alertness as atomoxetine can mask fatigue.
5. This drug may interact with medication prescribed by your dentist, so let him/her know the name of the drug you are taking.
6. Store your medication in a clean dry area at room temperature. Keep all medication out of reach of children.

If you have any questions regarding this medication, please ask your doctor, pharmacist, or nurse.

Patient Information on Clonidine

Clonidine, originally approved to treat high blood pressure, is used in the treatment of Attention Deficit Hyperactivity Disorder (ADHD) and tic disorder in children and adults. It has also been found effective for controlling some problematic behaviors in children and adults with autism, in decreasing symptoms in certain anxiety disorders as well as in schizophrenia, and in increasing patient comfort during heroin and nicotine withdrawal. Ask your doctor if you are not sure why you are taking this drug.

How quickly will the drug start working

Some response to clonidine is usually noted within the first week of treatment of ADHD and tends to increase over the next 3 weeks.

How does the doctor decide on the dosage?

Clonidine comes in both a tablet and a transdermal patch. The dose is based on the body weight. The tablet is usually given several times a day, while the patch is applied to the upper arm or chest and is left there for a period of one week.

Do not increase or decrease the dose without speaking to your doctor. Do not take off the patch mid-week unless you have been told to do so by your doctor.

How long should you take this medication?

Clonidine is usually prescribed for a period of several years for ADHD. The length of use for other indications varies.

What side effects may happen?

Side effects may happen with any drug. They are not usually serious and do not happen to everyone. Side effects may sometimes occur before beneficial effects of the medication are noticed. If you think you may be having a side effect, speak to your doctor or pharmacist as they can help you decrease it or cope with it.

Common side effects that should be reported to your doctor at the **NEXT VISIT** include:
- Feeling sleepy and tired – The problem goes away with time. Use of other drugs that make you drowsy will worsen the problem. Avoid operating machinery if drowsiness persist.
- Dry mouth – Sour candy and sugarless gum help increase saliva in your mouth. Do not drink sweet drinks like colas as they may give you cavities and help put on weight. Drink water and brush your teeth regularly.
- Dizziness – Get up from a lying or sitting position slowly; dangle your legs over the edge of the bed for a few minutes before getting up. Sit or lie down if dizziness persists or if you feel faint, then contact your doctor.
- Headache – This tends to be temporary and can be managed by taking pain medicine (e.g., acetaminophen) when required. If the headache persists or is "troubling", contact your doctor.
- Increased anxiety, agitation or excitability – Some individuals may feel nervous or have difficulty sleeping for a few days after starting this medication.

Rare side effects you should report to your doctor **RIGHT AWAY** include:
- Fast or irregular heart beat
- Skin rash with swelling, itching
- Sore mouth, gums or throat
- Any unusual bruising or bleeding, appearance of splotchy purplish darkening of the skin
- Nausea, vomiting, loss of appetite, feeling tired, weak, feverish or like you have the flu
- Yellow tinge in the eyes or to the skin; dark-colored urine (pee)
- Severe agitation, restlessness or irritability

Let your doctor know **right away** if you miss your period or think you may be **pregnant**, plan to become pregnant, or are breastfeeding.

What should you do if you forget to take a dose of your medication?

If you take clonidine more than once a day and you forget to take a dose by more than 6 hours, skip the missed dose and continue with your regular schedule. **DO NOT DOUBLE THE DOSE.**

Is this drug safe to take with other medication?

Because clonidine can change the effect of other medication, or may be affected by other medication, always check with your doctor or pharmacist before taking other drugs, including those you can buy without a prescription such as cold remedies and herbal preparations. Always inform any doctor or dentist that you see that you are taking clonidine.

Precautions/Considerations

1. Report to your doctor any changes in sleeping or eating habits or changes in mood or behavior.
2. Do not change your dose or stop the drug without speaking with your doctor.
3. Use caution while performing tasks requiring alertness as clonidine can cause fatigue.
4. Do not stop clonidine suddenly as it may result in withdrawal symptoms including insomnia and changes in blood pressure.
5. If taking transdermal clonidine and it begins to loosen from the skin after application, apply adhesive tape directly over the patch to make sure it stays on for the rest of the week.
6. Take off the used patch before applying a new patch to the skin. Handle used transdermal patches carefully; fold the patch in half with the sticky sides together, and place inside a baggie prior to discarding. Keep out of reach of children.
7. Store your medication in a clean dry area at room temperature. Keep all medication out of reach of children.

If you have any questions regarding this medication, please ask your doctor, pharmacist, or nurse.

Patient Information on Drugs for Treatment of Dementia

The name of your medication is _____.

What is this drug used for?

Cognition enhancers are primarily used to treat **symptoms of mild to moderate Alzheimer's dementia.**

How quickly will the drug start working?

Improvement in concentration and attention is noted over a period of several weeks. Because these drugs take time to work **do not decrease or increase the dose** without discussing this with the doctor.

How does the doctor decide on the dosage?

The drug is started at a low dose to minimize the chance of side effects. The dose can be increased after several weeks if minimal improvement is seen. The dose of the drug tacrine is determined by the results of tests of liver function, which the physician performs on a regular basis.

How long should you take this medication?

Cognition enhancers are usually prescribed for a period of several years.

What side effects may happen?

Side effects may happen with any drug. They are not usually serious and do not happen to everyone. Side effects may sometimes occur before beneficial effects of the medication are noticed. If you think you may be having a side effect, speak to your doctor or pharmacist as they can help you decrease it or cope with it.

Common side effects that should be reported to your doctor at the **NEXT VISIT** include:

- Energizing/agitated feeling, excitability – Some individuals may feel nervous or have difficulty sleeping for a few days after starting this medication. If you are taking the medication in the evening, the physician may decide to prescribe it earlier in the day.
- Nightmares or vivid dreams – let the doctor know; the time you take the drug or your dose may need to be adjusted
- Headache – This tends to be temporary and can be managed by taking pain medicine (aspirin, acetaminophen) when required. If the headache persists or is "troubling", contact your doctor.
- Nausea, vomiting, stomach pains, heartburn – If this happens, take the medication with food or milk.
- Diarrhea or constipation, flatulence.
- Loss of appetite, weight loss – Taking the medication after meals, eating smaller meals more frequently or drinking high calorie drinks may help.
- Feeling tired, weak
- Muscle aches or cramps – Can be managed by taking pain medicine when required.
- Nasal congestion.
- Hot flushes.

Rare side effects you should report to your doctor **RIGHT AWAY** include:

- Yellow tinge in the eyes or to the skin; dark-colored urine (pee)
- Sore mouth, gums, or throat
- Skin rash or itching, swelling of the face
- Nausea, vomiting, loss of appetite, fatigue, weakness, fever, or flu-like symptoms
- Severe agitation or restless

What should you do if you forget to take a dose of your medication?

If you take your total dose of the drug in the morning and you forget to take it for more than 6 hours, skip the missed dose and continue with your schedule the next day. **DO NOT DOUBLE THE DOSE.** If you take the drug several times a day, take the missed dose when you remember, then continue with your regular schedule.

Is this drug safe to take with other medication?

Because these drugs can change the effect of other medication, or may be affected by other medication, always check with your doctor or pharmacist before taking other drugs, including those you can buy without a prescription such as cold remedies and herbal preparations. Always inform any doctor or dentist that you see that you are taking a cognition enhancer.

Precautions/Considerations

1. Do not change your dose or stop the drug without speaking with your doctor.
2. Extended-release capsules of galantamine should not be broken, chewed or crushed, but should be swallowed whole.
3. The area where rivastigmine patch is applied should be rotated to other parts of the body routinely. If there is concern of the patch being removed prematurely or inadvertently, then it is suggested that a caregiver place the patch where the patient cannot easily remove it. Ensure the patch is removed after 24 hours and prior to applying the next dose. When removing the patch, fold it in half with the adhesive sides on the inside and dispose of in waste container; wash hands after handling.
4. Report to your doctor any changes in sleeping or eating habits or changes in mood or behavior.
5. Do not stop your drug suddenly as this may result in changes in behavior and/or concentration. If rivastigmine was stopped for more than 3 days, DO NOT restart without speaking to your doctor.
6. This drug may interact with medication prescribed by your dentist, so let him/her know the name of the drug you are taking.
7. Do not take any other medication (including drugs you can buy without a prescription and herbal products) without talking to your doctor or pharmacist.
8. Store your medication in a clean, dry area at room temperature. Keep all medication out of the reach of children.

If you have any questions regarding this medication, please ask your doctor, pharmacist, or nurse.

Practical recommendations for caregivers to decrease agitation and improve communication with patients with dementia

1. Decrease stimulation and change the environment to maintain safety.
2. Maintain physical comfort.
3. Slow down your pace and simplify your actions (i.e., one demand at a time).
4. Use simple direct statements; limit choices. Speak clearly and slowly and allow time for response.
5. Match verbal and nonverbal signals; maintain eye contact and relaxed posture.
6. Identify situations/actions that result in agitation; change these if possible.

Patient Information on Sex-Drive Depressants

The name of your medication is _____.

What is this drug used for?

These drugs are primarily used to **reduce sexual arousal and libido.**

How quickly will the drug start working?

These drugs interfere with the formation of the hormone testosterone in the body; their effect on sexual arousal and libido is noted over a period of several weeks. Because these drugs take time to work **do not decrease or increase the dose** without discussing this with the doctor.

How does the doctor decide on the dosage?

These drugs are available in different forms, including tablets and long-acting injections. For oral tablets, the dose of the drug is increased gradually until a good response is noted. A testosterone test, or your own report of the effects, can determine the correct dosage. The dose of the injection may also be related to whether the drug will be given every month or every 3 months.

How long should you take this medication?

Sex-drive depressants are usually prescribed for a period of several years.

What side effects may happen?

Side effects may happen with any drug. They are not usually serious and do not happen to everyone. Side effects may sometimes occur before beneficial effects of the medication are noticed. If you think you may be having a side effect, speak to your doctor or pharmacist as they can help you decrease it or cope with it.

Common side effects that should be reported to your doctor at the **NEXT VISIT** include:
- Sweating, hot flashes
- Impotence
- Muscle aches or spasms – can be managed by taking pain medicine when required (e.g., aspirin, acetaminophen).
- Swollen breasts
- Decrease in body hair
- Feeling tired, depressed mood
- Nervousness, problems sleeping

Rare side effects you should report to your doctor **RIGHT AWAY** include:
- Yellow tinge in the eyes or to the skin; dark-colored urine (pee)
- Sore mouth, gums, or throat
- Skin rash or itching, swelling of the face
- Nausea, vomiting, loss of appetite, feeling tired, weak, feverish, or like you have the flu
- Changes in your concentration
- Change in muscle movement or activity
- Swelling or pain in the legs

What should you do if you forget to take a dose of your medication?

If you take your total dose of the drug in the morning and you forget to take it for more than 6 hours, skip the missed dose and continue with your schedule the next day. **DO NOT DOUBLE THE DOSE**. If you miss your injection, contact your doctor and try to get an injection as soon as possible.

Is this drug safe to take with other medication?

Because these drugs can change the effect of other medication, or may be affected by other medication, always check with your doctor or pharmacist before taking other drugs, including those you can buy without a prescription such as cold remedies and herbal preparations. Always inform any doctor or dentist that you see that you are taking this medication.

Precautions/Considerations

1. Do not change your dose or stop the drug without speaking to your doctor.
2. Report to your doctor any changes in sleeping or eating habits or changes in mood or behavior.
3. Store your medication in a clean, dry area at room temperature. Keep all medication out of the reach of children.

If you have any questions regarding this medication, please ask your doctor, pharmacist, or nurse.

Patient Information on Disulfiram

What is this drug used for?

Disulfiram is primarily used as a **deterrent to alcohol use/abuse.** Disulfiram has been shown to maintain abstinence if taken, as directed, as part of a treatment program that includes counseling and support.

How quickly will the drug start working?

Disulfiram inhibits the breakdown of alcohol in the body, resulting in a build-up of a chemical called acetaldehyde; this results in an unpleasant reaction when alcohol is consumed. The reaction can occur 10–20 minutes after drinking alcohol and may last up to 2 hours.

 The reaction consists of: flushing, choking, nausea, vomiting, increased heart rate and decreased blood pressure (dizziness).

How long should you take this medication?

Disulfiram is usually prescribed for a set period of time to help the individual stop the use of alcohol. **Do not decrease or increase the dose** without discussing this with the doctor.

What side effects may happen?

Side effects may happen with any drug. They are not usually serious and do not happen to everyone. Side effects may sometimes occur before beneficial effects of the medication are noticed. If you think you may be having a side effect, speak to your doctor or pharmacist as they can help you decrease it or cope with it.

Common side effects that should be reported to your doctor at the **NEXT VISIT** include:

- Feeling sleepy, tired, depressed – This problem goes away with time. Use of other drugs that make you drowsy will worsen the problem. Avoid driving a car or operating machinery if drowsiness persists.
- Energizing/agitated feeling – Some individuals may feel nervous or have difficulty sleeping for a few days after starting this medication.
- Headache – Temporary use of pain medicine (e.g., acetaminophen, ASA).
- Skin rash – Contact your doctor.
- Garlic-like taste

Rare side effects you should report to your doctor **RIGHT AWAY** include:

- Yellow tinge in the eyes or to the skin; dark-colored urine (pee)
- Sore mouth, gums, or throat
- Skin rash or itching, swelling of the face
- Feeling tired, weak, feverish, or like you have the flu associated with nausea, vomiting, loss of appetite

Let your doctor know **right away** if you miss your period or think you may be **pregnant**, plan to become pregnant, or are breastfeeding.

What should you do if you forget to take a dose of your medication?

If you take your total dose of the drug in the morning and you forget to take it for more than 6 hours, skip the missed dose and continue with your schedule the next day. **DO NOT DOUBLE THE DOSE.**

Is this drug safe to take with other medication?

Because disulfiram can change the effect of other medication, or may be affected by other medication, always check with your doctor or pharmacist before taking other drugs, including those you can buy without a prescription such as cold remedies and herbal preparations. Always inform any doctor or dentist that you see that you are taking this medication.

Precautions/Considerations

1. Do not change your dose or stop the drug without speaking to your doctor.
2. Report to your doctor any changes in sleeping or eating habits or changes in mood or behavior.
3. Avoid all products (food and drugs) containing alcohol, including tonics, cough syrups, mouth washes and alcohol-based sauces. A delay in the reaction may be as long as 24 hours.
4. Exposure to alcohol-containing rubs or solvents (e.g., after-shave) may trigger a reaction.
5. Carry an identification card stating the name of the drug you are taking.
6. Store your medication in a clean, dry area at room temperature. Keep all medication out of the reach of children.

If you have any questions regarding this medication, please ask your doctor, pharmacist, or nurse.

What is this drug used for?

Acamprosate is primarily used in the treatment of alcohol dependence, where it reduces alcohol cravings and can prevent relapse.

How quickly will the drug start working?

Acamprosate is usually prescribed after an individual has been withdrawn from alcohol use. It is not effective if the person is actively drinking, nor will it treat withdrawal symptoms. It reduces cravings to alcohol.

Acamprosate has been shown to maintain abstinence if taken, as directed, as part of a treatment program that includes counseling and support.

How long should you take this medication?

Acamprosate is usually prescribed for a set period of time (months) to help the individual remain alcohol-free. Do not increase or decrease your dose of medication without discussing this with your physician.

What side effects may happen?

Side effects may happen with any drug. They are not usually serious and do not happen to everyone. Side effects may sometimes occur before beneficial effects of the medication are noticed. If you think you may be having a side effect, speak to your doctor or pharmacist as they can help you decrease it or cope with it.

Common side effect that should be reported to your doctor at the **NEXT VISIT** include:

- Upset stomach, nausea, gas, diarrhea – if these symptoms continue, the doctor may need to re-evaluate the dose
- Headache – this tends to be temporary and can be managed by taking pain medicine (aspirin, acetaminophen, ibuprofen) as required. If the headache persists or is "troubling", contact your doctor.
- Increased anxiety, sleeping difficulties – some individuals may feel nervous or have difficulty sleeping for a few days after starting this medication
- Itching, skin rash

Rare side effects you should report to your doctor **RIGHT AWAY** include:

- Severe anxiety, change in your mood or behavior, suicidal thoughts

Let your doctor know **right away** if you miss your period or think you may be **pregnant**, plan to become pregnant, or are breastfeeding.

What should you do if you forget to take a dose of your medication?

If you are taking the medication 3 times a day with meals, and miss taking your dose by more than 2 hours, skip the missed dose and continue with your next scheduled dose.

Is this drug safe to take with other medication?

Because acamprosate can change the effect of other medication, or may be affected by other medication, always check with your doctor or pharmacist before taking other drugs, including those you can buy without a prescription such as cold remedies and herbal preparations. Always inform any doctor or dentist that you see that are taking acamprosate.

Precautions/Considerations

1. This drug may impair the mental and physical abilities and reaction time required for driving or operating other machinery. Avoid these activities if you feel drowsy or slowed down.
2. Do not change your dose or stop the drug suddenly without discussing this with your physician.
3. Should you restart drinking during treatment, continue taking the acamprosate but notify your physician as soon as possible.
4. Report any changes in mood or behavior to your physician.
5. Store your medication in a clean, dry area at room temperature. Keep all medication out of reach of children.

If you have any questions regarding this medication, please ask your doctor, pharmacist, or nurse.

Patient Information on Naltrexone

What is this drug used for?

Naltrexone is mainly used as an aid in the treatment of alcohol dependence or addiction to opiates. Naltrexone has been shown to maintain abstinence if taken, as directed, as part of a treatment program that includes counseling and support.

Though not approved for this indication, naltrexone has also been used in the treatment of behavior and impulse-control disorders and obsessive-compulsive disorder. It is available as an oral tablet and (in the USA) as a monthly injection. Ask your doctor if you are not sure why you are taking this drug.

How quickly will the drug start working?

Naltrexone blocks the "craving" for alcohol and opiates. It does not suppress withdrawal symptoms that can occur in an opiate user and should not be used in anyone using narcotics in the previous 10 days; these individuals must undergo detoxification programs before starting naltrexone. Naltrexone is started at a low dose and increased gradually based on effectiveness. Onset of response is quick (within the hour).

How long should you take this medication?

Naltrexone is usually prescribed for a set period of time to help the individual discontinue the use of alcohol or opiates. Naltrexone is used for a prolonged period of time in the treatment of behavior and impulse-control problems and obsessive-compulsive disorder. **Do not decrease or increase the dose** without discussing this with the doctor.

What side effects may happen?

Side effects may happen with any drug. They are not usually serious and do not happen to everyone. Side effects may sometimes occur before beneficial effects of the medication are noticed. If you think you may be having a side effect, speak to your doctor or pharmacist as they can help you decrease it or cope with it.

Common side effects that should be reported to your doctor at the **NEXT VISIT** include:

- Feeling tired, confusion, depression – This problem goes away with time. Use of other drugs that make you drowsy will worsen the problem. Avoid driving a car or operating machinery if drowsiness persists.
- Nervousness, anxiety, problems sleeping – Some individuals may feel nervous or have difficulty sleeping for a few days after starting this medication.
- Headache – Temporary use of pain medicine (e.g., aspirin, acetaminophen) may be required; contact your doctor if headaches occur frequently or are "troubling".
- Joint and muscle pain or stiffness – Temporary use of pain medicine may be required (see #6 Precautions).
- Stomach pain, cramps, nausea and vomiting – If this happens take the medication with food or milk.
- Weight loss.
- Pain, tenderness itchiness at site of injection; occasionally a lump can be felt.

Rare side effects you should report to your doctor **RIGHT AWAY** include:

- Yellow tinge in the eyes or to the skin; dark-colored urine (pee)
- Sore mouth, gums, or throat
- Skin rash or itching, swelling of the face
- Nausea, vomiting, loss of appetite, fatigue, weakness, fever, or flu-like symptoms
- Shortness of breath, persistent coughing and wheezing

Let your doctor know **right away** if you miss your period or think you may be **pregnant**, plan to become pregnant, or are breastfeeding.

What should you do if you forget to take a dose of your medication?

If you take your total dose of the drug in the morning and you forget to take it for more than 6 hours, skip the missed dose and continue with your schedule the next day. **DO NOT DOUBLE THE DOSE.** If you take the drug several times a day, take the missed dose when you remember, then continue with your regular schedule.

Is this drug safe to take with other medication?

Because naltrexone can change the effect of other medication, or may be affected by other medication, always check with your doctor or pharmacist before taking other drugs, including those you can buy without a prescription such as cold remedies and herbal preparations. Always inform any doctor or dentist that you see that you are taking this medication.

Precautions/Considerations

1. Do not change your dose or stop the drug without speaking to your doctor.
2. Report to your doctor any changes in sleeping or eating habits or changes in mood or behavior.
3. Carry an identification card stating the name of the drug you are taking.
4. Store your medication in a clean, dry area at room temperature. Keep all medication out of the reach of children.
5. Do NOT use narcotic preparations while taking oral or injectable naltrexone as this may cause serious adverse effects including coma and death.
6. Limit the use of non-prescription pain medicine such as aspirin, acetaminophen (Tylenol) or non-steroidal anti-inflammatories (e.g., Motrin).

If you have any questions regarding this medication, please ask your doctor, pharmacist, or nurse.

What is this drug used for?

Methadone is primarily used as a substitute drug in the treatment of narcotic (opiate) dependent patients who desire maintenance therapy. It suppresses withdrawal symptoms of other narcotic analgesics as well as the craving for narcotics. It is part of a complete addiction treatment program that also includes behavior therapy and counseling.

On occasion it is prescribed for severe chronic pain. Ask your doctor if you are not sure why you are taking this drug.

How quickly will the drug start working?

Methadone blocks the "craving" and withdrawal reactions from narcotics/opiates immediately. Methadone is started at a low dose and increased gradually, based on effectiveness, to a maintenance dose. It is then prescribed once daily.

Why is methadone given on a daily basis?

Methadone is a narcotic and its dispensing and usage is governed by Federal regulations. It is prepared as a liquid, mixed with orange juice. Most patients receive their methadone, on a daily basis, from the Pharmacy and are required to drink the contents of the bottle in the presence of the pharmacist.

Some patients (who are stable on their medication) are permitted to carry several days' supply of methadone to use at home.

How long should you take this medication?

The length of time methadone is prescribed varies among individuals and depends on a number of factors, including their progress in therapy; most patients receive methadone for several months, while others may require it for several years. Any decreases in dose should be done very gradually under the direction of the physician. It has been shown that methadone helps patients avoid illicit narcotic use and helps them attain social stability.

What side effects may happen?

Side effects may happen with any drug. They are not usually serious and do not happen to everyone. Side effects may sometimes occur before beneficial effects of the medication are noticed. If you think you may be having a side effect, speak to your doctor or pharmacist as they can help you decrease it or cope with it.

Common side effects that should be reported to your doctor at the **NEXT VISIT** include:

- Feeling tired, confusion, depression – This problem goes away with time. Use of other drugs that make you drowsy will worsen the problem. Avoid driving a car or operating machinery if drowsiness persists.
- Energized feeling, insomnia – Some individuals may feel nervous or have difficulty sleeping for a few days after starting this medication.
- Dizziness, lightheadedness, weakness – This should go away with time.
- Joint and muscle pain – Temporary use of non-narcotic pain medicine may help (e.g. ASA, acetaminophen, ibuprofen).
- Nausea and vomiting – If this happens take the medication after eating.
- Loss of appetite, weight loss – Taking the medication after meals, eating smaller meals more frequently or drinking high calorie drinks may help.

- Changes in sex drive or sexual performance – Though rare, should this problem occur, discuss it with your doctor.
- Sweating, flushing – You may sweat more than usual; frequent showering, use of deodorants and talcum powder may help.
- Constipation – Drink plenty of water and try to increase the amount of fiber in your diet (like fruit, vegetables or bran). Some individuals find a bulk laxative (e.g., Metamucil, Fibyrax) or a stool softener (Colace, Surfak) helps regulate their bowels. If these remedies are not effective, speak to your doctor or pharmacist.

Rare side effects you should report to your doctor **RIGHT AWAY** include:

- Combination of symptoms that include dizziness, fainting spells, palpitations, nausea, and vomiting
- Yellow tinge in the eyes or to the skin; dark-colored urine (pee)
- Sore mouth, gums, or throat
- Skin rash or itching, swelling of the face
- Feeling tired, weak, feverish, or like you have the flu, associated with nausea, vomiting, loss of appetite

Let your doctor know **right away** if you miss your period or think you may be **pregnant**, plan to become pregnant, or are breastfeeding.

What should you do if you forget to take a dose of your medication?

It is important to take this medication at approximately the same time, on a daily basis. Missing a dose can result in a withdrawal reaction, consisting of restlessness, insomnia, nausea, vomiting, headache, increased perspiration, congestion, "gooseflesh," abdominal cramps, muscle and bone pain.

Is this drug safe to take with other medication?

Because methadone can change the effect of other medication, or may be affected by other medication, always check with your doctor or pharmacist before taking other drugs, including those you can buy without a prescription such as cold remedies and herbal preparations. Always inform any doctor or dentist that you see, that you are taking this medication. It is important to carry a card in your wallet, stating that you are on methadone, in cases of emergency.

Precautions/Considerations

1. Do not share this medication with anyone. If you receive "carries" of methadone, store them out of the reach of children (preferably in a lockable compartment in the refrigerator); methadone can be poisonous to individuals who do not take opiates.
2. Report to your doctor any changes in sleeping or eating habits or changes in mood or behavior.
3. This drug may impair the mental and physical abilities and reaction time required for driving or operating other machinery. Avoid these activities if you fell drowsy or slowed down.
4. Carry an identification card stating the name of the drug you are taking and ensure every doctor and dentist you visit is aware you are taking methadone.

If you have any questions regarding this medication, please ask your doctor, pharmacist, or nurse.

Patient Information on Buprenorphine

What is this drug used for?

Buprenorphine is primarily used as a substitute drug in the treatment of narcotic (opioid) dependent patients who desire maintenance therapy. It suppresses cravings for narcotics and can aid in the withdrawal process. Buprenorphine is part of a complete addiction treatment program that also includes behavior therapy and counseling.

How is it supplied?

Buprenorphine is available as two different preparations: Subutex, which is a sublingual tablet of buprenorphine, and Suboxone, which is a combination of sublingual buprenorphine and sublingual naloxone. The physician will determine which preparation is most appropriate for you.

Buprenorphine is a narcotic and its dispensing and usage is governed by Federal regulations.

How quickly will the drug start working?

Buprenorphine will be started once you have abstained from opioids for 12–24 hours and are in the early stages of withdrawal. The dose will be determined by your physician, and will be given once daily. Put the tablets under your tongue and let them melt; this will take 2–10 minutes. Do not chew or swallow the tablets, as this will change the effect of the drug.

Any changes in dosage of buprenorphine will be determined by your response, i.e., a decrease in cravings and no withdrawal symptoms. You should see a response within the first 2 weeks.

Follow your doctor's directions exactly; do not increase or decrease your dose as either severe adverse effects or withdrawal effects could occur.

How long should you take this medication?

The length of time buprenorphine is prescribed varies among individuals and depends on a number of factors, including how well they do in therapy. Most patients receive buprenorphine for several months, while others may require it for several years. Any decreases in dose should be done very gradually under the direction of the physician.

It has been demonstrated that buprenorphine is beneficial in helping patients avoid illicit narcotic use and helps them become socially stable.

What side effects may happen?

Side effects may happen with any drug. They are not usually serious and do not happen to everyone. Side effects may sometimes occur before beneficial effects of the medication are noticed. If you think you may be having a side effect, speak to your doctor or pharmacist as they can help you decrease it or cope with it.

Common side effects that should be reported to your doctor at the **NEXT VISIT** include:

- Energized feeling, insomnia – Some individuals may feel nervous or have difficulty sleeping for a few days after starting this medication.
- Nausea, stomach pain – If this happens take the medication after eating.
- Drowsiness – This problem goes away with time. Use of other drugs that make you sleepy will worsen the problem. Avoid driving a car or operating machinery if drowsiness persists.
- Constipation – Drink plenty of water and try to increase the amount of fiber in your diet (like fruit, vegetables or bran). Some individuals find a bulk laxative (e.g., Metamucil, Fibyrax) or a stool softener (Colace, Surfak) helps regulate their bowels. If these remedies are not effective, speak to your doctor or pharmacist.
- Sweating – You may sweat more than usual; frequent showering, use of deodorants and talcum powder may help.
- Pain in joints, muscles – Temporary use of non-narcotic pain medicine (e.g., ASA, acetaminophen, ibuprofen) may help.

Rare side effects you should report to your doctor **RIGHT AWAY** include:

- Feeling faint, dizzy and confused
- Slowed, difficult breathing
- Yellow tinge in the eyes or to the skin; dark-colored urine (pee)
- Sore mouth, gums, or throat
- Skin rash or itching, swelling of the face
- Nausea, vomiting, loss of appetite, accompanied by feeling tired, weak, feverish, or like you have the flu

Let your doctor know **right away** if you miss your period or think you may be **pregnant**, plan to become pregnant, or are breastfeeding.

What should you do if you forget to take a dose of your medication?

If you miss a dose, take it as soon as possible. If it is almost time for your next dose, skip the missed dose and go back to your regular dosing schedule. Do not take two doses at once unless told to do so by your doctor.

Missed doses as well as extra doses can cause withdrawal reactions which include: nausea/vomiting, diarrhea, muscle aches and cramps, sweating, tearing of the eyes, running nose, dilated pupils, yawning, craving, mild fever, irritability, and insomnia. If you have a combination of these symptoms, call your physician right away or your local hospital emergency number.

Is this drug safe to take with other medication?

Because buprenorphine can change the effect of other medication, or may be affected by other medication, always check with your doctor or pharmacist before taking other drugs, including those you can buy without a prescription such as cold remedies and herbal preparations. Always inform any doctor or dentist that you see, that you are taking this medication.

It is important to carry a card in your wallet, stating that you are on buprenorphine, in case of emergency.

DO NOT drink alcohol or take tranquilizers or sedatives while you are on buprenorphine, as serious reactions can occur.

Precautions/Considerations

1. Do not share this medication with anyone and store it out of reach of children (preferably in a locked cupboard or desk); buprenorphine can be poisonous to other individuals.
2. Do not change the dose or stop the drug suddenly without speaking to your doctor.
3. You can develop dependence from taking buprenorphine, so withdrawal symptoms can occur if you stop it suddenly.
4. Buprenorphine can cause death from overdose, or if it is injected.
5. You may feel drowsy while on buprenorphine; do not drive a car or perform tasks requiring alertness if you feel drowsy or slowed down.
6. Tell your doctor if you are planning to become pregnant.

If you have any questions regarding this medication, please ask your doctor, pharmacist, or nurse.

INDEX OF DRUGS*

Clinical Handbook of Psychotropic Drugs, 18th Edition, © 2009 Hogrefe & Huber Publishers

* Page numbers in **bold type** indicate main entries.

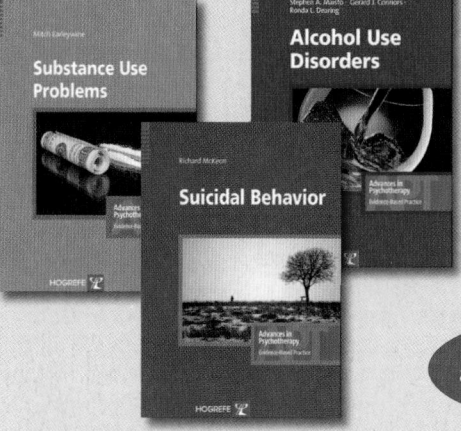

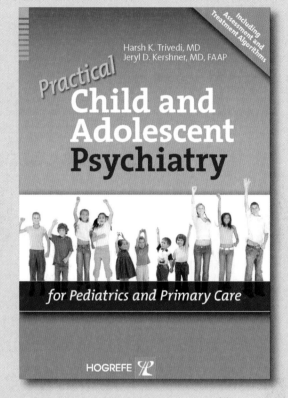
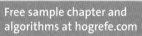
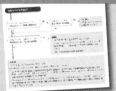
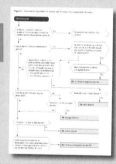
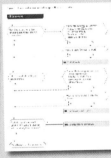
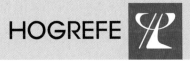

Order Forms

I would like to order:

QTY		Price	Total
	Clinical Handbook of Psychotropic Drugs, 18th edition	US $79.00 / € 57.00	
	Standing order for the Clinical Handbook – each new edition will be shipped automatically with an invoice		
	Clinical Handbook...for Children & Adolescents, 2nd edition	US $62.00 / € 49.95	
	Practical Child & Adolescent Psychiatry for Pediatrics & Primary Care	US $49.00 / € 34 .95	
	Advances in Psychotherapy – Evidence-Based Practice – Series Standing Order (Standing order price for min. 4 successive vols.: US $24.80 each)		
		Subtotal	

MA residents add 5% sales tax	

Postage & handling:
USA: 1st item US $6.00, each additional item US $1.25
Canada: 1st item US $8.00, each additional item US $2.00
South America: 1st item US $10.00, each additional item US $2.00
Europe: 1st item € 6.00, each additional item € 1.25
Rest of the World: 1st item € 8.00, each additional item € 1.50

Total

- Professor examination copies are available
- We offer discounts on bulk orders of 10 copies or more
  Call (800) 228-3749 for details

Call our order desk on (800) 228-3749 or order online at www.hogrefe.com

Shipping and Billing information

❑ Check enclosed   ❑ Charge my: ❑ VISA   ❑ MC   ❑ AmEx

Card # _____

CVV2/CVC2/CID # _____ Exp date _____

Cardholder's name _____

Signature _____

Shipping address:

Name _____

Address _____

City, State, ZIP _____

E-mail _____

Phone / Fax _____

Hogrefe Publishing · 30 Amberwood Parkway · Ashland, OH 44805 · Tel: (800) 228-3749 · Fax: (419) 281-6883
Hogrefe & Huber Publishers · Rohnsweg 25 · D-37085 Göttingen · Tel: +49 551 49 609-0 · Fax: +49 551 49 609-88
E-Mail: custserv@hogrefe.com

HOGREFE

I would like to order:

QTY		Price	Total
	Clinical Handbook of Psychotropic Drugs, 18th edition	US $79.00 / € 57.00	
	Standing order for the Clinical Handbook – each new edition will be shipped automatically with an invoice		
	Clinical Handbook...for Children & Adolescents, 2nd edition	US $62.00 / € 49.95	
	Practical Child & Adolescent Psychiatry for Pediatrics & Primary Care	US $49.00 / € 34 .95	
	Advances in Psychotherapy – Evidence-Based Practice – Series Standing Order (Standing order price for min. 4 successive vols.: US $24.80 each)		
		Subtotal	

MA residents add 5% sales tax	

Postage & handling:
USA: 1st item US $6.00, each additional item US $1.25
Canada: 1st item US $8.00, each additional item US $2.00
South America: 1st item US $10.00, each additional item US $2.00
Europe: 1st item € 6.00, each additional item € 1.25
Rest of the World: 1st item € 8.00, each additional item € 1.50

Total

- Professor examination copies are available
- We offer discounts on bulk orders of 10 copies or more
  Call (800) 228-3749 for details

Call our order desk on (800) 228-3749 or order online at www.hogrefe.com

Shipping and Billing information

❑ Check enclosed   ❑ Charge my: ❑ VISA   ❑ MC   ❑ AmEx

Card # _____

CVV2/CVC2/CID # _____ Exp date _____

Cardholder's name _____

Signature _____

Shipping address:

Name _____

Address _____

City, State, ZIP _____

E-mail _____

Phone / Fax _____

Hogrefe Publishing · 30 Amberwood Parkway · Ashland, OH 44805 · Tel: (800) 228-3749 · Fax: (419) 281-6883
Hogrefe & Huber Publishers · Rohnsweg 25 · D-37085 Göttingen · Tel: +49 551 49 609-0 · Fax: +49 551 49 609-88
E-Mail: custserv@hogrefe.com

HOGREFE